Lee's

IS of
HESIA

Commissioning Editor: *Natasha Andjelkovic*
Project Development Manager: *Hilary Hewitt*
Project Manager: *Kathryn Mason*
Production Assistant: *Gemma Lawson*
Designer: *Andy Chapman*
Illustration Manager: *Mick Ruddy*
Illustrator: *Richard Tibbitts*
Marketing Managers (UK/USA): *Brant Emery/Emily M. Christie*

Lee's SYNOPSIS of ANAESTHESIA

Edited by

N. J. H. Davies MA DM MRCP FRCA
Consultant Anaesthetist,
Southampton General Hospital, UK

J. N. Cashman BSc MD FRCA
Consultant Anaesthetist,
St George's Hospital, London, UK

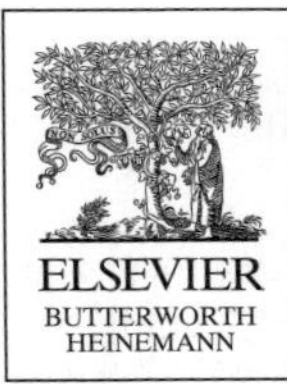

ELSEVIER
BUTTERWORTH
HEINEMANN

An imprint of Elsevier Limited

By J. Alfred Lee
First edition 1947,
Second edition 1950
Third edition 1953
Reprinted with minor amendments 1955
Reprinted 1956
Reprinted 1957
Fourth edition 1959
Reprinted 1960
Italian first edition 1963

By J. Alfred Lee and R. S. Atkinson
Fifth edition 1964
Spanish edition 1966
Sixth edition 1968
Seventh edition 1973
French edition 1975
Portuguese edition 1976
German edition 1977

By R. S. Atkinson, G. B. Rushman and J. Alfred Lee
Eighth edition 1977
Greek edition 1979
Reprinted 1979
Polish edition 1981
Ninth edition 1982
Spanish second edition 1981
Tenth edition 1987
Italian second edition 1986
German second edition 1986

By R. S. Atkinson, G. B. Rushman and N. J. H. Davies
Eleventh edition 1993
Reprinted 1993, 1994

By G. B. Rushman, N. J. H. Davies and J. N. Cashman
Twelfth edition 1999

By N.J.H Davies and J.N.Cashman
Thirteenth edition 2005

ISBN 0 7506 8834 3
ISBN 0 7506 8835 1 (International edition)

British Library Cataloguing in Publication Data
A catalogue record for this book is available from the British Library

Library of Congress Cataloging in Publication Data
A catalog record for this book is available from the Library of Congress

Notice
Medical knowledge is constantly changing. Standard safety precautions must be followed, but as new research and clinical experience broaden our knowledge, changes in treatment and drug therapy may become necessary or appropriate. Readers are advised to check the most current product information provided by the manufacturer of each drug to be administered to verify the recommended dose, the method and duration of administration, and contraindications. It is the responsibility of the practitioner, relying on experience and knowledge of the patient, to determine dosages and the best treatment for each individual patient. Neither the Publisher nor the author assume any liability for any injury and/or damage to persons or property arising from this publication.

The Publisher

Printed in the United Kingdom
Last digit is the print number:
9 8 7 6 5 4 3 2 1

CONTENTS

LIST OF CONTRIBUTORS

Julie Ashworth BSc FRCA
Consultant Anaesthetist
University Hospital of North Staffordshire
Stoke-on-Trent, UK 1.2

Simon Bricker MA FRCA
Consultant Anaesthetist
Countess of Chester Hospital
Chester, UK 3.1, 5.17

Ian Calder FRCA
Consultant Neuroanaesthetist
National Hospital for Neurology and Neurosurgery
London, UK 5.7

Charles Deakin MA MD FRCP FRCA
Consultant Anaesthetist
Department of Anaesthetics
Southampton General Hospital
Southampton, UK 2.9

Christopher Dodds MRCGP FRCA
Professor
Cleveland School of Anaesthesia
South Cleveland Hospital
Middlesbrough, UK 7.1

Simon Dolin PhD FRCA
Consultant in Pain Relief
King Edward VII Hospital
Midhurst, UK 6.1

Leslie Gemmell FRCA
Consultant Anaesthetist
Wrexham Maelor Hospital
Wrexham, UK 5.1

Ravi Gill FRCA
Consultant Anaesthetist
Southampton General Hospital
Southampton, UK 2.7

Sue Hill MA PhD FRCA
Consultant Anaesthetist
Southampton General Hospital
Southampton, UK 2.4

Anita Holdcroft MD FRCA
Reader in Anaesthesia
Imperial College London
Chelsea and Westminster Hospital
London, UK 5.5, 5.8

Ian Jenkins MRCP FRCA
Consultant in Paediatric Anaesthesia and Intensive Care
Royal Hospital for Children
Bristol, UK 5.6

Iain Levack MD FRCA
Consultant Anaesthetist
Ninewells Hospital and Medical School
Dundee, UK 5.15

Patrick Magee BSc FRCA
Consultant Anaesthetist
Royal United Hospital
Bath, UK 2.1, 2.2

Greg McAnulty FRCA
Consultant Anaesthetist
St George's Hospital
London, UK 5.14

Graeme McLeod MRCGP FRCA
Consultant Anaesthetist,
Senior Lecturer in Anaesthesia
Ninewells Hospital and Medical School
Dundee, UK 4.1, 4.2, 4.3

Peter Nightingale FRCP FRCA
Consultant in Anaesthesia and Intensive Care
Wythenshawe Hospital
Manchester, UK 2.8

Michael O'Connor FRCA ILTM
Consultant Anaesthetist
Great Western Hospital
Swindon, UK 3.3, 5.16

Nicholas Pace MPhil MRCP FRCA
Consultant Anaesthetist
Gartnavel General Hospital
Glasgow, UK 5.4

Adrian Pearce FRCA
Consultant Anaesthetist
Guy's Hospital
London, UK 2.6, 5.12

Ian Power MD FRCA FFPMANZCA FANZCA
Professor of Anaesthesia, Critical Care and Pain Medicine
University of Edinburgh
Royal Infirmary
Edinburgh, UK 3.2

Ralph Scott BSc MD FRCA
Consultant in Anaesthesia and Intensive Care Medicine
Salisbury District Hospital
Salisbury, UK 2.5

Ian Smith BSc MD FRCA
Senior Lecturer in Anaesthesia
University Hospital of North Staffordshire
Stoke-on-Trent, UK 5.3

Martin Smith FRCA
Consultant Neuroanaesthetist
National Hospital for Neurology and Neurosurgery
London, UK 5.7

Stephen Squires FRCA
Consultant Anaesthetist
Queen Victoria Hospital
East Grinstead, UK 5.13

Jane Stanford MA FRCA
Consultant Anaesthetist
St George's Hospital
London, UK 5.10

Brian Sweeney FRCA
Consultant Anaesthetist
Poole General Hospital
Poole, UK 1.1

Jean-Pierre van Besouw BSc FRCA
Consultant Anaesthetist and Honorary Senior Lecturer
St George's Hospital
London, UK 5. 2

Peter Venn FRCA
Consultant Anaesthetist
Queen Victoria Hospital
East Grinstead, UK 2.3

Christopher Wainwright FRCA
Consultant Anaesthetist
Southampton General Hospital
Southampton, UK 5.9

Lucy White MRCP FRCA
Consultant Anaesthetist
Southampton General Hospital
Southampton, UK 5.11

Andrew Wolf MA MD FRCA
Professor of Anaesthesia and Intensive Care
University of Bristol
Royal Hospital for Children
Bristol, UK 5.6

John Alfred Lee (1906–1989)

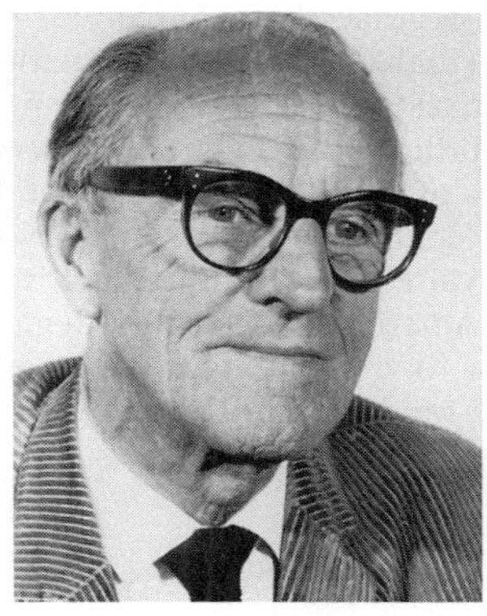

Alfred Lee was born near Liverpool in 1906 and qualified from Newcastle upon Tyne in 1927. His early experience of anaesthesia was that expected of the house surgeon of time, usually an open-drop method and occasionally a primitive Boyle's machine or a Clover's inhaler. After moving to Southend-on-Sea as a general practitioner, he continued to maintain an interest in anaesthesia and took up anaesthetic sessions at the hospital. In 1939, on the outbreak of hostilities, Alfred Lee became a wholetime specialist in the Emergency Medical Service, working at Runwell Hospital, near Southend. In 1948, the inauguration of the National Health Service enabled him to become a consultant anaesthetist, a post he held up to his retirement in 1971, when he became Honorary Consulting Anaesthetist. He continued his interest in anaesthesia and travelled extensively, attending many regional, national and international meetings right up to the month of his death in April 1989.

After the war years, there was a return of anaesthetists from the Services to civilian life. There were few texts on anaesthesia for them and Alfred Lee approached John Wright and Sons Ltd of Bristol who asked him to submit some specimen chapters. The result was the publication of *A Synopsis of Anaesthesia* in 1947. Alfred Lee was to participate in 11 editions over the next 40 years, some being translated into Italian, Spanish, French, Portuguese, German, Greek and Polish. He was also the author of many papers, wrote and edited a number of other texts and was, for a time, Assistant Editor and, later, Chairman of the Editorial Board of *Anaesthesia*. His special interests included preoperative care (he started an outpatient clinic for the preoperative assessment of patients), postoperative care (Southend was the first non-specialist hospital to have a Postoperative Observation Ward adjacent to the theatres), regional analgesia (he advocated and taught extradural block long before it became common practice) and history (he was the first President of the History of Anaesthesia Society).

He examined for the Final Fellowship Examination, was a member of the Board of Faculty of Anaesthetists, and President of the Association of Anaesthetists of Great Britain and Ireland. He served as President of the Section of Anaesthetics of the Royal Society of Medicine and in 1975 received the Hickman Medal. He was an Honorary Fellow of the Faculty of Anaesthetists of the Royal College of Surgeons in Ireland (1970), Gaston Labat Lecturer to the American Society of Regional Anesthesia (1985), Thomas Seldon Lecturer to the International Anesthesia Research Society (1985), and Koller Gold Medallist and Lecturer in Vienna (1984) to commemorate the centenary of local analgesia.

PREFACE TO THE THIRTEENTH EDITION

It is nearly 60 years since the first edition of *A Synopsis of Anaesthesia* was published. During this time it has been through 12 editions and been translated into seven different languages. Throughout this entire period *Synopsis* has been the work of only five authors. However, we acknowledge an increasing sub-specialisation in anaesthesia. It is for this reason we have invited authors with specialist interests and experience to modernise the text and ensure that it is consistent with current practice. In doing so we recognise that this is a major break with the tradition of previous editions of *Synopsis*.

There has been a complete change in layout. Every chapter has been substantially rewritten by its author to present as complete an account of the topic as possible in a book of this size. In particular, changes in surgery have necessitated major revision of Section 5. Furthermore, we consider that *Synopsis* should encompass not only clinical practice but also the importance of education in anaesthesia. We have, therefore, added a new section on training and standards.

The preface to the first edition stressed that *Synopsis* was not designed to take the place of larger textbooks of anaesthesia. This remains true. However, with the changes to this thirteenth edition we hope that *Synopsis* will continue to appeal to its traditional readership and also re-establish its position as a concise, general resource for anyone entering the specialty of anaesthesia.

NJHD
JNC

FROM THE PREFACE TO THE FIRST EDITION

This book is not designed to take the place of larger textbooks of anaesthesia and analgesia. It is a summary of current teaching and practice, and it is hoped that it will serve the student, the resident anaesthetist, the practitioner and the candidate studying for the Diploma in Anaesthetics as a ready source of reference and a quick means of revision.

January 1947
JAL

ACKNOWLEDGEMENTS

We would like to pay homage to J. Alfred Lee, Dick Atkinson and Geoff Rushman, our predecessors as authors of *Synopsis*. Never underestimate their massive contributions.

Section 1

Preparation of the Patient for Surgery

CHAPTER 1.1

ASSESSMENT AND PREPARATION

The essential first step in the assessment and preparation of a patient for anaesthesia and surgery is a preoperative visit. Ideally, for elective surgery, this should be carried out the day before surgery or as soon as possible after admission. The reasons for this visit are:

- to establish rapport, allay any fears or anxieties that the patient might have, and if necessary, prescribe premedication;
- to identify and assess existing medical conditions, note the patient's physical condition, and establish that the appropriate preoperative tests have been carried out;
- to assess the risks and benefits of the various options for anaesthesia and formulate a plan for the patient;
- to provide the patient with appropriate information and obtain consent for the anaesthetic procedures.

GENERAL ASSESSMENT

Pre-assessment clinics

Traditionally in the UK, anaesthetists carried out preoperative assessment for all surgical patients. Increasingly however, the need to optimise hospital facilities has led, at least in part, to the adoption of this task by nurses or other doctors.

For example, in many day units, nurses use a standard assessment protocol to screen patients for a wide range of relevant conditions and identify those who require few or no preoperative investigations. Non-medical staff are not qualified to determine whether a patient is fit for surgery, and so a consultant anaesthetist should should ideally be available for advice.

In addition, many hospitals have established consultant anaesthetist pre-assessment clinics where more complex patients may be evaluated.

Notwithstanding these developments, patients who have been screened in a pre-assessment clinic are normally seen by their anaesthetist in the immediate preoperative setting.

Preoperative assessment

Preoperative assessment usually begins with a careful reading of the case notes detailing key aspects of the patient's medical and surgical history, treatment and current medication. Previous anaesthetic charts may record important difficulties and complications. The case notes should also contain the results of current biochemical and haematological tests and other relevant investigations, such as electrocardiography (ECG), echocardiography, lung function tests and chest radiography.

Depending on the nature of the surgery, blood transfusion may be required during or after the operation. Blood must be ordered and its availability checked. In rare cases will it be necessary to contact the patient's general practitioner for additional information. The anaesthetist should be aware of the nature of the planned surgical procedure.

The anaesthetist should introduce him or herself to the patient and any relatives in a friendly and courteous manner, explaining the purpose of the visit and establishing whether the patient would like the interview to be conducted alone or in the presence of friends or relatives. It is best to have a systematic approach so that nothing is overlooked. Often the patient has failed to understand the nature of the planned surgery, usually as a result of anxiety, and a brief description will usually allay fears. The surgeon should be informed if more detailed information is required.

The history taken is dictated by the complexity of any problems encountered. In the case of a fit patient undergoing routine elective surgery, the discussion may be brief and a detailed examination superfluous. In the case of a patient with complex major co-morbidity, considerable time may be required to assimilate copious potentially relevant information before deciding which options are available and what further tests are necessary. The risks of proceeding with surgery should be balanced against those of postponement. In general, surgery should only be postponed if there is an opportunity to improve the patient's clinical status and thereby reduce overall risk.

Consent

Consent has been the focus of recent debate in the UK.[1] Anaesthetic consent used to be implied (i.e. part of the consent for surgery). However, it is now no longer acceptable for surgeons to accept responsibility for explaining the nature of the anaesthetic and its attendant risks. The anaesthetist should explain these to the patient in clear and simple terms. The consent is not valid if the patient has already received sedative premedication. In addition, the purpose and complications of regional anaesthetic blocks must be explained.

Although at present there is a lack of consensus regarding the amount of detail required for patients to make an informed choice, it is prudent for the anaesthetist to record any contentious discussion. Patients in the UK are often given information booklets about their anaesthetic before admission.

Box 1.1.1

Template for preoperative assessment

1. Assess general health – a detailed and careful assessment of effort tolerance and cardiovascular reserve is a most important determinant of risk. Patients may be vague and evasive. Only careful questioning will reveal limitations in physiological reserve.
2. Systematically enquire about current and past medical history and recent visits to the general practitioner. Current medications include oral contraceptives and regular ingestion of aspirin.
3. Note previous anaesthetics, with complications or unexpected outcomes, postoperative nausea and vomiting, and any family history of anaesthetic problems.
4. Establish daily nicotine and alcohol intake and for how long. Patients tend to underestimate these. Patients with a history of alcohol abuse may have liver dysfunction and be relatively resistant to the effect of sedative drugs.
5. Enquire about use of other recreational substances enjoyed on a regular basis. Drug addicts may be HIV and hepatitis B and C positive.
6. Assess body habitus with special reference to obesity, dentition and mental status.
7. Find out about allergies or drug sensitivities. Patients do not tend to differentiate between side-effects and true allergies.
8. Find out about the severity of any gastric reflux or hiatus hernia symptoms, especially when lying flat, and medications taken to control them.
9. Check for a history of thromboembolic disease.
10. Check for loose teeth, bridgework or crowns. This is especially important if intubation is planned.
11. Record the time of last intake of food and water. Standard regimens – based on American Society of Anesthesiologists (ASA) guidelines – permit solid food up to 6 h, breast milk up to 4 h, and clear fluids up to 2 h preoperatively.
12. Obtain consent for both the anaesthetic and the surgery.

Template for preoperative assessment

A template for areas that should be systematically covered is provided in Box 1.1.1. Depending on initial findings, more thorough questioning may be needed.

Preoperative investigations

Traditionally clinicians have seen admission to hospital as an opportunity to screen for biochemical, haematological and radiological abnormalities.

However, there is no benefit in this, and a test should only be ordered if it will change patient management. Recently, in an attempt to bring consistency to this area, the National Institute for Clinical Excellence (NICE) in the UK has introduced guidelines for preoperative investigations based upon consensus and best evidence.[2]

Risk assessment

There are several scoring systems to assess physical status and help quantify risk. The system most commonly used is the American Society of Anaesthesiologists (ASA) classification, which ranks physical status (Table 1.1.1). This is the simplest and most widely used system for describing a patient's physical condition, although there may be lack of consistency in its application. It does not accommodate the asymptomatic patient who, for example, may have severe coronary artery disease. It also ignores risks incurred by the proposed operation. It is therefore not synonymous with the risk of morbidity and mortality.

ASA classification[a]	Patient's condition
ASA 1	No organic, physiological, biochemical or psychiatric disturbance. The pathological process for which the operation is to be performed is localised and does not entail a systemic disturbance
ASA 2	Mild-to-moderate systemic disturbance caused by the condition to be treated surgically or other pathophysiology (e.g. mild heart disease, diabetes mellitus, mild hypertension, anaemia, old age, obesity, mild chronic bronchitis)
ASA 3	Limited lifestyle – severe systemic disturbance or disease from any cause; it may not be possible to define the degree of disability with any precision (e.g. angina, severe diabetes mellitus, and cardiac failure
ASA 4	Severe systemic disorder that is already life-threatening and not always correctable by operation (e.g. marked cardiac insufficiency, persistent angina, severe respiratory, renal or hepatic insufficiency)
ASA 5	Moribund. Little chance of survival, but submitted for operation in desperation. Little if any anaesthesia is required

[a]If the operation is an emergency, the letter E is placed after the numerical classification, and the patient is considered to be in a poorer physical condition

Table 1.1.1 ASA classification

Other useful preoperative scoring systems which may be employed, depending on the circumstances, are:

- Goldman index for cardiac disease;
- Glasgow Coma Scale for head injury;
- Pugh–Childs scoring index for liver disease;
- New York Heart Association (NYHA) scoring index for heart disease;
- Fleischer Risk Index for cardiac disease.

SYSTEMATIC ASSESSMENT

Cardiovascular system

Ischaemic heart disease and congestive cardiac failure are common in the elderly, but are also encountered in younger patients who have specific risk factors. Many such patients who present for surgery are on a variety of cardiac medications and have reasonably stable symptoms. Many of these will have had an intervention such as angioplasty or heart surgery, and an increasing number of patients have had heart transplantation. An important group of patients are those with a history of arrhythmias, including those with implanted pacemakers. Other conditions occasionally encountered include hypertensive and valvular heart disease, cardiomyopathies and pericarditis.

In the elderly, the murmur of aortic stenosis may be difficult to distinguish from a sclerotic murmur, and echocardiography may be useful. Irrespective of the pathology, it is important to establish the nature and severity of symptoms, whether the patient is stable, and which medications are currently being used.

A common scenario, particularly in children, is to be informed that there is a murmur. This is often a benign flow murmur in patients who are otherwise fit. Occasionally an asymptomatic valvular lesion will necessitate prophylactic administration of antibiotics. Usually the correct course of action can be determined by careful questioning of the parents and perusal of the notes.

The two cardinal symptoms of cardiac disease are exercise intolerance and chest pain, which typically has a crushing character and radiates to the left arm. Exercise intolerance may be assessed by asking about ability to perform everyday tasks, including capacity to walk on the flat or climb stairs etc. Patients with severe cardiac disease may have orthopnoea or paroxysmal nocturnal. The NYHA grades cardiac symptoms on a scale of 1 to 4 depending on whether the patient has symptoms that are absent, mild, severe, or occur at rest. Other symptoms of cardiac disease include ankle swelling, nocturia, palpitations and occasionally syncope.

Physical examination and investigations

Physical examination is extremely important and should include pulse (rate, rhythm and character) and blood pressure, and examination for engorgement of neck veins, hepatomegaly, ascites, ankle or sacral pitting oedema, basal crepitations in the lungs, cardiac murmurs and added heart sounds. An ECG should be obtained and chest radiography considered, together with routine haematology and biochemistry. Further tests are determined by the general condition of the patient and whether the symptoms are stable.

Risks of surgery

In patients with congestive cardiac failure, the risks of surgery are significant. A number of authors, including Goldman et al., [3] have tried using clinical indices to predict outcome in such patients undergoing non-cardiac surgery (Table 1.1.2).

Among the factors that consistently correlate with outcome are a history of myocardial infarct in the preceding 6 months, signs of heart failure and abnormal cardiac rhythm. A simplified and more recent analysis by Fleischer and Eagle has also implicated diabetes mellitus and impaired renal function as carrying a worse prognosis.[4] Fleischer's cardiac risk factors are:

- ischaemic heart disease (e.g. angina, previous myocardial infarct);
- congestive cardiac failure;
- poor cardiopulmonary functional status (e.g. exercise tolerance NYHA grade >3, recent non-Q-wave (subendocardial) myocardial infarction);
- diabetes mellitus;
- renal insufficiency.

A patient undergoing major surgery with three of these additional risk factors should be considered for further noninvasive testing of cardiac function.

A modified list has been described by Lee et al.[5] as follows:

- high-risk surgery (or age >70 years[6]);
- history of ischaemic heart disease;
- congestive cardiac failure;
- previous stroke;
- diabetes mellitus;
- renal failure.

These risk factors have been used to estimate risk of complications and the need for β-blockade.

A common further noninvasive test of cardiac function is the stress ECG. In most cases this is performed while the patient exercises. In patients for whom this is not possible (e.g. because of arthritis), it can be carried out using an inotrope such as dobutamine.

For some patients with more complex clinical findings, such as those with left bundle branch block or with persistent angina following coronary

A patient's score is totalled and used to calculate the risk of major complications associated with surgery	
Patient's score Criteria	**Points**
1. History	
Age >70 years	5
Myocardial infarct in preceding 6 months	10
2. Physical examination	
Third heart sound or gallop rhythm	11
Aortic stenosis	3
3. ECG	
Rhythm other than sinus, or atrial ectopic beats on ECG	7
>5 ventricular ectopics per minute	7
4. General status	
Po_2 <8 kPa (<60 mmHg) or Pco_2 >6.7 kPa (>50 mmHg)	3
K^+ <3.0 mmol/L or bicarbonate <20 mmol/L	
Blood urea nitrogen (BUN) >8.3 mmol/L or creatinine >270 µmol/L	
Abnormal liver enzymes or signs of chronic liver disease	
Patient bedridden from non-cardiac causes	
5. Operation	
Intraperitoneal, intrathoracic or aortic operation	3
Emergency operation	4
Total possible score	**53**

Risk of major complications associated with surgery		
Class (number of points)	**Cardiac death**	**Life threatening complications**
I (0–5)	0.2%	0.7%
II (6–12)	2%	5%
III (13–25)	2%	11%
IV (>26)	56%	22%

Table 1.1.2 Computation of cardiac risk (Goldman et al.[3])

revascularisation, radionuclide imaging or dobutamine stress echocardiography may be indicated.[7] Radionuclide stress testing can be carried out using a vasodilator such as adenosine or dipyridamole, which creates a coronary steal syndrome, whereas myocardial imaging is performed using thallium or technetium. Dobutamine stress echocardiography is a useful noninvasive test that gives baseline ejection fraction together with an indication of both abnormalities of regional wall motion and the response to inotropes. Cardiac catheterisation is usually indicated for patients in whom a noninvasive test is strongly positive or whose symptoms are unequivocal.

Patients who have cardiac prostheses and are on anticoagulant therapy should be changed from warfarin to heparin, so that their anticoagulation can be stopped for a minimum period of time. Patients with any form of valvular heart disease and those with intracardiac shunts require antibiotic prophylaxis against endocarditis before procedures known to cause bacteraemia.

Perioperative β-blockade

There is mounting evidence that patients with coronary ischaemia might benefit from perioperative β-blockade with agents such as atenolol and bisoprolol.[8] Despite most studies demonstrating a reduction in both infarction and mortality rates, there is still uncertainty about the best timing and duration of therapy[9] and there are no agreed recommendations. A number of authors have attempted to quantify perioperative cardiac risk and the effectiveness of β-blockade using, for example, Lee's revised cardiac risk index or Boersma's clinical risk score.[6] A suggested template based on these results is shown in Table 1.1.3.

Preoperative hypertension

Patients who have uncontrolled hypertension have a high perioperative morbidity. However, so-called 'white coat' hypertension is common. The patient should be carefully assessed and several blood pressure measurements should be obtained before surgery is needlessly postponed, which should probably only be considered if the blood pressure is higher than 180/110 mmHg. If necessary the patient's general practitioner should be contacted for further information regarding blood pressure control and current therapy.[10]

Apply one point per risk factor using Boersma's clinical risk score[6]

Points	Risk of adverse cardiac events (%)	Perioperative β-blockade
0	1.2	Not beneficial
1–2	3.0	Proven coronary artery disease – beneficial Unproven coronary artery disease – controversial
>3	6–33	Beneficial, except in small group of patients with abnormal ventricular wall motion on dobutamine stress echocardiography

Table 1.1.3 Perioperative β-blockade

Respiratory system

Lung disease is a major cause of intra- and postoperative complications, so a careful history and examination are needed. The degree of exercise intolerance should be established as well as factors that precipitate breathlessness or, in the case of patients who have asthma, factors that precipitate bronchospasm.

Cigarette smoking is important in the aetiology of chronic lung disease and lung cancer. Current consumption as well as previous smoking habits should be recorded. Despite recent trends, approximately 25% of the population continue to smoke. Although they may not be labelled as chronic bronchitics, many smokers have increased sputum production and airway sensitivity that can cause difficulties during and after anaesthesia. Together with the adverse effects of both nicotine and carbon monoxide, smokers are therefore advised to avoid smoking for as long as possible preoperatively.

Chronic bronchitis is usually defined as a recurrent productive cough for 3 months of the year over 2 consecutive years. Patients usually have seasonal fluctuations in symptoms, with characteristic winter exacerbations. The presence of a productive cough is important, as is the colour and consistency of the expectorate. Emphysema is dilatation of the air spaces distal to the terminal bronchioles with destruction of their walls. There is a clinical spectrum of chronic obstructive respiratory disease ranging from 'blue bloater' to 'pink puffer', but in practice most patients have features of both (Table 1.1.4).

Severe asthmatics require careful management, particularly if intubation is planned. This will require timed administration of bronchodilators preoperatively and a strategy such as topical application of local anaesthetic to prevent bronchospasm at induction.

Physical examination and investigations

Physical examination should include:

- initial assessment of cyanosis and finger clubbing;
- observation of the pattern of breathing and degree of chest expansion;
- auscultation of both lung fields for added sounds, mediastinal shift and localising signs.

If active infection is suspected, antibiotic therapy should be commenced after sampling of sputum. Patients who have an audible wheeze should be assessed using spirometry – not only to establish a baseline, but also to monitor the degree of airway reversibility and if possible optimise this using bronchodilator therapy.

Lung function tests are performed to quantify a number of physiological variables and by comparing these to a peer group, so estimates the severity of the underlying condition. The values can also be used as a control to

The classic features of the two ends of the spectrum of chronic obstructive airway disease — the pink puffer and the blue bloater		
Features	**"Pink puffer"**	**"Blue bloater"**
Clinical	Pink, dyspnoeic, thin, malnourished, heart disease uncommon, air trapping present, PEEP harmful	Central cyanosis, obese, excessive mucus production, sputum retention, intrapulmonary shunting usually present, PEEP may be helpful, cor pulmonale common
Haematology	Hb normal	Polycythaemia
Chest radiograph	Normal in early stages; later, overinflated lung fields, narrow mediastinum, horizontal ribs	Normal in early disease; later, cardiomegaly and upper lobe blood diversion
Lung function tests	Obstructive pattern, TLC increased, VC reduced	Obstructive pattern, TLC normal, VC reduced
Blood gases	Normal at rest, hypoxaemic on exercise	Hypoxaemic, hypercarbic
ECG	Normal	RA and RV hypertrophy

Hb, haemoglobin; PEEP, positive end-expiratory pressure; RA, right atrium; RV, right ventricle; TLC, total lung capacity; VC, vital capacity

Table 1.1.4 Chronic obstructive airway disease

measure the effects of treatment, and as a baseline should the patient deteriorate postoperatively (Table 1.1.5).

The three most commonly performed tests are PEFR, FVC and FEV_1. If FEV_1 is reduced, the response to bronchodilator therapy should be recorded. These tests can be carried out at the bedside. Flow rates can be measured by a handheld Wright's peak expiratory flow meter, and FEV_1 and FVC by a spirometer such as the Vitalograph. Diffusing capacity is less frequently measured. This is simply a measure of limited gas transfer across a thickened alveolar membrane using a gas such as carbon monoxide.

Arterial blood gas estimation may be advisable in patients with severe respiratory disease to act as a benchmark, particularly if postoperative intermittent positive-pressure ventilation (IPPV) is likely to be necessary, and to quantify the severity of impairment of gas exchange and detect carbon dioxide retention.

Test	Normal value	Use
Total lung capacity (TLC) – maximum lung volume	5–6 L	Distinguishes between restrictive (decreased TLC) and obstructive (increased TLC) lung disease
Forced vital capacity (FVC)	4–5 L	Measure of ventilatory reserve. Reduced in both obstructive and restrictive lung disease and in neuromuscular impairment
Residual volume (RV) – minimum lung volume	33% of TLC	Increased in emphysema
Forced expiratory volume in 1 second (FEV_1)	75% of FVC	Effort dependent. Reduced in both obstructive and restrictive lung disease
FEV_1/FVC ratio	>75%	Reduced in obstructive lung disease
Peak expiratory flow rate (PEFR)	450–650 L/ min	Good measure of respiratory obstruction. Severe obstruction if <120 L/min
Maximal voluntary ventilation (MVV)	70–100 L/min	Index of total cardiorespiratory function
Diffusion capacity for carbon monoxide (D_LCO)	>80%	Decreased in emphysema and in lung fibrosis. Represents the functional alveolar area

Table 1.1.5 Lung function tests

Upper airway

A cursory examination of the upper airway should always be carried out, and a more thorough examination should be carried out if intubation is planned. Mouth opening and neck mobility should be assessed. Dentition should be examined for the presence of prominent or loose teeth, caps, crowns, veneers and bridgework, especially at the front of the mouth. Their presence should be recorded, and the patient warned of possible damage.

A number of scoring systems have been developed in recent years to help predict difficult intubation. The most widely used is the Mallampati score, which assesses the extent to which intraoral structures can be visualised on maximal mouth opening:[11]

- grade 0 – tip of the epiglottis visible (Ezri et al.[12]);
- grade 1 – soft palate, faucial pillars and uvula visible;

- grade 2 – soft palate and faucial pillars visible, but uvula obscured by base of tongue;
- grade 3 – only soft palate visible;
- grade 4 – only hard palate visible.

This system has recently been modified as shown above.[12] Other indicators of difficult intubation include a thyromental distance less than 6.5 cm[13] and a sternomental distance less than 12.5 cm.[14] None of the published clinical tests provide either 100% sensitivity or 100% specificity. The combination of the Mallampati score with either the thyromental or the sternomental distance provides a positive predictive value of up to 100%.[15]

Gastrointestinal system

Liver

A history of jaundice should be noted. Often the underlying cause is clear (e.g. cholecystitis, gallstones or hepatitis). In the case of hepatitis, a more detailed history is required. A patient with a history of intravenous drug abuse may be HIV positive. Other causes of jaundice include adverse drug reactions. If this has occurred after anaesthesia, it may be related to the volatile agent, particularly halothane. Steps should be taken to determine the nature of the anaesthetic, the clinical course and whether a definitive diagnosis was made at the time. Volatile agents other than halothane may cause jaundice, and crossover reactions are well documented.[16]

Non-alcoholic fatty liver disease (NAFLD) encompasses a wide clinical and pathological spectrum from simple steatosis (fatty liver) to non-alcoholic steatohepatitis (NASH), which may advance to cirrhosis and end-stage liver disease. NASH is an advanced form of NAFLD associated with a syndrome comprising obesity, type 2 diabetes mellitus and elevated blood lipids. The prevalence of NAFLD in the USA is around 20%, and is increasing in the UK. In many cases of liver dysfunction patients remain asymptomatic.[17] There is therefore a wide spectrum of conditions where underlying liver disease may not be apparent, but which nevertheless constitute a perioperative risk.

Patients with asymptomatic liver dysfunction present for surgery with NASH, liver fibrosis or occasionally cirrhosis. Obstructive jaundice is usually caused by gallstones or occasionally by cancer of the head of pancreas. Rarely, patients with cirrhosis and severe liver dysfunction present for treatment of the complications of portal hypertension, such as bleeding varices.

Risk assessment

Risk assessment of patients with hepatic disease can be undertaken using the Child–Pugh Risk Index (Table 1.1.6). This is a useful guide to operative risk in a cirrhotic patient. The assessment is based on the sum of a number

	Child grade		
	A	B	C
Bilirubin (μmol/L)	<35	35–60	>60
Albumin (g/L)	>35	28–35	<28
Prothrombin time (seconds prolonged)	1–4	4–6	>6
Encephalopathy	0	1–2	3–4
Ascites	None	Easy	Difficult
Nutritional status	Excellent	Good	Poor
Operative mortality (approximate %)	0–10	4–31	19–76

Table 1.1.6 Child–Pugh scoring system for liver disease. Adapted from Pugh et al.[18]

of key clinical features. Grade A corresponds to low risk (0–10%). Grade B patients should be optimised preoperatively. Grade C patients should not undergo elective surgery if possible.

Preparation

Where necessary the jaundiced patient should be commenced on vitamin K. Ascites, due to a low serum albumin and retention of sodium and water, may impair respiration. The development of the hepatorenal syndrome is well documented in the jaundiced patient and prophylactic measures should be instigated, usually by preoperative administration of an osmotic diuretic such as mannitol. Patients with cirrhosis are particularly at risk from the effects of hypovolaemia, and central venous monitoring may be advisable. They may experience an exaggerated and prolonged effect of sedative drugs, and some are resistant to the effects of muscle relaxants due to an increased volume of distribution. Others are sensitive as a result of impaired metabolism.

Gastro-oesophageal reflux

Patients should be asked whether they have a hiatus hernia or symptoms of heartburn or acid reflux, and if so their severity, current treatment and precipitating factors should be assessed. In particular, obesity, inability to lie flat, or use of several pillows while sleeping will help in determining the need for antacid prophylaxis and rapid sequence intubation. In other cases, where symptoms are mild and especially if the anatomy suggests a possible difficult intubation, the inherent risks of a rapid sequence induction should be carefully considered.

Postoperative nausea and vomiting

Postoperative nausea and vomiting (PONV) is one of the most feared complications of anaesthesia. Many adults find PONV more distressing than postoperative pain.[19] Over the past decade its aetiology has become better understood, and new and more effective antiemetics have been introduced. Precipitating factors for PONV can be divided into:

- operative factors (e.g. ear, eye, gynaecological surgery);
- patient factors (e.g. women, children, people who suffer from travel sickness);
- anaesthetic factors (e.g. excess gas in the stomach, use of induction agents other than propofol, nitrous oxide, volatile agents and opioids).

Apfel et al.[20] have devised a simplified scoring system that gives a 20% risk to each of the following independent factors:

- female gender;
- non-smoker;
- history of PONV or motion sickness;
- predicted opioid use.

If more than one factor is present preoperatively, a prophylactic antiemetic should be administered.

Kidneys

Renal failure is normally treated with dialysis and renal transplantation, and so most patients presenting for elective surgery are well controlled. On the other hand, urgent surgical intervention is sometimes needed to relieve acute obstruction of the urinary tract. Plasma creatinine and urea levels remain within normal limits even if the glomerular filtration rate (GFR) is reduced to about 40 mL/min (one-third of normal). Thus a modest increase in creatinine may indicate a significant reduction in GFR, and a high value demonstrates a serious reduction in renal reserve.

Electrolytes (especially potassium), acid–base and fluid status must be carefully checked. Hyperkalaemia may cause serious cardiac arrhythmias, especially if suxamethonium is used. A patient with established renal failure should also be assessed for anaemia, evidence of weight loss and malnourishment, neuropathy and hypo- or hypercalcaemia. Uraemic pericarditis is a rare complication.

It is important to note the presence of any fistulae used for dialysis access, which must be carefully protected during surgery.

Finally, the renal excretion of some drugs and the metabolites of others that undergo hepatic metabolism is impaired in renal failure. For example, the glucuronated metabolites of morphine are active and may cause respiratory depression if normal dosage regimens are used.

Obesity

The body mass index (BMI) – weight in kg/square of height in m – should be recorded. A BMI above 35 represents morbid obesity, and a value above 27 for women and 28 for men represents a weight 25% above the ideal. This may cause difficulties with lifting and positioning in theatre. Special lifting equipment and an extra wide operating table may be required for the morbidly obese. The venous system should be examined for ease of cannulation.

Obese patients have an increased risk of death from stroke and cardiovascular disease, including thromboembolic disease. They are at risk of perioperative hypoxia because of hypoventilation and decreased FRC due to a position-dependent restriction of diaphragmatic excursion. Chest compliance is greatly reduced. Obese patients also commonly have a history of hypertension, sleep apnoea, gout, diabetes mellitus, hiatus hernia and gastric reflux. Obstructive sleep apnoea can progress to Pickwickian syndrome, daytime sleepiness and chronic right heart failure.

Endotracheal intubation may also be difficult, and provision should be made for this. Arterial cannulation is needed to measure blood pressure accurately because limb cuffs are difficult to apply correctly and are likely to lead to an overestimation of the true pressure.

If a neuraxial block is planned, check for a history of osteoarthritis, backache, disc prolapse or sciatica, and a history of surgery on the spine. Long spinal needles should be available. The volume of the epidural space is decreased, reducing the requirement for local anaesthetics.

Musculoskeletal system

Elderly patients and those with chronic illness may be frail and have exposed pressure points. This can lead to nerve damage if such patients are improperly positioned. Furthermore, many elderly patients have osteoporosis, which demands care when moving and positioning. This should be assessed for preoperatively.

Rheumatoid arthritis

Rheumatoid arthritis is a multisystem disorder that has a number of anaesthetic implications. Special attention should be paid to:

- the skin – which is delicate and easily traumatised;
- anaemia – which does not always respond to iron;
- the lungs – for nodules and fibrosis;
- the musculoskeletal system – for osteoporosis and painful joints.

The airway should be carefully assessed because it may be affected by poor mouth opening, an immobile neck and atlanto-occipital instability.

Patients with rheumatoid arthritis are usually on a number of drugs, including corticosteroids and immunosuppressive agents. These often have associated side-effects, such as:

- diabetes mellitus, hypertension, electrolyte imbalance (corticosteroids);
- folate deficiency and liver and pulmonary dysfunction (methotrexate);
- renal failure and hypertension (cyclosporin).

Neurological assessment

Dementia is common among the elderly and is normally apparent. However, in some patients the early stages may be subtle and the only manifestation may be short-term memory loss. It is not possible to take a medical history from patients with more severe dementia and consent for operation should be sought from a responsible relative or carer. Psychosis may be treated with lithium or monoamine oxidase inhibitors.

In a wide variety of neurological disorders, such as multiple sclerosis, myasthenia gravis and poliomyelitis, there are concerns about ventilatory function, which may be checked preoperatively by spirometry and used as a baseline for the postoperative period. Special attention should be paid to neuromuscular monitoring if relaxants are to be used.

Epilepsy

Patients with epilepsy should continue medication throughout the perioperative period. Enzyme induction and resistance to competitive neuromuscular blocking agents should be anticipated.[21] Patients with a history of fits should not be exposed to epileptogenic agents such as enflurane, methohexitone or ketamine. Propofol is not contraindicated in epileptics, although fits have been described after its use.

Parkinson's disease

Patients with Parkinson's disease should take their medication as normal until the time of surgery. Postoperative mobilisation may be difficult and care should be taken to avoid deep vein thrombosis (DVT) and pressure sores.

Haematological system

Anaemia

Anaemia should be sought by examination of the tongue, conjunctivae and mucous membranes, but mild anaemia is difficult to detect.

Iron deficiency is usually related to a poor diet or blood loss (e.g. menorrhagia or occult faecal loss).

In longstanding anaemia, as in chronic renal failure, there is little benefit in preoperative blood transfusion. Indeed, repeated transfusion in these patients may be disadvantageous owing to antibody formation, erythropoietin suppression and the risk of iron overload if transfusion is repeated. For a discussion on preoperative transfusion, see Chapter 1.2.

In a patient with cardiovascular disease, transfusion is unlikely to be indicated unless the haemoglobin level is less than 9–10 g/dL. This threshold may be set as low as 7 g/dL in a fit patient. Ideally, any preoperative transfusion should be completed 24 hours before surgery.

Clotting disorders

Abnormal or inappropriate bleeding or bruising should be asked about. Routine screening for clotting abnormalities is not recommended. The clotting status of patients on long-term warfarin therapy for whatever cause should be assessed with an INR (international normalised ratio). For major surgery, warfarin is normally stopped several days preoperatively and the operative period is covered with heparin.

Risk of thromboembolism

It should be established whether the patient has any added risk for thromboembolic disease that requires prophylaxis to be commenced preoperatively. Risk factors for thromboembolism are:

- history of previous thromboembolism;
- severe obesity;
- major orthopaedic, abdominal or gynaecological surgery;
- prolonged immobilisation;
- old age;
- malignancy;
- pregnancy;
- dehydration;
- polycythaemia;
- use of oral contraceptives;
- malignancy;
- presence of factor V Leiden (a congenital abnormality with resistance to the effect of the antithrombotic protein C).

A low-risk patient may only require prophylaxis with compressive stockings, whereas a high-risk patient may require prolonged anticoagulation with warfarin. A simplified approach to prophylaxis is as follows:

- low risk – compressive stockings with or without aspirin;
- medium risk – compressive stockings or an intermittent compressive device and low-molecular weight heparin (e.g. 20–40 mg enoxaparin subcutaneously);

- high risk – compressive stockings or an intermittent compressive device and low-molecular weight heparin. Maintain anticoagulation with warfarin.

Low molecular weight heparin should not be given less than 12 hours before the performance of neuraxial block to minimise the risk of epidural haematoma formation (see Ch. 4.3).

Sickle cell disease

Sickle cell disease is a congenital haemoglobinopathy in which sickle cell haemoglobin (HbS) leads to sickling of red cells under hypoxic, hypothermic or acidotic conditions. It is thought to confer a biological advantage against malaria and is prevalent among black Africans and their descendants. Individuals may be homozygous (sickle cell disease) or, more commonly, heterozygous (sickle cell trait). Patients of African or Afro-Caribbean descent should be screened before surgery, using a Sickledex test. If this is positive, haemoglobin electrophoresis is indicated to distinguish between the homozygous and the heterozygous state, and to exclude other haemoglobinopathies such as HbSC or HbS thalassaemia.

Diabetes mellitus

Overall control and stability of blood sugar should be assessed at the preoperative visit, together with current treatment, including amount and type of insulin, and the presence and severity of complications. Particular areas of concern are the cardiovascular, renal and nervous systems.

Autonomic dysfunction

Autonomic dysfunction should be excluded, particularly if the patient has peripheral neuropathy. This may be manifest by impotence, lack of sweating, postural hypotension, drop attacks, painless myocardial ischaemia and gastroparesis. A simple screening test is lack of R–R variability on an ECG strip and a lack of pulse rate change with deep inspiration. If autonomic dysfunction is suspected, it may be confirmed by observing an abnormal response to a Valsalva manoeuvre, particularly a lack of the characteristic bradycardia following release of the manoeuvre.

For details of the perioperative management of diabetes mellitus, see Chapter 1.2. It is often necessary to start an infusion of insulin and glucose preoperatively, with careful monitoring of blood sugar. The main aim is to avoid preoperative hypoglycaemia and perioperative ketoacidosis.

Inherited risk factors

Genetically determined risk factors for disease are increasingly being recognised. Some of these are single gene abnormalities, usually disclosed by a careful family history. Many have implications for the anaesthetist, including:

- malignant hyperpyrexia;
- suxamethonium sensitivity;
- factor V Leiden;
- sickle cell disease;
- haemophilia;
- Duchenne muscular dystrophy;
- dystrophia myotonica.

Malignant hyperpyrexia

Malignant hyperpyrexia, caused by an abnormality of the ryanodine gene, is a preventable cause of anaesthetic-related death. There is usually a family history and siblings should undergo screening before anaesthesia. The standard test is the in-vitro sensitivity of striated muscle to caffeine and halothane. Genotyping is likely to supplement this and avoid the need for muscle biopsy[22] (see Ch. 3.3).

PREMEDICATION

Anaesthetic premedication traditionally consisted of opioid analgesia combined with an antisialogogue such as atropine or hyoscine. There has been a gradual tendency in recent years to avoid intramuscular injections if possible, and oral premedication has become more popular. If only sedation is required, then a benzodiazepine such as temazepam is a popular choice.

In addition, a variety of conditions may merit prophylactic treatment (e.g. an antacid for a hiatus hernia or other tendency to regurgitation, or an anticoagulant for thromboembolism).

Some patients with ischaemic heart disease may benefit from preoperative β-blockade.

Children are a special group and require careful assessment. A sedative such as midazolam is a popular choice. In infants, the high vagal tone necessitates some form of anticholinergic agent, especially if intubation is planned.

Specific conditions for which premedication is advisable

Specific conditions for which premedication is advisable include the following:

- anxiety – to reduce fear and obviate the untoward effects of high sympathetic tone;
- planned endoscopic intubation – an antisialogogue to reduce saliva and bronchial secretions;

- to reduce vagal tone – atropine is advisable before laryngoscopy and intubation in infants and children, who have a high vagal tone; and anticholinergic agents may be used in all patients to inhibit vagal reflexes caused by either surgical stimulation (e.g. squint surgery, stretching of the anal sphincter) or medication such as β-blockers;
- needle phobia – topical application of local anaesthetic cream, such as EMLA®, or tetracaine (amethocaine) gel may be useful;
- for specific therapeutic effects – for example, corticosteroids, bronchodilators, antacids, H_2 blockers, transdermal glyceryl trinitrate patch dressings.

Drugs used for premedication

Sedatives

Benzodiazepines or phenothiazines are most commonly used. The sedative action is helped by the oral administration of a suitable benzodiazepine hypnotic the night before operation. Zopiclone 7.5 mg is a safe non-benzodiazepine alternative. Clonidine has a mild sedative effect, and has been used to reduce requirements for volatile anaesthetics.

Benzodiazepines

Benzodiazepines inhibit γ-aminobutyric acid (GABA) receptors and have anticonvulsant properties. These are good premedicants – they can be given orally and produce sedation, amnesia and freedom from anxiety. The amnesia is anterograde, and lasts some 10 minutes if given intravenously, but much longer after oral doses. They can also be given intramuscularly or rectally, and can be used singly or in combination.

Benzodiazepines can be combined with oral analgesics to add background analgesia. Effects on the cardiovascular and respiratory systems are minor, but they do potentiate propofol and thiopentone. Patients who regularly take benzodiazepines will be resistant to their action. The chief difference between them is their duration of action.

The action of benzodiazepines may be reversed with flumazenil. This is a specific antagonist, useful for reversing both therapeutic doses and overdoses. The dose is 100–200 μg intravenously up to total of 1 mg. This only lasts about 30 minutes, and so further infusion may be needed (100–400 μg/h). It can transiently increase pulse and blood pressure. Rarely, fits may occur.

Temazepam is a short-acting (4 hours) benzodiazepine. The adult dose is 10–30 mg. Temazepam is useful for night sedation or for premedication for all types of surgery, including day stay, and is suitable for the elderly. Temazepan syrup (2 mg/mL) is available for children and the dose is 0.5 mg/kg.

Midazolam is used as night sedation before surgery (15 mg orally) or as premedication. It can be given intramuscularly 70–100 μg/kg 30–60 minutes before surgery. It is commonly used as a sedative during endoscopy or regional analgesia (2–7.5 mg intravenously), sometimes combined with a short-acting opioid such as fentanyl. This is useful in patients with severe learning disabilities. It may also be used for induction in the elderly (up to 0.1 mg/kg), or as a co-induction agent with propofol.

Lorazepam is used in a dose of 1–4 mg (30–50 μg/kg) orally, sublingually or intramuscularly given 2 hours preoperatively. It is longlasting (4–24 hours) and causes appreciable anterograde amnesia. It abolishes the vasoconstriction that accompanies fear and attenuates the psychic sequelae of ketamine.

Diazepam is used in a dose of 10–20 mg orally or intramuscularly and has a duration of 4–8 hours. Combination with metoprolol greatly enhances its anxiolytic activity.

Phenothiazines

Promethazine is a sedative, anxiolytic, antihypertensive, antihistaminic and antiemetic, and is useful in combination with pethidine as a premedicant. The dose is 25–50 mg intramuscularly. Patients with alcoholic liver disease are very sensitive to all phenothiazines.

Trimeprazine tartrate is available as a syrup for oral administration to children. The dose is 2 mg/kg 2 hours preoperatively, although higher doses have been used with success. Many anaesthetists now use benzodiazepines in preference.

Analgesics

Opioids

Opioids usually produce euphoria, but at the price of some nausea in many patients. Preoperative analgesia is especially important when considerable postoperative pain is anticipated.

Non-steroidal anti-inflammatory drugs

Long-acting non-steroidal anti-inflammatory drugs (NSAIDs) give useful background analgesia for intraoperative and postoperative opioids to develop an enhanced analgesic effect, with fewer side-effects. Diclofenac (50–100 mg orally or rectally), ketoprofen (100–200 mg orally or rectally, up to 50 mg intramuscularly), and piroxicam (20–40 mg orally) will all give useful analgesia. Piroxicam is not licensed for postoperative use.

Anticholinergic agents

Atropine

From the Greek legend involving Atropos, the oldest of the three fates who spun the thread of life. Atropine is an alkaloid of *Atropa belladonna* or deadly nightshade. The atropine group of alkaloids are esters of tropic acid with organic bases – tropine (atropine) and scopine (hyoscine). Atropine is a racemic mixture, but the laevo isomer is the more active.

Effects on the nervous system Atropine has a competitive blocking action on muscarinic receptors supplied by postganglionic cholinergic nerves (e.g. smooth muscles and secretory glands). It has no effect on either production or destruction of acetylcholine, nor on its nicotinic effects. Complete vagal block requires a dose of 3 mg. Atropine also stimulates the medulla and higher centres and the respiratory centre, and causes auditory hyperacusis. It inhibits sweating and so may be best avoided in pyrexial children. Occasionally, restlessness and delirium are seen (central anticholinergic syndrome, see below).

Effects on the eye Topical atropine paralyses the sphincter of the iris, resulting in dilated pupils and loss of accommodation for up to 1 week. Parenteral atropine has little effect on the eye and is not contraindicated in a patient with glaucoma, even of the narrow-angle type, because significant dilatation of the pupil does not occur. Patients with Down's syndrome may show resistance to parenteral atropine and to sedatives.

Effects on the respiratory system Sweat, bronchial and salivary glands are inhibited by atropine. Bronchial muscle is relaxed, causing bronchodilation and a slight increase in anatomical dead space. If given intramuscularly 1 hour before anaesthesia, salivation is suppressed more efficiently than if given intravenously immediately before induction.

Effects on the circulatory system Atropine results in tachycardia due to inhibition of vagal influence on the sinoatrial node. The heart rate may slow initially due to the Bezold–Jarisch coronary chemoreceptor reflex. Atropine may cause nodal rhythm. The tachycardia decreases coronary filling time and increases myocardial oxygen consumption. Atropine should therefore be used with care in patients with coronary artery disease. Cardiac output and arterial pressure are usually increased, with a fall in central venous pressure (CVP). Tachycardia is less marked in the elderly. Bradycardia caused by vagal reflexes or neostigmine is prevented.

Atropine sometimes causes marked dilatation of the vessels of the face.

Atropine should be considered for asystole, although it is no longer recommended as first-line treatment.

Effects on the alimentary canal Tone and peristalsis of the gut and urinary tract are decreased by atropine. Like hyoscine and glycopyrronium, atropine lowers the opening pressure of the cardiac sphincter of the stomach and hence increases the chances of regurgitation.

Effects on the fetus Atropine crosses the placenta rapidly (as a tertiary amine), and may protect the fetus and newborn from vagal reflexes occurring during birth and resuscitation.

Pharmacokinetics The plasma half-life of atropine is 2–3 hours, and it is 50% protein bound. Elimination is slow in children under 2 years of age, and in the elderly. Excretion is partly renal, and it is partly destroyed in the tissues and liver, with the formation of tropine and tropic acid.

Dose The usual adult dose of atropine is 0.6 mg intramuscularly (in children 15–20 μg/kg) 1 hour before operation. The dose of atropine is 1–2 mg when coadministered with intravenous neostigmine.

Overdose may occur in small children, especially if septic, abolishing sweating and causing a febrile convulsion. In adults, the characteristic picture of overdose is mad (central effect), hot, blind (paralysis of accommodation), red (facial flushing) and dry (inhibition of secretions).

Hyoscine hydrobromide (scopolamine hydrobromide)

Hyoscine hydrobromide has similar actions to atropine. It is another belladonna alkaloid and is also a tertiary amine, so crosses the blood–brain barrier and causes drowsiness, sleep and amnesia in some patients. Occasionally it produces the central anticholinergic syndrome. Hyoscine hydrobromide is a mild respiratory stimulant, and its actions on the iris, the salivary, sweat and bronchial glands are stronger than those of atropine. It is a moderately powerful antiemetic. Its action on heart, intestine and bronchial muscle is weaker than that of atropine.

The adult dose of hyoscine hydrobromide is 0.3–0.6 mg intramuscularly. A combination of hyoscine 0.4 mg with pethidine 100 mg or papaveretum 20 mg has been widely used before surgery.

Hyoscine butylbromide

Used, like propantheline, as a gastrointestinal or urinary antispasmodic, hyoscine butylbromide can be absorbed from skin (e.g. posterior to the pinna). The dose is 10–30 mg orally, intramuscularly or intravenously.

Glycopyrronium bromide

Glycopyrronium bromide is a quaternary ammonium compound that does not readily cross the placental or blood–brain barriers, and so does not cause central anticholinergic effects. Like atropine and hyoscine it reduces the tone of the lower oesophageal sphincter (the opposite effect to metoclopramide). It suppresses gastric secretion better than atropine or hyoscine, and results in less tachycardia and arrhythmia. It is effective at preventing bradycardia after suxamethonium, and is more potent and longer lasting than atropine at drying salivary secretions. Emergence from anaesthesia is faster than after atropine. In clinical doses it does not affect the pupil size. Glycopyrronium bromide is not antiemetic, and is commonly used with neostigmine to reverse neuromuscular block.

The dose of glycopyrronium bromide for premedication is 0.2–0.4 mg for an adult and 4–8 μg/kg for a child. The dose to prevent bradycardia is 0.2 mg for an adult and 4 μg/kg for a child.

Central anticholinergic syndrome

Excitement, drowsiness or even coma may be seen, especially in the elderly, after treatment with atropine or hyoscine. There may also be thought impairment, memory disturbances, hallucinations, ataxia and behavioural abnormalities. The patient may be slow to wake up in recovery. Treatment is with physostigmine salicylate, an anticholinesterase derived from the Calabar bean that has a tertiary amine, allowing it to cross the blood–brain barrier (neostigmine has a quaternary amine that prevents this). The dose of physostigmine is 2 mg intravenously, repeated if necessary. Physostigmine has also been used in the treatment of depressant effects on the central nervous system by tricyclic antidepressants and phenothiazines, and also modifies the psychotic side-effects of ketamine.

PRE-EXISTING DRUG THERAPY

Antihypertensive drugs

Antihypertensive drugs are normally continued up to the time of surgery, which maintains a normal blood volume and minimises the risk of a dangerous hypotension at induction. Some prefer to omit angiotensin-converting enzyme (ACE) or angiotensin-II receptor blockers, which both may nevertheless cause significant hypotension.

Anti-anginal drugs

Anti-anginal drugs such as calcium channel blockers or nitrates should be continued up to the time of surgery or angina may recur. If the oral route is impossible, transdermal glyceryl trinitrate patch dressings placed on the chest wall last about 24 hours. Reapplication should be at a fresh site. Sublingual glyceryl trinitrate spray may be used for a fast onset of action.

Lithium

Lithium should be stopped 2 days before major surgery because it potentiates non-depolarising relaxants. In emergencies, suxamethonium and regional blocks should be considered as alternatives. Lithium toxicity may occur when the patient is dehydrated. It is generally safe to continue lithium therapy before minor surgery provided that due attention is paid to fluid and electrolyte balance.

Monoamine oxidase inhibitors

There are two types of monoamine oxidase (MAO) – type A, which is mainly in the brain, and type B, which is mainly in the lungs and liver.

The older non-selective drugs such as phenelzine, isocarboxazid, and especially tranylcypramine, should be discontinued 2 weeks before elective surgery. They irreversibly inhibit MAO-A and B. Their mode of action cannot be explained solely in terms of MAO inhibition. They also have anticholinergic properties. Reactions to pethidine, and to a much lesser extent to fentanyl and morphine, have been reported in patients taking these drugs, causing fits, coma, muscle twitching, hypertension, ataxia and ocular palsies. Deaths have occurred. Relief has been obtained following administration of 25 mg chlorpromazine. Not all patients show adverse reactions, and small test doses of pethidine have been given while monitoring pulse and blood pressure. A combination of chlorpromazine and codeine has been successfully used for postoperative analgesia, as have regional blocks and NSAIDs. Severe hypertension and even death may occur when pressor drugs (e.g. epinephrine (adrenaline) in local analgesic solutions) are given to patients on MAO inhibitors, but may be treated with phentolamine. The same reaction occurs when tyramine is ingested, as in cheese.

The reversible specific MAO-A inhibitors (moclobemide) and MAO-B inhibitors (selegiline) are much less dangerous during anaesthesia and may be continued up to the day before surgery. Caution is still needed. Pethidine and sympathomimetic drugs should be avoided. Selegiline is used in the treatment of Parkinson's disease.

Selective serotonin uptake inhibitors

Selective serotonin uptake inhibitors (e.g. fluoxetine, paroxetine, sertraline, fluvoxamine) are commonly prescribed for depression and obsessive–compulsive disorders. The half-life is several days. Selective serotonin uptake inhibitors inhibit the P450 enzymes and may prolong the actions of other drugs metabolised by this system (e.g. warfarin). They are relatively free of side-effects relevant to the anaesthetist, although it has been reported that the metabolism of ropivacaine is reduced by fluvoxamine.

Levodopa

Levodopa should be continued up to the time of surgery to prevent the recurrence of severe parkinsonism, dysphagia and the risk of aspiration pneumonia.

Corticosteroid therapy

Normal secretion of cortisol (hydrocortisone) from the adrenal cortex is about 25 mg/day, but can rise as high as 300–500 mg/day in response to the stress of trauma or surgery. Corticosteroid therapy suppresses adrenocorticotrophic hormone (ACTH) production by the anterior pituitary. In time the adrenal cortex atrophies and is therefore unable to increase its secretion in response to stress. This can result in profound hypotension during and after anaesthesia, with a decreased sensitivity to catecholamines. A course as short as 1 week may produce this cortical depression. It usually recovers by 2 months after stopping the corticosteroid, but may last over 1 year, and in some cases of prolonged therapy may never recover. This risk is present whatever route of administration is used. For example, more than 1.5 g (6 puffs) per day of betamethasone may cause adrenal suppression.

Adrenal cortical function can be tested by giving tetracosactide (Synacthen, synthetic ACTH) and measuring the plasma cortisol response, but this is not a routine preoperative test. It is normally assumed that low-dose corticosteroid therapy (<10 mg prednisone per day) has little effect. For higher-dose therapy it is safe to give extra hydrocortisone over the period of surgery (e.g. hydrocortisone 25 mg at induction, followed by 25 mg 6-hourly for 24 hours for intermediate or 48 hours for major surgery). The intramuscular route gives more sustained plasma levels than intravenous administration.

Corticosteroids may be contraindicated in patients with active infections, tuberculosis or peptic ulcers, and are likely to make blood sugar control more difficult in patients who have diabetes mellitus.

Oral contraceptives

Oestrogen-containing (combined) oral contraceptives increase the risk of DVT, although the magnitude of this risk is uncertain. Surgery and the combined pill both reduce the activity of antithrombin III. The risk is greatest following major pelvic, cancer and orthopaedic operations, and in patients with factor V Leiden mutation. Combined pills should, if possible, be discontinued 4 weeks before major elective surgery or leg surgery, such as for varicose vein stripping or ligation, and started again at the first menstrual period following an interval of 2 weeks after the operation, providing the patient is fully mobile. If this is not possible (e.g. because of urgent surgery), prophylactic heparin should be considered. Additional risk factors are older age, obesity and cigarette smoking.

References

1. The Association of Anaesthetists of Great Britain and Ireland. Information and Consent for Anaesthesia. London: The Association of Anaesthetists of Great Britain and Ireland; 1999.
2. National Institute for Clinical Excellence. Preoperative tests. Summary of guidance issued to the NHS in England and Wales. 2003; Issue 7:285–302.

3. Goldman L, Caldera DL, Nussbaum R, et al. Multifactorial risk index of cardiac risk in noncardiac surgical procedures. N Engl J Med 1977; 297:845–850.

4. Fleischer LA, Eagle KA. Clinical practice: lowering cardiac risk in non-cardiac surgery. N Engl J Med 1995; 333:1750–1756.

5. Lee TH, Marcantonio ER, Mangione CM, et al. Derivation and prospective validation of a simple index for prediction of cardiac risk of major noncardiac surgery. Circulation 1999; 100:1043–1049.

6. Boersma E, Poldermans D, Bax JJ, et al. Predictors of cardiac events after major vascular surgery: role of clinical characteristics, dobutamine echocardiography and beta blocker therapy. JAMA 2001; 285:1865–1873.

7. Lee TH, Boucher CA. Clinical practice: non-invasive tests in patients with stable coronary artery disease. N Engl J Med 2001; 344:1840–1845.

8. Mangano DT, Layug EL, Wallace A, et al. Effect of atenolol on mortality and cardiovascular morbidity after noncardiac surgery. N Engl J Med 1996; 335:1713–1721.

9. Piccard BM. Perioperative beta blockade and haemodynamic optimisation in patients with coronary artery disease and decreasing exercise capacity presenting for non-cardiac surgery. Anaesthesia 2004; 59:60–68.

10. Howell J, Sears JW, Foex P. Hypertension, hypertensive heart disease and perioperative cardiac risk. Br J Anaesth 2004; 92:570–583.

11. Mallampati SR, Gatt SP, Gugino LD, et al. A clinical sign to predict difficult tracheal intubation: a prospective study. Can Anaesth Soc J 1985; 32:429–434.

12. Ezri T, Warters D, Szmuk P, et al. The incidence of class zero airway and the impact of Mallampati score, age, sex and body mass index on prediction of laryngoscopy grade. Anaesth Analg 2001; 93:1073–1075.

13. Patil VU, Stehling LC, Zaunder HL. Fibreoptic endoscopy. Chicago, USA: Chicago Year Book; 1983, p. 111.

14. Savva D. Prediction of difficult intubation. Br J Anaesth 1994; 73:149–153.

15. Iohom G, Ronayne M, Cunningham AJ. Prediction of difficult tracheal intubation. Eur J Anaesth 2003; 20:31–36.

16. Hasan F. Isoflurane hepatotoxicity in a patient with a previous history of halothane-induced hepatitis. Hepatogastroenterology 1998; 45:518–522.

17. Gronbaek H, Eivindson MV, Hamilton-Dutoit S, et al. Non-alcoholic steatohepatitis – a new hepatic disease. Ugeskr Laeger 2003; 165: 1115–1118.

18. Pugh RNH, Murray-Lyon IM, Dawson JL, et al. Transection of the oesophagus for bleeding oesophageal varices. Br J Surg 1973; 60:646–649.

19. Koivuranta M, Laara E, Snare L, Alahuhta S. A survey of postoperative nausea and vomiting. Anaesthesia 1997; 52:443–449.

20. Apfel CC, Laara E, Koivurantu M, et al. A simplified risk score for predicting postoperative nausea and vomiting. Anesthesiology 1999; 91:693–700.

21. Wright P, McCarthy G, Szenorhadszadsky J, et al. Influence of phenytoin use on pharmacokinetics, pharmacodynamics of vecuronium. Anesthesiology 2004; 100:626–633.

22. Nelson TE, Rosenberg H, Muldoon M. Genetic testing for malignant hyperthermia in North America. Anesthesiology 2004; 100:212–213.

CHAPTER **1.2**

MEDICAL DISEASES INFLUENCING ANAESTHESIA

CARDIOVASCULAR DISEASE

Cardiovascular disease is a frequent finding in patients presenting for anaesthesia and may be associated with an increased risk of perioperative cardiovascular complications, including myocardial infarction, which carries a high mortality rate.

Assessment of cardiac risk

The evaluation of risk factors[1,2] is of little benefit in predicting the outcome for an individual patient, but may be useful in assessing the need for further investigations and in planning anaesthetic management. Consideration should be given to:

- clinical factors that indicate the presence, severity and stability of cardiovascular disease as shown in Box 1.2.1;
- the functional capacity of the patient – poor functional capacity (e.g. inability to climb a flight of stairs) is associated with an increased risk of perioperative cardiovascular complications (although as an assessment of cardiovascular function, this may be of limited value where function is impaired by other conditions such as arthritis or respiratory disease);
- the surgical procedure, which may be categorised as high, intermediate or low risk, as shown in Box 1.2.2.

Coronary artery disease

The severity and stability of coronary artery disease and the efficacy of current treatment should be determined preoperatively. An ECG should be performed, but is normal in many cases. Further noninvasive investigations, such as exercise or pharmacological stress testing, dipyridamole thallium scanning and echocardiography, may be indicated in patients with predictors of increased risk, but should only be carried out if the results will affect perioperative management. Referral for assessment and optimisation by a cardiologist may be required, but there is no justification for performing revascularisation purely to facilitate elective non-cardiac surgery.[2]

Box 1.2.1

Clinical risk factors for perioperative cardiovascular complications. Compiled from Eagle et al.[1] and Chassot et al.[2]

Major risk factors

Recent myocardial infarction (<6 weeks)

Unstable or severe angina (class III–IV)

Decompensated/symptomatic heart failure

Malignant arrhythmias

Severe valvular heart disease

Recent myocardial revascularisation (<6 weeks) by either coronary artery bypass grafting surgery (CABG) or percutaneous transluminal coronary angioplasty (PTCA)

Intermediate risk factors

Previous myocardial infarction (>6 weeks)

Stable angina (class I–II)

Compensated heart failure

Diabetes mellitus

Minor risk factors

Age >70 years

ECG abnormalities (e.g. left ventricular hypertrophy, bundle branch block, ST segment abnormalities)

Uncontrolled systemic hypertension

Rhythm other than sinus (e.g. atrial fibrillation)

Family history of coronary heart disease

Hypercholesterolaemia

Smoking

Renal dysfunction

Previous myocardial infarction

The risk of a perioperative cardiac event is high during the first 6 weeks after myocardial infarction and only emergency, life-saving surgery should be performed during this period. The same applies to patients who have undergone revascularisation by CABG or PTCA with or without a coronary stent.[2]

Box 1.2.2
Surgical predictors of increased perioperative cardiovascular risk (excluding cardiac surgery). Compiled from Eagle et al.[1] and Chassot et al.[2]
High risk (cardiovascular complication rate often >5%)
Emergency major or intermediate surgery, particularly in elderly patients
Aortic and other major vascular surgery
Peripheral vascular surgery
Prolonged procedures, with large fluid shifts or blood loss
Procedures associated with unstable haemodynamic situations
Intermediate risk (cardiovascular complication rate generally 1–5%)
Carotid endarterectomy
Head and neck surgery
Abdominal or thoracic surgery
Orthopaedic surgery
Prostatectomy
Low risk (cardiovascular complication rate generally <1%)
Endoscopic procedures
Breast and superficial surgery
Eye surgery

Beyond 6 weeks, the time elapsed after infarction is less important than the history or presence of complications. The period between 6 weeks and 3 months is generally considered a time of intermediate risk when non-urgent elective surgery should be postponed. A patient with ongoing ischaemia, cardiac failure or ventricular arrhythmias may still be at increased risk more than 3 months after infarction, and in all cases both the risks and benefits of surgery and the consequences of delaying surgery should be considered.

Anaesthesia

Cardiac medications should be continued into the perioperative period, with the possible exception of angiotensin-converting enzyme (ACE) inhibitors, which have been implicated in severe intraoperative hypotension and are withheld for 24 hours by some anaesthetists.

High-risk patients undergoing major surgery may benefit from preoperative admission to a high-dependency area for goal-directed optimisation of cardiac output with fluids and inotropes. There is evidence that selected high-risk patients may benefit from acute perioperative β-blockade, which should be continued for at least 72 hours postoperatively.[3] Premedication should be adequate to allay anxiety.

The main aim of intraoperative management should be to preserve the balance of myocardial oxygen supply and demand to avoid ischaemia. Oxygen supply is maintained by ensuring an adequate haemoglobin level, oxygen saturation and arterial blood pressure. Tachycardia and excessive hypertension are associated with increased oxygen demand and should be avoided.

The haemodynamic response to laryngoscopy and intubation may be obtunded using opioids or short-acting β-blockers.

The choice of anaesthetic agent and technique does not significantly affect the incidence of complications provided the above haemodynamic goals are achieved. Regional techniques may be of benefit in providing effective analgesia and reducing the stress response to surgery, so long as an adequate perfusion pressure can be maintained. Prevention of hypothermia and tight blood glucose control may also reduce morbidity and mortality rates.[4]

Myocardial ischaemia is best detected by monitoring a five-lead ECG, and invasive monitoring of arterial, central venous and pulmonary artery pressures may be considered in those at high risk. The gold standard for detecting intraoperative ischaemia, as well as assessing volume status and valvular function, is probably transoesophageal echocardiography, but it is expensive, not widely available and requires considerable expertise to interpret.

Most perioperative myocardial infarctions occur in the first 3 days postoperatively. The same haemodynamic goals apply as for the intraoperative period. All patients require effective analgesia and should receive humidified oxygen therapy for at least 72 hours after major surgery. High-risk patients are best managed in a high-dependency or intensive care unit.

Hypertension

Hypertension is a major risk factor for coronary heart disease, congestive cardiac failure, renal failure and cerebrovascular disease, and the risk rises with increasing arterial pressure. Hypertension may be classified according to severity, as shown in Table 1.2.1.

There is little evidence to suggest that patients with isolated stage 1 or 2 hypertension are at increased risk of perioperative cardiac complications and therefore no justification for postponing surgery in such cases.[5]

Severe hypertension, however, has been associated with an increased incidence of perioperative haemodynamic instability, silent myocardial ischaemia and arrhythmias. As a result it is usually recommended that surgery in patients with grade 3 hypertension is postponed to allow treat-

Category	Systolic arterial pressure (mmHg)	Diastolic arterial pressure (mmHg)
Grade 1	140–159	90–99
Grade 2	160–179	100–109
Grade 3	≥180	≥110

Table 1.2.1 Classification of hypertension[5]

ment.[1] The evidence for a clinically significant increase in adverse outcome is lacking however, and the potential risks of delaying surgery should be borne in mind.[5] The presence of target organ damage, such as coronary artery disease, congestive cardiac failure, renal dysfunction and cerebrovascular disease, is of far greater importance in terms of perioperative risk than the blood pressure per se.

Anaesthesia

An accurate assessment of blood pressure should be obtained preoperatively. A single reading taken on admission may be artificially elevated, particularly in the anxious patient. Evidence of hypertension-associated comorbidities should be sought, and if present, evaluated and treated where possible. Antihypertensive medication should be continued into the perioperative period, although there are some concerns regarding intraoperative hypotension in association with ACE inhibitors and angiotensin II antagonists.

Haemodynamic instability should be anticipated. Hypotension on induction may be managed with judicious use of fluids and vasoconstrictors. The cardiovascular responses to laryngoscopy and intubation may be attenuated by short-acting opioids, β-blockers and lidocaine (lignocaine). Ideally the blood pressure should be maintained within 20% of the best estimate of preoperative pressure.

Cardiac failure

Cardiac failure may occur due to ischaemic heart disease, hypertension, valvular heart disease, cardiomyopathy and pulmonary disease. Symptoms include dyspnoea, orthopnoea, cough, wheeze and peripheral oedema.

Anaesthesia

Decompensated or symptomatic heart failure is a major risk factor for perioperative complications and warrants thorough investigation and optimisation of medical treatment before elective surgery is considered.[1] In an emergency, invasive cardiovascular monitoring should be used to guide therapy, which may include diuretics, inotropes and vasodilators.

Intermittent positive-pressure ventilation (IPPV) with or without positive end-expiratory pressure (PEEP) reduces cardiac work and pulmonary oedema, but both may reduce cardiac output.

Arrhythmias and conduction disorders

Arrhythmias may be associated with cardiopulmonary disease, drug toxicity or metabolic abnormality. Treatment is indicated in the presence of symptoms or haemodynamic disturbance and should be directed first at correcting any underlying cause. The indications for antiarrhythmic therapy are identical to those in the non-surgical population.[1]

Supraventricular arrhythmias

The rate of atrial fibrillation should be controlled preoperatively with digoxin. If rapid control is required, intravenous β-blockers (e.g. esmolol), amiodarone, verapamil or DC cardioversion may also be used. Paroxysmal supraventricular tachycardia may respond to vagal manoeuvres, adenosine, β-blockers and verapamil, but the best treatment in an emergency situation is DC cardioversion.

In Wolff–Parkinson–White syndrome there is an accessory pathway between the atria and ventricles (bundle of Kent), which permits the development of re-entry tachycardias and atrial fibrillation. Flecainide, disopyramide, procainamide and amiodarone may all be used in treatment. DC cardioversion should be considered early in acute attacks of atrial fibrillation and adenosine may be useful in the emergency treatment of supraventricular tachycardia. Digoxin and verapamil may exacerbate Wolff–Parkinson–White syndrome and are contraindicated.

Ventricular arrhythmias

Ventricular ectopic beats occur in a significant proportion of the normal population. There is no evidence that the presence of frequent ventricular ectopics or asymptomatic non-sustained ventricular tachycardia is associated with an increased incidence of perioperative myocardial infarction or death.[1] Symptomatic ventricular arrhythmias should be treated with antiarrhythmics or cardioversion as appropriate.

Sick sinus syndrome

Also known as bradycardia/tachycardia syndrome, this is a general term for various disorders of sinoatrial node function. It affects mainly elderly patients and results in a sinus bradycardia with periods of sinus arrest and escape rhythms, and sometimes intermittent episodes of tachyarrhythmias. Symptoms, which may include syncope, dizziness, palpitations and extreme tiredness, are treated with a permanent atrial pacemaker. These patients have a high incidence of thromboembolism and may be anticoagulated.

Anaesthesia

Sick sinus syndrome is associated with a risk of brady- or tachyarrhythmias during anaesthesia and those who do not have a permanent pacemaker should have a temporary pacing wire inserted preoperatively.

Heart block

An abnormality of conduction at the atrioventricular node results in atrioventricular block, the classification of which is shown in Box 1.2.3.

Anaesthesia

General anaesthesia may result in deterioration of the heart block because most volatile agents prolong cardiac conduction. In particular, type II second-degree heart block may progress to complete heart block. The indications for the preoperative insertion of a permanent or temporary pacemaker are sometimes debatable, but would include complete heart block, type II second-degree atrioventricular block, and lesser degrees of heart block in the presence of symptoms or cardiac failure. Chronotropic drugs such as atropine and isoprenaline and facilities for external pacing should be readily available during anaesthesia.

Pacemakers

Pacemakers[6] are classified using a five-letter code, as shown in Box 1.2.4.

Anaesthesia

The indication for insertion and mode of function of the pacemaker should be determined preoperatively and its function checked. Rate-responsive

Box 1.2.3
Classification of atrioventricular block
First degree block PR interval >0.2 s
Second degree block Type I Wenckebach's phenomenon – progressive lengthening of the PR interval until conduction fails and a beat is dropped Type II Intermittent failure of atrioventricular conduction without preceding prolongation of the PR interval.
Third degree block (complete heart block) Complete dissociation of the atria and ventricles as atrial impulses fail to be transmitted

Box 1.2.4

Code for the classification of pacemaker functions

1 – chamber paced – V ventricle, A atrium, D dual
2 – chamber sensed – V ventricle, A atrium, D dual, O none
3 – mode of response – T triggered, I inhibited
4 – programmable functions
5 – anti-tachycardia functions

pacemakers respond to physiological variables and are best converted to a fixed rate for the perioperative period.

Modern pacemakers with bipolar electrodes are less liable to interference by electromagnetic sources, but precautions concerning diathermy should still be taken. Bipolar diathermy is preferable, but if unipolar must be used then the ground plate should be placed on the same side as the operating site, as far away from the pacemaker as possible. The frequency and duration of use should be limited and the lowest possible current used.

Magnetic resonance imaging is contraindicated because it may cause serious pacemaker malfunction and permanent damage. Magnets should not be placed over pacemakers during surgery because they have an unpredictable effect on the programming of modern pacemakers. A backup pacing system and chronotropic drugs such as atropine, epinephrine (adrenaline) and isoprenaline should be available in case of pacemaker failure.

Automatic implantable cardioverter defibrillator (AICD)[6]

An automatic implantable cardioverter defibrillator (AICD)[6] is used in the treatment of recurrent tachyarrhythmias unresponsive to medical treatment. It senses ventricular tachycardia or fibrillation and responds with countershocks to the heart. The AICD may be triggered by any form of electromagnetic radiation, including diathermy. The anti-tachycardia and defibrillation functions should be switched off before surgery where the use of diathermy is anticipated, and also before lithotripsy and electroconvulsive therapy. The use of transcutaneous electrical nerve stimulation (TENS) for pain management is contraindicated.

Hypertrophic obstructive cardiomyopathy

Hypertrophic obstructive cardiomyopathy[7] is a genetic disorder that causes myocardial hypertrophy, affecting the ventricular septum in particular. Dynamic left ventricular outflow tract obstruction results, often with secondary mitral regurgitation. Many patients are asymptomatic, but others are prone to arrhythmias and sudden cardiac death. An ejection systolic murmur is usually present and the ECG shows evidence of left ventricular hypertrophy. The diagnosis is confirmed by echocardiography. The condition is worsened by hypovolaemia, vasodilatation and the use of catecholamines. Anaesthesia constitutes a significant risk.

Constrictive pericarditis

Constrictive pericarditis results from chronic fibrous thickening and/or calcification of the pericardial sac. It classically presents with debilitating chronic right heart failure.[8] Vasodilatation (e.g. at induction of anaesthesia) is poorly tolerated.

Valvular heart disease

All patients with valvular heart disease, a prosthetic heart valve or a congenital lesion such as ventricular septal defect and patent ductus arteriosus are at risk of bacterial endocarditis. Antibiotic prophylaxis (according to local guidelines) is required before dental surgery and some surgical procedures, particularly those involving instrumentation of the upper respiratory tract and genitourinary system.

Many patients are also anticoagulated, particularly in the presence of a mechanical prosthetic valve or mitral valve disease. Management of their anticoagulation in the perioperative period depends on the risk of bleeding associated with the procedure and the risk of thromboembolism. Before minor surgery, it may be sufficient to omit warfarin preoperatively until the international normalised ratio is in the low therapeutic range, but more major procedures usually require conversion to heparin therapy during the perioperative period.

Severe valvular heart disease is a major risk factor for anaesthesia, and successful anaesthetic management of these patients is based on an understanding of the appropriate haemodynamic goals for the particular lesion.

Aortic stenosis

Significant aortic stenosis is a major risk factor for perioperative complications.[6] Symptoms tend to appear late in the disease, therefore all ejection systolic murmurs warrant careful preoperative examination and judicious use of echocardiography. Anaesthesia should be administered cautiously and the use of invasive monitoring is highly recommended. Extremes of heart rate and atrial fibrillation are not well tolerated and should be promptly treated. Ventricular filling must be maintained by avoiding hypovolaemia and maintaining systemic vascular resistance. Vasodilatation may result in profound hypotension, subendocardial ischaemia and even sudden death.

Aortic regurgitation

Bradycardia and vasoconstriction increase the degree of regurgitation and should be avoided. A mild tachycardia, moderate fluid loading, a degree of vasodilatation and avoidance of myocardial depression will usually improve forward flow. Invasive monitoring is recommended for those with severe disease. Acute aortic regurgitation is usually a surgical emergency; these patients may respond poorly to vasodilatation.

Mitral stenosis

Patients with mitral stenosis are prone to develop congestive cardiac failure and pulmonary oedema. Atrial fibrillation may result in acute deterioration and should be treated preoperatively. Tachycardia, myocardial depression and excessive vasodilatation should be avoided. Careful attention to fluid balance is required because hypovolaemia compromises ventricular filling, but fluid overload can easily precipitate pulmonary oedema. The use of invasive monitoring is advisable for patients with severe disease, but the pulmonary capillary wedge pressure, as an estimate of left atrial pressure, may be inaccurate in the presence of pulmonary hypertension. The use of inotropes may be required. Nitrous oxide should be avoided if there is evidence of pulmonary hypertension.

Mitral regurgitation

In patients with mitral regurgitation, bradycardia and vasoconstriction increase the regurgitant fraction and should be avoided. During anaesthesia a mild tachycardia, a slight reduction in systemic vascular resistance and avoidance of myocardial depression are desirable. Hypovolaemia should be avoided, but a cautious approach to fluid loading is recommended.

PULMONARY DISEASE

Acute upper respiratory tract infection

Patients, especially children, presenting for elective surgery commonly have, or are recovering from, an acute upper respiratory tract infection (URTI). Whether anaesthesia and surgery should be postponed in such patients has been the subject of debate. There is little evidence that general anaesthesia in adults with URTI is associated with an increased risk of adverse respiratory events, although upper airway reactivity may be increased.[9]

In children with URTI, increased airway reactivity and a higher incidence of intraoperative adverse respiratory events have been demonstrated, particularly in association with intubation, surgical procedures involving the airway and a history of reactive airway disease.[10] Few of these adverse events result in postoperative sequelae, however, and it has been suggested that surgery need not necessarily be postponed in children with mild URTI, and that an individual approach, taking into account whether the child is actually unwell, the child's past history and the nature of the surgery is preferable. Increased airway reactivity may persist for from 4 to 6 weeks and therefore if surgery is postponed, it should be for a period of at least 6 weeks.[10]

Chronic obstructive pulmonary disease

Chronic obstructive pulmonary disease (COPD)[11] may be defined as predominantly fixed airflow obstruction accompanied by features of chronic bronchitis, emphysema or both.

Chronic bronchitis is characterised by airway inflammation and mucus hypersecretion with productive cough.

In emphysema there is dilatation of the air spaces distal to the terminal bronchioles and overinflation of the lungs.

Smoking is by far the most important aetiological factor, followed by occupational exposure to dusts and atmospheric pollution.

Implications for anaesthesia

The implications of COPD for anaesthesia are:

- hypersensitivity of the airways and increased risk of bronchoconstriction in response to airway instrumentation, irritant vapours and histamine-releasing drugs;
- increased sensitivity to respiratory depressants;
- increased risk of barotrauma with artificial ventilation;
- increased risk of postoperative pulmonary complications.

Preoperative assessment should aim to evaluate the severity of respiratory impairment based on clinical signs, symptoms and reported exercise tolerance. Lung function tests such as spirometry and arterial blood gas analysis should be performed in those with significant disease. A recent chest radiograph provides limited information with regard to function, but is a useful baseline investigation and allows the detection of emphysematous bullae. The presence of hypercapnia, hypoxia and a reduced forced expiratory volume in 1 second (FEV_1), are all associated with increased risk of pulmonary complications postoperatively.[12]

Smoking and obesity also increase the perioperative risk, and advice regarding weight loss and cessation of smoking should be given before contemplating elective surgery.

Anaesthesia

The patient's condition should be optimised preoperatively. Bronchodilators are of benefit where a reversible element has been demonstrated, infection should be treated with antibiotics, and physiotherapy will aid the clearance of secretions. Sedative premedication may cause respiratory depression and should be avoided. Anxious patients may benefit from the judicious use of benzodiazepines. The use of anticholinergic agents in patients with copious secretions is not recommended because it may make it difficult to clear the secretions.

Regional or local anaesthesia has the advantage of avoiding the respiratory complications of general anesthesia, but is not suitable for all procedures or all patients. Some patients may be unable to lie supine without coughing or may become hypoxic and uncooperative, particularly if sedated. Most patients, even those with quite severe COPD, may be managed safely under carefully conducted general anaesthesia.

The risk of bronchoconstriction is minimised by ensuring deep anaesthesia before attempting airway instrumentation, and avoiding histamine releasing drugs where possible.

Minor procedures of short duration may be performed with spontaneous ventilation, but hypoventilation and hypercapnia may result and the use of opioids should be kept to a minimum.

For more major surgery controlled ventilation is preferable. The risk of gas trapping and barotrauma is minimised by the use of pressure-controlled or pressure-limited ventilation with a low ventilation rate and prolonged expiratory phase.[13] Nitrous oxide should be avoided in patients with emphysema, particularly where there is evidence of bullae.

The provision of good-quality analgesia is important, particularly after thoracic or abdominal surgery. Postoperative pain is a major cause of hypoventilation and inadequate clearance of secretions, leading to atelectasis and pneumonia. Epidural analgesia has been shown to improve postoperative pulmonary function and reduce the incidence of pulmonary complications after thoracic and upper abdominal surgery. Postoperative chest physiotherapy also plays an important role in the prevention of pulmonary complications.

Asthma

Asthma is characterised by hyperreactivity of the airways leading to recurrent, reversible airways obstruction, bronchial mucosal oedema and the formation of mucous plugs. The mainstay of treatment is with anti-inflammatory agents such as inhaled corticosteroids and bronchodilators, usually β_2-agonists. Leukotriene antagonists are also now available and have anti-inflammatory and bronchodilator properties.[14]

Implications for anaesthesia

The implications of asthma for anaesthesia are:

- increased airway reactivity, particularly in response to airway manipulation and histamine-releasing drugs;
- increased risk of barotrauma with positive-pressure ventilation;

- exacerbation of asthma by non-steroidal anti-inflammatory drugs (NSAIDs) in some patients;
- long-term corticosteroid therapy (including high-dose inhaled corticosteroids) may necessitate perioperative corticosteroid cover.

Anaesthesia

Lung function should be optimised preoperatively with appropriate anti-inflammatory and bronchodilator therapy. An anxiolytic premedication should also be considered. Adequate depth of anaesthesia and muscle relaxation before intubation reduces the incidence of bronchospasm. Administration of lidocaine (lignocaine) intravenously at a dose of 1–1.5 mg/kg may also suppress the response to intubation, but topical lidocaine (lignocaine) spray is not effective and may induce bronchoconstriction in some patients.

The use of a laryngeal mask airway is associated with a lower incidence of bronchospasm than intubation.

The choice of anaesthetic agents should aim to avoid histamine-releasing drugs where possible. Volatile anaesthetics are bronchodilators and are therefore generally well tolerated. Ketamine also has bronchodilator properties and may be useful in emergency circumstances.

Regional techniques may provide a useful alternative to general anaesthesia and should be considered where appropriate.

Acute bronchospasm may be treated by deepening anaesthesia using a volatile agent and the administration of a bronchodilator, usually salbutamol 250 μg, by slow intravenous injection. Aminophylline 250 mg given intravenously over 20 minutes may also be used. For severe bronchospasm unresponsive to the above, epinephrine (adrenaline) 1 in 10 000 may be given in 1 mL increments.

Smoking

In addition to the many long-term hazards to health associated with smoking, there are adverse effects in the perioperative period. Smoking causes an increase in carboxyhaemoglobin and consequent impairment of oxygen carriage and delivery, and this effect may persist for 12 hours or more. There is also a greater likelihood of perioperative adverse respiratory events due to increased airway reactivity, mucus hypersecretion and impaired ciliary function. Coronary artery disease, hypertension, thromboembolism and chronic pulmonary disease are all more likely in smokers and further increase the perioperative risk.

Patients should be advised to stop smoking preoperatively. Abstinence for 6–8 weeks is required to significantly improve respiratory function, but oxygen carriage will be improved after 24 hours.

ENDOCRINE DISEASE

See also Chapter 5.4 Endocrine surgery.

Diabetes mellitus

Diabetes mellitus is the most common endocrine abnormality encountered in surgical patients and is associated with increased perioperative morbidity and mortality rates, due mainly to the complications of the disease. Diagnosis is made by a fasting plasma glucose level greater than 7.0 mmol/L or a random plasma glucose level of greater than 11.1 mmol/L. Diabetes may be classified into four types, as shown in Box 1.2.5.

Implications for anaesthesia

The complications of diabetes may increase perioperative risk (Box 1.2.6).

Perioperative blood glucose management must take into account the following:

- starvation may cause hypoglycaemia, particularly in the presence of long-acting hypoglycaemic agents;
- general anaesthesia or sedation mask the symptoms of hypoglycemia;
- the stress response to surgery results in increased catabolic hormone secretion, which may worsen hyperglycaemia;
- circulatory disturbance during anaesthesia and surgery may affect the absorption of subcutaneous insulin.

Box 1.2.5
Classification of diabetes. Compiled from Porter and McCirrick.[16]
Type I (insulin-dependent diabetes)
Associated with a lack of endogenous insulin secretion caused by autoimmune or viral destruction of the β cells of the islets of Langerhans in the pancreas
Type II (non insulin-dependent diabetes)
Associated with reduced secretion of the active form of the insulin molecule, usually in combination with peripheral insulin resistance
Type III
Hyperglycaemia due to certain drugs (thiazide diuretics, corticosteroids and β-blockers) or concurrent disease
Type IV
Gestational diabetes, which affects 4% of pregnancies, usually in the third trimester

Box 1.2.6
Complications of diabetes mellitus
Hyperglycaemia Leading to dehydration, acidaemia, poor wound healing and increased susceptibility to infection
Cardiovascular Accelerated atherosclerosis and generalised microvascular disease leading to coronary heart disease, hypertension, peripheral vascular disease
Neurological Autonomic neuropathy (postural hypotension, gastroparesis, bladder dysfunction), peripheral neuropathy (typically glove and stocking distribution)
Renal Diabetic nephropathy is the commonest cause of end-stage renal failure
Ophthalmic Cataract, exudative and proliferative retinopathy
Respiratory Increased incidence of infections, including tuberculosis
Stiff joint syndrome Increased incidence of infections, including tuberculosis

Perioperative blood glucose control

Optimal glycaemic control minimises metabolic disturbance and end-organ damage and may result in better wound healing, lower morbidity and shorter hospital stay.[15] Blood glucose levels should be measured at least every 2 hours and ideally should be maintained between 6 and 10 mmol/L.[16] The regimen used to achieve this depends on the type of diabetes, the adequacy of preoperative control and the nature of the proposed surgery.

Type II diabetics with good glucose control undergoing minor surgery should omit their oral hypoglycaemics on the morning of surgery (or 24 hours before surgery in the case of long-acting agents). The blood glucose should be monitored regularly and oral hypoglycaemic therapy restarted once oral intake is resumed.

Type II diabetics who are poorly controlled or who are to undergo major surgery should be converted to a dextrose and insulin regimen as for type I diabetics.

Type I diabetics undergoing anything other than minor surgery are best managed with an intravenous insulin and dextrose regimen. There are two main types of regimen in use:

- glucose–insulin–potassium systems such as the Alberti regimen, whereby insulin is added to a 500 mL bag of 10% dextrose which contains potassium and the contents of the infusion are altered according to the blood glucose measurement. Such systems are inherently safe because the insulin and glucose are in the same solution, but may be considered inconvenient because a new infusion must be prepared if the blood glucose level falls outside the accepted range;
- separate infusions of insulin and 5% or 10% dextrose which contains potassium. This gives greater flexibility because the infusions may be controlled independently, but creates the potential to administer insulin without glucose resulting in hypoglycaemia.

Type I diabetics with good glucose control undergoing minor surgery where an early return to oral intake is anticipated are managed with a variety of regimens, including:

- no insulin/no glucose;
- omission of short-acting insulin and administration of one-third of the dose of intermediate or mixed insulin on the morning of surgery;
- administration of one-half of the normal insulin dose on the morning of surgery followed by 5% dextrose infusion.

Each has advantages and disadvantages – careful glucose monitoring is essential and the patient should be early on the morning list.

Anaesthesia

Regional anaesthesia has a number of advantages for the diabetic patient. Preservation of consciousness allows detection of hypoglycaemic symptoms and permits earlier oral intake postoperatively, minimising the metabolic disturbance.

Epidural and spinal anaesthesia also reduce the stress response to surgery. There are disadvantages, however:

- profound hypotension may occur in patients with autonomic neuropathy;
- there may be an increased risk of infection and epidural abscess formation;
- regional anesthesia may be implicated in any subsequent deterioration of diabetic neuropathy.

A detailed discussion with the patient and accurate documentation of any existing neurological deficit is necessary for medicolegal reasons.

General anaesthesia masks the early signs of hypoglycaemia and the blood glucose should be closely monitored. Rapid sequence induction is indicated in the presence of autonomic neuropathy, but the potential for difficult intubation should be considered, particularly in type I diabetics with stiff joint syndrome. The blood pressure should be maintained within reasonable limits to reduce the risk of further end-organ damage.

Lactate-containing fluids such as Hartmann's solution should be avoided because they may increase blood glucose and worsen lactic acidosis in the presence of hyperglycaemia.

Care should be taken to protect pressure areas because diabetics are at risk of skin trauma, ulceration and nerve injury.

Thyroid disease

Hypothyroidism

Hypothyroidism (myxoedema) is most commonly due to autoimmune thyroiditis (Hashimoto's disease) and iatrogenic causes. There is a generalised reduction in metabolic rate and clinical features include fatigue, intolerance of cold, weight gain, mental slowing and dry skin. Treatment is usually with oral levothyroxine sodium (thyroxine sodium), which may take 7–10 days to produce a clinical effect. Tri-iodothyronine may also be used; it has a shorter half-life and may be given intravenously for emergency treatment.

Anaesthesia

Hypothyroid patients often present for surgery incidental to their thyroid problem and should be rendered euthyroid before elective surgery.[17] Undiagnosed mild or subclinical hypothyroidism is common, particularly in the elderly. The presence of a hypometabolic state necessitates careful perioperative cardiovascular monitoring and judicious use of anaesthetic agents. There may be increased sensitivity to respiratory depressants, and controlled ventilation may be the preferred technique. Temperature monitoring and measures to protect against hypothermia are recommended.

Hyperthyroidism

The commonest cause of hyperthyroidism is Graves' disease, an autoimmune disorder. The classic clinical features include restlessness, heat intolerance, weight loss and tremor. Cardiovascular effects include atrial fibrillation and congestive cardiac failure. Treatment is with drugs that block thyroxine synthesis, such as carbimazole and propylthiouracil, or with radioactive iodine. β-Blockers such as propranolol may be used to alleviate symptoms.

Anaesthesia

Hyperthyroid patients should be rendered euthyroid before surgery because a thyroid crisis may be precipitated by any major physical stress, such as surgery, trauma or infection.[17] Thyroid crisis is characterised by tachycardia, arrhythmias, hyperpyrexia and heart failure, and can be fatal if untreated. Supportive treatment includes hydration, cooling, β-blockade and inotropes.

Diseases of the adrenal glands

Primary adrenocortical insufficiency (Addison's disease)

Addison's disease[18] may be caused by autoimmune disease, tuberculosis, haemochromatosis, and infiltration with metastatic tumour or amyloid. Clinical features result from glucocorticoid and mineralocorticoid deficiency and include fatigue, weight loss, postural hypotension, increased pigmentation, hyponatraemia, hyperkalaemia and hypoglycaemia. Treatment is with oral hydrocortisone or prednisolone and fludrocortisone.

Secondary adrenocortical insufficiency

Secondary adrenocortical insufficiency is due to absent or low levels of adrenocorticotrophic hormone (ACTH), caused either by disease of the anterior pituitary or suppression of the hypothalamopituitary axis by long-term exogenous corticosteroid administration.

Addisonian crisis

Acute addisonian crises may be precipitated by physiological stress and are characterised by abdominal pain, vomiting, dehydration and hypotension. Acute adrenal failure may also be caused by adrenal haemorrhage or infarction secondary to septicaemia (Waterhouse–Friedrichsen syndrome) although this is rare.

Anaesthesia

All patients with adrenocortical insufficiency and patients on long-term exogenous corticosteroids should receive corticosteroid supplementation in the perioperative period. Surgery in undiagnosed or inadequately treated patients may precipitate an addisonian crisis. Such crises may present as cardiovascular collapse during anaesthesia or postoperatively and are treated with intravenous saline and hydrocortisone 100 mg every 6 hours.[18]

Cushing's syndrome

In Cushing's syndrome[18] there is excess circulating glucocorticoid. The commonest causes are therapeutic administration of synthetic corticosteroids and increased ACTH secretion by the pituitary (Cushing's disease). Other causes include ectopic ACTH secretion by tumours and adrenal adenoma or carcinoma. Clinical features include weakness, thin skin, obesity, striae, osteoporosis, hypertension, hypokalaemia and hyperglycaemia.

Primary hyperaldosteronism (Conn's syndrome)

Conn's syndrome[18] is usually caused by a unilateral adrenal adenoma, but may result from bilateral hyperplasia of the zona glomerulosa of the adrenal cortex. The main clinical features are severe hypertension and hypokalaemia. Treatment is with the aldosterone receptor antagonist spironolactone. Secondary hyperaldosteronism may result from excessive renin secretion by a tumour or renal artery stenosis.

Phaeochromocytoma

See Chapter 5.4 Endocrine surgery.

Disorders of the pituitary gland

Most pituitary disorders[19] are caused by adenomas of the anterior pituitary or the effects of their treatment. The tumours may secrete prolactin, ACTH or growth hormone. An excess of growth hormone in adults causes acromegaly and in children, before epiphyseal closure, causes gigantism.

Acromegaly

Elevated growth hormone levels result in an overgrowth of bone, connective tissue and viscera. Clinical features include enlargement of the jaw, hands and feet, thickening of the soft tissues of the pharynx and larynx, hypertension, cardiomegaly and impaired left ventricular function. Diabetes mellitus and obstructive sleep apnoea are common. Medical treatment is with bromocriptine, a dopamine receptor agonist, and/or octreotide, a somatostatin analogue, but many patients require surgery, usually trans-sphenoidal hypophysectomy. Treatment with octreotide in advance of surgery may reduce the perioperative risk. Potential problems for the anaesthetist include difficult airway management, difficult intubation, cardiac complications and postoperative respiratory problems.

Hypopituitarism (Simmonds' disease)

Hypopituitarism is usually due to a pituitary tumour or iatrogenic ablation. Ischaemic necrosis of the anterior lobe of the pituitary in labour (Sheehan's syndrome) is now rare. The clinical picture depends on which of the anterior pituitary hormones are deficient and treatment is with appropriate hormone replacement therapy. Anaesthesia and surgery in patients with unrecognised hypopituitarism is associated with a greatly increased risk of hypoglycaemia, hypothermia, water intoxication and respiratory failure.

Carcinoid disease

Carcinoid tumours

Carcinoid tumours[20] arise from enterochromaffin cells and can be found in any tissue derived from endoderm. Most are slow growing, although some may be very aggressive with widespread metastases. Carcinoid tumours have traditionally been classified by embryonic site of origin as foregut (including thymus and lung), midgut and hindgut. Midgut tumours, particularly in the region of the appendix, are the most common.

Carcinoid tumours may secrete many types of vasoactive amine and neuropeptide, most commonly serotonin (5-hydroxytryptamine – 5HT), bradykinin and the tachykinins. The liver normally metabolises these substances before they reach the systemic circulation, so clinical effects are seen only in the presence of liver metastases or tumours with venous drainage directly into the systemic circulation.

Carcinoid syndrome

The clinical manifestations of carcinoid syndrome[20] depend on the substances released and may include cutaneous flushing, tachycardia, hypotension or hypertension, bronchoconstriction and diarrhoea. Carcinoid heart disease develops in around 50% of patients, with plaque formation and fibrosis affecting particularly the right-sided heart valves. Medical treatment may include antihistamines, 5HT antagonists and the somatostatin analogue octreotide.

Anaesthesia

Serious respiratory and cardiovascular complications may occur intraoperatively due to the release of vasoactive substances by the carcinoid tumour in response to mechanical and pharmacological stimuli. Severe bronchoconstriction and hypotension, resistant to conventional therapy, may occur. Intravenous octreotide has been successfully used to manage such events, as has aprotinin. Delayed emergence from anaesthesia has been reported and is thought to be related to high serotonin levels. Anxiolytic premedication, avoidance of histamine-releasing drugs and invasive cardiovascular monitoring are recommended. The use of regional techniques is controversial because they may exacerbate any hypotension.

METABOLIC AND BIOCHEMICAL DISORDERS

Porphyria

The porphyrias[21] are a group of disorders resulting from defects of enzymes involved in the synthesis of haem. Haem is produced mainly in the liver and bone marrow. The first enzyme in the pathway of haem synthesis is δ-aminolaevulinic acid (ALA), and its production is controlled by the concentration of haem, through feedback inhibition.

Acute attacks of porphyria are usually precipitated by a decrease in haem concentration, which stimulates ALA production. In the presence of a defect further down the pathway this leads to the accumulation of ALA and other porphyrinogen precursors, the nature of which depends on the particular enzyme deficiency. Acute exacerbations may be provoked by hormonal fluctuations, stress, dehydration, fasting and infection. Clinical features include abdominal pain, vomiting, pyrexia, tachycardia and usually hypertension, but sometimes hypotension. Peripheral neuropathy, cranial nerve palsies, autonomic disturbance, epilepsy and neuropsychiatric symptoms may also occur. Variegate porphyria causes blistering skin lesions and photosensitivity. The excretion of porphyrins causes the urine to turn red or dark brown on standing.

The hepatic porphyrias are of particular importance to the anaesthetist because they affect the synthesis of the cytochrome P450 enzyme system. Certain drugs, particularly those that cause enzyme induction, may trigger acute attacks by increasing the metabolic demand for haem.

There are three acute hepatic porphyrias:

- acute intermittent porphyria is an autosomal dominant disorder, that is relatively common in Sweden and Finland and results from a defect of porphobilinogen deaminase;
- hereditary coproporphyria is a rare disorder of coproporphyrinogen oxidase;
- variegate porphyria is common in certain regions of South Africa and results from a deficiency of protoporphyrinogen oxidase.

Anaesthesia

The identification of drugs likely to be hazardous in porphyria is far from clearcut[21] and it is advisable to seek expert guidance before anaesthesia.

Barbiturates are contraindicated and etomidate should probably also be avoided because it is potentially porphyrinogenic in animals, although reports in humans are conflicting.

Pentazocine is considered unsafe, but other opioids, including morphine, codeine, pethidine, fentanyl, alfentanil and naloxone, have been used safely. Propofol, benzodiazepines, muscle relaxants, neostigmine, atropine, aspirin, indomethacin, naproxen, lidocaine (lignocaine) and bupivacaine are all considered safe.

Of the inhalational agents, nitrous oxide and halothane are considered safe; isoflurane is probably also safe, but there are insufficient data for the remaining agents, which should therefore be used with caution.

ELECTROLYTE DISTURBANCES

Hyponatraemia

Hyponatraemia[22] is defined as a serum sodium level less than 135 mmol/L. There are three main types:

- isotonic (hyperproteinaemia, hyperlipidaemia);
- hypertonic (hyperglycaemia);
- hypotonic – which may be further classified as hypovolaemic (gastrointestinal losses, diuretics, and Addison's disease), hypervolaemic (cardiac failure, cirrhosis and nephrotic syndrome) and isovolaemic (inappropriate antidiuretic hormone [ADH] secretion).

Neurological symptoms occur with severe hyponatraemia, and cerebral oedema, convulsions and coma may develop. In addition to correction of the underlying cause, management includes fluid restriction and loop diuretics if there is hypervolaemia, or administration of normal or hypertonic saline in the presence of low or normal volume status. The rate of correction should not exceed 1–2 mmol/L per hour because rapid correction may cause central pontine myelinosis.

Hypernatraemia

Hypernatraemia[22] in hospital patients is often iatrogenic owing to insufficient water intake or excessive sodium administration. Treatment involves intravenous fluid therapy to replace the volume deficit. Correction should be undertaken slowly to avoid precipitating cerebral oedema and convulsions.

Diabetes insipidus (DI) results in the production of inappropriately dilute urine, raised serum osmolality and hypernatraemia due to reduced ADH secretion (central DI) or reduced responsiveness of the kidney to ADH (nephrogenic DI). Treatment is with desmopressin and fluid replacement.

Hypokalaemia

Hypokalaemia[22] may result from a shift of potassium into the cells or a deficiency of intracellular potassium. Causes of potassium depletion include inadequate intake, excessive gastrointestinal losses and increased renal excretion.

Hyperpolarisation of cell membranes results and may cause cardiac, neuromuscular, renal and endocrine sequelae. Characteristic ECG changes include flattened T waves, ST segment depression and U waves. Digitalis toxicity is enhanced and can induce life-threatening ventricular arrhythmias.

Hypokalaemia should be corrected using oral supplements, potassium-sparing diuretics or potassium-containing intravenous fluids. If urgent correction is required potassium may be given intravenously with continuous ECG monitoring.

Hyperkalaemia

Hyperkalaemia[22] may result from redistribution of potassium out of the cells and into the extracellular compartment as a result of acidosis, insulin deficiency, drugs (including suxamethonium) and muscle damage or diseases. Retention of potassium occurs in renal failure, aldosterone deficiency, and Addison's disease and due to the use of drugs such as NSAIDs, ACE inhibitors and potassium-sparing diuretics.

Hyperkalaemia may cause paralysis, acidosis and hypotension, but the primary concern is the increased risk of cardiac arrhythmias. Characteristic ECG changes include flattened P waves, widened QRS complexes and tented T waves.

Emergency management is aimed at minimising the risk of cardiac toxicity with intravenous calcium preparations and shifting potassium back into the cells. The latter may be achieved with an infusion of insulin and dextrose, sodium bicarbonate and β-agonists. Subsequent treatment is aimed at removing the cause and eliminating excess potassium from the body with a cation exchange resin.

Hypercalcaemia

The commonest causes of hypercalcaemia are primary hyperparathyroidism and malignancy.[23]

Severe hypercalcaemia can seriously disrupt gastrointestinal, neurological, cardiovascular and renal functions. Complications of particular relevance to the anaesthetist include dehydration, muscle weakness, impaired renal function, hypertension and cardiac arrhythmias. Characteristically there is a shortened QT segment on the ECG.

Initial treatment is by rehydration with intravenous saline and is often very effective. If additional measures are required, administration of large volumes of saline with furosemide (frusemide) to produce a forced saline diuresis may be of benefit, but the cardiovascular status and electrolyte levels must be closely monitored.

Hypocalcaemia

The commonest cause of hypocalcaemia is renal failure; other causes include vitamin D deficiency, magnesium deficiency, acute pancreatitis, hypoparathyroidism and massive transfusion with citrate-anticoagulated blood. Hypocalcaemia may also occur following parathyroidectomy, thyroidectomy and cardiopulmonary bypass. Ionised calcium levels should be measured to exclude an apparent hypocalcaemia due to hypoalbuminaemia.

Severe hypocalcaemia[23] causes increased neuronal irritability, which may result in neurological, respiratory, cardiovascular and psychiatric disturbances. Complications of particular relevance to the anaesthetist include hypotension, impaired cardiac contractility, cardiac arrhythmias, tetany, muscle weakness, laryngeal spasm, bronchospasm and convulsions.

Treatment is by intravenous administration of calcium and correction of any coexisting hypomagnesaemia or alkalosis.

LIVER AND GASTROINTESTINAL DISEASE

Acute liver disease

Acute liver disease is most commonly due to viral hepatitis, which in the early stages may be asymptomatic or associated with jaundice and vague malaise. There is a high perioperative mortality rate in the acute phase and elective surgery should be postponed until the liver function tests return to normal.[24]

Chronic liver disease

Chronic hepatitis

Most cases of chronic hepatitis follow infection with the hepatitis B and hepatitis C viruses. Other causes include autoimmune hepatitis, Wilson's disease, α_1-antitrypsin deficiency and other viral infections. Patients with milder forms of the disease (chronic persistent hepatitis) are usually asymptomatic and generally tolerate anaesthesia well. More severe disease (chronic active hepatitis) may cause progressive liver fibrosis and, in some cases, cirrhosis. The aetiology and degree of hepatic impairment require evaluation before anaesthesia and surgery to determine the perioperative risk and the potential for infection of healthcare staff.

Alcoholic liver disease

Excessive alcohol intake may result in fatty liver, alcoholic hepatitis and cirrhosis. Patients with fatty liver generally tolerate surgery well, but hepatitis and cirrhosis are associated with increased perioperative morbidity and mortality rates.

Chronic alcoholism may also be associated with malnutrition, particularly B vitamin deficiencies, cardiomyopathy, peripheral or autonomic neuropathy and immunocompromise. Enzyme induction may increase the doses of anaesthetic agents required. Acute withdrawal in the perioperative period may result in agitation, sweating and tremor, progressing in severe cases to delirium tremens with hallucinations, grand mal convulsions and hyperthermia. Benzodiazepines such as chlordiazepoxide and diazepam are most commonly used to treat the symptoms of alcohol withdrawal and prevent seizures.

Cirrhosis

The commonest causes of cirrhosis are alcohol abuse and chronic active hepatitis. The risk associated with anaesthesia and surgery depends on the severity of the disease, as assessed by liver function tests, and the presence of complications such as ascites and encephalopathy. Pugh's modification of the Child classification of severity of liver disease[25] provides a useful scoring system for preoperative risk and has been validated in more recent studies[26] (Table 1.2.2). Patients are classified as:

- grade A (score 5 or 6) – good risk with predicted mortality around 5%;
- grade B (score 7–9) – moderate risk with a predicted mortality of 10%;
- grade C (score 10–15) – poor risk with a predicted mortality of over 50%.

Implications for anaesthesia

The implications of cirrhosis for anesthesia are[27]:

- coagulopathy – due to reduced hepatic synthesis of clotting factors, cholestasis, impaired clearance of activated clotting factors and

	Child grade		
	A	B	C
Bilirubin (μmol/L)	<35	35–60	>60
Albumin (g/L)	>35	28–35	<28
Prothrombin time (seconds prolonged)	1–4	4–6	>6
Encephalopathy	0	1–2	3–4
Ascites	None	Easy	Difficult
Nutritional status	Excellent	Good	Poor
Operative mortality (approximate %)	0–10	4–31	19–76

Table 1.2.2 Child–Pugh scoring system for liver disease. Adapted from Pugh et al.[25]

increased factor consumption, disorders of fibrinolysis, thrombocytopenia secondary to hypersplenism, platelet dysfunction;

- hypoalbuminaemia – due to altered protein binding of some drugs;
- impaired drug metabolism – enhanced or prolonged effects of some drugs, including opioids, possible reduction in plasma cholinesterase, prolonging the action of suxamethonium;
- renal dysfunction – there is an increased risk of postoperative renal dysfunction, particularly with obstructive jaundice (hepatorenal syndrome);
- ascites – may lead to atelectasis and respiratory compromise, hypoxia due to a mismatch of ventilation and perfusion, and an increased risk of infection;
- encephalopathy – precipitated by constipation, infection, upper gastrointestinal bleeding, uraemia, alkalosis and overuse of sedative drugs.

Anaesthesia

Coagulopathy should be corrected preoperatively using vitamin K, fresh frozen plasma and cryoprecipitate as required. Ascites may be treated with diuretics and possibly paracentesis. Anaesthetic agents with minimal hepatic metabolism, such as isoflurane and sevoflurane, are preferred, and atracurium is the muscle relaxant of choice. Opioids should be administered cautiously at a reduced dose and other sedatives avoided where possible. Drugs that are potentially hepatotoxic or nephrotoxic, including NSAIDs, should be avoided. Regional anaesthetic techniques may be of benefit in the absence of coagulopathy or thrombocytopenia.

GASTROINTESTINAL DISORDERS

Hiatus hernia

Hiatus hernia is associated with an increased risk of regurgitation and aspiration on induction of anaesthesia. Patients who are symptomatic may be taking H_2-receptor blockers or proton pump inhibitors, and these should be continued in the perioperative period. There is no evidence of benefit, however, from the routine use of pharmacological prophylaxis, such as antacids or prokinetic agents (e.g. metoclopramide).[28] Rapid sequence induction and tracheal intubation are recommended to minimise the risk of airway soiling during anaesthesia.

Intestinal obstruction

Intestinal obstruction is a common condition that may be complicated by perforation, ischaemia and sepsis. The clinical features vary enormously depending on the site and duration of obstruction, the presence of complications and any co-morbid conditions. External fluid losses such as vomiting and third space losses due to sequestration of fluid within the bowel lumen lead to dehydration, which may be severe and accompanied by disturbances of electrolyte and acid–base balance. Careful preoperative assessment, fluid resuscitation and correction of electrolyte imbalance are required before anaesthesia. Rapid sequence induction of anaesthesia is indicated and insertion of a nasogastric tube to decompress the stomach is recommended.

RENAL DISEASE

Chronic renal failure

Causes of chronic renal failure include diabetes mellitus, hypertension, glomerulonephritis, polycystic kidney disease, pyelonephritis and obstructive uropathy. The presence of renal failure increases the risk associated with anaesthesia and surgery both directly and indirectly due to the sequelae of the disease[29] (Box 1.2.7). There is an increased likelihood of perioperative cardiovascular complications, postoperative infection and impaired wound healing. Furthermore, deterioration in renal function may result from reduced renal blood flow or drug-induced nephrotoxicity during the perioperative period.

Anaesthetic drugs and renal failure

Renal failure affects the pharmacokinetics of some drugs[30] owing to:

- changes in protein binding associated with hypoalbuminaemia;
- associated changes in hepatic metabolism;
- impaired elimination of renally excreted drugs.

Box 1.2.7
Sequelae of chronic renal failure relevant to anaesthesia
Hypertension
Cardiomyopathy
Anaemia (normochromic, normocytic)
Platelet dysfunction
Metabolic acidosis
Fluid and electrolyte imbalance (fluid overload, oedema, hyperkalaemia, hypocalcaemia, hyperphosphataemia, hypermagnesaemia)
Delayed gastric emptying, oesophageal sphincter dysfunction
Autonomic neuropathy
Altered pharmacokinetics

The free fraction of benzodiazepines is increased and the dose should be reduced. The effect of thiopental sodium may be enhanced owing to decreased protein binding, and propofol is considered a more suitable induction agent. Inhalational agents have the advantage of being eliminated primarily by the lungs rather than the kidneys, but some volatile agents are metabolised to fluoride, which is potentially nephrotoxic. Isoflurane, halothane and desflurane are considered the safest agents in renal failure. Enflurane produces the highest fluoride levels and is probably best avoided. Sevoflurane is also metabolised to fluoride and degrades in soda lime to form compound A, which is nephrotoxic in rats, although there has been no evidence of this in humans.

Atracurium and cisatracurium are the muscle relaxants of choice because their elimination is independent of renal function. Vecuronium and rocuronium are also considered safe, but the predominantly renal excretion of pancuronium means it should be avoided. Suxamethonium causes a rise in serum potassium of around 0.5 mmol/L, but should be safe in the absence of hyperkalaemia.

Opioid analgesics are largely metabolised in the liver, but problems may arise because of the accumulation of metabolites. The action of morphine may be prolonged due to the active metabolite morphine-6-glucuronide, and accumulation of norpethidine, a metabolite of pethidine, may result in CNS excitation and convulsions. NSAIDs may result in further deterioration of renal function and should be avoided.

Anaesthesia

Regional techniques may be preferable in the absence of coagulopathy. For general anaesthesia, a rapid sequence induction may be indicated because of the increased risk of regurgitation, but suxamethonium should be avoided in the presence of hyperkalaemia. Drugs should be given slowly and titrated to response. Careful attention to fluid balance and maintenance of blood pressure are required to preserve renal blood flow.

End-stage renal failure

Patients with end-stage renal failure have a high incidence of coronary artery disease and congestive cardiac failure.[29] Haemodynamic instability is common during anaesthesia and these patients are particularly sensitive to the vasodilating effects of anaesthetic drugs. Fluid overload and hyperkalaemia are common and should be corrected by dialysis preoperatively. Coagulopathy may be present due to platelet dysfunction or the residual effect of heparin after dialysis. Care should be taken to protect the sites of any arteriovenous fistulae.

NEUROLOGICAL DISEASES

Epilepsy

Epilepsy is a clinical diagnosis based on the occurrence of at least two seizures. Treatment is with anticonvulsants and these drugs should be continued throughout the perioperative period. Most anticonvulsants cause enzyme induction, which affects the metabolism of other drugs. Sodium valproate may interfere with haemostasis.

Many anaesthetic drugs appear to have both pro- and anticonvulsant activity, making the choice of suitable agents somewhat controversial. It is advisable to avoid those agents that have been particularly implicated in the production of clinical excitatory events or EEG excitation, such as methohexitone, etomidate, propofol and enflurane, particularly in those patients who hold a driving licence.[31] Thiopental sodium is a good choice of induction agent and isoflurane is suitable for maintenance.

Status epilepticus is defined as seizure activity lasting 30 minutes or more without recovery of consciousness. Rapid treatment is required to prevent neuronal damage and systemic complications. Lorazepam is considered to be the most effective initial treatment, followed by phenytoin and/or phenobarbital according to response. General anaesthesia using thiopental or propofol has been used successfully in severe cases.[32]

Parkinson's disease

Parkinson's disease[33] is associated with a loss of dopaminergic neurons in the substantia nigra of the basal ganglia and is characterised by resting tremor, muscle rigidity and bradykinesia. Treatment is usually with levodopa in combination with a peripheral dopa-decarboxylase inhibitor to minimise peripheral side-effects. Dopamine agonists (bromocriptine) and type B monoamine oxidase inhibitors (selegiline) may also be used. Surgical treatments for Parkinson's disease have also been developed.

Anaesthesia

Levodopa must be continued perioperatively to prevent the patient from becoming rigid and immobile, but can only be given orally or via a nasogastric tube. Patients with pharyngeal dysfunction have an increased risk of regurgitation and aspiration. Postoperative atelectasis and respiratory infection may occur owing to impaired clearance of secretions. Patients with advanced disease may have autonomic dysfunction. Phenothiazines, butyrophenones and metoclopramide should be avoided because they may exacerbate extrapyramidal symptoms. A higher than normally expected incidence of postoperative confusion and hallucinations has been reported.[33]

Multiple sclerosis

Multiple sclerosis is a demyelinating disease affecting the CNS. It is thought to be autoimmune in nature, but viral and genetic factors have also been implicated. The optic nerve, brainstem and spinal cord are most commonly affected and progression is very variable, marked by remissions and relapses. Pregnancy, particularly the third trimester, is often associated with an improvement in symptoms, but an increased relapse rate has been reported during the first 3 months postpartum.[34]

There is no evidence to suggest that general anaesthesia is associated with relapse, but there has been much debate regarding the safety of regional anaesthesia. It has been suggested that spinal anaesthesia is associated with an increased incidence of neurological complications, but uneventful use of the technique has been reported. Epidural anaesthesia may be preferable and does not appear to be associated with an increase in complications or relapse rate, although it has been suggested that a concentration of no greater than 0.25 % bupivacaine is used.[34] All existing signs and symptoms must be documented before performing a regional technique, and the patient must be fully involved in the decision-making process. Local anaesthetic toxicity may be more likely due to disruption of the blood–brain barrier.

Motor neuron disease

Motor neuron disease (amyotrophic lateral sclerosis) is a progressive disease of upper and lower motor neurons that usually presents in middle age. Clinical features include muscle cramps, weakness, wasting, fasciculations, spasticity and hyperreflexia. Bulbar palsies are common and may lead to impairment of speech, swallowing and laryngeal reflexes. Respiratory failure develops due to inspiratory muscle weakness and inability to cough and clear secretions effectively.

Anaesthesia

Patients with advanced motor neuron disease are at considerable risk from general anaesthesia. Suxamethonium may cause severe hyperkalaemia and there is increased sensitivity to non-depolarising muscle relaxants. Bulbar involvement increases the risk of regurgitation and aspiration. These patients are prone to postoperative respiratory failure because of an increased sensitivity to respiratory depressants and an impaired ability to clear secretions. Despite concerns that exacerbations of the disease may follow the use of regional anaesthetic techniques, epidural anaesthesia has been used successfully.

PSYCHIATRIC DISORDERS

Depressive illness

Anaesthesia has no effect on the course of depressive illness, but some antidepressant medications may interact with drugs used during anaesthesia.[35]

Tricyclic antidepressants have anticholinergic effects and there have been isolated reports of arrhythmias with halothane.

Monoamine oxidase inhibitors (MAOIs) may interact with sympathomimetics to produce severe hypertensive crises, and also with pethidine, causing hyperpyrexia, hypertension and rigidity. Ideally MAOIs should be stopped at least 2 weeks before elective surgery.

Selective serotonin reuptake inhibitors (SSRIs) such as fluoxetine and paroxetine have become the first-line agents in the treatment of depression and do not appear to have any specific interactions with anaesthetic agents. Abruptly stopping SSRIs may result in a severe withdrawal, however, and they should be continued throughout the perioperative period where possible.

Lithium is used as a mood stabilising drug and may cause ECG changes such as T-wave inversion, and rarely sinus node dysfunction and ventricular irritability. It can prolong the action of muscle relaxants, but this is not usually of any clinical significance.

Schizophrenia

Antipsychotic medication such as phenothiazines and butyrophenones may enhance the CNS depression caused by barbiturates and opiates. Occasionally ECG abnormalities may occur, and rarely these drugs may cause ventricular irritability with premature ventricular complexes. Another rare side-effect is neuroleptic malignant syndrome, characterised by muscle rigidity, profound hyperthermia and autonomic instability. These drugs should be continued perioperatively where possible because abrupt withdrawal can cause dyskinesia or rebound agitation.

NEUROMUSCULAR DISORDERS

Myasthenia

Myasthenia gravis

Myasthenia gravis is an autoimmune disorder affecting the neuromuscular junction and is characterised by impaired neuromuscular transmission and muscle weakness. Most patients have circulating autoantibodies to the post-synaptic nicotinic acetylcholine receptors. A thymoma is found in approximately 10% of patients and hyperplasia of the thymus is common in younger patients, although the precise aetiology is often unknown.

The characteristic feature of myasthenia gravis is weakness on exertion that improves with rest. Ocular, bulbar and facial muscles are commonly involved, and clinical features include ptosis, reduced facial expression, dysarthria and dysphagia. Limb weakness, when present, is usually proximal, although specific weakness of the small muscles of the hand may occur. Myasthenia may be unmasked by anaesthesia with neuromuscular blockade, resulting in hypoventilation or apnoea postoperatively.

Symptomatic treatment is with oral anticholinesterases such as pyridostigmine, and immunosuppression using corticosteroids or azathioprine is often effective in eliminating the antibody. Thymectomy may be performed in young-onset, antibody-positive patients and in those with a thymoma. Plasmapheresis may be considered in an emergency, when it often produces a dramatic, albeit temporary, improvement.

Implications for anaesthesia

The implications of myasthenia gravis for anaesthesia are:

- increased sensitivity to non-depolarising muscle relaxants;
- resistance to depolarising muscle relaxants;
- increased sensitivity to the neuromuscular effects of volatile agents;
- risk of aspiration with bulbar weakness;
- risk of postoperative respiratory failure with respiratory muscle weakness;
- risk of cholinergic crisis with excessive doses of anticholinesterases;
- effects of immunosuppressant therapy.

Anaesthesia

The management of anaesthesia depends on the severity of the disease, the type of surgery and the requirement for muscle relaxation. A short-acting non-depolarising relaxant administered in increments or by infusion with careful monitoring of the neuromuscular blockade is advised for patients in whom muscle relaxation is deemed necessary.

Many surgical procedures, including thymectomy, may be performed without the use of muscle relaxants and this may facilitate early extubation.[36]

Volatile agents, particularly isoflurane, decrease the availability of acetylcholine at the neuromuscular junction and potentiate the effects of non-depolarising muscle relaxants. Sevoflurane is rapidly eliminated and is probably the volatile agent of choice.[36]

Maintenance of anaesthesia with propofol has the advantage of avoiding the neuromuscular effects of volatile agents, and in combination with thoracic epidural analgesia has been reported to reduce the requirement for postoperative ventilatory support after thymectomy.[37]

Cautious use of other respiratory depressants such as opiates is recommended. Non-opioid analgesics and local anaesthesia should be used where possible. Neostigmine should be used cautiously because of the risk of precipitating a cholinergic crisis.

All patients with myasthenia gravis should be closely monitored in a high-dependency area postoperatively, and some may require ventilatory support.

Myasthenic emergencies

Respiratory failure may be caused by either a myasthenic or a cholinergic crisis. Myasthenic crises are life-threatening episodes of respiratory or bulbar paralysis. Cholinergic crises result from excessive anticholinesterase medication leading to a depolarising block of neuromuscular transmission. The patient should be ventilated and anticholinergic medication withheld until the nature of the crisis can be ascertained.

Myasthenic syndrome (Eaton–Lambert syndrome)

Myasthenic syndrome is an autoimmune disorder, originally described in association with small cell carcinoma of the lung. Autoantibodies to the presynaptic calcium channels cause impaired neuromuscular transmission, which shows little response to anticholinesterases. Clinical features include weakness of the proximal lower limbs and trunk, loss of lower limb reflexes, ptosis and autonomic dysfunction. There is marked sensitivity to both depolarising and non-depolarising neuromuscular blockers and prolonged paralysis may occur.

Myotonia

Myotonia is defined as delayed relaxation of muscle after voluntary contraction or mechanical stimulation. The myotonic muscle disorders, caused by abnormalities of the voltage-gated ion channels of the muscle membrane, include hyperkalaemic periodic paralysis, paramyotonia congenita, myotonia congenita and myotonic dystrophy.

Myotonic dystrophy

Myotonic dystrophy (dystrophia myotonica) is an autosomal dominant disorder that differs from the other myotonic disorders in that it is a multisystem disease. Clinical features include myotonia, progressive muscle weakness and wasting, along with cataracts, frontal balding, facial weakness with loss of expression, ptosis, atrophy of the gonads and low IQ. A progressive cardiomyopathy with impaired cardiac conduction and arrhythmias may develop.

Implications for anaesthesia

The implications of myotonic dystrophy for anaesthesia are:

- respiratory muscle weakness – with an increased risk of postoperative respiratory complications;
- pharyngeal muscle weakness and tendency to obstructive sleep apnoea;
- oesophageal dysfunction – with a risk of regurgitation and aspiration;
- cardiovascular disease – arrhythmias, conduction defects and heart failure;
- suxamethonium may produce prolonged contraction;
- surgical manipulation, diathermy, hypothermia, shivering and potassium may all cause myotonia;
- myotonia is not necessarily abolished by muscle relaxants, local or regional anaesthesia.

Anaesthesia[38]

The severity of any respiratory dysfunction must be evaluated preoperatively. Arrhythmias and conduction defects may require treatment. Precautions are required against regurgitation and aspiration. Suxamethonium should be avoided, but co-induction with alfentanil and propofol may be a good alternative to the standard rapid sequence induction. Response to induction agents is variable and cautious administration in increments or by infusion is recommended. The response to non-depolarising muscle relaxants is also difficult to predict and the use of short-acting agents, given in increments and monitored with a nerve stimulator, is recommended. Regional anaesthetic techniques have been used successfully, but do not abolish myotonia during surgery. Cataract surgery is usually performed under local anaesthesia. The patient must be kept warm, and close observation in a high-dependency or intensive care unit is recommended postoperatively.

Muscular dystrophy

The muscular dystrophies are a group of inherited muscle disorders characterised by progressive muscle wasting and weakness.

Duchenne muscular dystrophy

Duchenne muscular dystrophy is the commonest and most severe of the muscular dystrophies. It is an X-linked recessive condition that presents in early childhood with weakness of the lower limb and pelvic muscles.

Cardiac muscle involvement results in hypertrophic cardiomyopathy and progressive respiratory muscle weakness leads to respiratory failure. Scoliosis is common.

Implications for anaesthesia

The implications of Duchenne muscular dystrophy for anaesthesia are:

- abnormal metabolic responses to suxamethonium and volatile agents may lead to a clinical syndrome of rhabdomyolysis and hypermetabolism, which resembles, but is often unrelated to, malignant hyperpyrexia. Although suxamethonium is considered to be contraindicated in these patients, the position regarding the use of volatile agents is more controversial. Their use is not always accompanied by complications, but in the presence of suitable alternatives such as continuous propofol infusion it may be safer to avoid them;[39]
- perioperative cardiac events, including arrhythmias, cardiac failure and cardiac arrest, may occur due either to cardiomyopathy or more usually to metabolic disturbance, particularly hyperkalaemia;
- the response to non-depolarising muscle relaxants is variable, but the duration of action may be prolonged. Administration of incremental doses and neuromuscular monitoring are recommended;
- respiratory complications are more common late in the disease, with an increase in the incidence of postoperative chest infection and respiratory failure.

MUSCULOSKELETAL DISORDERS

Scoliosis

Scoliosis is a lateral curvature of the spine with rotation of the vertebral body and spine in the direction of the concavity of the curve. It may be idiopathic, congenital, or secondary to a variety of neuromuscular and connective tissue disorders.

Implications for anaesthesia

The implications of scoliosis for anaesthesia are:

- there may be anaesthetic problems associated with the underlying cause of secondary scoliosis;
- respiratory impairment – usually a restrictive defect, an abnormal response to hypercapnia often made worse by anaesthesia, and an increased risk of postoperative respiratory insufficiency and retention of secretions;
- pulmonary hypertension and right ventricular failure in severe cases;

- regional techniques may be technically difficult because of the anatomical distortion.

Ankylosing spondylitis

Ankylosing spondylitis is an inflammatory arthropathy with systemic involvement. The spine and sacroiliac joints are primarily, but not exclusively, affected and a proportion of patients develop ophthalmic, cardiovascular, respiratory and neurological complications.

Implications for anaesthesia

The implications of ankylosing spondylitis for anaesthesia are:

- difficult intubation as a result of cervical immobility and/or limited mouth opening due to temporomandibular joint involvement;
- increased risk of cervical fracture with hyperextension;
- increased risk of postoperative respiratory complications due to limited chest expansion and pulmonary fibrosis;
- cardiovascular complications, including aortic regurgitation and conduction defects;
- increased incidence of vertebrobasilar insufficiency;
- technical difficulties with spinal and epidural techniques.

Anaesthesia

Difficult intubation should be anticipated. The laryngeal mask airway (LMA) or intubating LMA may be useful, and awake fibreoptic intubation may be indicated in severe disease. In some circumstances preliminary tracheostomy under local anaesthesia may be appropriate. Postoperative respiratory support may be required.

CONNECTIVE TISSUE DISEASES

Connective tissue diseases are often multisystem disorders and require careful preoperative assessment. Many are treated with long-term corticosteroid therapy and perioperative corticosteroid cover is required. The more common disorders are discussed in more detail below.

Rheumatoid arthritis

Rheumatoid arthritis is a relatively common autoimmune connective tissue disorder, primarily affecting joints but with widespread systemic effects. Characteristically there is a symmetrical peripheral polyarthritis, and systemic complications, which may affect the lungs, heart, kidneys, blood vessels and nervous system, occur in more than 50% of patients.

Implications for anaesthesia

The implications of rheumatoid arthritis for anaesthesia are:

- cervical instability, most commonly atlantoaxial subluxation due to involvement of the cervical vertebrae – there is a risk of cord damage with cervical manipulation, particularly flexion;
- temporomandibular joint involvement resulting in limited mouth opening;
- laryngeal deviation and cricoarytenoid joint involvement;
- pulmonary fibrosis and restrictive lung defect;
- renal dysfunction;
- pericarditis, pericardial effusion, aortic regurgitation;
- chronic anaemia;
- autonomic and peripheral neuropathy.

Anaesthesia

Careful preoperative assessment is required to identify potential airway and intubation problems and determine the extent of any systemic involvement. Awake fibreoptic intubation may be indicated in the presence of cervical instability.[40]

Systemic lupus erythematosus

Systemic lupus erythematosus (SLE) is an autoimmune connective tissue disorder that occurs mainly in females. Arthritis, often affecting the hands, and skin lesions are the commonest presenting features, but cardiac, respiratory, renal, haematological and neurological complications may occur. The presence of antiphospholipid antibodies is associated with thrombosis formation. SLE may be exacerbated by pregnancy and there is an increased risk of pre-eclampsia and fetal loss.

Implications for anaesthesia

The implications of SLE for anaesthesia are:

- cardiac complications, including conduction abnormalities, noninfective endocarditis of the mitral valve, myocarditis and an increased incidence of coronary artery disease;
- pulmonary involvement with a restrictive lung defect;
- pulmonary hypertension may develop;
- renal dysfunction due to glomerulonephritis;
- anaemia, leucopenia, thrombocytopenia and coagulopathy may occur;
- risk of thrombosis.

Scleroderma

Scleroderma (systemic sclerosis) is the name given to a spectrum of diseases involving abnormal collagen deposition and microvascular changes in the skin and other organs. Characteristically, the skin becomes taut and shiny with a loss of skin folds. Contractures of the joints and around the mouth may develop. Raynaud's phenomenon is common, and oesophageal, pulmonary, cardiac and renal complications may also occur.

Implications for anaesthesia

The implications of scleroderma for anaesthesia are:

- difficult venous access due to skin changes;
- limited mouth opening due to contractures, potential difficult intubation;
- oesophageal motility disorders may occur and increase the risk of regurgitation;
- cardiovascular complications, which may include hypertension, arrhythmias, conduction defects, left ventricular failure and pulmonary hypertension;
- pulmonary fibrosis and limited chest wall expansion owing to contractures, which may increase the risk of postoperative respiratory insufficiency;
- renal involvement is common and may progress to renal failure.

HAEMATOLOGICAL DISORDERS

Anaemia

Common causes of chronic anaemia include dietary iron or folate deficiency, chronic blood loss, renal failure, chronic illness and malignancy. Anaemia causes a reduction in oxygen-carrying capacity, and the extent to which it causes adverse effects depends on the capacity of the individual to compensate for this.

Physiological adaptations to anaemia, designed to improve oxygen delivery to the tissues, include an increase in the 2,3-diphosphoglycerate (2,3-DPG) level of red blood cells, which shifts the oxygen dissociation curve to the right, and an increase in cardiac output.

Chronic anaemia, developing slowly, is better tolerated than acute anaemia due to sudden haemorrhage. Clinically acceptable oxygen transport has been shown to be sustained at haemoglobin levels of 7–8 g/dL, in the presence of normal intravascular volume, a normal coronary circulation and normal haemodynamic responses.[41]

Before elective surgery, anaemia should be treated medically where possible. Nutritional deficiencies are treated with iron, folate or vitamin B_{12}

therapy, and erythropoietin may be useful for anaemia due to radiotherapy, chemotherapy or chronic renal failure.

In view of the potential hazards of blood transfusion and shortage of blood products, a rational approach to the transfusion of red cells in the perioperative period is recommended. The decision to transfuse should take into account the duration of anaemia, intravascular volume, likely intraoperative blood loss, and co-morbidity, such as impaired pulmonary function and ischaemic heart disease. A transfusion threshold of 7 g/dL may be adequate for haemodynamically stable and otherwise fit patients, whereas patients with cardiovascular disease may benefit from a higher haemoglobin level of around 9–10 g/dL.[41] Preoperative transfusion, if required, should ideally be completed 24 hours before surgery, to allow time for depleted 2,3-DPG in stored red cells to be restored. In an emergency situation, however, blood replacement therapy may be required immediately to help maintain intravascular volume and minimally acceptable haemoglobin levels.

Polycythaemia

Polycythaemia is a general term for an increased haemoglobin level, red cell count or haematocrit. The commonest type is apparent polycythaemia due to chronic hypoxia, smoking, obesity, fluid loss and hypertension. Absolute polycythaemia is associated with an increased red cell mass and may be primary (polycythaemia vera) or secondary to pulmonary disease, cyanotic heart disease and inappropriate production of erythropoietin.

Polycythaemia vera is a chronic myeloproliferative disorder. In addition to an increase in haemoglobin level, red cell mass and packed cell volume, there is often a leucocytosis, raised platelet count and splenomegaly. There is raised blood viscosity and an increased risk of thrombotic events, but paradoxically, bleeding problems may also occur due to impaired platelet function.

Elective surgery should be postponed until the condition has been medically controlled. Treatment is with hydroxyurea, radioactive phosphorus or alkylating agents.

If emergency surgery is required, venesection should be performed and the blood replaced with an equal volume of colloid until a satisfactory haematocrit is reached. Despite an adequate platelet count platelet transfusion may be required if bleeding problems arise.

Haemoglobinopathies

Sickle cell disease

Sickle cell disease is an autosomal recessive abnormality of haemoglobin synthesis. The substitution of valine for glutamic acid at the sixth position in the β-chain of the globin molecule results in the formation of haemoglobin S (HbS) rather than normal adult haemoglobin A (HbA). This occurs mainly in people of African descent, but also in some Mediterranean races.

The homozygous form of the disease results in sickle cell anaemia, whereas heterozygotes are said to possess the sickle cell trait. In homozygotes 75–95% of the haemoglobin is HbS, whereas in sickle cell trait HbS accounts for 20–45%.

The solubility of deoxygenated HbS is much lower than that of HbA and it undergoes a conformational change in the presence of low oxygen tension, which results in the red cell adopting a sickle shape. Sickle cells may damage the vascular endothelium and tend to aggregate in the microcirculation, increasing blood viscosity and obstructing small vessels, causing tissue infarction.

A chronic haemolytic anaemia results from premature destruction of the abnormal red cells. Painful vaso-occlusive crises may affect any organ. They are precipitated by dehydration, cold, infection and systemic illness, but may also occur spontaneously. Recurrent splenic infarction results in hyposplenism and immunocompromise, and progressive bone infarction may cause skeletal abnormalities. Gallstones, renal dysfunction, lung disease, pulmonary hypertension and heart failure may also occur.

Anaesthesia

Sickle cell screening should be performed in at-risk populations before surgery. A Sickledex test will detect the presence of HbS, but haemoglobin electrophoresis is required to differentiate between the disease and the trait. Sickle cell trait does not significantly increase anaesthetic risk except in the presence of severe hypoxia, but it is prudent to pay close attention to oxygenation, fluid balance and temperature.

Patients with sickle cell disease have an increased perioperative risk as a result of anaemia, sickle-related organ damage, the potential for vaso-occlusive crises and susceptibility to infection.

Preoperative transfusion of red cells is usually performed in an attempt to reduce perioperative complications. A conservative transfusion regimen aims to raise the haemoglobin level to around 10 g/dL regardless of the proportion of HbS present, whereas the aggressive regimen involves exchange transfusion to raise the haemoglobin and reduce the proportion of HbS to less than 30%.

The conservative regimen has been shown to be equally effective in preventing perioperative complications while resulting in fewer transfusion-associated complications,[42] but this may not apply to high-risk patients.

Preoperative administration of intravenous fluids is advisable to ensure optimum hydration.

Careful perioperative monitoring of temperature, acid–base status and fluid balance is required to prevent hypothermia, acidosis and dehydration.

Controlled ventilation is recommended to maintain a mild respiratory alkalosis.

Conditions that promote local stasis of blood, such as vasoconstrictors and tourniquets, should generally be avoided, although tourniquets have been used without complications in the presence of normal oxygenation and acid–base status.[43]

Thalassaemia

Thalassaemia is an inherited haemoglobinopathy characterised by an imbalance of globin chain synthesis. It is prevalent across a wide geographical area that extends from the Mediterranean, across North Africa, the Middle East, and into India and China.

β-Thalassaemia is the most common form of thalassaemia and results from reduced or absent production of β chains. In homozygotes (thalassaemia major), there is anaemia due to ineffective erythropoiesis and haemolysis. Bone marrow expansion and extramedullary erythropoiesis occur, and characteristically lead to skull and facial deformities. There is usually gross hepatosplenomegaly and splenectomy may be required. Increased iron absorption often produces iron overload, and iron deposits result in many of the complications of the disease, including cardiac hypertrophy and dilatation, pulmonary hypertension, cirrhosis and hypogonadism. Treatment is with regular blood transfusion and desferrioxamine to chelate iron. Heterozygous patients (thalassaemia minor) are usually asymptomatic.

Methaemoglobinaemia

In methaemoglobinaemia the ferrous iron in haemoglobin is oxidised to the ferric state, resulting in a loss of oxygen-carrying capacity and a shift of the oxygen dissociation curve to the left. Causes include genetic abnormalities, toxins, and drugs such as sulphonamides and prilocaine. Characteristically, the patient has slate-grey cyanosis and the pulse oximeter reading tends towards 85%. Reducing agents such as intravenous methylthioninium chloride (methylene blue) may be required to treat severe cases.

Sulphaemoglobinaemia

Cyanosis may also be due to sulphaemoglobinaemia, which is a side-effect of some drugs, particularly sulphonamides.

Abnormalities of haemostasis

Acquired disorders

Causes of acquired coagulopathy include liver disease, vitamin K deficiency, anticoagulant drugs and massive blood transfusion.

The coagulopathy associated with vitamin K deficiency, liver disease and warfarin therapy may be treated by administration of vitamin K and/or fresh frozen plasma (FFP), which contains clotting factors V, VIII and IX.[41]

Coagulopathy following massive blood transfusion is usually due to a combination of clotting factor deficiency and thrombocytopenia. Treatment may include FFP, platelets and, in the presence of low fibrinogen levels, cryoprecipitate which contains fibrinogen, factor VIII and von Willebrand factor.

The effect of intravenous heparin is usually reversed within 2–4 hours of stopping the infusion, but more rapid reversal may be achieved using protamine.

Disseminated intravascular coagulation

Disseminated intravascular coagulation (DIC) is a syndrome characterised by systemic activation of the coagulation system, which results in the widespread deposition of fibrin and microvascular thrombus formation. Consumption of clotting factors and platelets may lead to severe bleeding.

DIC usually results from either a systemic inflammatory response (as in sepsis or major trauma) or the release of procoagulant material into the circulation (as in amniotic fluid embolism or malignancy).

The management of DIC involves transfusion of appropriate blood products (FFP, cryoprecipitate and platelets) and treatment of the underlying cause.

Inherited disorders

Haemophilia

The haemophilias are sex-linked recessive disorders of coagulation. The commonest type, haemophilia A, is associated with a deficiency of factor VIII. Haemophilia B (Christmas disease), although clinically indistinguishable, is associated with a deficiency of factor IX

Haemophiliacs should only undergo essential surgery, and management should be guided by a haematologist. Factor levels are measured preoperatively and appropriate factor concentrate is administered throughout the perioperative period, as guided by the factor assay. Desmopressin gives a short-term increase in von Willebrand factor and factor VIII and may be used in those with mild haemophilia A undergoing minor surgery.[41]

Von Willebrand disease

Von Willebrand disease results from an autosomal dominant inherited deficiency or abnormality of von Willebrand factor – which is required for platelet adhesion and aggregation – resulting in a prolonged bleeding time. Desmopressin is recommended for diagnostic procedures, but factor VIII concentrate is required before surgery.[41]

COMMON PROBLEMS

The elderly patient

The elderly patient is difficult to define in terms of age alone and there is considerable variation between individuals of the same chronological age. The conventional social definition is people aged over 65 years, but in terms of physiological parameters 80 years is probably a more relevant definition.

Surgery in the elderly is associated with greater perioperative morbidity and mortality rates due to both an increased incidence of co-morbidity and the physiological consequences of ageing[44] (Box 1.2.8). The ageing process is associated with a loss of functional reserve and reduced ability of the cardiovascular and endocrine systems to respond to external stress. The elderly also tend to be sicker by the time they present and are more likely to require emergency surgery. With careful management, however, many of these patients can be treated safely and it is no longer considered acceptable to deny patients surgical treatment on the basis of age alone.

A thorough preoperative assessment is required and should include an assessment not only of the risks and benefits of the procedure, but also of the risks associated with not performing surgery.

Implications for anaesthesia

The implications of elderly patients for anaesthesia are:

- implications of coexisting diseases and long-term medication;
- increased risk of adverse drug reactions due to altered pharmacokinetics;
- increased haemodynamic instability under anaesthesia due to loss of compensatory mechanisms;
- fluid overload may easily precipitate pulmonary oedema and cardiac failure;
- impaired temperature regulation increases the risk of hypothermia;
- increased risk of postoperative pulmonary complications;
- postoperative cognitive dysfunction and delirium are common – risk factors include increasing age, coexisting disease, pre-existing cognitive dysfunction, metabolic abnormalities and a history of alcohol abuse;
- increased risk of pressure sores and thromboembolism, especially with prolonged procedures and postoperative immobility;
- increased risk of postoperative infection.

Anaesthesia

The choice of anaesthetic technique is probably less important than the skill with which it is given. Drugs should be administered slowly and

Box 1.2.8
Physiological and anatomical consequences of ageing
Cardiovascular
Fibrosis in the myocardium and conducting system results in an increased incidence of arrhythmias, heart block and congestive cardiac failure with diastolic dysfunction
Calcification of the heart valves
Decreased response to catecholamines
Reduced arterial compliance – elevated systolic blood pressure, slight reduction in diastolic pressure
Respiratory
Reduction in lung and chest wall compliance
Closing volume may exceed functional residual capacity, particularly when supine, leading to alveolar and small airway collapse
Increased physiological dead space
Increased ventilation–perfusion mismatch, resulting in lower arterial oxygen tension
Reduced laryngeal sensitivity – silent aspiration may occur
Renal
Reduced renal blood flow and glomerular filtration rate
Reduced number of functioning nephrons
Loss of renal reserve
Neurological
Progressive loss of neurones
Increased incidence of cognitive impairment
Autonomic dysfunction (postural hypotension, impaired temperature regulation, tendency to urinary retention and constipation)
Deafness
Locomotor
Osteoarthritis
Osteoporosis
Pharmacokinetics
Impaired metabolism due to a decline in renal and hepatic function
Altered volume of distribution due to decreased total body water and decreased lean muscle mass
Altered protein binding to due decreased serum albumin

according to response because it is likely that a reduced dose will be required. Agents associated with rapid recovery should be used where possible to minimise postoperative impairment. Care of pressure areas, maintenance of body temperature and careful attention to fluid balance are all important.

Local anaesthesia is associated with fewer postoperative sequelae and should be used where appropriate. Regional techniques may also be useful, but require careful management because profound hypotension may occur.

The pregnant patient

Only essential surgery should be performed during pregnancy, and delayed where possible until the second trimester. The anaesthetist must consider the safety of two patients – the mother and the fetus – and should take into account the physiological and anatomical changes associated with pregnancy.[45]

Pregnancy is associated with increased metabolic demands, resulting in a rise in oxygen consumption and increased minute ventilation. Anatomical changes result in a reduced residual volume and functional residual capacity, decreasing the oxygen reserve and increasing the risk of hypoxia with hypoventilation and apnoea. Airway management may be technically difficult owing to weight gain, breast enlargement and laryngeal oedema. Plasma volume and cardiac output increase, whereas peripheral vascular resistance decreases. From around mid-pregnancy onwards there is a risk of aortocaval compression by the gravid uterus when the woman is supine. Mechanical and hormonal changes reduce lower oesophageal sphincter tone and increase the risk of regurgitation and aspiration.

Preoxygenation and rapid sequence induction is indicated from the start of the second trimester onwards. Lateral displacement of the uterus to prevent aortocaval compression may be required after around 20 weeks of gestation. The minimum alveolar concentration of volatile agents decreases and there may be increased axonal block by local anaesthetics.

Potential hazards for the fetus include intraoperative hypoxaemia or asphyxia, exposure to teratogenic drugs, and the risk of spontaneous abortion or preterm delivery.

Fetal hypoxaemia may result from reduced uterine blood flow, maternal hypotension or hypoxia, and depression of the fetal cardiovascular or central nervous systems by drugs that cross the placenta. Maternal hypotension should be promptly managed by postural changes, fluids and ephedrine. The use of vasoconstrictors should be avoided because they may further compromise uterine blood flow.

Despite concerns about the potential teratogenic effects of anaesthetic agents, there is no evidence to date to suggest that they are associated with deleterious effects on embryonic or fetal development in humans.[45] An increased risk of spontaneous abortion, growth restriction and low birth weight has been demonstrated in association with surgery during pregnancy, but the reasons for this are more likely to be attributable to the requirement for surgery than to the administration of anaesthesia.

The patient with HIV and AIDS

Acquired immune deficiency syndrome (AIDS) was first described in 1981 and since then there has been an exponential rise in the number of people infected with the human immunodeficiency virus (HIV) worldwide. Transmission of the virus is via blood and blood products, sexual contact and perinatally. Impaired cell-mediated immunity renders infected individuals susceptible to infections and malignant disease.

AIDS is a multisystem disorder and may be associated with cardiovascular, respiratory, haematological, neurological, gastrointestinal, renal and metabolic complications. Treatment with antiretroviral drugs delays the progress of the disease and improves survival. It is estimated that 20–25% of HIV-positive patients will require surgery during the course of their illness.[46]

The status of the disease, the presence of complications and the side-effects of antiretroviral therapy should be determined preoperatively. Strict aseptic technique should be observed to minimise the risk of infection to the patient and universal precautions adopted to prevent the spread of infection to healthcare staff.

Regional anaesthesia has the advantages of not interfering with the immune system or interacting with antiretroviral drugs, but is contraindicated in the presence of sepsis or coagulopathy. The presence of neuropathy may also be a concern, but there is no evidence so far of adverse outcomes from regional techniques in AIDS patients.

Substance abuse

Substance abuse may be defined as the use of a drug or chemical in a way that was not intended and/or to excess. The range of abused substances is diverse and increasing. Chronic substance abuse may result in tolerance, addiction, and complications due to both the substance itself and to the route of administration. Inhalational administration is associated with the complications of smoking and the intravenous route may result in thrombophlebitis, infection with bloodborne viruses such as hepatitis B, hepatitis C and HIV, and infective endocarditis. The lifestyle associated with chronic substance abuse may also have health consequences as a result of an inadequate diet, poor hygiene and a reluctance to seek medical help.

Opioid addiction, most commonly to diamorphine (heroin), is associated with the highest morbidity and mortality rates. No attempt should be made to withdraw the drug during the perioperative period. Patients on withdrawal programmes should receive their usual dose of methadone. The use of local anaesthetic techniques and non-opioid analgesics for post-operative pain is recommended where possible, but there is no justification for withholding opioid analgesia and increased doses may be required.

Stimulant drugs such as cocaine, amphetamines and Ecstasy cause hypertension and tachycardia, often with ventricular extrasystoles. Where possible, anaesthesia should be postponed if there is evidence of recent intake. Adverse reactions associated with hyperthermia may occur and the principles of management are similar to those for malignant hyperpyrexia.

References

1. Eagle KA, Berger PB, Calkins H, et al. ACC/AHA guideline update for perioperative cardiovascular evaluation for non-cardiac surgery – executive summary. J Am Coll Cardiol 2002; 39:542–553.
2. Chassot PG, Delabays A, Spahn DR, et al. Preoperative evaluation of patients with, or at risk of, coronary artery disease undergoing non-cardiac surgery. Br J Anaesth 2002; 89:747–759.
3. Biccard BM. Perioperative β blockade and haemodynamic optimisation in patients with coronary artery disease and decreasing exercise capacity presenting for major non-cardiac surgery. Anaesthesia 2004; 59:60–68.
4. Moyna Bill K. Anaesthesia for patients with cardiac disease undergoing non-cardiac surgery. Anaesth Intens Care Med 2003; 4:297–300.
5. Howell SJ, Sear JW, Foex P. Hypertension, hypertensive heart disease and perioperative cardiac risk. Br J Anaesth 2004; 92:570–583.
6. Shammash JB, Ghali WA. Preoperative risk evaluation and perioperative management of the patient with non-ischaemic heart disease. Med Clin North Am 2003; 87:137–152.
7. Nishimura RA, Holmes DR Jr. Clinical practice: hypertrophic obstructive cardiomyopathy. N Engl J Med 2004; 350:1320–1327.
8. Troughton RW, Asher CR, Klein AL. Pericarditis. Lancet 2004; 363:717–727.
9. Nandwani N, Raphael JH, Langton JA. Effect of an upper respiratory tract infection on upper airway reactivity. Br J Anaesth 1997; 78:352–355.
10. Tait AR, Malviya S, Voepel-Lewis T, et al. Risk factors for perioperative adverse respiratory events in children with upper respiratory tract infections. Anaesthesiology 2001; 95:299–306 and Editorial 283–285.
11. Henzler D, Rossaint R, Kuhlen R. Anaesthetic considerations in patients with chronic pulmonary disease. Curr Opin Anaesthesiol 2003; 16:323–330.
12. McAlister FA, Khan NA, Straus SE, et al. Accuracy of the preoperative assessment in predicting pulmonary risk after non-thoracic surgery. Am J Respir Crit Care Med 2003; 167:741–744.

13. Hillier J, Gillbe C. Anaesthesia for lung volume reduction surgery. Anaesthesia 2003; 58:1210–1219.
14. Lipworth BJ. Modern drug treatment of chronic asthma. Br Med J 1999; 318:380–384.
15. McAnulty GR, Robertshaw HJ, Hall GM. Anaesthetic management of patients with diabetes mellitus. Br J Anaesth 2000; 85:80–90.
16. Porter AL, McCirrick A. Anaesthetic management for the diabetic patient. Anaesth Intens Care Med 2002; 3.9:316–319.
17. Farling PA. Thyroid disease. Br J Anaesth 2000; 85:15–28.
18. Heald A. Adrenocortical hormones. Anaesth Intens Care Med 2002; 3.9:327–329.
19. Smith M, Hirsch NP. Pituitary disease and anaesthesia. Br J Anaesth 2000; 85:3–14.
20. Dierdorf SF. Carcinoid tumor and carcinoid syndrome. Curr Opin Anaesthesiol 2003; 16:343–347.
21. James MFM, Hift RJ. Porphyrias. Br J Anaesth 2000; 85:143–153.
22. Caskey F, Pickett T. Fluid and electrolyte problems. Anaesth Intens Care Med 2003; 4:214–216.
23. Aguilera IM, Vaughan RS. Calcium and the anaesthetist. Br J Anaesth 2000; 55:779–790.
24. Lentschener C, Ozier Y. What anaesthetists need to know about viral hepatitis. Acta Anaesthesiol Scand 2003; 47:794–803.
25. Pugh RNH, Murray-Lyon IM, Dawson JL, et al. Transection of the oesophagus for bleeding oesophageal varices. Br J Surg 1973; 60:646–649.
26. Mansoor A, Watson W, Shayani V, et al. Abdominal operations in patients with cirrhosis: still a major surgical challenge. Surgery 1997; 122:730–735.
27. Rizvon MK, Chou CL. Surgery in the patient with liver disease. Med Clin North Am 2003; 87:211–227.
28. Engelhardt T, Webster NR. Pulmonary aspiration of gastric contents in anaesthesia. Br J Anaesth 1999; 83:453–460.
29. Gilder FJ. Anaesthetic problems in renal transplantation. Anaesth Intens Care Med 2003; 4.6:179–182.
30. Joseph AL, Cohn SL. Perioperative care of the patient with renal failure. Med Clin North Am 2003; 87:193–210.
31. Sneyd JR. Propofol and epilepsy. Br J Anaesth 1999; 82:168–169.
32. Chapman MG, Smith M, Hirsch NP. Status epilepticus. Anaesthesia 2001; 56:648–659.
33. Nicholson G, Pereira AC, Hall GM. Parkinson's disease and anaesthesia. Br J Anaesth 2002; 89:904–916.

34. Confavreux C, Hutchinson M, Hours MM, et al. Rates of pregnancy related relapse in multiple sclerosis. N Engl J Med 1998; 339:285–291.
35. Mercado DL, Petty BG. Perioperative medication management. Med Clin North Am 2003; 87:41–57.
36. Della Rocca GD, Coccia C, Diana L, et al. Propofol or sevoflurane without muscle relaxants allow the early extubation of myasthenic patients. Can J Anaesth 2003; 50:547–552.
37. Chevalley C, Spiliopoulos A, de Perrot M, et al. Perioperative medical management and outcome following thymectomy for myasthenia gravis. Can J Anaesth 2001; 48:446–451.
38. Imison AR. Anaesthesia and myotonia – an Australian experience. Anaesth Intens Care 2001; 29:34–37.
39. Goresky GV, Cox RG. Inhalation anesthetics and Duchenne's muscular dystrophy. Can J Anaesth 1999; 46:525–528.
40. Halaka P, Randell T. Intubation difficulties in patients with rheumatoid arthritis. A retrospective analysis. Acta Anaesthesiol Scand 1998; 42:195–198.
41. Armas-Loughran B, Kalra R, Carson JL. Evaluation and management of anemia and bleeding disorders in surgical patients. Med Clin North Am 2003; 87:229–242.
42. Vichinsky EP, Haberkern CM, Neumayr L, et al. A comparison of conservative and aggressive transfusion regimens in the perioperative management of sickle cell disease. N Engl J Med 1995; 333:206–213.
43. Tobin JR, Butterworth J Sickle cell disease: dogma, science and clinical care. Anesth Analg 2004; 98:283–284.
44. Beliveau MM, Multach M. Perioperative care for the elderly patient. Med Clin North Am 2003; 87:273–289.
45. Rosen M. Management of anesthesia for the pregnant surgical patient. Anaesthesiology 1999; 91:1159–1163.
46. Evron S, Glezerman M, Harow E, et al. Human immunodeficiency virus: anaesthetic and obstetric considerations. Anesth Analg 2004; 98:503–511.

Further reading

Mason R. Medical disorders and anaesthetic problems. Anaesthesia databook: a perioperative and peripartum manual, 3rd edn. London: Greenwich Medical Media; 2001:3–520.

Section 2

General anaesthesia

CHAPTER 2.1

ANAESTHETIC EQUIPMENT

THE ANAESTHETIC MACHINE

The principles of gas delivery in a modern anaesthetic machine are basically unchanged since the days of the Boyle's machine. In other aspects, however, such as in monitoring and safety devices, the modern apparatus has evolved a long way. Gases are delivered from pipelines or cylinders via pressure-reducing valves to the flowmeters, where the needle valves reduce pressure further and control flow. In the backbar are one or more vaporisers. Gases then pass through the common gas outlet to a breathing system. Modern anaesthetic machines, usually with integrated monitoring, are complex items of equipment that are increasingly dependent on electronic hardware and software. This provides a high level of redundancy in fault detection, but may diminish clinical watchfulness.

THE PREANAESTHETIC CHECKLIST

The third edition of the Association of Anaesthetists 2004 recommendations for checking anaesthetic equipment are as follows:[1]

- check the anaesthetic machine is connected to the electricity supply, and switched on. Some workstations may enter a self-test programme;
- check all monitors are operating, with appropriate alarm limits set. Sampling lines should be connected and unobstructed;
- check each gas pipeline is connected to the appropriate supply terminal using a tug test and that all pipeline pressures are 400–500 kPa. There should be an adequate supply of oxygen connected to the machine and a reserve cylinder. Supplies of other gases should be checked. Carbon dioxide cylinders should not normally be present and an empty cylinder yoke should be fitted with a blanking plug;
- check that flowmeters and flow valves function adequately, and that the oxygen flush valve works. If nitrous oxide is to be used, there must be a functioning antihypoxic linkage device;
- vaporisers should be checked for adequate (but not excessive) filling and for correct seating on the backbar. A leak test should be performed, with vaporiser on and off, by occluding the common gas outlet;

- the breathing system should be checked for correct configuration, secure connections (push and twist), correctly functioning valves, and patency of gas flow throughout. The system should be pressure tested and coaxial systems tested by occluding the inner tube. A single-use filter should be attached for each patient;
- the ventilator should be checked for correct configuration, including appropriately secured tubing, correct pressure, volume and alarm settings. An alternative means of ventilation should be available.;
- all ancillary equipment should be checked.

SUPPLY OF ANAESTHETIC GASES

In medically advanced countries, medical gases are usually supplied in hospitals by pipeline, with cylinders available as backup.

Oxygen

Vacuum insulated evaporator (VIE)

Oxygen is usually supplied and stored on the hospital site in liquid form in a VIE. One volume of liquid yields 840 volumes of gaseous oxygen at 15°C. The VIE consists of an insulated container in which the liquid oxygen is stored at about –160°C, at a pressure between 700 and 1200 kPa. There is a vapour withdrawal line at the top of the VIE, from which oxygen vapour is heated towards ambient temperature and delivered to the pipeline. Continual evaporation keeps the VIE cold. There is also a liquid withdrawal line from the bottom of the VIE, from which liquid oxygen can be withdrawn and superheated to a vapour.

Oxygen vapour is passed through a series of pressure regulators to drop the pressure down to the distribution pipeline pressure of 410 kPa. There is a pressure relief valve on top of the VIE in case lack of demand and gradual temperature rise result in a pressure rise. There is considerable wastage during filling of the VIE. The whole device is situated outside the hospital building on a hinged weighing device, protected by a caged enclosure, which also houses two banks of reserve cylinders. These take over automatically if the VIE output falls.

Cylinder banks

In a smaller hospital, banks of large cylinders can be used to deliver piped oxygen. Appropriate valves, monitoring and alarms need to be in place to ensure that the supply automatically switches to a full cylinder. Gas pressure in a full cylinder, including the E size on the anaesthetic machine, is around 135 atmospheres (13 700 kPa). The ISO (International Standards Organisation) colour for oxygen cylinders, indicated on the cylinder shoulder, is white, while the body is black.

Oxygen concentrator

An oxygen concentrator is used in some countries. Ambient air is compressed, then passed through zeolite, an aluminium hydroxide lattice,[2] which adsorbs nitrogen, leaving a 95% oxygen mixture at the outlet. On depressurisation the nitrogen is desorbed and released to the environment. Efficiency depends on the pressure change available and the need to adsorb water vapour from air using silica before entering the zeolite. Other methods of oxygen production, including chemical means, have been used in military and field anaesthesia.[3]

Oxygen failure alarm

The oxygen failure alarm is activated when oxygen delivery pressure falls below 200 kPa. The ideal device should:

- not depend on the pressure of any gas other than the oxygen itself;
- have an alarm system that does not use battery or mains power, and sounds an audible signal of sufficient length, volume and character;
- warn of impending failure, and warn again that failure has occurred;
- open the breathing system to the atmosphere to give an oxygen concentration prevent other gases flowing, and minimise the retention of carbon dioxide. It should be impossible to resume anaesthesia until the oxygen supply has been restored.

Nitrous oxide

Nitrous oxide is stored as a liquid in pressurised cylinders, either in a bank or on the anaesthetic machine. It is released as vapour. The pressure of a full cylinder is therefore the saturated vapour pressure at room temperature – usually between 4400 and 5400 kPa. If the gas flow is high, freezing and possible obstruction of the regulator outlet can occur unless thermostatically controlled. The ISO colour for a nitrous oxide cylinder is blue.

Entonox

Entonox is a safe and effective analgesic gas mixture of 50% each of oxygen and nitrous oxide. The mixture is stored and delivered to the patient using a two-stage pressure regulator, the second incorporating a demand valve.

If the cylinder temperature falls below –6°C – the pseudocritical temperature – the oxygen and nitrous oxide separate into layers (a process known as lamination, or the Poynting effect). The effects of lamination may be minimised either by storing the cylinders horizontally at a temperature of 5°C or more for 24 hours, or by the presence of a tube from the valve housing at the top of the cylinder to a point near the bottom, which prevents the withdrawal of pure nitrous oxide. The pressure in an Entonox cylinder is 135 atmospheres. Its ISO colour is blue and white quarters on the cylinder shoulder and a blue body.

Medical compressed air

Medical compressed air requires no trace of oil to be present, mainly because of the risk of explosion. Medical air for breathing devices is supplied from the pipeline at 410 kPa. When supplied at 700 kPa it is used to power operating tools, when the oil lubricant should be re-added. These two sources of compressed air must not be confused. If supplied by cylinder, the pressure is 135 atmospheres, and the ISO colour is black and white quarters on the cylinder shoulder and a black body.

GAS PIPELINES

The union between gas hoses and the anaesthetic machine should be permanent. The connection of hoses to the appropriate wall outlet is via a gas-specific, non-interchangeable Schräder valve, making it theoretically impossible to connect hoses incorrectly. The routine anaesthetic machine check will detect any such faults. Hoses are colour coded – white for oxygen, blue for nitrous oxide, black for air. When repairs are necessary a complete hose assembly is provided. A 'permit to work' system in the UK requires a six-part certificate to be signed when the action of one group of workers could expose others to hazard. Three levels of hazard are identified:

- high – work involves cutting an in-service pipeline, with danger of cross-connection or pollution;
- medium – work on a terminal unit where more than one gas is supplied, with danger of cross-connection;
- low – only one gas is involved.

Piped medical vacuum

A medical suction device is connected to a vacuum source by a yellow colour-coded hose. The outlet on the wall supplying a vacuum is one of many on a ring main, whence the pipe work goes via drainage, filtering and valve mechanisms towards a vacuum reservoir. Materials that have been suctioned then go through bacterial filters towards a vacuum pump. Flexible hoses are used for this transmission to reduce noise. Duty and standby pumps are in the system. The pump output is passed through a silencer.

Gas cylinders

Gas cylinders are made from a steel alloy of molybdenum, which is resistant to corrosion. Cylinders are subject to regular testing.

	Cylinder size					
	C	D	E	F	G	J
Oxygen capacity (L)	170	340	680	1360	3400	6800
Nitrous oxide capacity (L)	450	900	1800	3600	9000	–
Entonox capacity (L)	–	500	–	2000	5000	–
Air capacity (L)	–	–	–	–	3200	6400
Carbon dioxide capacity (L)	450	900	1800		–	–

Table 2.1.1 Cylinder sizes and capacities

Oxygen, nitrogen, air and helium are stored in cylinders as gases. Nitrous oxide, carbon dioxide and cyclopropane (no longer available for anaesthesia in the UK) are stored as liquids in equilibrium with saturated vapour.

A 'full' nitrous oxide cylinder contains liquid in up to 80% of its volume. The ratio of the weight of nitrous oxide to the weight of water that would fill the cylinder is the filling ratio – usually 0.75 in temperate climates, 0.67 in tropical climates.

Cylinder outlet valves use the pin index system (British Standard 1319, 1955) which makes it impossible to connect cylinders to the wrong yokes. Yokes are connected to flowmeters via non-interchangeable screw-threaded (NIST) connectors.

Before connection to the yoke, the cylinder valve is opened briefly to flush out inflammable dust and the presence of a Bodok seal checked.

After connection, the cylinder valve is slowly opened 2.5 turns. Machine backflow check valves prevent cross-filling of cylinders, but if a cylinder yoke is empty, it must be blanked off to prevent leakage from other cylinders. Table 2.1.1 shows cylinder sizes and capacities in current use.

Pressure-reducing valves (pressure regulators) and other valves

Pressure-reducing valves minimise danger to patients and damage to the downstream flowmeters. Between an oxygen cylinder and the anaesthetic machine, the pressure is reduced from 13 700 to 420 kPa, and on some makes (Ohmeda) there is a further reduction to 140 kPa.

The classic reducing valve is the Adams valve, in which a toggle mechanism occludes the high-pressure outlet when the downstream pressure rises.

The pressure is further reduced at the entrance to the flowmeter by the needle valve operating the flow controller to the flowmeter (see below).

Distal to the flowmeters, backbar pressure ranges from 1 to 8 kPa. The backbar has a pressure-relief valve, which activates at about 40 kPa.

Automatic pressure-limiting (APL) valves and expiratory valves on breathing systems are springloaded valves designed to open at preset pressures.

Flowmeters

When flow is laminar, the flow rate is directly proportional to the pressure gradient causing it. When flow is turbulent, the flow rate is proportional to the square root of the pressure gradient. In terms of the physical properties of the flowing gas, laminar flow depends on viscosity, and turbulent flow depends on density.

Rotameters

A rotameter is a variable-orifice, constant-pressure flowmeter. Gas is led to the base of a machined glass tube with a tapering cross-section.

A metal bobbin rides the gas jet, rotating in the flow, the gas escaping between the bobbin and the walls of the glass tube. As the bobbin rises with increased flow, the size of the annular gap between it and the glass tube increases. The height to which the bobbin rises indicates the flow rate.

Calibration accounts for both gas density and viscosity. At low flows, gas flow round the bobbin behaves like laminar flow through a tube (width of annulus less than length). At high flows, it is turbulent through an orifice (width of annulus greater than length). Hence, a rotameter calibrated for carbon dioxide will not read true for cyclopropane, because although their densities are similar (44:42), their viscosities are different (1:0.6).

The needle valve control knob carries the name of the gas and is colour coded. The oxygen control knob commonly protrudes further than the others to assist recognition.

The needle valve may be upstream of the rotameter (UK), or downstream (USA), which maintains a more constant pressure in the glass tube, and avoids error due to ventilator backpressure. The bank of tubes may have oxygen on the left (UK) or on the right (USA).

Antihypoxic device

The antihypoxic device limits the flow of nitrous oxide if the delivery pressure or flow of oxygen falls or fails, to prevent delivery of a hypoxic mixture. Such devices include the Ohmeda chain link between the oxygen and nitrous oxide flowmeter controls, and the Dräger device, which uses a hydraulically coupled valve.

Oxygen flush button

A button connected directly to the high-pressure oxygen source allows delivery of oxygen (oxygen flush) at more than 35 L/min. Safety dictates that the button should not be lockable in the depressed position.

Effect of barometric pressure

Rotameters are calibrated for use at sea level. They are inaccurate at high altitudes and in hyperbaric chambers. Similarly, if the outlet is restricted, as when a ventilator is used, the pressure rises and flow is greater than indicated with variable orifice rotameters. These inaccuracies can be corrected by placing the control valve distal to the orifice, when the pressure in the flowmeter is the same as that in the supply line. The flowmeter is calibrated in terms of litres the gas will occupy after discharge to atmospheric pressure.

Inaccuracies and dangers of rotameters

A variety of inaccuracies and dangers are associated with rotameters, thus:

- static electricity and dirt can cause sticking of the bobbin, especially when low flows are used, leading to inaccuracy as high as 35%. The bobbin must rotate freely;
- a leak through a cracked glass tube may cause a hypoxic mixture. This is less likely if the oxygen enters the backbar last. An internal baffle at the top of the rotameter bank achieves this even when the oxygen rotameter is upstream on the left;
- a defect in the top sealing washer of a rotameter can cause hazardous hypoxia;
- the rotameter tube must be vertical;
- backpressure from a ventilator can give a falsely low flow reading;
- a wire stop at the top keeps the bobbin in sight. This prevents a small bobbin jamming there with the anaesthetist unaware that gas is flowing.

Solenoid valve flow controllers

Modern anaesthetic machines with integrated electronic control systems simply have a rotameter icon on a monitoring screen. The manually operated flow control knob appears the same, but is connected to a series of eight solenoid valves, each of which double the flow of the previous one.[4]

VAPORISERS

Plenum vaporisers

When carrier gas enters a vaporiser, part of it goes through the vaporisation chamber while the remainder bypasses it. The control knob determines the ratio of these two flows – the splitting ratio. Thus the anaesthetic agent vapour, with a partial pressure equal to its saturated vapour pressure (SVP) at room temperature, is diluted by the carrier gas so the emerging mixture contains an accurate fractional vapour concentration. Full vaporisation within the chamber may be ensured by use of a wick, a cowl, multiple baffles and a nebuliser. A keyed filling port prevents filling with the wrong agent. The vaporiser should not be overfilled.[5]

Modern vaporisers include the Ohmeda Tec 5 or the Dräger Vapor. In each case the user has access to calibration curves. Output has been shown to vary by more than ± 15%.[6] In anaesthetic machines incorporating integral agent monitoring, a servo-controlled closed-loop feedback mechanism changes the splitting ratio if the measured output differs from the dialled output.

Temperature compensation

The SVP is kept constant by attaching the vaporiser to a metal jacket to minimise the temperature fall. Other methods of temperature compensation, to prevent a fall in output if temperature falls, include:

- a bimetallic strip, acting as a cap over the gas entry port to either the bypass or the vaporising chamber;
- aneroid bellows in the vaporisation chamber, which reduces the bypass flow if temperature falls.

Pressure compensation

If downstream pressure increases (e.g. owing to the presence of a ventilator), there may be retrograde movement of vapour-rich gas into the vaporiser. This pumping effect will increase the resultant vapour concentration. It may be prevented by including either a one-way valve or an additional length of tubing downstream of the vaporiser.

Altitude

At altitude the fractional output from a vaporiser is increased because the carrier gas is less dense. However, the SVP is independent of ambient pressure, so its partial pressure is unchanged for a given position of the control knob. This is the important variable pharmacologically in determining its clinical effect.

Drawover vaporisers

Plenum vaporisers are mounted on a continuous-flow anaesthetic machine with a pressurised gas supply, and resistance to gas flow is not considered important. When the patient inhales air through a vaporiser, either spontaneously or with intermittent positive-pressure ventilation (IPPV), the resistance to gas flow must be designed to be as low as possible. This is called a drawover vaporiser. For use in a military or field setting, see Chapter 5.15.

ANAESTHETIC BREATHING SYSTEMS

A breathing system consists of a fresh gas limb, inspiratory and expiratory limbs, expiratory valve, and reservoir bag, and may also have one or more unidirectional valves and a CO_2 absorber. The simpler systems have fewer components and usually involve some rebreathing. The ability to minimise rebreathing at a low fresh gas flow is a measure of the breathing system's efficiency, and depends on design and whether the patient is breathing spontaneously or being ventilated. More complex systems ensure minimum rebreathing by the use of unidirectional valves and CO_2 absorption while allowing more economical use of fresh gas and volatile agent.

Semi-closed rebreathing systems

Mapleson A system

The Mapleson A system (Fig. 2.1.1) is also known as the Magill system, and is very economical in spontaneous breathing. The last gas inhaled on inspiration is fresh gas, which therefore resides in the patient's deadspace, becomes the first gas exhaled on expiration, and is stored for the next breath. As expiration proceeds, the expiratory valve opens and alveolar gas is preferentially vented. No significant rebreathing occurs when the fresh gas flow falls as low as alveolar ventilation (70 mL/kg/min or 70% of minute ventilation). This efficiency is unrelated to the respiratory pattern.[7]

Efficiency during controlled ventilation is relatively poor. The design, which preferentially vents alveolar gas and stores fresh gas in spontaneous breathing, does the opposite when intermittent positive pressure ventilation (IPPV) is used. When the reservoir bag is squeezed, the partially closed expiratory valve opens and fresh gas is preferentially vented, although some will go to the patient. On expiration, the system preferentially fills with alveolar gas, ready to be rebreathed on the next inspiration. The Mapleson A system is the least appropriate for IPPV when a fresh gas flow of up to three or four times minute ventilation is required to prevent rebreathing.[8]

The efficiency of the Mapleson A system during IPPV can be improved with the Miller modification,[9] which prevents the escape of fresh gas during inspiration by enclosing the expiratory valve in a shroud, pressurised by the positive pressure used to compress the reservoir bag. This is an example of an enclosed afferent rebreathing (EAR) system.

Lack system

The Lack system (Fig. 2.1.2) is a coaxial variant of the Mapleson A system. It allows inspiration to occur through the outer tube and expiration down the inner tube. Therefore the diameter of the tubing is wider than standard 22 mm tubing. It is functionally identical to the Magill, and probably as efficient. In the parallel Lack system the tubes lie side by side.[10]

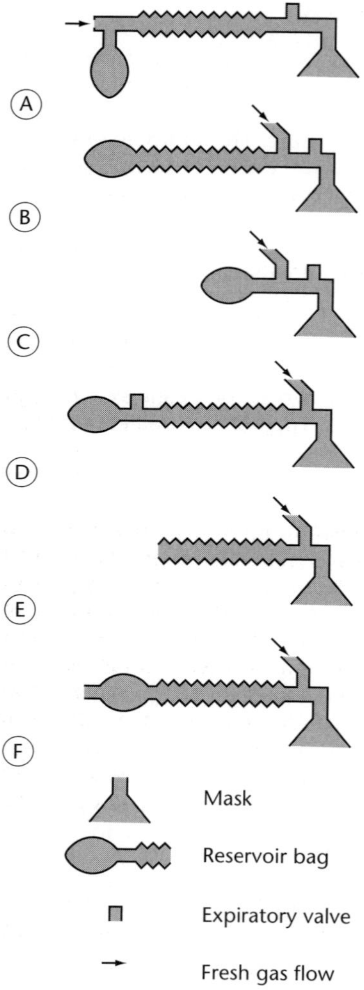

A

B

C

D

E

F

Mask

Reservoir bag

Expiratory valve

Fresh gas flow

Figure 2.1.1 Mapleson classification of semi-closed rebreathing systems.

Mapleson B and C systems

The Mapleson B and C systems are seldom used these days, except occasionally for resuscitation purposes.

Mapleson D, E and F systems

The Mapleson D, E and F systems are all known as T pieces because fresh gas is delivered at a T junction close to the patient. Functionally, all T pieces

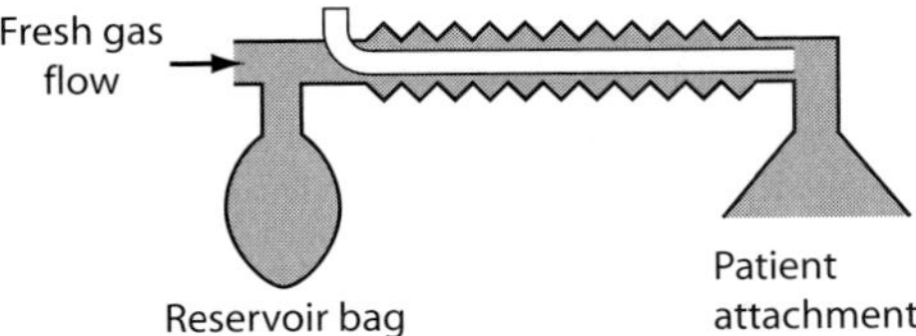

Figure 2.1.2 Coaxial Mapleson A system — the Lack system.

have common performance characteristics. In the early part of inspiration, fresh gas flow exceeds the inspiratory requirement, allowing some to be stored in the system. Their performance is highly dependent on a long expiratory pause.[7] They are much less efficient than Mapleson A systems for spontaneous breathing, when a fresh gas flow of at least twice minute ventilation is needed. For IPPV, a fresh gas flow of 70–100 mL/kg/min will give normocapnia, provided minute ventilation is sufficiently high (120–150 mL/kg/min).

Bain system

The Bain system (Fig. 2.1.3) is a coaxial variant of the Mapleson D system. Although superficially it resembles the Lack system, fresh gas is delivered down the relatively narrow-bore inner tube to a point close to the patient. Expiration occurs down the standard 22 mm diameter outer tube. Care must be taken that the inner coaxial tube does not become detached at either end or the circuit deadspace becomes much larger. It may not be as efficient as the orthodox Mapleson D system, because the coaxial arrangement at the patient end may encourage gas mixing. If it is necessary to ventilate patients from a distance, as for magnetic resonance imaging, a long Bain system may be used. The additional length increases its compliance and resistance, so smaller tidal volumes and higher end-expiratory pressures result.[11]

Mapleson E and F systems

Mapleson E and F systems are otherwise known respectively as the Ayre's T piece and its Jackson Rees modification. A reservoir tube with a volume

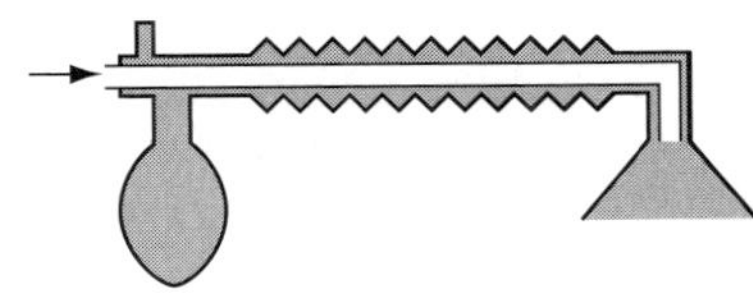

Figure 2.1.3 Coaxial Mapleson D system — the Bain system.

one-third of the patient's tidal volume is needed to prevent both rebreathing and dilution. The valveless system is simple and provides low resistance to spontaneous breathing for small children.

The Jackson Rees modification is the addition of an open-tailed reservoir bag to allow visible monitoring of breathing, as well as a means of manual controlled ventilation. During spontaneous respiration, the fresh gas flow required to avoid rebreathing is twice the child's minute ventilation. During IPPV, as with the Mapleson D system, much less is needed, e.g. 1000 mL/min + 200 mL/kg/min.

Humphrey ADE system

The Humphrey ADE system was designed so that, at the turn of a lever, a system with Mapleson A characteristics could be used for spontaneous ventilation, and a system with D and E characteristics is available for controlled ventilation. It may also be used in children.[12]

The circle system

The circle system (Fig. 2.1.4) is a more complex system in which exhaled gas is recirculated to enhance economy and to reduce pollution. It incor-

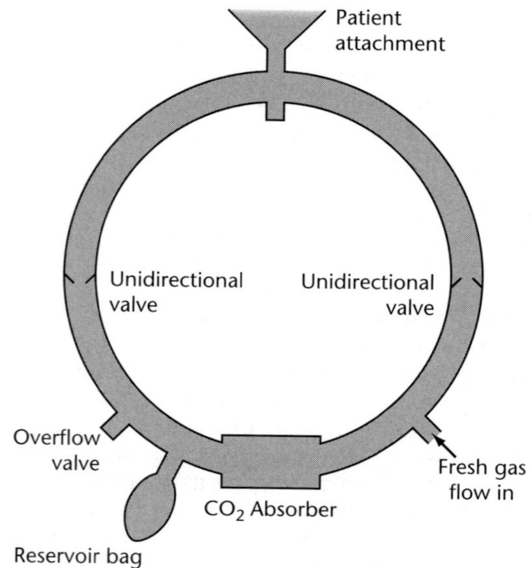

Figure 2.1.4 Circle system.

porates unidirectional valves and a means of absorbing CO_2. The fresh gas flow can be quite low, say 500 mL/min or less of both oxygen and nitrous oxide. Its complexity may be a disadvantage. There are a number components and connections. Inspired anaesthetic gas and vapour concentrations are lower than those in the fresh gas input, particularly at low fresh gas flows, because of uptake into the patient's tissues. Gas and vapour monitoring is particularly important. At higher fresh gas flows, above about 3 L/min, a circle system behaves more like a semi-closed rebreathing system and the CO_2 absorber may be unnecessary. High fresh gas flows at the beginning of an anaesthetic enhance gas uptake and denitrogenation, after which they may be reduced. The response time of a circle system is inversely proportional to gas inflow and directly proportional to system volume.

Circle systems can be used for paediatric anaesthesia, using a 1 L reservoir bag and smaller-bore tubing. The work of breathing is acceptable.

Carbon dioxide absorption

A low-resistance absorber is an important part of a circle system. Two absorbents in common use are soda lime and baralyme.

Soda lime consists of 4% sodium hydroxide, 1% potassium hydroxide, 14–19% water, and the balance is calcium hydroxide. There are also small amounts of silica for drying, kieselguhr for hardening and dye indicators to show when the crystals are spent. Ethyl violet is one such indicator, although its activity can be impaired by fluorescent lighting. The water is essential for CO_2 absorption, thus:

- $CO_2 + H_2O \rightarrow H_2CO_3$;
- $2NaOH + 2H_2CO_3 + Ca(OH)_2 \rightarrow CaCO_3 + Na_2CO_3 + 4H_2O$.

The heat and water liberated by these reactions provide useful warmth and humidity for the patient.

Baralyme is a mixture of 20% barium hydroxide, 80% calcium hydroxide and a small amount of potassium hydroxide. The water for the reaction is present as the octahydrate of barium hydroxide.

In both cases, the monovalent hydroxides are more reactive than the divalent $Ca(OH)_2$. Where the absorbent crystals have been allowed to dry out, these highly reactive monovalent hydroxides can also produce significant amounts of carbon monoxide and formaldehyde. An absorbent consisting of only $Ca(OH)_2$ has been produced to counteract this.[13]

Absorbents also tend to absorb volatile agents, which was hazardous when the (now obsolete) volatile agent trichloroethylene was used. This reacted with soda lime to produce dichloroacetylene gas or phosgene, a neurotoxin. Sevoflurane reacts with soda lime to produce Compound A, a renal toxin. This is not clinically significant,[14] although regulations in the USA recommend a minimum fresh gas flow of 3 L/min to minimise this.

SCAVENGING SYSTEMS

Scavenging systems transport waste anaesthetic gases from the breathing system to the atmosphere to avoid local pollution. Systems can be active or passive. They consist of a collecting system, a transfer system, a receiving system and a disposal system.

Active scavenging

With active scavenging the patient should be protected from negative pressures greater than 100 Pa (1 cm H_2O). This may be achieved by an open T-piece reservoir or an air break.

Passive scavenging

With passive scavenging total flow resistance should not exceed 50 Pa (0.5 cm H_2O) at 30 L/min. Copper pipes of 28–35 mm outer diameter are satisfactory. The discharge point should avoid wind pressures. A T termination with a downward right-angle bend at each end is preferred, placed above a flat roof.

VENTILATORS

Modern ventilators can act as constant or non-constant generators of either pressure or flow. The ventilator has to execute an inspiratory phase, cycle from inspiration to expiration, allow expiration and an expiratory pause, and then cycle back to inspiration.

Pressure generator

A pressure generator delivers a preset pressure to the patient. The flow (and hence the tidal volume) depends on the resistance and compliance of the respiratory system. It may be thought of as a weighted bellows.

Flow generator

A flow generator delivers a preset flow pattern, which is maintained whatever the resistance and compliance of the respiratory system. Under adverse circumstances, airway pressure may rise high enough to cause barotrauma.

Constant flow generation may be achieved by forcing gas at high pressure through a nozzle, whereas other flow patterns may be achieved by a sinusoidal or positive displacement pump.

Power

Power is required during the inspiratory phase, typically about 20 W. Peak power production must exceed peak airway pressure times peak flow rate, plus any energy losses. A high proportion of the required power is spent overcoming the internal resistance of the ventilator, which can be as much as 200 W.

The power provided may be from the fresh gas flow itself in minute volume dividers (e.g. Manley ventilator), electrical power or compressed gas, usually oxygen.

Cycling

Cycling is initiated by time, volume, pressure, flow or patient triggering.

Expiration

Expiration is generally passive release to the atmosphere. Patients with acute lung injury often benefit from positive end-expiratory pressure (PEEP) to recruit alveoli and improve oxygenation.

Safety features

All users of ventilators should have a low threshold of suspicion for faults. Numerous variables are monitored on a ventilator and there should be appropriate alarms on these monitors, especially to detect inadequate or excessive volume or airway pressure before the patient is harmed. The function of low-pressure (disconnection) alarms should be checked by disconnecting at the patient end of the circuit, in case the threshold pressure is set inappropriately low.

Testing

Before being put into clinical use, all ventilators are rigorously tested on a lung model. Testing to an ISO standard includes tests of endurance, waveform and volume performance, and internal compliance.

Paediatric ventilators

Paediatric ventilators need to offer respiratory rates between 15 and 40 per minute, and tidal volumes between 16 and 500 mL. Lung compliance and airways resistance in babies can vary tenfold. Neonates may require an inspiratory time as short as 0.5 seconds, inspiratory flow as low as 2 L/min and peak airway pressure limited to 6–7 cm H_2O. Appropriate alarms should be available and used to respond to the tight constraints of excessive or inadequate measured values of important variables. Adequate humidification is mandatory.

AIRWAY MANAGEMENT DEVICES

See Chapter 2.6, Airway management.

INTRAVENOUS PUMPS AND SYRINGE DRIVERS

Programmable volumetric intravenous pumps and syringe drivers are use to deliver intravenous anaesthesia, patient-controlled anaesthesia and epidural infusions. Some pumps control the flow rate by a photoelectric drip-rate detector in conjunction with a microprocessor-controlled occlusion device.

Syringe drivers give a continuous, pulsatile flow to an accuracy of 2–5%. Some syringe drivers are driven by clockwork motors, others by a battery-powered motor, which is intermittently on and off. The syringe driver should not be positioned above the patient to avoid siphoning. Modern syringe drivers are usually sufficiently accurate, but there may be a delay before the infusion is initiated. Where the bolus to be delivered is small, say 0.5 mL from a patient-controlled analgesia (PCA) pump, the accuracy of the delivered bolus becomes questionable.[15]

Volumetric pumps enable constant volumetric delivery despite variation in resistance to flow, and use either a peristaltic pump, a reservoir or syringe-type cassettes to drive the flow, and have an accuracy of 5–10%. Safety problems with these devices include infusion of air, power failure, disturbance of the infusion by a secondary infusion, and software corruption.

Target-controlled infusion pumps with advanced software have been developed which allow patient characteristics and desired drug plasma concentration to be entered. A pharmacokinetic model is used to control the pump.

STERILISATION OF EQUIPMENT

Disinfection is the killing of non-sporing microorganisms. Sterilisation is the killing of all microorganisms, including viruses, fungi and any spores. Disposable equipment meant for single use only is increasingly used in anaesthetic and even surgical practice.

Methods of sterilisation

Moist heat

Moisture increases cellular permeability and heat coagulates protein.

Boiling (100°C) for 15 minutes kills bacteria, but spores may escape destruction. Increased pressure makes it possible to produce higher temperature.

In the modern autoclave, air is replaced by steam at 134°C and 2 bar pressure for 3½ min. To remove moisture, the steam is evacuated and replaced by sterile air. The cycle takes about 10 minutes. It is useful for metal objects and fabrics. This will kill all living organisms provided the material treated is properly wrapped to allow penetration. Deterioration of rubber and plastics is hastened by this method and exposure for 15 minutes to a temperature of 121°C may be substituted. Sharp instruments may become dulled.

Low-temperature (73°C) steam sterilisation (290 mmHg pressure) takes just over 2 hours. If formaldehyde is added spores are also killed. This may be used for materials harmed by steam at higher temperatures.

Chemical sterilisation

Chemical sterilisation is useful for objects that will not withstand heat (e.g. endoscopes). Chemicals kill by coagulation or alkylation of proteins. Non-sporing bacteria, viruses, the tubercle bacillus and spores are resistant to destruction (in ascending order). Chemicals only act on exposed surfaces, some react with metals, and some impregnate materials (e g. rubber) and remain as a source of mucosal irritation.

Formaldehyde

Formaldehyde can be used for endoscopic equipment, catheters etc. Residual formaldehyde may persist after prolonged airing and harm the skin or irritate the operator's eye.

Ethylene oxide

Ethylene oxide (C_2H_4O) is a colourless gas and is a good bactericidal agent, although very toxic to inhale. It has good penetrability and few materials are harmed; it is effective against all organisms, but is slow (8–12 hours).

Ethylene oxide is explosive at a concentration above 3% in air, and it is necessary to use 10% in CO_2 at a relative humidity of 30–50%. This is a good method for sterilising complicated and delicate apparatus (e.g. oxygenators, prostheses, ventilators, respiratory equipment), although expensive and time consuming.

The accepted method of removing adsorbed ethylene oxide by allowing 7 days' shelf-life is inadequate, and the pulling of six post-sterilisation vacuums is advised. The cylinders containing the mixture are identified by aluminium paint: the shoulder is red and below it is a circular band of yellow paint.

Liquids

Liquids used for chemical sterilisation are as follows:

- phenol (1–5%) – used to clean surfaces of apparatus. It should not be used on equipment that comes into contact with the patient, and does not kill spores;
- iodine (0.5–2% in alcohol) – which may irritate or burn the skin. Povidone-iodine 10% is less irritant;
- ethyl alcohol 70–80% is more efficient than absolute (100%) alcohol. Isopropyl alcohol 50–70% can be used;

- chlorhexidine 0.5% in 70% ethyl alcohol for skin sterilisation. Cetrimide may be added;
- glutaraldehyde – commonly used for endoscopes – a 2% solution made alkaline by the addition of 0.3% sodium carbonate. This will kill bacteria in 15 minutes and spores in 3 hours.

Gamma rays (ionising radiation)

2.5 Mrad is bactericidal.

Filtration

Filters are used to prevent contamination by organisms, and can remove 99.99% of particles over 0.5 μm diameter. The filters themselves can be autoclaved. Disposable filters are used for bolus injections or infusions through epidural catheters.

References

1. Association of Anaesthetists of Great Britain and Ireland. Checking anaesthetic equipment. 3rd edn. 2004, London.
2. Li YY, Perera SP, Crittenden BD. Zeolite monoliths for air separation. Trans I Chem E 1998; 76A:921–930.
3. Bhisman NR, Rout CC, Murray WB. Laboratory assessment of oxygen delivery from a portable chemical generator. Anaesthesia 1996; 51:1127–1128.
4. Boaden RW, Hutton P. The digital control of anaesthetic gas flow. Anaesthesia 1986; 41:413–418.
5. Palayiwa E, Hahn CEW. Overfill testing of anaesthetic vaporizers. Br J Anaesth 1991; 74:100–103.
6. Nielsen J, Pedersen FM, Knudsen F, et al. Accuracy of 94 anaesthetic agent vaporisers in clinical use. Br J Anaesth 1993, 71:453–457.
7. Cook LB. The importance of the expiratory pause. Comparison of the Mapleson A, C and D rebreathing systems using a lung model. Anaesthesia 1996; 51:453–460.
8. Tyler CKG, Barnes PK, Rafferty MP. Controlled ventilation with a Mapleson A (Magill) breathing system: reassessment using a lung model. Br J Anaesth 1989; 62:462–466.
9. Bruce WE, Soni NC. Preliminary evaluation of the enclosed Magill breathing system. Br J Anaesth 1989; 62:144–149.
10. Ooi R, Lack JA, Soni N, Whittle J, Pattison J. The parallel anaesthetic Lack breathing system. Anaesthesia 1993; 48:409–414.
11. Sweeting CJ, Thomas PW, Sanders DJ. The long Bain system: an investigation into the implications of remote ventilation. Anaesthesia 2002; 57:1183–1186.
12. Orlikowski CE, Ewart MC, Bingham RM. The Humphrey ADE system: evaluation in paediatric use. Br J Anaesth 1991; 66:253–257.

13. Bedi A. The in vitro performance of carbon dioxide absorbent with and without strong alkali. Anaesthesia 2001; 56:546–550.

14. Baxter A, Garton K, Kharasch ED. Formation of carbon monoxide from difluoro-methyl ether anaesthetics. Anesthesiology 1998; 89:937–940.

15. Jackson IJB, Semple P, Stevens JD. Evaluation of the Graseby patient controlled analgesia pump. Anaesthesia 1991; 46:478–481.

CHAPTER **2.2**

MONITORING

GENERAL PRINCIPLES

Monitoring is intended to measure and record deviations from normal values and warn of adverse events. Standards have been agreed in many countries, and those in the UK are published and updated by the Association of Anaesthetists.[1] It is necessary to monitor both the patient and the anaesthesia delivery system.

Clinical monitoring

The most important factor for clinical monitoring is the continual presence of a trained and competent anaesthetist. This applies to general and regional anaesthesia, sedation with multiple drugs and the early phase of recovery. The experienced anaesthetist will monitor:

- the circulation – pulse rate, rhythm and quality, vein filling, skin elasticity and temperature, and urine output (if catheterised);
- respiration – effort, pattern, tidal volume, frequency, reservoir bag movement;
- oxygenation – skin, mucous membrane and blood colour;
- depth of anaesthesia – pupillary signs (after Guedel), lacrimation, sweating, muscle movement.

Instrumental monitoring

Of the patient

In this age of numerical recording of variables, it is important to make use of simple and well-established technology to monitor the patient's physiology, which should be applied from immediately before the induction of anaesthesia and maintained until the patient has recovered, as follows:

- circulation – noninvasive blood pressure, electrocardiogram (ECG), pulse oximetry;
- respiration – pulse oximetry, airway pressure, especially during intermittent positive-pressure ventilation (IPPV), ventilatory volume,

inspired and expired carbon dioxide and volatile agent concentrations, expired carbon dioxide waveform;

- neuromuscular transmission – nerve stimulators when relaxants are used;
- metabolic monitoring – sometimes indicated (e.g. temperature, blood glucose, acid–base balance).

Of the anaesthetic machine

Instrumental monitoring of the anaesthetic machine is also necessary to ensure patient safety. Some of the monitors already listed as physiological monitors perform some of these functions, but others are also needed as follows:

- loss or reduction of gas supply – gas pressure, gas concentration (particularly oxygen), oxygen failure warning device;
- breathing system disconnection or ventilator failure – airway pressure, inspired and expired carbon dioxide concentrations, gas volumes;
- vaporiser malfunction – inspired and expired volatile agent concentrations.

Additional monitoring

In many major surgical operations invasive monitoring of the circulation is sometimes required, such as:

- invasive measurement of arterial pressure, central venous pressure, and occasionally pulmonary arterial catheterisation to monitor left atrial pressure and cardiac output. Noninvasive monitoring of cardiac output using transthoracic electrical bioimpedance or echocardiography is now preferred; the probe for echocardiography can be usefully incorporated in the tip of an endotracheal tube;
- catheter to measure urine output;
- coagulation testing;
- haemoglobin and electrolytes, which are readily obtainable with modern blood gas analysers.

Monitors all have limitations

Pulse oximeter probes become detached, gas sampling lines become blocked, a gas-pressure alarm can fail to detect a disconnection if the sensor is placed inappropriately. The anaesthetist's clinical sense and experience should always be paramount.

Noninvasive and minimally invasive monitoring are preferred if they give information that is as accurate or useful as invasive monitors. It is difficult to determine with certainty the effect that additional instrumental monitoring has on patient safety. No study to do this would be ethical.

An extensive Australian study[2] concluded that more than 70% of critical incidents occurring during anaesthesia are detectable by monitor, and that of these, over 80% would be detectable by correct use of pulse oximetry. When used in conjunction with a capnometer, over 90% of such incidents are detectable. This strongly supports the combined use of these two monitors. Nonetheless, if resources are limited a high level of safety may be achieved by a careful, conscientious anaesthetist.

The information available from clinical observation and monitors must be accurately and contemporaneously recorded. This is usually done manually, but can be now automatically downloaded to a printer.

Transfers

Critically ill or anaesthetised patients who need to be transferred within or between hospitals should be monitored to the same standards outlined above.

Alarms

Alarms should always be enabled and appropriate limits set by the anaesthetist. This includes infusion pumps, if used to administer anaesthetic drugs.

Monitors have vastly increased the amount of information available to the anaesthetist. This can result in multiple alarm noises, making alarm systems unpopular and risking their non-use.

There are international standards relating to the nature and hierarchy of alarms.[3] It is important that alarms are designed with their intended users in mind.[4]

CARDIOVASCULAR MONITORING

Pulse oximetry

The human eye has difficulty in detecting cyanosis, and the pulse oximeter has undoubtedly improved the ability to monitor oxygenation. It uses both plethysmography and infrared spectroscopy.

The pulse oximeter probe consists of a light source on one side, capable of delivering both red and infrared light, and a photodetector on the other side. The probe is placed either on a digit or an earlobe.

The light source emits alternating red and infrared light separated by a gap, at a frequency of 400 Hz. The wavelengths used are 660 nm and 940 nm, these being wavelengths on the absorption spectra of reduced and oxygenated haemoglobin at which the absorptions of these two haemoglobins are, respectively, widely separated and nearly equal. This allows the device to take account of the total amount of haemoglobin present as well the proportion of oxygenated haemoglobin present.

Signals from non-pulsatile sources are electronically filtered out. The software contains a calibration curve constructed from a series of blood samples from volunteers, which calculates arterial oxygen saturation from the absorption data.

The amplitude of the plethysmographic signal should not be thought of as a quantitative indicator of the pulse signal because it is variably amplified by the device.

Sources of error in pulse oximetry

These include the following:

- a poorly fitting probe;
- poor pulsatile arterial flow (e.g. vasoconstriction);
- pulsatile venous flow (e.g. tricuspid regurgitation);
- electrical or mechanical interference (e.g. strong ambient light, diathermy, vibration and movement);
- presence of other haemoglobin variants. For example carboxyhaemoglobin (which has a similar absorption spectrum to oxygenated haemoglobin in red light) and sulphaemoglobin or methaemoglobin – perhaps caused by drugs such as prilocaine (which have similar absorption spectra to reduced haemoglobin and cause the oximeter to read around 85%). Fetal haemoglobin does not alter the accuracy of pulse oximetry;
- dyes, such as methylthionium chloride (methylene blue). Bilirubin does not significantly absorb light in this bandwidth to corrupt pulse oximetry, but does affect the accuracy of a co-oximeter that uses a greater range of wavelengths. Dark nail polish interferes with the probe, but skin colour does not;
- there is a delay in the response to changes in arterial saturation, which is longer for digital probes than for ear probes. There is a further delay caused by electronic averaging of several heart beats;
- readings outside the calibrated range (usually down to 85%) are extrapolated and therefore should not be relied upon.

Arterial blood pressure

Blood pressure was first measured invasively by arterial cannulation in an animal by Hales in 1733. Noninvasive methods were introduced into clinical practice in the late 19th century, and remain a primary means of monitoring the circulation. All monitors can measure systolic and diastolic pressures and deduce mean arterial pressure.

Noninvasive measurement

A single compression cuff or double cuff is wrapped around a limb, usually the upper arm, and inflated above systolic pressure. The onset of pulsations is detected as the cuff is deflated. This can be either a manual or an automatic process.

The dimensions of a single compression cuff are important in determining the accuracy of measurement, particularly in children or in obese patients. The American Heart Association stipulates that the width (of the inflatable bladder part) of the cuff should be 40% of the mid-circumference of the limb, and the length of the cuff should be twice this width. Recommended cuff widths are:

- neonate 2.5 cm;
- 1–4 years 6.0 cm;
- 4–8 years 9.0 cm;
- adult 12–14 cm (15 cm for the adult leg).

A narrow cuff gives a falsely high reading whereas a wide cuff gives a falsely low reading. A cuff reading may not correlate with intra-arterial measurement across the whole range of pressures because there is a non-linear relationship between the pressure in a cuff and its internal diameter around a limb.

Morbidity from cuffs includes skin and underlying tissue damage, and possible ulnar nerve damage when used on the arm too close to the elbow.

Manual measurement

The cuff is compressed by inflating a bulb that is connected to the cuff and to either a mercury column or an aneroid barometer and a pressure gauge. As the system is decompressed, the return of pulsations in the downstream artery is detected, usually by palpation or auscultation of the Korotkoff sounds.

The Von Recklinghausen oscillotonometer has a double cuff. The upper cuff is a narrower, occluding cuff connected to the inside of a sealed box, the pressure inside which is measured by an aneroid barometer. The lower cuff is wider for sensing the return of pulsations on deflation of the occluding cuff, and is connected to a more sensitive aneroid barometer inside the sealed box. An inflation bulb and a small lever allow inflation and deflation of the cuff, and detection of the onset of systolic and diastolic pressures.

Automatic measurement

Oscillometry uses a single cuff, which allows the process to be automated using microprocessor technology. Automated, controlled hydraulics allow the cuff to be inflated to above systolic pressure, and then deflated in a stepwise fashion.

Arterial pulsations are detected by the cuff as the systolic value is reached. As mean pressure is reached, these pulsations reach maximum amplitude. At diastolic pressure the pulsations diminish and disappear.

A single pressure transducer continuously detects both the cuff pressure and the arterial pulsations. These signals are digitised and electronically processed to display systolic, mean and diastolic pressures. The electronic algorithm crosschecks the relationship between the three pressures. The original Dinamap measured only mean arterial pressure.

Accuracy is maximised if the system volume is kept to a minimum. Extreme hypotension, excessive cuff movement, rapid changes in blood pressure, abnormal pulse rhythms and interchanging cuffs can all be causes of inaccurary. Otherwise, these devices have been shown to be convenient and reasonably accurate.

Finapres

The Finapres uses the principle of arterial volume clamp plethysmography developed by Peñaz and Slurer. A small, low-volume, noncompliant cuff is placed around a finger. The cuff contains an infrared light source and photodetector, so that the finger is transilluminated. The cuff is attached to a small pump and a solenoid valve, which allows rapid small-amplitude pressure changes to be applied. This is linked to a servo-control mechanism with a fast response time.[6]

After inflation, the cuff is initially deflated until cuff oscillations are maximum, corresponding to mean pressure. This forms a set-point based on the amount of infrared light transmitted through the finger to the photodetector.

Subsequently the cuff pressure is adjusted rapidly to maintain constant light transmission through the finger. It does this as the pressure rises and falls between systolic and diastolic, around the mean arterial pressure set-point. Thus the device tracks arterial pressure and the output is displayed as an arterial waveform.

For accuracy, all components of the compressible volume, including the noncompliant cuff, must be kept to a minimum. There have been variable reports of the accuracy of the Finapres under different clinical circumstances.[5]

Invasive measurement

Direct measurement of blood pressure using an arterial cannula allows a continuous, real-time arterial waveform to be obtained. It is potentially the most accurate method, and is indicated in the following circumstances:

- critically ill patients;
- where the cardiovascular system may be compromised or unstable;
- in patients who require physiological or pharmacological manipulation of blood pressure (e.g. cardiopulmonary bypass or hypotensive anaesthesia);
- as a convenient means for analysing blood gases.

The radial artery is usually cannulated, using a 20 G or 22 G cannula connected to the transducer system. Although the vessel might become partially thrombosed, the hand is protected by the arterial arcade supplied by both radial and ulnar arteries. Other arterial choices include the brachial artery and the dorsalis pedis artery.

A fluid-filled catheter connects the arterial cannula to the transducer and a means of processing and displaying the resulting electronic signal. The catheter must be reasonably stiff and straight. The fluid is assumed to be incompressible and must not contain any air bubbles.

The pressure transducer consists of a diaphragm separating the catheter connecting system from the electronic measuring system. The diaphragm usually contains four strain gauges, which transduce the mechanical movement of the diaphragm into an electrical signal. These are connected to a bridge circuit to minimise errors.

The accuracy of this system depends on its natural frequency being well above those of the waveform to be measured to avoid resonance, as well as providing optimal damping to the waveform displayed. The whole system must be properly calibrated, usually at manufacture, and then levelled and zeroed at the chosen reference level (usually the heart) by the user.

Cardiac filling pressures

Central venous pressure

Normal central venous pressure (CVP) when the patient is breathing spontaneously is just a few mmHg, and therefore accurate zeroing of the measurement system is important. A mean value is usually quoted because the pulsatile component is relatively small. A U-tube manometer often suffices. The CVP represents the filling pressure of the right side of the heart. Nevertheless, unless there is heart or lung disease a relationship is assumed to exist between right atrial pressure and left ventricular filling pressure. In general, CVP measurements are interpreted in the light of trends in values rather than the actual values themselves. Problems with CVP measurement occur when:

- the catheter is too short and therefore does not reach the thoracic cavity;
- the catheter is too long and therefore in the right ventricle, where it may also cause arrhythmias;
- the catheter is being used simultaneously to deliver fluids;
- there is compression of intrathoracic veins by IPPV, especially if positive end-expiratory pressure (PEEP) is applied, when vein compression gives falsely high readings.

Pulmonary artery and pulmonary capillary wedge pressure

When more precise knowledge of left ventricular filling pressure is needed, a pulmonary artery (PA) catheter may be used, introduced via either the internal jugular or the subclavian vein. The route via the internal jugular vein has the lowest incidence of misdirection.

Progress of the catheter tip through the right side of the heart to the PA is monitored by observation of the pressures being measured at the tip. Most pass into the right lower lobe artery. Measurements should be made in the lower zone of the lung for best accuracy.

A small balloon at the tip of the Swan–Ganz PA catheter allows it to be flow directed and wedged in a small PA. On wedging, flow in that artery is brought temporarily to a standstill, and so the manometer looks at the pulmonary vasculature towards the left atrium, a vascular system with a relatively low pressure drop from one end to the other. Thus the pressure then measured (pulmonary capillary wedge pressure, PCWP) can be considered to represent left atrial pressure or left ventricular filling pressure. Normal values during spontaneous ventilation are about 5–10 mmHg, and are higher during IPPV or if left ventricular function is poor.

The balloon should not be overinflated to avoid rupturing the PA. Once the measurement has been made, the balloon should be deflated so that the PA waveform is once again visible, if necessary withdrawing the catheter a little to achieve this. Failure to do so may result in ischaemia. If the patient is undergoing artificial ventilation the wedge pressure (PCWP) must be measured at end-expiration.

The PA catheter becomes a less accurate estimate of left ventricular filling pressure if:

- there is pulmonary vascular disease, such as pulmonary hypertension;
- there is mitral valve disease;
- the catheter is placed in the apical zone of a lung, especially during IPPV.

It is also possible to sample mixed venous blood from the PA to measure the mixed venous oxygen saturation. This gives useful information about oxygen usage by cells and is characteristically low in sepsis.

Complications of PA catheters

Many complications are associated with the use of PA catheters, including:

- arrhythmias (as with any intracardiac catheter);
- damage to the PA and lung tissue;
- infection and thromboembolism;
- obstruction of venous return during cardiopulmonary bypass;
- balloon rupture, knotting or migration of the catheter.

Cardiac output

Thermodilution

If a PA catheter has a thermistor at its tip it may also be used to measure cardiac output by thermodilution.

A bolus of cold dextrose is introduced into the circulation through a proximal hole in the catheter situated in the right atrium, mixes with the circulation, and the change in blood temperature is measured by the thermistor. The associated microprocessor plots a curve of blood temperature with respect to time, and the cardiac output is inversely proportional to the area under this curve. Room temperature fluid can be as accurate as iced infusate.

An average of three estimates is normally taken. A change of more than 15% suggests a real change of cardiac output.

A variant on this technique allows continuous cardiac output measurement by using a constant infusion instead of a bolus injection.

Errors in the method include variations in temperature of the PA blood and overestimation of a low cardiac output due to the increase in cardiac preload caused by the injectate bolus.

For many years the PA catheter was the gold standard for cardiac output measurement against which all other methods were compared. More recently, factors that have contributed to its lesser use include:

- possible damage to the right ventricular wall, PA wall or tricuspid or pulmonary valves;
- difficulty demonstrating significant improvement in outcome from life-threatening conditions such as septic shock after years of use of the PA catheter;
- the development of noninvasive methods of assessing cardiac output, in particular echocardiography.

Echocardiography

Doppler ultrasound measures the velocity of blood through the aorta, and multiplication by the aortic cross-sectional area gives blood flow or cardiac output. The technique can also be used to measure blood flow in vessels other than the aorta.

There are several approaches to using a Doppler probe to measure cardiac output. One route is to insert or swallow it into the oesophagus. It is also possible to use such a transducer situated on the tip of an endotracheal tube, thus allowing continuous intraoperative cardiac output monitoring. The noninvasive transthoracic or suprasternal approach is another route.

The ultrasonic waves from the end of the probe are produced by a piezoelectric crystal in the range 2.5–5.0 MHz. The same transducer alternately transmits the wave for 1 μs and detects the reflected waves for 250 μs. Cardiac output measured by Doppler can be as accurate as thermodilution[14] even when used intraoperatively in the presence of cardiac disease,[15] although the user must be appropriately trained

Echocardiography can also be used to look at cardiac structure and function (e.g. valvular area) or dysfunction, abnormal wall movement in ischaemic regions, end-diastolic and systolic volumes, ejection fraction, and the detection of thrombus, air embolus and aortic dissection. Bernoulli's theorem is used to calculate any pressure gradient across the aortic valve.

Transthoracic electrical bioimpedance

An electrical signal of 100 kHz frequency is applied across electrodes attached round the body at the upper and lower limits of the thorax. The output signal from the thorax is amplified and processed to give electrical impedance. Some change occurs with respiration, but the majority is associated with changes in blood distribution within the thorax. The method has a variance of more than 20%, which may explain why it is not in common use.

Pulse contour analysis

A newer technique for cardiac output measurement is the use of algorithms to analyse the pulse contour obtained from an arterial waveform.[7]

Electrocardiogram

The ECG is a noninvasive monitor of cardiac rate and rhythm and especially of unexpected cardiac events. It also monitors R–R interval variability, which is a useful index of autonomic activity.

The ECG is a surface reflection of the depolarising and repolarising electrical activity of various parts of the heart. It does not measure the heart's mechanical activity. In fact, normal electrical activity may occur when there is no cardiac output.

Excitation of the atria gives rise to the P wave, but an atrial recovery wave is rarely seen because it is obscured by ventricular excitation, which is signalled by the QRS wave. Recovery of the ventricles is preceded by the T wave.

For routine operating room monitoring three electrodes are placed on the chest, as near to the heart as convenient to increase the signal-to-noise ratio. Because about 75% of ischaemic ECG patterns are best detected in the V5 lead, the positive electrode should be placed in this position (CM5) if possible. Electrical interference from the mains can be minimised by ensuring good electrode contact, high-quality lead screening, and a high common mode rejection ratio in the associated differential amplifier. Electronic filtering can give a bandwidth of 0.5–40 Hz, which removes most interference and is usually adequate for operating room use.

Measurement of blood loss

Gravimetric method

The gravimetric method is the simplest and most commonly used method for measuring blood loss. Blood loss is estimated by measurement of the gain in weight of swabs, together with the measurement of the contents of suction bottles. It is assumed that 1 mL of blood weighs 1 g. The weight gain of swabs is said to underestimate blood loss by 25%. In operations involving complex exchanges of blood (e.g. extracorporeal circulation), it may be useful to weigh the whole patient before and after operation.

Colorimetric method

In the colorimetric method swabs and towels are mixed thoroughly with a large known volume of water, and the change in colour is estimated by infrared absorption. Errors may occur owing to incomplete extraction of blood or contamination with bile. The patient's haemoglobin must be known.

RESPIRATORY MONITORING

Respiratory gas analysis

Different gas analysers capitalise on different physicochemical properties of the gas or vapour.[8]

The response time of any analyser depends on the time taken for the gas to be sampled (delay time), and the time taken for the device to measure the gas concentration (response time).

The sampling flow rate is usually about 100–200 mL/min.[9]

Response time is often expressed as the time taken to produce a 90 or 95% response to a step or square wave input change. Zeroing and calibration of the analyser are important because they are all prone to drift in both zero and gain.

Breath-by-breath analysis of respiratory gases has a number of clinical uses.

Oxygen analysis at the common gas outlet of the anaesthetic machine identifies adequate oxygen delivery and oxygen supply failure. In the breathing system it fulfils the same role, which is particularly important in low-flow anaesthesia, and also gives data on oxygen consumption.

Volatile agent analysis confirms correct functioning of the vaporiser, and is particularly useful in low-flow anaesthesia.

Carbon dioxide analysis (capnography) has particularly important applications, including clinical decision-making in:

- confirming successful tracheal intubation, and avoiding unintentional oesophageal or endobronchial intubation;
- detection of breathing system or ventilator disconnection, or failure of other breathing system components, such as unidirectional valves or coaxial tubing;
- determining the adequacy of ventilation or the presence of rebreathing;
- detecting changes in the circulation, such as a fall in cardiac output, the presence of a pulmonary embolus, or other causes of ventilation–perfusion mismatch;
- the presence of metabolic changes, such as malignant hyperpyrexia or the respiratory response to metabolic acidosis;

- detecting bronchospasm;
- detecting the offset of neuromuscular blockers.

Oxygen

Paramagnetic oxygen analyser

In contrast to most other molecules, which are diamagnetic, oxygen and nitric oxide are attracted into a magnetic field and are paramagnetic. This enables oxygen concentration to be analysed breath by breath.

A paramagnetic oxygen analyser contains a pair of glass spheres filled with nitrogen, suspended between the poles of a magnet by a thread. Zeroing is carried out in the carrier gas destined to have oxygen added to it later.

When a gas mixture containing oxygen is drawn through the analyser, oxygen is attracted into the magnetic field, resulting in a measurable displacement of the nitrogen-filled spheres. The detection system can either be a deflection measurement or a null deflection type.

These devices are accurate to within 0.1% oxygen, but are adversely affected by pressurisation, vibration, water vapour and high flow rates. There is also a slow response time of up to 1 minute.

A modern development of the analyser contains an electromagnet, which produces an alternating magnetic field at a frequency of 110 Hz. A bifurcated gas sample tube passes through the field. A reference gas enters one arm of the sample tube, the gas for analysis enters the opposite arm. Vibrations in the gas molecules caused by the alternating magnetic field are detected and measured by a pressure transducer. The difference between them causes 2–5 Pa pressure oscillations, which are transduced into a sound signal, the amplitude of which is directly proportional to the oxygen concentration. Desflurane interferes with the accuracy of this type of analyser.

Polarographic electrodes and fuel cells

The Clarke polarographic electrode consists of a cellophane-covered platinum cathode and Ag/AgCl anode in a phosphate and KCl electrolyte, between which a potential difference of –0.6 V is applied by a battery. The gas sample is separated from the device by a membrane permeable to oxygen. At the cathode the following reaction takes place:

- $O_2 + 2H_2O + 4e^- \rightarrow 4OH^-$

At the anode the following reactions take place:

- $4Ag \rightarrow 4Ag^+ + 4e^-$;
- $4Ag^+ + 4Cl^- \rightarrow 4AgCl$.

The current generated is proportional to the Po_2 of the gas sample.

A fuel cell consists of a gold cathode and a lead anode. The same reaction occurs at the cathode as in the polarographic electrode and no polarising voltage is required.

For both devices the response time is comparatively slow, making them acceptable but less suitable for breath-by-breath analysis than other methods.

Carbon dioxide and volatile anaesthetic agents

Infrared absorption spectroscopy

The interatomic bonds between dissimilar atoms of polyatomic molecules such as nitrous oxide (N_2O), carbon dioxide (CO_2), water vapour and the volatile anaesthetic agents absorb infrared (IR) radiation, whereas oxygen, nitrogen and helium do not.

Different polyatomic species absorb maximally at characteristic wavelengths, making it possible to identify the gas molecule as well as quantify the gas concentration.

In a typical Luft analyser a source emits IR with wavelengths between 1 and 15 μm, and filters allow through IR to match the wavelength of maximum absorption of the gas under study. For example, the filters transmit a wavelength of 3.3 μm for halothane, isoflurane and enflurane, 4.3 μm for CO_2, and 4.5 μm for N_2O.

The light passes through to a reference chamber and a sample chamber. Transmitted (non-absorbed) light is passed to a pair of air-filled detector chambers, separated by a diaphragm. The diaphragm oscillates and produces a signal proportional to the gas concentration.

Although CO_2, N_2O and carbon monoxide (CO) absorb IR light maximally at 4.3, 4.5 and 4.7 μm, respectively, there is considerable overlap in their absorption spectra, which can result in error.

There is also the phenomenon of collision broadening, where the presence of one gas may broaden the IR absorption spectrum of another. Electronic correction factors in the analysers try to allow for this. For example, in a gas mixture containing 79% helium in oxygen, an IR analyser under-reads CO_2 values.[10] Desflurane, cyclopropane, acetone and alcohol all produce errors in IR spectroscopy.

Water is a strong absorber of IR across the bandwidths of interest and must be eliminated in the sampling process, which produces some inaccuracy.

Some analysers use the 10–13 μm bandwidth to detect volatile agents where there is less chance for interference between absorption spectra.

Infrared spectroscopy is a means for determining partial pressure, so error can be introduced if the pressure of the gas sample changes or if ambient pressure changes. If the gas sample pressure changes, the partial pressure of the gas being analysed will change, without there being a real change in the fractional concentration. Similarly, if the device is calibrated at sea level and subsequently used at altitude, there will be an error in calculating gas concentration.

The 90–95% response time of IR analysers to a step change is 150 ms.

Most devices either have a water trap or use sample tubing, which absorbs water vapour.

IR capnographs are accurate to about 0.1% in a range of CO_2 up to 10%.

A variant of the IR analyser described above uses a combination of IR and photo-acoustic spectroscopy. Oscillating pressure waves from the IR heated gas sample, separated into its components by a chopper wheel and filters, produce audible pressure waves detectable by microphone. The advantages of photo-acoustic IR spectroscopy over conventional IR spectroscopy include stability, zero drift, reduced need for calibration over prolonged periods and fast response time.

All gases

Mass spectrometry

Mass spectrometry identifies gas molecules by bombarding them with electrons and separating them in a magnetic field according to the ratio of mass and charge. The method can identify and quantify all molecular species. It is considered the gold standard of gas monitoring techniques.

The device consists of three stages:

- in the first, the gas sample is drawn into a very low-pressure chamber (about 1 mmHg);
- in the second, which is the main part of the device, the sample diffuses into an ionisation chamber with an even lower pressure (about 10^{-6} mmHg), where the gas molecules are bombarded with electrons and the resulting ions are accelerated into a dispersion chamber;
- in the third stage, the ions are deflected by a magnetic field, the separated beams of ions are detected, and the signal is processed and displayed.

The respiratory mass spectrometer is accurate and requires only 20 mL/min gas sampling rate, with a 100 ms response time. However, if the device itself is at some distance from the sampling site, significant delay time may be added to the response time. Water condensation can be avoided by heating the sampling tube.

Some molecules lose two electrons rather than one in the ionisation process, and therefore become doubly charged ions. They then behave within the magnetic field like an ion with half the mass, which can make interpretation difficult. Furthermore, ionisation can lead to fragmentation of a molecule, so that a mass spectrum appears at the output rather than a single peak.

This anomaly is useful to distinguish gas components with the same molecular weight, such as N_2O and CO_2 (44 Da), or N_2 and CO (28 Da). N_2O is fragmented into NO, O_2, N_2, N and O, and can be detected at the subordinate peak for NO (30 Da). CO_2 is fragmented into O_2, C_2, C and O, and can be detected at the peak for C (12 Da). Because the fragmentation is predictable, the amplitude of the subordinate peak can be used to measure gas concentration.

Raman spectroscopy

A small fraction of incident light reflected from the surface of a molecule, about 10^{-6}, is scattered with a loss of energy and a change of wavelength characteristic of the molecule off which the light is being reflected. This is Raman scattering.

To be useful in a clinical setting Raman spectroscopy requires powerful laser light sources and sensitive photocell detectors . A Raman spectroscope incorporates an argon laser source of wavelength 485 nm, high reflectance mirrors to concentrate the laser beam, a gas sampling chamber, appropriate optics, a detection system, and a microprocessor and display system. If plotted graphically, the amplitudes of the frequency shifted peaks are proportional to the gas concentrations.

In Raman spectroscopy each gas is analysed independently, including CO_2, N_2O, volatile agents, O_2, N_2 and water vapour. The response time is 100 ms. The sample is not altered by the process and can therefore be returned to the breathing system, an advantage in low-flow anaesthesia, although there is some overlap between gas species. However, the devices are power consumptive and noisy.

Respiratory gas volumes and flow rates

Wright's respirometer

Wright's respirometer allows expired gas to flow past some stationary vanes to ensure unidirectional flow, and past some moving vanes, calibrated in air, to measure expired volume and indicate its value by a pointer. Inertia and friction of the moving vane spindle can result in over-reading and under-reading at high and low flow rates, respectively. It is accurate to within 10%. Inaccuracy can occur in the presence of N_2O.

Fleisch pneumotachograph

The Fleisch pneumotachograph is a variable pressure drop, fixed-orifice flowmeter. It depends on a reasonably linear relationship between pressure and flow during laminar flow. Gas flow through the device is divided into a large number of parallel small-diameter tubes, thus ensuring laminar flow through each. Accuracy depends on the extent to which this has been achieved. The pressure difference between the inlet and outlet is measured and is directly related to flow. Variations use a mesh rather than tubes, which does not result in laminar flow but is adequate for clinical use. The flow signal is integrated to give volume. Further software uses airway pressure measurement and the volume calculation to draw a pressure–volume loop for each breath.

Hot wire anemometry

If a heated wire is placed in a gas stream, the degree of its cooling by the gas flow depends on gas temperature, specific heat and flow rate.

Ultrasonic flow transducer

The ultrasonic flow transducer is based on ultrasonic detection of vortex formation behind a partial obstruction to gas flow. It is not affected by temperature or gas composition, but may only detect vortices above a critical flow rate.

Respiratory inductance plethysmography

A pair of electrical inductance coils are wrapped around the chest and abdomen. Respiration and change in chest volume alters the inductance between them, a change which is therefore related to tidal volume.

Positive displacement flowmeter

The positive displacement flowmeter consists of a pair of low-friction cogwheels within the gas volume measurement tube. The gas flow rotates the cogwheels and a small metal button on one of them acts as a magnetic revolution counter.

Blood gas analysis

A heparinised blood sample, 100–300 μL, is passed through four electrodes simultaneously. Partial pressure of blood O_2 is measured using a Clarke electrode, CO_2 using a Severinghaus electrode and pH with a conventional glass electrode. The fourth electrode is a reference electrode.

A blood gas analyser frequently measures haemoglobin concentration and biochemical parameters,[11] as well as deriving such values as O_2 saturation and content, bicarbonate, base excess and total CO_2. The sample is usually from an artery, but might also be capillary, or taken from a PA catheter as a mixed venous sample. Intravascular, microminiaturised versions of these devices are being developed.

Clarke polarographic electrode

The Clarke polarographic electrode for measuring Po_2 has been described in the section on gas analysers (see p. 112). It is suitable for both gas and blood analysis. The membrane covering the electrode is designed to allow only oxygen to cross it, rather than blood.

pH electrode

The pH electrode consists of two half electrochemical cells. One half consists of an Ag/AgCl electrode and the other of a Hg/$HgCl_2$ (calomel) electrode, each maintaining a fixed potential. The Ag/AgCl electrode is immersed in a buffer solution of known pH, surrounded by pH-sensitive glass. Outside the glass membrane is the blood sample. The potential difference across the glass, between these two solutions, is variable. The blood sample is separated from the calomel electrode by a porous plug and a potassium chloride salt bridge to minimise diffusion. The potential difference across the system is about 60 mV per unit of pH change at 37°C. The electrode is calibrated against standard buffer solutions of pH 6.841 and 7.383.

PCO₂ (Severinghaus) electrode

The $P\text{CO}_2$ (Severinghaus) electrode is similar to a pH electrode. The H^+-sensitive glass membrane is itself covered with a membrane, which is selectively permeable to CO_2. There is a dynamic equilibrium between H^+ and CO_2, described by the Henderson–Hasselbalch equation:

$$\text{pH} = \text{p}K_a + \log_{10} \frac{[HCO_3^-]}{\alpha \,.\, P\text{CO}_2}$$

This electrode therefore allows a change in $P\text{CO}_2$ to generate a change in pH, which is measured by the electrode.

Temperature and blood gas analysis

Analysers measure blood gas variables at 37°C. Hypothermia itself does not alter blood gas values at 37°C, and arterial blood taken at lower temperatures should be corrected by the analyser software to 37°C before clinical decisions are made on the results.

Transcutaneous blood gas analysers

Modified electrodes can be used to measure $P\text{O}_2$ and $P\text{CO}_2$ transcutaneously. A common O_2 and CO_2 permeable membrane and electrolyte solution is used, ensuring a common pH for both measurements. Measured values are not particularly accurate, but trends are clinically useful, especially in babies.

OTHER MONITORING

Neuromuscular junction monitoring

A supramaximal electrical stimulus of between 10 and 50 mA is applied to an accessible peripheral motor nerve (e.g. ulnar or facial nerve) and the response of the appropriate muscle group is assessed. The stimulus may be delivered as a single stimulus, a train-of-four stimuli at 2 Hz, a tetanic stimulus at 50 Hz, or a double burst stimulation, which is two 40 ms tetanic bursts 750 ms apart. The stimulus has a square waveform of width 0.2 ms. The nerve stimulator should have a constant current output.

Assessment of the responding muscle group is usually visual (e.g. levator palpebrae superioris in the case of the facial nerve, or adductor pollicis longus with the ulnar nerve).

Electromyographic assessment is now more commonly available.

Electroencephalography

Electroencephalography (EEG) is a surface recording of cortical neuronal activity and is made up of frequencies up to around 40 Hz, often described as δ (<4 Hz), θ (4–7 Hz), α (8–13 Hz) and β (13–40 Hz).

α Activity occurs during relaxation with the eyes closed. Mental activity or eye opening results in a higher-frequency, lower-amplitude waveform. The normal EEG amplitude is 10–50 μV, with the range 1–100 μV. Anaesthetics affect the EEG, as do other factors such as blood pressure, $P\text{O}_2$, $P\text{CO}_2$, temperature and stimulation.

The raw EEG signal can be analysed with respect to time or frequency. Frequency analysis by Fourier transform yields a frequency spectrum and the power within each frequency band. It is quantified by indices such as the median power frequency and spectral edge frequency. These have been studied during single drug anaesthesia and correlate well with drug levels and clinical effect.

One commercial device examines the bispectral index (BIS), which includes consideration of the phase relationships of the different component waves of the EEG. The device uses three frontotemporal electrodes and calculates a dimensionless number between 0 (deeply unconscious) and 100 (wide awake), which is meant to be drug independent.[12] A value of 40–60 correlates with surgical anaesthesia, and a value of 60–85 with sedation.

Instead of monitoring the spontaneous EEG, it is possible to input a sensory stimulus to the patient and monitor the evoked potential. The stimulus can be visual, auditory or somatosensory, and is repeated to allow temporal summation of the evoked potentials. The early cortical waves, Pa and Nb, occurring 10–50 ms after an auditory stimulus, seem to be most suitable when attempting to monitor depth of anaesthesia.[13] Increasing depth lowers their amplitude and increases their latency.

Temperature

Formerly temperature was measured using a glass thermometer containing either mercury or alcohol. A thermistor is a semiconductor device whose electrical resistance changes with temperature, and is the basis of the nasopharyngeal temperature probe.

A thermocouple generates a potential difference between the two junctions formed at the connections of two dissimilar metals, proportional to the difference in temperature between them. This is the Seebeck effect.

The infrared tympanic thermometer consists of a thermopile, a series of thermocouples that detect the infrared radiation from the tympanic membrane. The thermopile generates a potential difference proportional to tympanic membrane temperature.

Liquid crystal displays may be made of materials that change colour with temperature. They exhibit hysteresis and are sensitive to draughts.

References

1. Birks RS (chairman) Recommendations for standards of monitoring during anaesthesia and recovery – 3. Association of Anaesthetists. 2000.

2. Webb RK, van der Walt J, RuncimanWB, et al. Which monitor? The first 2000 AIMS reports. Anaesth Intens Care 1993; 21:529–542.
3. ISO standard 9703-3; Anaesthesia and respiratory care alarm signals part 3 – guidance on application of alarms. Geneva, 1998.
4. Nazir T, Beatty PCW. Anaesthetists' attitudes to monitoring instrument design options. Br J Anaesth 2000; 85:781–784.
5. Dorlas JC, Nijboer JA, Butijn WT, et al. Effects of peripheral vasoconstriction on the blood pressure in the finger, measured continuously by a new noninvasive method (the Finapres). Anesthesiology 1985; 62:342.
6. Farquhar IK. Continuous direct and indirect blood pressure measurement (Finapres) in the critically ill. Anaesthesia 1991; 46:1050–1055.
7. Wiseley NA, Cook LB. Arterial flow waveforms from pulse oximetry compared with Doppler flow waveforms. Anaesthesia 2001; 56:556–561.
8. Davey A, Diba A. Physiological monitoring of gases. In: Magee PT, ed. Ward's anaesthetic equipment. 5th edn. London: Elsevier; 2004. In press.
9. Chan KL, Chan MTV, Gin T. Mainstream vs sidestream capnometry for prediction of $P\text{aCO}_2$ during supine craniotomy. Anaesthesia 2003; 58:149–155.
10. Ball JAS, Grounds RM. Calibration of three capnographs for use with helium and oxygen mixtures. Anaesthesia 2003; 58:156–160.
11. King R, Campbell A. Performance of the Radiometer OSM 3 and ABL 505 blood gas analysers for the determination of Na, K, and Hb concentrations. Anaesthesia 2000; 55:65–69.
12. Johansen JW, Sebel PS. Development and clinical application of the electroencephalographic bispectrum monitoring. Anesthesiology 2000; 93:1336–1344.
13. Tooley MA, Stapleton CL Greenslade GL, Prys-Roberts C. The auditory evoked response during propofol and alfentanil anaesthesia. Br J Anaesth 2004; 92:25–32.
14. Lefrant JY, delaCoussaye JE, Aya G el al. Cardiac output measurement: comparison of esophageal Doppler vs. thermodilution. Br J Anaesth 1993; 70, suppl 1:9.
15. Ryan T, Page R, Boucher Hayes D et al. Transoesophageal pulsed Doppler wave measurement of cardiac output during major vascular surgery: comparison with thermodilution technique. Br J Anaesth 1992; 69:101–104.

CHAPTER **2.3**

ADMINISTRATION OF VOLATILE ANAESTHETICS AND GASES

HISTORY

Nitrous oxide (N_2O) was first prepared by Priestley (1733–1804) in 1772. In 1799 Sir Humphrey Davy inhaled N_2O and noted strange effects that included euphoria mixed with uncontrollable laughter and sobbing, finally leading to loss of consciousness. He called it 'laughing gas'. This was the year in which 'anaesthesia' was born, although the term did not enter common usage until the 1840s. In 1844, Horace Wells, a dentist in Connecticut, had one of his teeth extracted painlessly by Dr John Riggs and the great value of 'laughing gas ' in surgery was thus established.

In 1846, just 2 years after Wells' success with N_2O, William Morton constructed the first anaesthetic machine for the delivery of ether, and on 16 October that year, Morton demonstrated ether anaesthesia at Massachusetts General Hospital in Boston for the surgical removal of a lump from under the jaw of a patient named Gilbert Abbott. So although the anaesthetic properties of both N_2O and ether were discovered in England, the Americans first realised the practical use of both substances in clinical medicine. Word spread, and before the end of 1846, ether was demonstrated in both Scotland and London on the same day – 19 December.

Dr James Simpson, a well-known Edinburgh gynaecologist, was the first to use ether in obstetric practice, but he found it unsatisfactory, not only because it was irritant to his eyes as well as being flammable, but also because it appeared clinically unstable. He looked for other agents, and considered chloroform to be superior to both N_2O and ether. Simpson demonstrated chloroform in 1847, but although easier to use than ether, it soon exhibited complications, including unexpected death in anxious patients. Despite its drawbacks, it became widely used after 1853, when Queen Victoria was given chloroform for the birth of her eighth child, Prince Leopold, leading to its nickname of 'anaesthesia à la Reine'.

During the course of the 20th century, inhalational anaesthetic agents were constantly developed to enhance their safety and ease of use. Ethyl chloride was introduced for induction of anaesthesia in the 1920s, followed by trichloroethylene and cyclopropane in the 1930s. Other innovations of the period included the development of routine endotracheal intubation by

Magill and Rowbottom, as well as intravenous induction of anaesthesia using barbiturates. The introduction of halothane (1956), methoxyflurane (1960), enflurane (1973), isoflurane (1980), sevoflurane (1990) and finally desflurane (1994) has brought inhalational anaesthesia to its present stage of development.

At the time of writing there are no new agents planned, and although inhalational agents remain at the centre of general anaesthesia worldwide, total intravenous techniques are slowly displacing them, at least in westernised countries.

GENERAL PRINCIPLES OF INHALATIONAL ANAESTHESIA

Uptake of anaesthetic gases and vapours

The uptake and distribution of an inhaled anaesthetic from the inspired gas through the body to a site of action is principally determined in any individual by the physicochemical properties of the agent.[1,2] Ultimately, general anaesthesia is the result of a rise in the partial pressure of the agent in the central nervous system (CNS). Provided the partial pressure of the agent is higher in the alveoli than it is in the brain, the flux of the agent will be down a pressure gradient in that direction. If the partial pressure in the alveoli is reduced below that in the brain, the flux is reversed. To study this flux, three areas require consideration:

- partial pressure of the agent in the alveoli;
- partial pressure of the agent in the circulation;
- partial pressure of the agent in the brain and other organs.

Partial pressure of anaesthetic agent in the alveoli

Concentration of the agent in the inspired gas

According to Dalton's Law of Partial Pressures, the concentration by volume of the agent in inspired gas determines its partial pressure. The concentration and partial pressure of the agent in the alveoli are slightly less than in the inspired fresh gas because:

- of dilution by carbon dioxide (CO_2) and nitrogen;
- the agent is removed into the pulmonary capillary circulation.

Increasing the inspired concentration will speed induction of anaesthesia provided that it does not cause breath-holding or laryngeal spasm.

If the inspired concentration requirement of the agent is high, such as with N_2O, rapid uptake into the blood allows more fresh gas to enter the lungs. This shortens the time of induction and is called the concentration effect. The alveolar partial pressure of any accompanying volatile agent also rises more quickly – the second gas effect – and induction with a volatile agent is therefore more rapid in the presence of N_2O.

Alveolar ventilation

The alveolar concentration of anaesthetic agent will rise more quickly if alveolar ventilation is increased, and more slowly if it is reduced by respiratory depression or airway obstruction.

Partial pressure of anaesthetic agent in the circulation

Blood/gas partition coefficient

The blood/gas partition coefficient is the ratio of the concentration of agent in blood to that in gas at equilibrium.

A high value indicates high solubility in blood, and that the partial pressure of the agent in blood will therefore rise slowly owing to the agent being continuously dissolved. In consequence, the alveolar partial pressure will also rise slowly because the agent continues to be absorbed and dissolved.

Correspondingly, the alveolar concentration of a poorly soluble agent will rise towards the inspired value more rapidly, and also decay more rapidly when withdrawn at the end of surgery.

In summary, agents with low blood/gas partition coefficients are characterised by alveolar, arterial, and hence brain partial pressures that respond rapidly to changes in the inspired vapour concentration and vice versa.

Cardiac output or pulmonary blood flow

An increased cardiac output removes agent from the lungs more quickly, thus reducing the alveolar partial pressure. This delays induction of anaesthesia. This effect is compounded where more soluble agents are concerned. Correspondingly, a low cardiac output will decrease induction time (within the limitations of the increased lung/brain circulation time) although this may be offset by the longer lung/brain circulation time.

Ventilation–perfusion relationships

Where pulmonary ventilation and perfusion are within normal limits, there is no barrier to the diffusion of anaesthetic agents from alveolar gas into pulmonary capillary blood. The agents are then distributed in the arterial circulation. Areas of ventilation–perfusion mismatch and certain lung diseases, such as pulmonary fibrosis and emphysema, delay the uptake of anaesthetic agents from the alveoli into the circulation and slow the induction of anaesthesia.

Partial pressure of anaesthetic agent in the brain and other tissues

Cerebral blood flow

Although the brain comprises only 2% of the body weight, it receives 14% of the cardiac output. Depth of anaesthesia depends on the partial pressure of agent in the brain and rises more quickly with increased cerebral blood flow (CBF). In health the CBF is maintained until the mean blood pressure has fallen to 40–50 mmHg. However, CBF then assumes a greater proportion of the cardiac output, and equilibration of the partial pressures of agent in the blood and brain is reached more quickly. A similar situation occurs with intravenous anaesthetics.

Oil/gas partition coefficient

The oil/gas partition coefficient is the ratio of the concentration of agent in fat to that in gas and is a measurement of fat solubility, and therefore solubility in the fat-rich tissues of the CNS. This equates with the potency of individual agents. There is a direct relationship between the minimum alveolar concentration (MAC) value of inhaled anaesthetic agents and lipid solubility in terms of the oil/gas partition coefficient according to the Meyer–Overton theory (1899) (Fig. 2.3.1).

Relative blood supply to different tissues.

Under basal conditions 75% of the cardiac output goes to the brain, heart, liver, kidneys and endocrine glands – the so-called vessel-rich group of organs, although collectively these account for only 7% of the body weight.

Muscle and skin receive less than 20% of the cardiac output and constitute an intermediate group.

The vessel-poor group of tissues – fat, bone, ligament and cartilage – comprise 25% of the body weight, but receive only a small blood flow. However, fat has a great affinity for anaesthetic vapours because of their

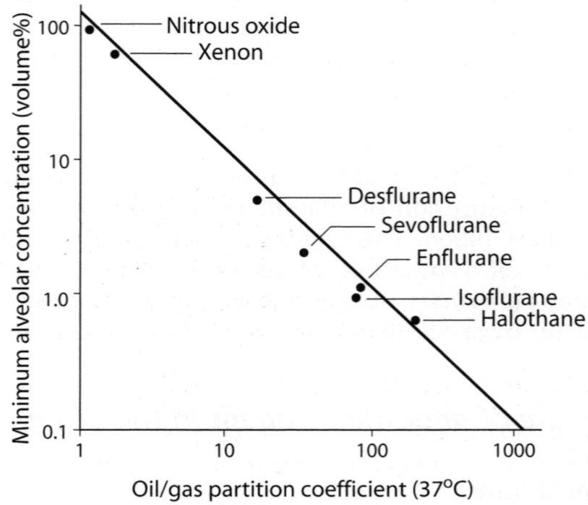

Figure 2.3.1 The Meyer–Overton theory was proposed independently by Hans Horst Meyer and Charles Overton in 1899. The oil/gas partition coefficient as a measurement of lipid solubility is related to anaesthetic potency when both are plotted logarithmically.

high oil/gas partition coefficients. This slows induction and recovery from anaesthesia in obese patients.

In general, the speed of equilibration of an anaesthetic agent between the alveolar concentration and any tissue of the body depends upon a rich blood supply combined with a low agent solubility in that tissue. The time constant for N_2O in brain tissue is just over 1 minute, but is 100 minutes in fat. For halothane the respective figures are 3.3 and 2720 minutes.

Minimum alveolar concentration

The potency of anaesthetic vapours may be compared by determining the MAC of an anaesthetic agent, which produces a lack of reflex movement in 50% of non-paralysed subjects when skin is incised.

Alveolar partial pressure rather than inspired concentration is the important factor because alveolar vapour concentration alters with changes in total barometric pressure at different altitudes, whereas minimum alveolar partial pressure (MAP) remains constant. Therefore MAC values are quoted under steady state conditions at 1 atmosphere pressure.

MAC has limited usefulness and the median anaesthetic dose to obtund reflex movement in 95% of subjects (AD_{95}) is more useful. The AD_{95} is about 1.5 times the MAC value.

When more than one agent is used their separate MAC fractions may be simply added together to estimate the total effect on the patient.

Other drugs that depress the CNS, such as opioids, sedatives and alcohol, reduce MAC values. MAC values are also reduced by hypothermia, hypoxaemia, hypotension and old age.

MAC values are higher in children, in states of excessive anxiety, hyperthermia, hyperthyroidism and in chronic ingestion of alcohol.

Two other derivatives of MAC are sometimes quoted:

- MAC-BAR refers to the blockade of the adrenergic response causing a rise in heart rate and blood pressure in 50% of subjects due to surgical stimulus;
- MAC-awake refers to the value at which 50% of subjects fail to respond to command during inhalational induction, and may be related to the value required to prevent awareness.

Clinical signs of anaesthesia

Classic stages of anaesthesia are rarely seen now with the routine use of intravenous induction agents and inhalational agents with low blood/gas partition coefficients.

In 1937, Guedel described a series of physical signs describing the onset of anaesthesia and its subsequent depth.[3] This was based on observations made on unpremedicated patients inhaling diethyl ether causing prolonged induction. The signs were classified into stages of progressive depth (Box 2.3.1).

Box 2.3.1
Stages of anaesthesia
Stage 1 – Analgesia
Normal reflexes maintained until loss of consciousness
Abolition of the eyelash reflex
Stage 2 – Excitement
Excitement
Breathing is irregular
Struggling and resisting
Regurgitation, coughing and laryngeal spasm
Pupillary dilatation
Stage 3 – Surgical anaesthesia
Plane I
Eyes centrally placed, loss of conjunctival reflex
Swallowing, vomiting depressed
Pupils normal or small
Increased lacrimation
Plane II
Beginning of intercostal muscle paralysis
Regular deep breathing
Loss of corneal reflexes
Pupillary dilatation
Further increase in lacrimation
Plane III
Complete intercostal muscle paralysis
Shallow breathing
Depression of laryngeal reflexes
Depression of lacrimation
Plane IV
Complete diaphragmatic paralysis
Depression of carinal reflexes
Stage 4 – Overdose
Apnoea
Pupils maximally dilated

Excitement is still seen in very light planes of anaesthesia, and ocular movements occur in light anaesthesia as does lacrimation. Autonomic responses can still occur in the presence of full muscular relaxation, and neuroendocrine responses occur in response to surgery or trauma.

General anaesthesia has three basic components:

- narcosis;
- analgesia (and associated suppression of reflexes and the neuroendocrine stress response);
- muscle relaxation.

With appropriate selection of drugs, these three components can be varied individually.

Properties of an ideal inhalational anaesthetic agent

The desirable properties for an ideal inhalational anaesthetic agent would include the following:

- a stable molecule, not broken down by light or soda lime, not requiring preservatives, and with a long shelf-life;
- non-flammable in air, O_2 or N_2O;
- potent enough to allow use with high concentrations of O_2;
- saturated vapour pressure (SVP) high enough to allow easy vaporisation, but not so high as to boil at room temperature;
- low solubility in blood to allow rapid induction and recovery, and rapid response to changes in inhaled concentration;
- pleasant and non-irritating to inhale;
- devoid of organ-specific toxicity;
- lack of toxic effect when inhaled in low doses by theatre staff;
- should not undergo metabolism in the body;
- minimal cardiovascular and respiratory side-effects;
- should provide some analgesia;
- no stimulant effects on the nervous system;
- no sensitisation of the heart to catecholamines;
- no interactions with other drugs;
- cheap to manufacture.

Environmental effects

There has been interest in the possible effects of gaseous and volatile anaesthetic agents on the environment. Chlorine-containing molecules are probably more destructive than those with fluorine.[4] Anaesthesia contributes at most 0.01% to the total atmospheric burden of chlorine-containing compounds and will have a negligible impact on global warming.[4]

PHARMACOLOGY OF INHALATIONAL AGENTS

The pharmacology of some of the more modern inhalational anaesthetic agents is reviewed here, together with diethyl ether, which is regarded as of historical importance (Table 2.3.1).

Nitrous oxide

Although the use of N_2O quickly became overshadowed by ether in the 1840s, Gardner Quincy Colton revived its use in dentistry in 1863. It was introduced into dental practice in London in 1868 by TW Evans, initially supplied compressed into cylinders, and then available 2 years later as liquefied N_2O in cylinders.

Nitrous oxide is a weak anaesthetic agent, with a MAC value between 100 and 105%. It is a potent analgesic. Unplanned awareness may occur if it is used as the sole anaesthetic.

Tolerance to the analgesic effects has been demonstrated in volunteers, which can develop in 2 hours, and may make awareness more likely.

Nitrous oxide may cause the release of endorphins in the CNS. There is evidence of reversal of its analgesia by naloxone. N_2O 25% has compared favourably with morphine for relief of postoperative pain despite having little general effect on consciousness. Psychomotor performance is not affected at concentrations below 8%.

Nitrous oxide is a very useful agent that has been in use for over 150 years, although its undesirable properties may now outweigh its benefits (see below).

Manufacture

Although colloquially referred to as a gas, N_2O is actually a vapour at room temperature, made by heating a solid or aqueous solution of 83% ammonium nitrate to 240°C:

- $NH_4NO_3 \rightarrow 2H_2O + N_2O$

At higher temperatures the percentage of impurity increases. The issuing vapour is collected, purified and compressed into liquid in metal cylinders at 5200 kPa. The cylinders are painted blue in the UK and USA and under the International Standard System for colour coding of medical gas cylinders (ISO:32, 1977). Common sizes are C (450 L), D (900 L) and E (1800 L), the volumes being measured at room temperature and pressure.

Nitric oxide (NO) and nitrogen dioxide (NO_2) are produced as impurities so the gases evolved must be washed with water and caustic soda in turn, before being passed through activated alumina to remove water vapour. At various stages, monitors are used to detect the presence of higher oxides of nitrogen.

Metabolism	Molecular weight	Boiling point (°C)	SVP (kPa) @ 20°C	Specific gravity @ 20°C	Oil/gas partition coefficient	Blood/gas partition coefficient	MAC (%) (in adults)	Metabolism (%)
Nitrous oxide (N_2O)	44.01	–88.5	5200	1.2	1.4	0.47	104	0
Halothane ($CF_3.CHClBr$)	197	50	32	1.87	220	2.3	0.75	20
Enflurane ($CHF_2–O–CF_2.CHFCl$)	184.5	56.5	24	1.52	98.5	1.9	1.68	3
Isoflurane ($CHF_2–O–CHCl.CF_3$)	184	48.5	33	1.50	98.5	1.4	1.15	0.2
Sevoflurane ($CFH_2–O–CH(CF_3)CF_3$)	200	58.5	21	1.52	53.0	0.69	2.0	3
Desflurane ($CF_2H–O–CHF.CF_3$)	168	23.5	88	–	19.0	0.42	6.0	0.2
Diethyl ether ($CH_3CH_2–O–CH_2CH_3$)	74	36.5	55	–	–	12	1.92	10–15

Table 2.3.1 Physical properties of some inhalation anaesthetic agents

The effects of contamination with NO has recently been reviewed and may be beneficial to the oxygenation of arterial blood.[5,6] As a further check, regular random sampling of cylinders is carried out.

The amount of N_2O present in the cylinder can only be ascertained by weighing to calculate the mass of the contents, which are in liquid form. The SVP above the liquid phase only varies with temperature.

Using Avogadro's hypothesis – that one mole of a gas occupies 22.4 L at standard temperature and pressure (STP) – and knowing the molecular weight of N_2O (44.01 Da), the volume of emerging gas at STP can easily be calculated. In fact, some fall in pressure may occur due to a fall in temperature as the liquid N_2O evaporates, removing the latent heat of vaporisation from the liquid.

Up to four-fifths of the contents of a full cylinder is in the liquid state, so when in use the valves of the cylinder must be elevated above the horizontal.

Just before exhaustion of the cylinder, when all the liquid is vaporised, the pressure quickly drops to zero.

Cylinders are filled to a filling ratio (ratio of the mass of N_2O in the cylinder to the mass of water required to completely fill it) of 0.75 in temperate and 0.67 in tropical climates. The weight of the cylinder, full and empty (tare weight), is stamped on the side.

Physical properties

Nitrous oxide is a sweet-smelling, non-irritating, colourless gas with a boiling point of –88.5°C, molecular weight 44.01 Da, critical pressure 72.5 bar, critical temperature 36.5°C, blood/gas partition coefficient 0.47 and oil/gas partition coefficient 1.4.

The vapour pressure of N_2O at 15°C is 44 bar and 52 bar at room temperature. The vapour density at 15°C is 1.875 g/L (1.5 times that of air).

The velocity of sound in N_2O is 262 m/s (compared with 317 m/s for O_2) and a suitable whistle can be used to differentiate the two gases. Change from O_2 to N_2O causes the pitch to fall $1\frac{1}{2}$ tones.

Nitrous oxide is neither flammable nor explosive, but supports the combustion of other agents even in the absence of oxygen, if a high temperature (above 450°C) is supplied to initiate decomposition into nitrogen and oxygen.

Nitrous oxide is eliminated unchanged from the body, mostly via the lungs, but partly through the skin. It is unaffected by soda lime.

Impurities in nitrous oxide

Two cases of poisoning in the UK were reported in detail by Clutton-Brock,[7] in which there was contamination with NO and NO_2. Both are toxic, and one patient died. There was methaemoglobinaemia and cardiorespiratory failure. Higher oxides of nitrogen can cause respiratory distress above 100 ppm, but clinical features may be delayed for several hours.

A crude test for contamination is to put a piece of moistened starch iodide paper into a large syringe and then fill this with the suspected N_2O mixed with 25% O_2. If the gas is contaminated by over 300 parts per million, the starch iodide will turn blue after 10 minutes.

Undesirable effects of nitrous oxide

Nitrous oxide is an extremely safe nontoxic anaesthetic agent, provided it is administered with a sufficient concentration of O_2. Undesirable effects may, however, sometimes occur, as discussed below.

Diffusion into gas-containing spaces

There is a 35-fold difference in the blood/gas partition coefficients of N_2O (0.47) and nitrogen, (0.013), so for every molecule of nitrogen removed from gas-containing spaces, 35 molecules of N_2O will enter. The diffusion of N_2O between blood, tissue and gas is more rapid than that of nitrogen. This causes an increase in the volume of the gas space if the space can expand (pneumothorax, gut, air embolus) and an increase in pressure if the space cannot expand (sinuses, middle ear, pneumoencephalocoele).

In surgery for retinal detachment where sulphur hexafluoride is used, N_2O diffusion can cause a rise in intraocular pressure. N_2O should be discontinued up to 15 minutes before the bubble is injected. The changes in middle ear pressure may cause postoperative hearing loss, and problems in otological surgery (e.g. myringoplasty) when tympanic grafts are used. It may be preferable to avoid N_2O in these cases.

Interaction with vitamin B_{12}

Nitrous oxide inactivates the cobalt in vitamin B_{12} and so irreversibly inactivates the enzyme methionine synthetase. This has recently been reviewed. The time course of this interaction is much slower in humans than in rodents, in which it has been most extensively studied. A period of at least 8 hours of N_2O anaesthesia is needed to demonstrate a significant fall in plasma methionine concentrations which interferes with the metabolism of folate and the synthesis of DNA and proteins. Megaloblastic anaemia and peripheral neuropathy have been reported after exposure of patients to N_2O for periods of from 6 to 12 hours. Pretreatment with folinic acid prevents these megaloblastic changes.

In 1956 HCA Lassen, a Copenhagen physician, reported that very prolonged N_2O and O_2 anaesthesia, as in the treatment of poliomyelitis or tetanus, could cause bone marrow aplasia.

Prolonged occupational exposure to N_2O may result in subacute combined degeneration of the cord.[9] This emphasises the need to avoid pollution in the operating room.

Teratogenicity

Although teratogenic changes have been observed in pregnant rats exposed to N_2O for prolonged periods, there is no evidence of harm to the fetus in humans.

Cardiorespiratory effects

Nitrous oxide causes a small reduction in myocardial contractility, but this is more than compensated for by an increase in catecholamine release, and is more marked under hyperbaric conditions.

Nitrous oxide is non-irritant to the airway, and causes a small reduction in minute volume.

Diffusional hypoxia

Immediately following N_2O anaesthesia hypoxaemia may occur because N_2O diffuses into alveolar gas faster than nitrogen (from inspired room air) can diffuse into the blood, causing a reduction in alveolar O_2 tension. This may be prevented by giving 100% O_2 for a few minutes at the end of anaesthesia, and continuing administration of O_2 in the recovery room.

Postoperative nausea and vomiting

Postoperative nausea and vomiting is more likely with N_2O than when it is not used, possibly associated with its diffusion into the middle ear. Eexpansion of the gut and effects on opioid receptors have also been implicated

Advantages of nitrous oxide in anaesthesia

Advantages of nitrous oxide in anaesthesia include its potent analgesic and non-irritant properties, its low solubility in blood, and additive effects, allowing lower doses of volatile agents. Nitrous oxide also speeds induction with volatile agents owing to the second gas effect (see above)

Nitrous oxide is useful to supplement continuous or intermittent intravenous anaesthesia to reduce the chances of awareness. When using a mainly inhalational technique, it is common practice to prevent awareness by adding a volatile agent to a mixture of O_2 and N_2O.

Premixed nitrous oxide/oxygen

Certain mixtures of N_2O and O_2 will remain in the gaseous phase at pressures and temperatures at which N_2O by itself would normally be a liquid (Poynting effect).

Entonox

Entonox is the trade name for a 50:50 mixture of gaseous N_2O and O_2. The cylinder shoulder is painted white and blue in quarters and the body is blue under ISO 32 classification.

If cylinders are exposed to temperatures of less than −7°C, the N_2O component can separate as a liquid (lamination) and may lead to delivery of uneven mixtures, too much O_2 at the beginning and too much N_2O at the end of the cylinder life. Danger of lamination can be avoided by immersing the cylinder in water at 52°C and inverting it three times, or by keeping it above a temperature of 10°C for 2 hours before use.

Uses of Entonox include obstetric analgesia and analgesia for dressing wounds, chest physiotherapy, removal of chest drains, coronary infarction and dental surgery. It is often carried by ambulances. The English National Board for Midwifery permits its use by midwives on their own responsibility.

Entonox may be supplied by pipeline from large cylinders via a manifold, and is usually delivered to patients through a demand valve.

Isoflurane

Isoflurane (1-chloro-2,2,2-trifluoroethyl difluoromethyl ether) was synthesised by Ross Terrell in 1965, who had synthesised its isomer, enflurane, in 1963. However, due to a misleading study, which showed hepatic carcinogenicity in mice, it was not introduced into clinical practice until 1980.

Physical properties

Isoflurane is a colourless volatile liquid with a pungent vapour. Its molecular weight is 184.5 and its boiling point is 49°C. Its SVP is 33 kPa at 20°C which is similar to that of halothane, and it could theoretically be used in the same vaporiser as halothane, although this is not recommended.

Induction and recovery are rapid, partly because of the low blood/gas partition coefficient of 1.4, but also because of a fairly low fat solubility. The oil/gas partition coefficient is 98.5.

The MAC in O_2 ranges from 1.68% in children to 1.05% in patients over 60 years of age. The MAC falls to 0.66 in 70% N_2O.

Isoflurane is stable and no preservatives are necessary to prevent its decomposition. It does not react with metal in breathing systems, but can react with dry soda lime to produce carbon monoxide.

Pharmacodynamics

Cardiovascular system

Isoflurane is a direct myocardial depressant, but less so than either halothane or enflurane. Isoflurane lowers arterial blood pressure less than halothane or enflurane, principally as a result of reduced systemic vascular resistance. The cardiac rhythm is stable, and the myocardium is not sensitised to catecholamines. Tachycardia is common, especially in young patients.

Isoflurane is a powerful coronary vasodilator at normal concentrations. Therefore coronary steal may occur in patients with some types of coronary artery disease, where the healthy myocardium receives increased blood flow at the expense of myocardium supplied by the stenosed vessels. On the other hand, isoflurane with N_2O has improved the tolerance to pacing-induced myocardial ischaemia in patients with coronary artery disease. Animal work on this subject has yielded conflicting results.

Respiration

Isoflurane decreases tidal volume and increases respiratory rate. Isoflurane depresses respiration more than halothane but less than enflurane. It blunts the ventilatory response to hypercapnia, being 30% of the awake value at 1 MAC and 14% at 1.5 MAC. The ventilatory response to hypoxia is abolished at just 0.1 MAC (as with all volatile agents).

The incidence of coughing and laryngeal spasm during induction with isoflurane is greater than with halothane because the vapour is irritant, which limits its value for gaseous induction. Bronchodilatation and a reduction in hypoxic pulmonary vasoconstriction both occur.

Nervous system

Low concentrations up to 1 MAC do not increase CBF in normocapnia, so isoflurane is widely used in neurosurgical anaesthesia. Larger concentrations do increase CBF. At 2 MAC the electroencephalogram (EEG) may become isoelectric, and therefore afford some protection in cerebral hypoxia.

Isoflurane has anticonvulsive properties, and does not affect the development of cerebral oedema after trauma. It has poor analgesic properties.

Muscle tone is reduced with isoflurane, as with other volatile agents, and isoflurane potentiates non-depolarising muscle relaxants.

Uterus

Isoflurane causes a dose-related relaxation of the pregnant uterus, but is suitable for caesarean section in a concentration of 0.75%.

Liver

Repeated isoflurane administrations have failed to produce measurable changes in liver function. However, isolated cases of fatal hepatic necrosis have occurred after the use of isoflurane.[10] Isoflurane causes a reduction in hepatic portal blood flow, but hepatic arterial blood flow is maintained.

Kidneys

Isoflurane decreases renal blood flow by 50% and glomerular filtration rate by 30%. Both return to normal when the drug is withdrawn. Serum fluoride concentrations after 3 MAC hours of exposure amount to 5% of the levels associated with renal toxicity.

Other

There is a fall in intraocular pressure with isoflurane, and isoflurane may precipitate malignant hyperpyrexia.

Pharmacokinetics

Inhaled isoflurane is almost 100% excreted through the lungs, and only about 0.2% can be recovered as urinary metabolites. The likelihood of renal or hepatic toxicity following isoflurane anaesthesia is considered to be minimal.

Indications

Of the various inhalation agents available, isoflurane has the advantage of providing a stable cardiac rhythm and lack of sensitisation of the heart to exogenous and endogenous epinephrine (adrenaline).

Rapid awakening is an advantage in the day-stay patient. Isoflurane is stable and is unlikely to be toxic. It produces hypotension with little cardiac depression. For maintenance with spontaneous breathing 1–2% is usually required.

Sevoflurane

Sevoflurane (1,1,1,3,3,3-hexafluoroisopropyl fluoromethyl ether) was first described in North America in 1971, and was first given to human volunteers in 1981. As with isoflurane, introduction into clinical use was delayed because of fears about toxicity, in this case related to high levels of organic and inorganic fluoride, together with reports that breakdown products when used with CO_2 absorbents were nephrotoxic in rats. This delayed its introduction until 1990.

Physical properties

Sevoflurane is a colourless liquid with a pleasant-smelling non-pungent vapour. It has a molecular weight of 200 Da, a boiling point 58.5°C, and specific gravity of 1.52.

The SVP for sevoflurane is 21 kPa at 20°C.

The blood/gas partition coefficient is 0.69 for sevoflurane (the second lowest of the volatile agents after desflurane, for which the blood/gas partition coefficient is 0.4) and the oil/gas partition coefficient is 53. The MAC ranges from 3.3% in neonates to 1.4% at 80 years of age.

Pharmacodynamics

Cardiovascular system

Vasodilatation and hypotension may occur with sevoflurane, but blood pressure is better preserved than with isoflurane. There is no evidence of coronary steal, and coronary vasodilator properties are similar to those of isoflurane at equivalent MAC values. Sevoflurane is also less likely to cause tachycardia than isoflurane. Heart rhythm is stable and there is no myocardial sensitisation to catecholamines.

Respiratory system

Sevoflurane vapour is sweet smelling and easy to breathe, making it ideal for gaseous induction in small children. Respiratory rate increases slightly, but tidal volume is reduced enough to decrease minute volume overall.

Bronchodilatation and reduced hypoxic pulmonary vasoconstriction occur, as with isoflurane.

Nervous system

Sevoflurane produces a smooth and rapid onset of general anaesthesia at concentrations of between 4 and 8%. There is no increase in CBF or intracranial pressure below 1 MAC. It has anticonvulsant properties with no excitatory phenomena. Muscle tone is reduced, potentiating non-depolarising muscle relaxants. Cerebral oxygen consumption is halved at 2 MAC. Analgesic properties are very poor.

Effects on the uterus

The effects of sevoflurane on the uterus are similar to those of isoflurane, with a dose-related relaxation of the pregnant uterus. It may be used in caesarean section.

Toxicity

There is no known hepatic or renal toxicity with sevoflurane, even after repeated administration. It may trigger malignant hyperpyrexia in susceptible individuals.

About 5% of sevoflurane is metabolised by cytochrome P450 2E1 in the liver with the production of hexafluoro-isopropanol and inorganic fluoride. The former is rapidly glucuronidated and excreted by the kidneys. The rest is excreted by the lungs. Concentrations of inorganic fluoride are only likely to reach 50 μmol/L (the proposed threshold at which renal impairment may occur) after about 8 MAC-hours of sevoflurane anaesthesia. In clinical practice sevoflurane does not cause renal damage, and the raised inorganic fluoride levels return to normal after the drug is withdrawn. However, some workers still caution against its use if renal function is significantly impaired.

Sevoflurane is absorbed into soda lime and baralyme, and degraded by them, particularly where potassium hydroxide is present in the lime. Five breakdown compounds have been identified – compounds A to E. This degradation is more marked at higher temperatures. Compound A (PIFE, pentafluoroisopropenyl fluoromethyl ether) is the only one likely to be produced in clinical use, and is toxic to the liver, kidneys and CNS in rats. The concentrations of compound A found in patients have been generally less than 10 ppm, and are higher if baralyme is used. Concentrations over 30 ppm have been recorded after very prolonged exposure using low fresh gas flows. These values are substantially less than the 200 ppm that seems to be the minimum dose needed to cause renal damage in rats. Compound A is almost certainly of no clinical significance except when sevoflurane is used for a very long time with fresh gas flows under 2 L/min. For example, transient changes in renal function, attributed to compound A, have been noticed in volunteers after administration of 1.25 MAC of sevoflurane for 8 hours with fresh gas flows of 2 L/min.

There is also evidence that production of compound A, fluoride, methanol and formaldehyde is more likely to occur where sevoflurane is passed over dry baralyme, with an increased risk of inhalation of these noxious substances by the patient. Moist baralyme should therefore always be used, and it has been recommended that baralyme should not be allowed to dry out when not used over weekends. This effect does not occur with dry soda lime, where the production of compound A actually decreases.[11]

Indications

Inhalational induction using sevoflurane is rapid (1–2 min), smooth and well tolerated in both children and adults.

Sevoflurane is poorly soluble in blood, pleasant smelling and fairly non-irritant to the upper airways. It therefore has a useful place as an induction agent. Various techniques have been used with success, either increasing the inspired concentration rapidly from 0.5% up to 4–8% by taking a single vital capacity breath of 4.5% or higher, or by immediately breathing a high concentration (8%). The incidence of coughing is extremely low.

The trachea may be intubated under deep sevoflurane anaesthesia, and a laryngeal mask airway inserted at about 1 MAC. Sevoflurane is often recommended as an induction agent when maintaining the airway may be difficult using a facemask, although its superiority over halothane for this purpose is not fully established.

Emergence from anaesthesia is more rapid than with isoflurane, and is comparable to that seen after continuous propofol anaesthesia. This makes it suitable for day surgery.

Desflurane

Desflurane (1-fluoro-2,2,2-trifluoroethyl difluoromethyl ether) was developed in the USA and introduced to the UK in 1994. The chemical structure is the same as that of isoflurane, but with fluorine substituted for chlorine.

Physical properties

Desflurane is a colourless liquid with a pungent vapour and a molecular weight of 168 Da. Its SVP at 20°C is 88 kPa owing to its low boiling point of 23.5°C. Its blood/gas partition coefficient is 0.42 and oil/gas partition coefficient 19. MAC values range from 5–7% in adults to 10% in children. No preservative is required, but desflurane can react with dry soda lime to produce carbon monoxide.

Vaporiser (Datex-Ohmeda Tec 6)

Because the boiling point of desflurane is so close to room temperature, standard vaporisers are unsatisfactory and electrically heated vaporisers are used to heat the liquid desflurane to 39°C (above its boiling point), thus vaporising it completely. The internal vaporiser pressure at this temperature is about 200 kPa, and the vapour is then injected into the fresh gas flow, rather than the fresh gas flow passing over the surface of the vapour. Electronic sensors monitor the fresh gas flow and adjust the vapour output automatically.

Pharmacodynamics

Cardiovascular system

Desflurane has similar effects on the cardiovascular system to isoflurane, with a reduction in systemic vascular resistance causing hypotension. However, some sympathetic hyperactivity has been reported when the inspired concentration is increased rapidly, and tachycardia and hypertension can then result. The myocardium is not sensitised to catecholamines and there are no reports of coronary steal.

Respiratory system

Although desflurane vapour is not unpleasant to inhale, desflurane is much more irritant to the airways than sevoflurane, with a higher incidence of coughing and laryngeal spasm at induction in both adults and children, making its use unsuitable for inhalational induction. There is a dose-dependent reduction in tidal volume and a compensatory increase in breathing rate.

Nervous system

There is an increase in CBF and intracranial pressure with desflurane, together with a reduction in cerebral oxygen consumption. EEG changes are similar to those produced by isoflurane, with anticonvulsive properties. Very little analgesia is produced. Muscle relaxation occurs and non-depolarising neuromuscular blocks may be potentiated.

Other

Desflurane causes a dose-dependent relaxation of the pregnant uterus. Malignant hyperthermia is a potential risk.

Pharmacokinetics

0.02% of desflurane is metabolised, the rest being excreted unchanged by the lungs. There are no reports of significant liver or kidney toxicity.

Indications

Because of the extremely low blood/gas partition coefficient, induction, change of depth of anaesthesia and recovery are rapid. Desflurane is therefore particularly suitable for day surgery. Desflurane solubility in body tissues is also low, so that in a closed breathing system the concentration of vapour in the system will approach that in the basal flow more rapidly than in the case of other agents.

Enflurane

The first clinical account of enflurane (2-chloro-1,1,2-trifluoroethyl difluoromethyl ether) appeared in 1966. It was developed by Ross Terrell in the USA in 1963.

Physical properties

Enflurane is a colourless volatile liquid with a halogenated hydrocarbon-like smell. Its molecular weight is 184.5 Da and boiling point is 56.5°C, giving an SVP of 24 kPa at 20°C.

The MAC for enflurane is 1.68% in O_2 and 1.28% in 70% N_2O for adults, but up to 2.4% in children. Its blood/gas partition coefficient is 1.9 and oil/gas partition coefficient is 98.5.

Concentrations of enflurane above 4.25% are flammable in 20% O_2 with N_2O.

Enflurane is stable with soda lime and metals and does not require preservative.

Pharmacodynamics

Cardiovascular system

As the depth of anaesthesia is increased, there is a reversible fall in arterial pressure with enflurane due to myocardial depression with some vasodilatation. Arrhythmias are uncommon and there is only slight sensitisation of the myocardium to catecholamines. The safe dose of epinephrine (adrenaline) is up to three times that permitted with halothane.

Respiratory system

Minute volume is reduced more with enflurane than with halothane or isoflurane because of a reduction in tidal volume, often with a slight compensatory rise in respiratory rate. Airway reflexes are well maintained, and tracheal intubation is more difficult than with halothane. Salivary and bronchial secretions are not increased. Bronchodilatation occurs and there may be occasional deeper inspirations.

Nervous system

The main disadvantage of enflurane is that EEG changes of an epileptiform nature often occur. These are more common during hypocapnia and may persist for several weeks. Convulsions may occur at 2 MAC and enflurane should be used with extreme caution in patients who have a history of epilepsy. Cerebral blood flow is doubled at 1 MAC.

Muscle relaxation is greater with enflurane than with halothane or isoflurane, enhancing the action of non-depolarising relaxants.

Enflurane has weak analgesic properties.

Uterus

Enflurane is satisfactory for caesarean section in a concentration of 1%. There is a dose-related relaxation of the uterus.

Other

Postoperative nausea and vomiting are uncommon with enflurane. There is a reduction in intraocular pressure. Enflurane has been reported to trigger malignant hyperpyrexia.

Toxicity

Enflurane is eliminated mostly via the lungs, although about 3% is metabolised in the body and the resultant fluoride ions are excreted by the kidney. Peak fluoride concentrations are similar to those seen after sevoflurane anaesthesia, and are usually well below the possible toxic level of 50 μmol/L. Changes in renal function are not clinically significant, and enflurane seems to produce no further impairment of renal function, even when this is impaired preoperatively. However, caution should be exercised when potentially nephrotoxic drugs such as isoniazid are also being administered.

There have been reports of hepatitis following enflurane anaesthesia, and cross-sensitivity with halothane has been suggested.

Emergence from anaesthesia is smooth and reasonably rapid, and shivering is infrequent.

Halothane

Halothane (2-bromo-2-chloro-1,1,1-trifluoroethane) is a potent, non-flammable, relatively non-toxic anaesthetic agent. Its ease of use revolutionised anaesthesia following its introduction in 1956.

Physical properties

Halothane is a colourless liquid with a relatively non-pungent vapour. Its molecular weight is 197 Da, with a liquid density at 20°C of 1.87. The boiling point of halothane is 50°C, and its SVP at 20°C is 32 kPa.

The MAC for halothane is 0.75%, although up to 1.5% may be required in spontaneously breathing patients.

Partition coefficients for halothane are blood/gas 2.3, oil/gas 220, fat/blood 60.0, and brain/blood 2.6.

Halothane is decomposed by light and stabilised by 0.01% thymol, but is stable when stored in amber-coloured bottles. It can be used safely with soda lime. The vapour is absorbed by rubber (rubber/gas partition coefficient at 20°C is 120). In the presence of moisture it attacks tin, brass and aluminium in vaporisers and circuits.

Halothane is non-flammable and non-explosive when its vapour is mixed with O_2 in any concentration (including hyperbaric conditions) used clinically.

Halothane is decomposed by an open flame, liberating free bromine.

Pharmacodynamics

Cardiovascular system

Arterial pressure falls with halothane owing to myocardial depression and significant vasodilatation. Sinus or nodal bradycardia is common due to increased vagal tone and can be reversed by atropine. Coronary arteries dilate, but there is an increase in myocardial oxygen demand.

Myocardial excitability is significantly increased, causing ventricular extrasystoles. These are more likely when there is CO_2 retention, sensory stimulation in light anaesthesia, and with the use of β-stimulant drugs and catecholamines. Ventricular fibrillation has occurred following epinephrine (adrenaline) infiltration during halothane anaesthesia. Intravenous infusion of more than 10 μg/min of epinephrine (adrenaline) is likely to provoke an arrhythmia.

CNS

Halothane produces a smooth and relatively rapid onset and emergence of anaesthesia. It increases CBF threefold at 1 MAC and abolishes autoregulation. It should only be introduced in neurosurgery if the $P\text{CO}_2$ has previously been lowered by hyperventilation to about 3.5 kPa. With halothane there is a moderate degree of muscle relaxation and a potentiation of non-depolarising muscle relaxants.

Respiratory system

Halothane depresses respiration by decreasing tidal volume and increasing respiratory rate. It causes bronchodilatation and has been used as an adjunct to ventilation in severe asthma in intensive care.

Halothane is not irritant to the airway, but depresses pharyngeal and laryngeal reflexes. Deep halothane anaesthesia allows relatively easy laryngoscopy and intubation where the airway is difficult and muscle relaxants are contraindicated.

Uterus

Halothane causes a dose-related relaxation of the uterus. A concentration as low as 0.5% may increase blood loss during termination of pregnancy, even when oxytocin is administered.

Temperature

Induction of anaesthesia with halothane is soon followed by a drop of up to 1°C in core temperature, together with a rise of up to 4°C in skin temperature, owing to redistribution of blood flow between deep and peripheral tissues. Later, skin temperature may fall as peripheral vasodilatation aids heat loss.

Shivering

Shivering (halothane shakes) and tremor are both common during the immediate postoperative period following halothane anaesthesia. They may be associated with a generalised increase in muscle tone – clonic or tonic.

Although a fall in core temperature during anaesthesia may precipitate shivering, it has also been postulated that decreased descending inhibitory control of spinal reflexes may be important.

Shivering can increase oxygen demand threefold, and supplemental oxygen should be administered if it occurs. Increased muscle tone can cause biting, and damage to teeth and crowns is possible if an oral airway is in place. Treatment with pethidine is sometimes helpful.

Other

Halothane classically produces malignant hyperpyrexia in susceptible individuals. There is a reduction in intraocular pressure.

Pharmacokinetics

About 20% of the halothane taken up by the body is metabolised by the liver. This is mainly by oxidative pathways, but hypoxia may cause metabolism by alternative reductive pathways, leading to the possibility of liver damage. Metabolites include bromine, chlorine and trifluoroacetic acid, with very small numbers of fluoride ions.

Liver toxicity

Massive hepatic necrosis following halothane anaesthesia was first reported in 1958, though widespread attention was not drawn to the problem until 1963. Subclinical 'halothane hepatitis' (a lesser degree of liver dysfunction, with a hepatocellular pattern of elevated transferases) may also occur in up to 20% of patients. The most susceptible patients are middle-aged women and the obese, and there may a genetic predisposition.[12,13]

The incidence of halothane hepatitis is low, between 1 in 6000 and 1 in 30 000, making it difficult to study. The National Halothane Study in the USA (1969) reported on 850 000 cases of hepatitis within 6 weeks of anaesthesia, but less than 30% had received halothane.[12,13]

Metabolites of halothane are slowly cleared from the body for up to 3 weeks. The pathways are complex, but the products of the reductive pathways appear more toxic and may cause direct damage to hepatocytes. There is also evidence, however, for an immune-mediated reaction, with the production of antibodies that react with liver cells altered by halothane.

The Committee on Safety of Medicines (1986) recommends that:

- a careful history should be taken relating to previous halothane anaesthetics and any adverse effects;

- halothane should not be used within 3 months of a previous halothane anaesthetic without 'overriding clinical circumstances';
- unexplained jaundice or fever after a previous halothane anaesthetic is an absolute contraindication to further use of halothane.

Many anaesthetists consider that the second point should not apply to children, in whom liver toxicity has been extremely rare.

Pre-existing liver disease unrelated to halothane is not a specific contraindication to the use of halothane. Severe liver damage is unlikely to follow a single administration of halothane. Hepatitis has been reported after the use of enflurane and isoflurane, but repeat anaesthetics with these agents are thought to be safe.

Other causes of postoperative jaundice include side-effects of drugs (phenothiazines, monoamine oxidase inhibitors), blood transfusion, sepsis, hypotension and coincidental viral hepatitis.

Stress and starvation may produce overt jaundice in patients with Gilbert's syndrome (familial unconjugated hyperbilirubinaemia), but the serum transaminases remain normal.

Xenon

Xenon was isolated in 1898 by William Ramsey (1852–1916), winner of the 1904 Nobel Prize for chemistry.

Xenon was first used in 1951. It is a weak anaesthetic agent with a MAC of 70%, and it has been suggested that xenon compares favourably with N_2O in terms of haemodynamic, neuroendocrine and analgesic properties. Radioactive Xenon^{133} can be used to study regional cerebral blood flow.

Diethyl ether

Diethyl ether is of historical importance but is also still a widely used anaesthetic agent in several continents. It was introduced by WTG Morton in Boston on 16 October 1846.

Diethyl ether is a safe anaesthetic used by open-drop technique on to a gauze mask, or in plenum or drawover vaporisers. Sympathetic stimulation maintains the blood pressure with a low incidence of arrhythmia, but may increase blood sugar levels.

Disadvantages of diethyl ether include flammability, a high blood/gas partition coefficient of 12, and irritation of the airway, with laryngeal spasm, both of which lengthen induction time. There is also increased salivation, with nausea and vomiting postoperatively.

Physical properties

The SVP of diethyl ether at 20°C is 55 kPa, and the blood/gas partition coefficient 12 results in a very slow induction and recovery. The MAC is 1.92.

Diethyl ether has an irritant vapour, which can readily induce laryngeal spasm and make induction even slower. It is flammable in air and explosive in O_2.

Diethyl ether stimulates salivary and bronchial secretions, and so anticholinergic premedication is advisable.

Diethyl ether is commonly given from an EMO drawover vaporiser. Spontaneous respiration may be maintained and the concentration of diethyl ether slowly increased, or the same apparatus may be used in conjunction with an Oxford inflating bellows for intermittent positive-pressure ventilation (IPPV) using air in field environments. Muscle relaxants are unnecessary because diethyl ether itself produces excellent relaxation.

The use of a concomitant regional block with local anaesthetic greatly reduces the concentration of ether needed, lessens the side-effects and speeds recovery. The typical maintenance concentration is 5% without local block, and 2% with local block. The use of opiates will also reduce the necessary concentration of diethyl ether, but will make postoperative nausea and vomiting much worse. These respond to antiemetics.

Diethyl ether liberates catecholamines and tends to maintain blood pressure. There is little cardiac depression. Arrhythmias are rare. Epinephrine (adrenaline) is relatively safe with diethyl ether. Bronchial smooth muscle is relaxed.

The products of the metabolism of ether (alcohol, acetaldehyde and acetic acid) are relatively non-toxic.

Diethyl ether should not be used when diathermy is needed in the airways because of the risk of fire or explosion, although these have not occurred when air is used to carry the diethyl ether vapour.

GASES USED IN ASSOCIATION WITH ANAESTHESIA

Oxygen

Antoine Lavoisier and Pierre Laplace coined the term 'oxygène' (oxy, acid; gene, producer) in 1779. They were the first to compare the heat produced by respiration in animals with that from the combustion of carbon.

Medical O_2 is manufactured by the fractional distillation of liquid air, nitrogen boiling off first at −195°C followed by oxygen at −183°C.

Oxygen cylinders are painted black with white shoulders in the UK, blue in some European countries and green in the US. The recommended ISO 32 colour code is white. The cylinders contain gaseous O_2 compressed to 137 bar. Oxygen is also supplied as a liquid at about −183°C in vacuum-insulated evaporators with a vapour pressure above the liquid of around 10.5 bar: 1 mL of liquid O_2 gives 842 mL of gas at 15°C. Hospital pipeline pressure is set at 4.1 bar.

The oxygen concentrator produces O_2 from ambient air by preferential absorption of nitrogen on zeolites (crystalline aluminosilicates). It behaves like a molecular sieve with a pore size of 0.5 nm. The resultant gas contains 6% of harmless impurities, mostly argon, and is suitable for use in hospitals and homes, remote areas, developing countries and in the military. Small machines producing about 2 L/min are cheaper than cylinders for domestic use.

Properties

Oxygen has a molecular weight of 32 Da. Its solubility in water is 0.024 mL/mL at 37°C, 0.031 mL/mL at 20°C and 0.049 mL/mL at 0°C.

The boiling point of O_2 is –183°C, its critical temperature is –118.4°C and its critical pressure is 50.8 bar.

The specific gravity of O_2 is 1.1 (air is 1.0) and its density is 1.35 kg/m^3 at 15°C.

Electric sparks convert O_2 into ozone (O_3).

When rapidly compressed, O_2 may ignite grease or oil, which should not therefore be used in cylinder pressure gauges. It encourages fires, although it is not in itself flammable.

Oxygen (and N_2O) cylinders should be turned on momentarily before being fitted to the anaesthetic machine yoke to allow any dirt in the valve to escape. They should then be turned on slowly after fitting to the yoke to prevent sudden surges of pressure into the reducing valve and pressure gauge.

Medical air

Atmospheric air contains 78.08% nitrogen, 20.95% O_2, 0.93% argon, 0.03% CO_2, and traces of neon, helium, krypton, hydrogen and xenon in descending order of abundance.

Medical air is supplied in the UK in grey cylinders with black and white shoulder quadrants, compressed to 137 bar. In hospitals it is also supplied through two sets of pipelines at 4 and 7 bar.

Medical air is used as a respired gas and to drive ventilators at 4 bar, and drives surgical drills and saws at a pressure of 7 bar. Medical air has fewer impurities than industrial compressed air, contains no water and less than 0.5 mg/m^3 of oil mist.

Carbon dioxide

Carbon dioxide was discovered by Jean Baptiste von Helmont and isolated by Joseph Black in 1757, who showed that it was produced by respiration, combustion and fermentation. It was used to produce 'suspended animation' and surgical anaesthesia in animals in 1824 by Henry Hill Hickman; 30% CO_2 was used by Ralph Waters to render humans unconscious in 1928.

Properties

Carbon dioxide is a colourless gas with a pungent odour in high concentration. It has a molecular weight of 44 Da, a boiling point of –78.5°C and a solubility in water of 0.88 mL/mL at 20°C. Its critical temperature is 31°C and critical pressure 73.8 bar.

The specific gravity of CO_2 is 1.52 and it has a density of 1.87 kg/m^3 at 15°C.

Preparation and storage

In the UK CO_2 is obtained from four sources:

- fermentation in the brewing of beer;
- as a byproduct from the manufacture of hydrogen in petroleum refining;
- combustion of other fuels;
- by heating magnesium and calcium carbonate in the presence of their oxides.

Only a small fraction of the CO_2 manufactured is used for medicinal purposes. It is stored in grey cylinders under the ISO 32 recommendation. Solid CO_2 is stored and transported in insulated containers. The filling ratio in cylinders is 0.75 in temperate climates and 0.67 in the tropics. The liquid phase disappears when about 83% of the gas by mass has been discharged.

Anaesthetic machines should no longer have CO_2 cylinders attached, and modern machines do not have a yoke provided for it.

Effects

Inspired air contains 0.03% CO_2, mixed expired gas 3.5–4% CO_2 and alveolar gas 5.3% CO_2 in health. Breathing 5% CO_2 in air or O_2 causes a tolerable rise in minute volume, but higher amounts cause dyspnoea, headache and increased sympathetic discharge. Above 10% CO_2 the narcotic effect becomes noticeable, and at 30% CO_2 the EEG becomes isoelectric as coma ensues. Muscle twitching, a flap of the hands and fits may occur before coma supervenes. At 40% CO_2 respiration is directly depressed. Carbon dioxide has frequently been used to anaesthetise small laboratory animals.

Hypercapnia by itself is a direct myocardial depressant, but this is masked by a rise in plasma catecholamines causing multifocal ventricular extrasystoles. The blood concentration of CO_2 is the major physiological factor influencing CBF.

In the past CO_2 has been used to hasten inhalational induction of anaesthesia, especially with agents of high blood solubility, to facilitate blind intubation, and to facilitate the onset of spontaneous breathing after IPPV. It is still used as a cerebral vasodilator in studies of CBF and to insufflate the abdomen for laparoscopy.

Water vapour

Water has a high specific heat of 4.2 kJ/kg/°C or ten times that of copper. Inspired air is warmed to body temperature and fully saturated with water vapour by the time it reaches the trachea. If the trachea is intubated and dry air is inspired this important process is bypassed and has to take place in the tracheobronchial tree, with consequent drying of the mucosa. Air saturated with water vapour at 15, 20 and 37°C has partial pressures of water vapour of 12, 18 and 47 mmHg and water contents of 13, 19 and 50 mg/L, respectively.

Helium

Helium was isolated by Sir W Ramsey (1852–1916), a British chemist and winner of the 1904 Nobel Prize for his work on the inert gases, in 1895.

Preparation

Collected as a natural gas, from gas wells in Poland, Texas and New Mexico which contain air with 1% Helium by volume. Natural gas from the North Sea contains only 0.01–0.03%. Air contains 0.0005%.

Helium cylinders are brown and helium–oxygen cylinders are brown with brown/white shoulder quadrants. The pressure in a full cylinder is 137 bar.

Properties

Helium is an inert, colourless, odourless gas with a molecular weight of 4 Da, a boiling point of –269°C, and solubility in water of 0.0088 mL/mL at 20°C. Its critical temperature is –268°C, specific gravity 0.14, critical pressure 2.3 bar and density 0.17 kg/m^3 at 15°C. Only hydrogen has a lower mass.

A mixture of 21% O_2 and 79% helium has a low density which enables flow through an orifice three times that air for the same pressure gradient. It may therefore be used for therapeutic benefit in patients with upper airways obstruction. Because its viscosity is very similar to that of O_2 it will make no difference to the laminar flow in smaller airways, but the lower Reynolds number for helium mixtures will encourage laminar flow in the larger airways.

Helium has a low solubility that enables it to be used in the measurement of lung volumes by gas dilution.

High diffusibility and low solubility make helium less likely than nitrogen to be responsible for decompression sickness. Its high thermal capacity encourages loss of body heat.

References

1. Kety SS. The physiological and physical factors affecting the uptake of anesthetic agents by the body. Anesthesiology 1950; 11:517–526.
2. Eger EJ. Anesthetic Uptake and Action. Baltimore: Williams & Wilkins; 1974.
3. Guedel AE. Inhalation Anesthesia 1937 and 2nd edn. Macmillan, London, 1951.

4. Brown AC, Canosa-Mas CE, Parr AD, et al. Tropospheric lifetimes of halogenated anaesthetics. Nature 1989; 341:635.
5. Hess WC. et al. Contamination of anaesthetic gases with nitric oxide and its influence on oxygenation: study in patients undergoing open heart surgery. Br J Anaesth 2003; 93:629–33.
6. Marczin N. Tiny wonders of tiny impurities of nitrous oxide during anaesthesia. Br J Anaesth 2004; 93(5):619–23.
7. Clutton-Brock J. Two cases of poisoning by contamination of nitrous oxide with higher oxides of nitrogen during anaesthesia. Br J Anaesth 1967; 39:388.
8. Weinmann J. Toxicity of nitrous oxide. Best Prac Res Clin Anaesthesiol 2003; 17(1):47–61.
9. Ahn SC, Brown AW. Cobalamin deficiency and subacute combined degeneration after nitrous oxide anesthesia: a case report. Arch Phys Med Rehabil 2005; 86(1):150–53.
10. Weitz J, Kienle P, Bohrer H, et al. Fatal hepatic necrosis after isoflurane anaesthesia. Anaesthesia 1997; 52:884.
11. Eger EI 2nd, Ionescu P, Laster MJ, et al. Baralyme dehydration increases and soda lime dehydration decreases the concentration of compound A resulting from sevoflurane degradation in a standard anesthetic circuit. Anesth Analg 1997; 85:892–898.
12. Bunker JP, Forrest WH, Mostella F. (Eds) The National Halothane Study. A Study of the possible association between halothane anesthesia and post-operative hepatic necrosis. Washington US Government Press Office 1966.
13. McCaughey W. A summary of the National Halothane Study. Br J Anaesth 1972; 44(9):918.

CHAPTER **2.4**

INTRAVENOUS ANAESTHESIA

This chapter describes those drugs given by the intravenous route for induction of anaesthesia. They may also be used for maintenance of anaesthesia, or at subanaesthetic doses as sedatives. Other intravenous drugs used as adjuvants to anaesthesia are discussed in Chapters 2.5 and 3.2.

The groups of drugs considered are:

- those with actions at γ-aminobutyric acid ($GABA_A$) receptors – barbiturates, benzodiazepines, etomidate and propofol;
- ketamine, which acts at the *N*-methyl-D-aspartate (NMDA) receptor.

They differ physicochemically and in their pharmacodynamic and pharmacokinetic properties. The important common property is good lipid solubility, which enables them to penetrate the blood–brain barrier, particularly when largely unionised at pH 7.4 (Table 2.4.1).

General anaesthesia may be maintained after intravenous induction either by converting to inhalation anaesthesia or by continuing intravenous administration of the induction agent using an infusion device.

There is an increasing number of microprocessor-controlled drug delivery systems for maintenance of the required effect site concentration either directly or indirectly through control of plasma concentration.

Total intravenous anaesthesia (TIVA) and the more sophisticated target-controlled intravenous anaesthesia (TCI) are discussed later in this chapter.

PROPERTIES OF AN IDEAL INDUCTION AGENT

These include pharmaceutical, physicochemical, pharmacodynamic and pharmacokinetic properties (Box 2.4.1). Maintenance of anaesthesia, particularly with TIVA or TCI, also introduces cost as an important consideration.

None of the currently available induction agents is ideal, although propofol comes closest. There is a new agent, THRX-918661,[1] undergoing clinical evaluation which is an ester that undergoes rapid hydrolysis. This results in a short constant context-sensitive half-time that may be advantageous for maintenance of anaesthesia or long-term sedation without accumulation. Like thiopental, propofol and etomidate it is a positive allosteric modulator at the $GABA_A$ receptor.

Agent	Molecular weight	Acid–base status	pK_a	% Un–ionised at pH 7.4
Thiopental	264	Weak acid	7.6	61
Thioamylal	286	Weak acid	7.6	61
Methohexital	284	Weak acid	7.9	75
Etomidate	342	Weak base	4.24	99.9
Propofol	178	Weak acid	11	99.97
Midazolam	326	Weak base	6.2	94.1
Ketamine	237.5	Weak base	7.5	55.7

Table 2.4.1 Physicochemical properties of induction agents

HISTORICAL PERSPECTIVE

Barbiturates were the first intravenous induction agents used clinically; hexobarbital was superseded by thiopental, which had fewer unwanted effects. Methohexital, an ultra-short-acting barbiturate, was popular, but propofol has replaced it.

Steroid-based induction agents have been used, but are now withdrawn: althesin, a 3:1 mix of alphaxalone and alphadolone, had several advantages compared to thiopental, but produced severe allergic reactions to its solvent Cremophor EL. In the 1990s, following the successful introduction of propofol, another steroid-based induction agent, eltanolone or 5β-pregnanolone, was presented in soyabean oil but withdrawn owing to a high incidence of urticaria. It had few advantages over propofol. The eugenol derivative propanidid, which had a very short duration of action and minimal accumulation due to rapid metabolism by tissue and hepatic esterases, was also solubilised in Cremophor EL. It was also withdrawn because of allergic reactions.

CURRENTLY AVAILABLE INTRAVENOUS INDUCTION AGENTS

The structure of agents currently available to anaesthetists in the UK is shown in Figure 2.4.1.

Thiopental

In the UK the only available barbiturate for induction of anaesthesia is thiopental (sodium 5-ethyl-5′-(1-methylbutyl)-2-thiobarbiturate; thiopentone). It was first used in 1934 by Lundy and Waters. Other barbiturates used outside the UK as induction agents are methohexital and thiamylal.

Box 2.4.1
Properties of an ideal induction agent
Pharmaceutical
Needs no mixing or diluting
Long shelf-life without refrigeration
pH close to plasma
No preservatives needed
Pharmacodynamic
Affects only CNS
No excitatory phenomena
No unwanted effects, particularly respiratory or cardiovascular
Good correlation between plasma concentration and clinical effects
High therapeutic index
Analgesic
No important drug interactions
No pain on injection
No histamine release or anaphylactic reactions
Pharmacokinetic
No organ-based metabolism
Rapid onset and offset of action
No active metabolites
Economic
Cheap to produce
Sustainable supply at low cost
Physicochemical
High lipid solubility
High proportion unionised at plasma pH

Anaesthetic barbiturates are derivatives of barbituric acid, formed by a condensation reaction between urea and malonic acid. They are weak acids and have p*K*a values above plasma pH, making them largely unionised and hence able to cross the blood–brain barrier. They differ in substitutions on the carbon at position 5 in the heterocyclic ring. Thiobarbiturates have oxygen replaced by suphur on the urea-derived carbon at position 2

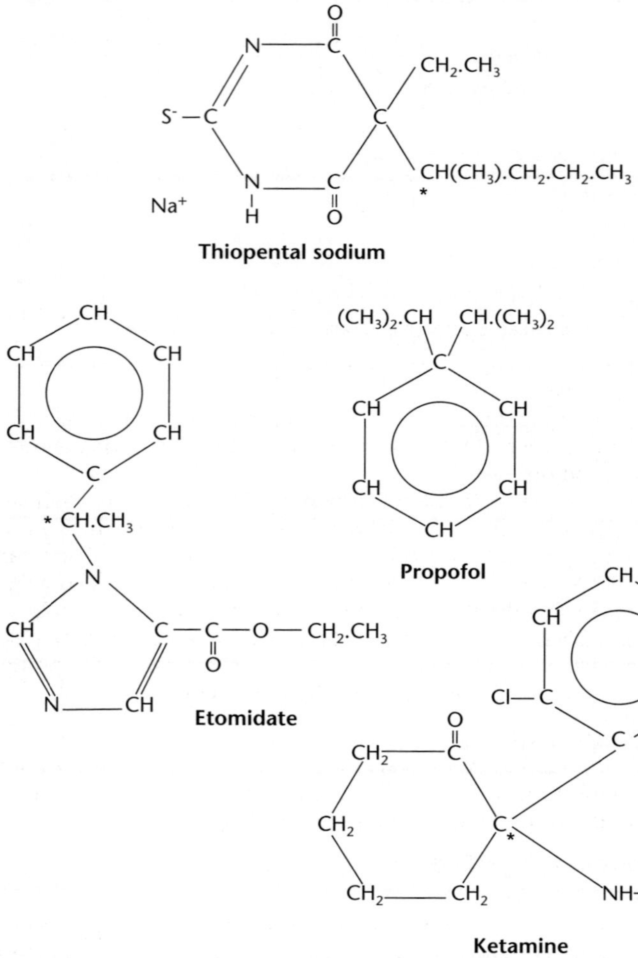

O
N—C
S^-—C
C
$CH_2.CH_3$
N—C
Na^+
H
O
$CH(CH_3).CH_2.CH_2.CH_3$
*

Thiopental sodium

CH
CH CH
CH CH
C
* $CH.CH_3$
N
CH C—C—O—$CH_2.CH_3$
O
N CH

Etomidate

$(CH_3)_2.CH$ $CH.(CH_3)_2$
C
CH CH
CH CH
CH

Propofol

CH
CH CH
Cl—C CH
C
O
CH_2—C
CH_2
C*
CH_2—CH_2 NH—CH_3

Ketamine

Figure 2.4.1 Structure of common intravenous anaesthetic agents. All have one chiral centre (indicated by *), except propofol, which is achiral.

Barbiturate	C2 (O or S)	N1	R1	R2
Thiopental	S	H	Ethyl ($-CH_2.CH_3$)	1-methyl butyl ($-CH(CH_3).CH_2.CH_2.CH_3$)
Thiamylal	S	H	Propenyl (allyl) ($-CH_2.CH{:}CH_2$)	1-methyl butyl
Methohexital	O	Methyl	Propenyl (allyl)	1-methyl penten-2-yl ($-CH(CH_3).CH{:}CH.CH_2.CH_3$)

Table 2.4.2 Structures of barbiturate induction agents

(Table 2.4.2). Short duration of action is associated with the thio substitution and a branched group on C5. Larger, unbranched groups prolong duration of action and increase convulsant activity.

Thiopental is the sulphur derivative of pentobarbital, both of which have a single chiral carbon.

Barbiturates are almost water insoluble, but are weak acids in the tautomeric enol form (–C(OH):N– rather than –CO.NH–). This allows formation of the sodium salt.

Presented as a yellow powder containing 6% anhydrous sodium carbonate, thiopental is prepared and stored under nitrogen, which prevents release of free thiobarbituric acid in the presence of atmospheric carbon dioxide. It is dissolved in water for injection and usually diluted to give a 2.5% (25 mg/mL) alkaline solution, pH 11, which may be stored for up to 48 hours if refrigerated. Injection into a vein may cause precipitation because the lower pH of blood increases the proportion in the unionised form. Once in the blood, thiopental is highly protein bound.

Dose of thiopental

The dose of thiopental varies between 3 and 5 mg/kg, with an effective plasma concentration of 15 μg/mL. Thiopental can also be given rectally, using a 5 or 10% solution and a dose of 50 mg/kg.

Pharmacodynamic effects

Mechanism of action

Barbiturates are positive allosteric modulators at $GABA_A$ and glycine receptors. They cause increased channel opening time for chloride, which increases inhibitory effects. Evidence of stereoselective differences between the enantiomers, *S*- more potent than *R*-thiopental, suggests specific binding sites. Other inhibitory activity can be demonstrated at central sodium and calcium channels, particularly neuronal nicotinic receptors.

Central nervous system

Central effects of thiopental include sedation, anaesthesia, respiratory depression, anticonvulsant action, retrograde amnesia and depression of the vasomotor centre.

Thiopental has no analgesic action and may be antanalgesic in low dose.

Thiopental, like other intravenous general anaesthetic agents, is a cerebral vasoconstrictor, causing a reduction in cerebral blood flow and intracranial pressure and depression of cerebral metabolism. These are features of neuroprotection (see Ch. 5.7). Burst suppression of the EEG can be induced with high doses when used in the treatment of status epilepticus or intractable rises in intracranial pressure following head injury.

Respiratory system

Thiopental causes centrally mediated respiratory depression and reduced sensitivity to raised CO_2, which is dependent on dose and rate of injection. Transient apnoea is common and may require supportive manual ventilation. Laryngeal reflexes remain intact. Coughing, laryngeal spasm and mild bronchoconstriction can occur, particularly in asthmatics.

Cardiovascular system

Myocardial contractility is depressed in a dose-dependent manner with thiopental. Peripheral vascular resistance falls, leading to reduced preload and cardiac output. There is hypotension and tachycardia. Hypotension will be exaggerated if there is hypovolaemia, and may be dramatic if the myocardium cannot compensate for abnormalities such as autonomic dysfunction, tight aortic stenosis and tamponade.

Other actions

Pupils initially contract but then dilate with thiopental. Pupillary response is lost with surgical anaesthesia. Loss of the eyelash reflex is commonly used as a clinical endpoint for an adequate induction dose. Skeletal muscle tone falls more than that of smooth muscle. Uterine tone is unaffected. Lipid solubility allows passage across the placenta, with peak fetal plasma levels lower and delayed compared to maternal levels.

Pharmacokinetics

The pharmacokinetic parameters of thiopental are summarised in Table 2.4.3 for comparison with other induction agents.

The effect compartment equilibration half-life for thiopental is very short – 1.2 minutes, which is faster than for propofol.

Thiopental is highly protein bound depending on pH: binding falls as pH rises. Clearance is by hepatic metabolism, not renal excretion (<1%). Plasma concentration falls rapidly after a bolus dose of thiopental owing to uptake by vessel-rich tissues, not metabolism. Hepatic extraction ratio is low – 0.15 – with saturable metabolism by oxidation to the carboxylic

Agent	Protein bound %	Clearance (mL/kg/min)	Vd_{ss} (L/kg)	$t_{1/2}\beta$ (h)	Active metabolites
Thiopental	85	4	2.5	10	Pentobarbital
Thiamylal	85	3	4	14	Quinalbarbital
Methohexital	85	11	2.2	4	Hydroxymethohexital
Etomidate	76	18	2.5	3	None
Midazolam	98	7	1	2	1- and 4-Hydroxymidazolam
Propofol	98	30	2–3	6	None
Ketamine	60	19	3	3	Norketamine, dehydronorketamine

Vd_{ss}, steady state volume of distribution; $t_{1/2}\beta$, elimination half-time

Table 2.4.3 Pharmacokinetic parameters for induction agents

acid derivative, 5-ethyl-5′(4-carboxyl-1-methylbutyl)-2-thiobarbituric acid, which is inactive, and to a lesser extent by *S*-oxidation to pentobarbital, an hypnotic oxybarbiturate with slow elimination.

After a single bolus dose or short infusion pharmacodynamic decay curves follow typical first-order kinetics. With longer, high-dose infusions hepatic metabolic capacity may be exceeded and zero-order kinetics may be seen. Desulphuration may then become a significant metabolic pathway. Recovery will be prolonged as a result of both reduced metabolism and the presence of an active metabolite.

The elderly show reduced metabolism and a smaller volume of distribution, and a reduced dosage is needed.

Barbiturates are able to induce hepatic metabolism by several isoforms of the cytochrome P450 system. This is of importance only after repeated dosage or with prolonged infusion. CYP 1A2 (warfarin) and CYP 3A3/4 (midazolam, fentanyl, alfentanil, hydrocortisone) may be of importance to anaesthetists.

Adverse effects

Inadvertent intra-arterial injection

Inadvertent intra-arterial injection of thiopental requires prompt recognition and treatment. Surgery should be postponed if possible.

Immediate pain, blanching of the hand and loss of the radial pulse occur, followed by secondary thrombosis.

The cannula should be left in the artery to effect immediate sympathetic blockade using intra-arterial phentolamine or another vasodilator such as papaverine. This should be followed by brachial plexus or stellate ganglion block. A bolus of heparin should be given and longer-term anticoagulation instituted as soon as possible.

Extravasation

Infiltration with lignocaine and hyaluronidase should reduce the pain caused by extravasation of thiopental.

Hypersensitivity

Anaphylactoid reactions are very rare with thiopental (1 in 15 000), but are severe.

Contraindications

Thiopental is contraindicated in porphyria, status asthmaticus, severe shock, pericardial tamponade and uncompensated myocardial disease.

Thiamylal

Thiamylal is an intravenous barbiturate that is unavailable in the UK. It is equipotent with and has properties very similar to those of thiopental.

Methohexital

Methohexital sodium (sodium 5-allyl-5′(1-methylpenten-2-yl)-*N*1-methylbarbiturate; methohexitone) is presented as a white powder mixed with anhydrous sodium carbonate, as for thiopental. It is water soluble with pH of 10–11. The methyl group on the nitrogen in position 1 of the heterocyclic ring confers an ultra-short duration of action.

Unlike thiopental, methohexital has two chiral carbons and is presented as a racemic mix of just the two α-isomers. The β-isomers produce excitation.

Metabolism of methohexital is by oxidation at the *N*1 position to hydroxymethohexital, which has some hypnotic activity. Intrinsic hepatic clearance of methohexital is far higher than for thiopental and saturation kinetics are not seen.

Dose of methohexital

The dose of methohexital is 1–2 mg/kg of a solution containing 10 mg/mL.

Methohexital is more potent than thiopental, and has a shorter onset and duration of action. Induction is often accompanied by pain on injection and involuntary myoclonic movements, particularly of the hands. Methohexital is proconvulsant.

There is less risk of tissue damage than with thiopental following extravasation or inadvertent intra-arterial injection owing to its lower concentration.

Etomidate

The sulphate of etomidate (*R*-1-(methybenzyl)-imidazole-5-ethylcarboxylate sulphate) is water soluble and is presented as a 0.2% solution with pH 7 in 35% propylene glycol.

Etomidate has a single chiral carbon; the *R*- and *S*-isomers have very different potencies and the clinical preparation is just the *R*-enantiomer.

Dose of etomidate

The dose of etomidate is 0.3 mg/kg. It may cause pain on injection. Etomidate does not release histamine.

Pharmacodynamic effects

Mechanism of action

Etomidate is a selective positive allosteric modulator at the $GABA_A$ receptor and, unlike thiopental, does not appear to affect other pentameric ion channels. A single point mutation on the β_2-subunit can alter the sensitivity of the $GABA_A$ receptor to etomidate.

Central nervous system

As with thiopental, cerebral blood flow and metabolism, intracranial and intraocular pressure all fall with etomidate.

As with methohexital, excitatory phenomena may be seen on induction, which can be prevented by benzodiazepine premedication or concomitant use of opioids.

Central sympathetic outflow is stimulated, which maintains haemodynamics.

Respiratory system

Respiratory depression is increased with etomidate in the presence of opioids, but is less than with thiopental.

Cardiovascular system

Etomidate has no effect on mean blood pressure, cardiac output or coronary perfusion. Myocardial oxygen consumption may fall.

Pharmacokinetics

Etomidate has a rapid onset and offset of action owing to redistribution (see Table 2.4.3). Metabolism is mainly by ester hydrolysis in the liver, with a clearance that is flow limited, unlike thiopental. Metabolites undergo both renal (78%) and biliary excretion. None are active.

Owing to its pharmacokinetics etomidate is suitable for maintenance of anaesthesia by continuous infusion, but adverse effects have restricted its use to bolus dose only.

Adverse effects

Adrenocortical suppression

Synthesis of both mineralo- and glucocorticoids is inhibited in the adrenal cortex following continuous infusion of etomidate, leading to higher-than-predicted mortality in the critically ill.

It has been suggested that a single dose of etomidate is sufficient to cause suppression in susceptible patients. The mitochondrial P450 enzymes inhibited are responsible for 11-β and 17-α hydroxylation of the steroid nucleus.

Nausea and vomiting

Etomidate is more likely to be associated with nausea and vomiting than other induction agents.

Propofol

Propofol (2,6-di-isopropylphenol) has replaced thiopental as the most commonly used induction agent in the UK. It is highly lipid soluble but insoluble in water, so is presented as a 1% or 2% emulsion in 10% soyabean oil with 1.2% egg phosphatide as the emulsifying agent.

Ampoules of 20 mL and 50 and 100 mL bottles of 1% propofol are available, together with 1% and 2% 50 mL prepackaged electronically tagged syringes for use in Diprifusor™ TCI devices.

Propofol may be used as an induction agent alone or for both induction and maintenance of anaesthesia.

Dose of propofol

The dose of propofol is 1–2.5 mg/kg for induction. The lower dose should be used in the elderly.

The effective blood concentration for anaesthesia (ED_{90} – the dose at which the effect is seen for 90% of patients) is 3.4 μg/mL when used with 67% nitrous oxide.

Sedation may be produced with a 0.2 mg/kg bolus dose intravenously or an infusion of 1 mg/kg/h, which produces a blood concentration of about 1.5 μg/mL.

Co-induction with either an opioid or midazolam enables the induction dose and initial target level for TCI to be reduced.

Myoclonic movements are common on induction, especially with slow injection. Emergence is more rapid than with thiopental, with less 'hangover'.

Pharmacodynamic effects

Mechanism of action

Propofol binds to the β-subunit of the $GABA_A$ receptor, leading to an increased hyperpolarisation owing to increased channel opening time.

A point mutation resulting in replacement of methionine by tryptophan at position 286 on the β-subunit abolishes indirect receptor activation by propofol. This site is distant from that for benzodiazepines.

Other centrally located ion channels are depressed by propofol, particularly nicotinic cholinergic Na^+ and $5\text{-}HT_3$ channels, but often at higher doses than for the GABA effect.

Central nervous system

Like thiopental, propofol is a cerebral vasoconstrictor. It reduces cerebral blood flow and metabolism, and intracranial pressure.

A central anticholinergic response may be responsible for bradycardia.

Propofol causes dose-dependent burst suppression of the EEG and is used to treat status epilepticus. Myoclonic movement is associated with increased δ-waves on the EEG during induction.

Respiratory system

Central respiratory depression occurs with propofol. Laryngeal tone is reduced more than with thiopental, making it easier to insert a laryngeal mask. There is less risk of coughing and laryngospasm than with thiopental.

Cardiovascular system

Myocardial depression is dose dependent with propofol and seen more commonly in ischaemic heart disease. Systemic vascular resistance is reduced – up to 30% – without compensatory tachycardia. Associated arterial hypotension is more pronounced in the hypertensive patient. Centrally mediated bradycardia can lead to heart block. Prior administration of glycopyrrolate or atropine may be helpful. Slow, low-dose induction maintains cardiac output in hypertrophic obstructive cardiomyopathy.

Other effects

Propofol has been used as a low-dose infusion (target 1 μg/mL) to reduce pruritus due to epidural morphine.

Nausea and vomiting are very uncommon after propofol-based anaesthesia.

Placental transfer of propofol is rapid and causes fetal depression.

Propofol is an antioxidant and may act as a free radical scavenger.

Pharmacokinetics

Propofol is lipophilic (see Table 2.4.3) and a weak acid with a p*K*a of 11, existing in the unionised form, which allows fast onset of action. Effect compartment concentrations rise rapidly, but not quite as fast as for thiopental. The rapid distribution to tissues and high hepatic clearance account for rapid recovery after a bolus dose. Steady-state volume of distribution is large, but clearance is high.

Hepatic metabolism of propofol is by glucuronidation (40%) through the hydroxyl group and oxidation (60%) to 4-hydroxypropofol, a quinol derivative thought to be responsible for the green colour of urine. CYP 2B6 and, to a lesser extent, CYP 2C9, are the hepatic isoforms of the cytochrome P450 system involved in metabolism. The quinol undergoes 4-glucuronidation (85%) or sulphation. The metabolites are inactive and renally excreted. Hepatic metabolism is flow limited. Extrahepatic metabolism has been demonstrated.

After continuous infusion, terminal elimination half-life is long but context-sensitive half-time is short, being 20 minutes after a 12-hour infusion. This is due to rapid metabolism and slow redistribution.

Adverse effects

Unwanted movements

There are reports of persistent epileptiform activity in myotonic dystrophy following propofol. Myoclonic movements are commonly seen. Fits have also been reported up to several hours postoperatively.

Pain on injection

Pain on injection of propofol is often severe, may extend to the upper arm and shoulder, and most common when a rapid bolus is given into too small a vein. Addition of lignocaine may reduce pain. A new preparation of propofol in a 50:50 mixture of medium- and long-chain triglycerides (propofol-lipura) is associated with less pain on injection. Thrombophlebitis is rare.

Hypersensitivity

The incidence of hypersensitivity to propofol is low and less than for etomidate. Initial reports attributed the sensitivity to the preparation in the solvent Cremophor EL. Few hypersensitivity reactions attributable to the emulsion have been reported.

Support of bacterial growth

Support of bacterial growth was demonstrated with earlier preparations of propofol. Newer formulations contain ethylenediaminetetraacetic acid (EDTA) or sodium metabisulphite as preservatives.

Propofol infusion syndrome

Propofol infusion syndrome is a very rare but potentially lethal syndrome of metabolic acidosis, acute cardiomyopathy and skeletal myopathy associated with prolonged (> 48 hours) high-dose (> 5 mg/kg/h) infusion. It appears to be due to failure of free fatty acid (FFA) metabolism secondary to inhibition of both FFA entry into mitochondria and specific sites in the respiratory chain. It was first identified in paediatric intensive care.

Midazolam

Midazolam exists as two dynamic isomers – the open diazepine ring form is water soluble, but the closed-ring form is not. It is presented as a solution at pH 4, favouring the ionised, open-ring isomer. On intravenous injection, a rise in pH alters the equilibrium that favours ring closure and passage across the blood–brain barrier.

Dose of midazolam

The dose of midazolam is 0.15–0.3 mg/kg for induction. The onset of anaesthesia is slower than for other agents and less predictable.

Midazolam is more frequently used as a sedative agent by infusion (2–5 μg/kg/min) in intensive care.

Co-induction with a small intravenous dose (1–3 mg of midazolam) allows a reduction in the dose of propofol required for induction and adds to the hypnotic and amnesic effect.

A combination of midazolam and opioids with nitrous oxide can also be used for intravenous anaesthesia.

Use as a premedicant

Midazolam can be administered by the intranasal (0.2 mg/kg), oral (0.5 mg/kg) or rectal (0.3–0.5 mg/kg) routes. It has an unpleasant bitter taste that needs masking, particularly for children.

Pharmacodynamic effects

Mechanism of action

Midazolam is a full agonist at the benzodiazepine site on the γ-subunit of the $GABA_A$ receptor complex. It augments hyperpolarisation by increasing the frequency of channel opening (unlike thiopental, propofol and etomidate, which all increase the duration of channel opening). Its actions are reversed by the benzodiazepine antagonist flumazenil.

Central nervous system

Midazolam produces sedation and hypnosis, and is anticonvulsant. The amnesic effect is greater than that of diazepam. Intranasal midazolam (0.3 mg/kg) has been demonstrated to be more effective at terminating seizures in children than rectal diazepam.

Respiratory system

Respiratory depression occurs at a relatively low dose of midazolam, which is useful in intensive care. During induction, apnoea commonly occurs before anaesthesia is established.

Cardiovascular system

Midazolam is stable when used in combination with opioids for anaesthesia. Overdose in the elderly can cause hypotension, but in low doses blood pressure is relatively well maintained. Reflex tachycardia compensates for any fall.

Pharmacokinetics

Midazolam has a short terminal elimination half-life and a low steady-state volume of distribution, although its clearance is not high (see Table 2.4.3).

Effect compartment concentration rises more slowly than for other induction agents, accounting for a slower onset time for hypnosis.

Hepatic metabolism is by hydroxylation by CYP 3A4 and CYP 2A19 isoforms of cytochrome P450 to active compounds – 1- and 4-hydroxymidazolam. These are then glucuronidated for renal excretion.

Adverse effects

Confusional state

A confusional state is commonly encountered in intensive care after stopping a prolonged infusion of midazolam.

Ketamine

Ketamine – 2-(2-chlorophenyl)-2-methylaminocyclohexanone hydrochloride – is a phencyclidine derivative presented as a racemic mixture of *R*- and *S*-ketamine. The *S*-enantiomer is three times more potent and is associated with fewer unwanted effects. It is lipophilic but more water soluble than thiopental. It is available as a 1%, 5% or 10% solution (pH 4), with benzethonium chloride as a preservative. An enantiopure preparation of *S*-ketamine is available in some countries.

Dose of ketamine

The dose of ketamine is 1–2 mg/kg intravenously for induction. Ketamine can also be used to induce anaesthesia using the intramuscular (4–6 mg/kg) or rectal (8–10 mg/kg) routes.

Onset of anaesthesia is rapid, but recovery from a bolus dose is slower than for propofol and thiopentone.

An infusion of ketamine at 25–100 μg/kg/min may be used for maintenance of anaesthesia. Ketamine, unlike other induction agents, is an analgesic agent even at subanaesthetic dosage.

Ketamine produces a different form of anaesthesia from other agents, known as dissociative anaesthesia. Muscle tone is maintained, spontaneous respiration is preserved and there is profound analgesia and amnesia. Patients appear to keep their eyes open and involuntary movement is common. It is useful in the asthmatic patient and for children undergoing short, painful procedures.

Unpleasant emergence phenomena restrict the usefulness of ketamine.

Pharmacodynamic effects

Mechanism of action

Ketamine is a non-competitive inhibitor at the *N*-methyl-D-aspartate (NMDA) receptor. It is also a ligand at opioid receptors, both μ and κ, where *S*-ketamine is more potent than *R*-ketamine.

Central nervous system

Unlike propofol and thiopental, ketamine increases cerebral blood flow and metabolism and intracranial pressure, making it unsuitable for neuroanaesthesia. Central sympathetic stimulation and inhibition of catecholamine (and serotonin) reuptake leads to increases in catecholamine levels. These can be prevented by premedication with 2 μg/kg clonidine intramuscularly. Movement of the eyes and limbs may occur spontaneously during anaesthesia.

Respiratory system

Respiratory depression is much less with ketamine than with other induction agents. Pharyngeal reflexes are preserved. Ketamine is a powerful bronchodilator owing to its indirect sympathomimetic activity.

Cardiovascular system

Heart rate, blood pressure, cardiac output and myocardial oxygen consumption all increase on induction with ketamine. Indirect sympathomimetic effects predominate over direct negative inotropic and vasodilatatory effects. Ketamine sensitises the heart to small doses of epinephrine (adrenaline) and can precipitate arrhythmias in the anxious patient.

Pain

Ketamine reduces central sensitisation after tissue injury and secondary hyperalgesia. It prevents growth of new pain pathways by inhibition of c-*fos* oncogene induction. Pre-emptive analgesic effects and opioid sparing are seen at low doses (0.15 mg/kg).

Reports suggest that ketamine is useful in the treatment of neuropathic pain. Ketamine appears to have found a useful role at low doses as part of a multimodal analgesic plan. A pure preparation of *S*-ketamine may replace the racemic mix for analgesic use.

Other effects

Mood and memory disturbance may be seen.

Ketamine readily crosses the placenta and fetal levels exceed maternal within 1.5–2 minutes. Apgar scores may be lower.

Pharmacokinetics

Onset of action for ketamine is less rapid than for other agents. Recovery is slower than for propofol by infusion. Metabolism of the racemate is slower than for either enantiomer, suggesting mutual inhibitory effects. *S*-ketamine is metabolised more rapidly and recovery is faster than with *R*-ketamine. High-affinity, low-capacity *N*-demethylation is associated with the CYP 2B6 isoform and high-capacity, low-affinity demethylation with CYP 3A4 and CYP 2C9 isoforms. In vivo, CYP 3A4 is probably the most important route for *N*-demethylation. Elimination follows a three-compartment model, with clearance slower than for propofol but similar to that of etomidate (see Table 2.4.3).

Adverse effects

Emergence phenomena

Emergence phenomena can occur for up to 24 hours with ketamine, and include hallucinations and vivid dreams that are very unpleasant for the patient. Their incidence is less in children. These may be reduced by premedication with a benzodiazepine or clonidine, using propofol as the maintenance agent, and by allowing a slow wake-up with minimal disturbance.

Drug of abuse

Ketamine may produce psychosis.

Contraindications

Ketamine should be avoided in patients with intracranial pathology, particularly raised intracranial pressure or penetrating eye injury. It should be used with caution in patients with hypertension.

TOTAL INTRAVENOUS ANAESTHESIA (TIVA)

Induction and maintenance of anaesthesia using the intravenous route is gaining popularity. Advantages are both clinical and environmental. Short-acting opioids and nitrous oxide may be used as adjuncts for analgesia and to reduce infusion requirements.[2]

Suitable drugs

A drug suitable for TIVA should ideally have the following pharmacokinetic profile:

- rapid onset of action – short effect compartment half-life ($t\frac{1}{2}\ k_{eo}$) (i.e. rapid equilibration between blood and brain);
- rapid offset with a constant context-sensitive half-time (CSHT, the time taken for plasma concentration to fall to half its value when the infusion is stopped) – rapid elimination, not by organ metabolism, and slow redistribution from tissues compared with metabolism;
- not accumulative – small steady-state volume of distribution.

Propofol

The pharmacokinetic profile of propofol is suited to TIVA because the combination of high lipid solubility and rapid clearance ensures plasma levels fall rapidly, even after long infusions.

Context-sensitive half-time is not a fixed value but varies according to its context (i.e. the duration of the infusion). Although the CSHT for propofol does increase with the duration of infusion, it never exceeds about 20 minutes. The time to wake-up is therefore dependent on both the duration of the infusion and the plasma concentration reached. A patient will wake up once plasma levels fall below about 1–1.2 μg/mL. Wake-up time is also affected by residual effects of any other hypnotic and analgesic drugs. There is variation between patients, which is to be expected when elimination depends on hepatic metabolism, although there do not appear to be major pharmacogenetic influences.

Propofol and remifentanil

A combination of propofol and remifentanil infusions is ideally suited to TIVA.

Remifentanil is a very short-acting opioid with a CSHT that varies very little regardless of infusion duration. It undergoes rapid ester hydrolysis with a clearance in excess of 3 L/min. Its use reduces the plasma concentration of propofol required for adequate anaesthesia by about 50%.

Remifentanil is rapidly eliminated, so awakening is much faster than with other opioids. It is important to give longer-acting analgesics before the patent awakens fully, or the analgesic effect of remifentanil will have disappeared, leaving the patient in severe pain.

Propofol and alfentanil

Alfentanil has also been used in combination with propofol for TIVA. Alfentanil has a longer CSHT than remifentanil, with a maximum of 40 minutes after a 90-minute infusion, longer than for propofol. The combination is useful for short procedures, but not for prolonged surgery.

Unsuitable drugs

Fentanyl is unsuitable for use by continuous infusion during anaesthesia. Although it has a rapid clearance its intercompartmental clearance is such that the CSHT of fentanyl rapidly escalates with increasing duration of infusion (Fig. 2.4.2).

Clinical application of TIVA

Manually controlled infusion

The Bristol infusion regimen[2] for propofol ('10–8–6') based on lean body weight, produces an approximate plasma concentration of 3.5 μg/mL, which is adequate for body surface surgery (Fig. 2.4.3). Higher infusion rates may be required for other surgery.

The technique involves premedication, induction with 3 μg/kg of fentanyl and a 1.0 mg/kg bolus of propofol. This is followed by an infusion of 10 mg/kg/h for 10 minutes then 8 mg/kg/h for the next 10 minutes with a final maintenance level of 6 mg/kg/h using 67% nitrous oxide in oxygen.

Recovery after procedures lasting up to 90 minutes is within 5–10 minutes, with minimal airway irritability and coughing.

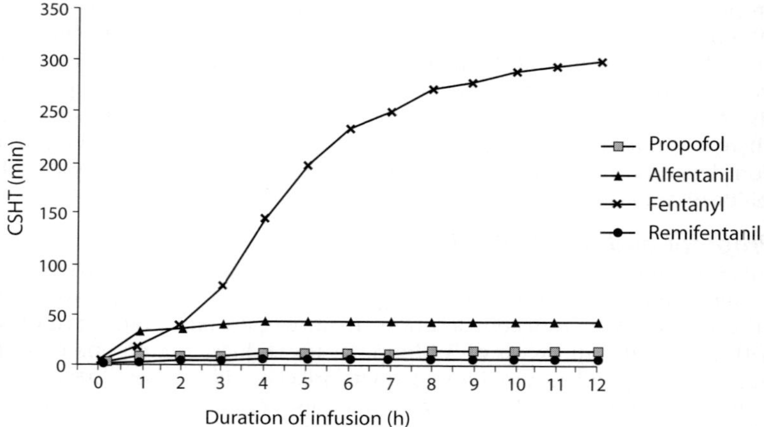

Figure 2.4.2 Context-sensitive half-times (CSHT) for propofol, remifentanil, alfentanil and fentanyl. Fentanyl is unsuitable for infusions of long duration, but has a shorter CSHT than alfentanil for infusions of less than 2 hours.

Target-controlled infusion

The manual technique described above has some disadvantages, particularly for use in surgery with great variations in stimulus intensity and for long procedures. TCI devices have been available for propofol since 1996. These use microprocessor technology incorporating a pharmacokinetic model to control the rate of infusion to maintain a given target concentration.[3] It is possible to target either plasma or site of action (effect compartment) concentration of propofol and remifentanil. Patient body weight and required target concentration are entered by the user. A visual display shows calculated concentrations for both plasma and effect compartment, together with actual infusion rate in mg/h. Often the decrement time is also displayed (i.e. time to reach predicted wake-up concentration), and there is a record of total dose infused.

The longer-established technique targets plasma concentration. The device first gives a bolus dose of propofol followed by a decreasing infusion rate according to the model. The effect compartment is in communication with plasma, but there is a rate constant for equilibration, k_{eo}, so the effect compartment concentration lags behind plasma. Onset of anaesthesia using propofol alone is therefore slower than using a single induction dose.

More recent devices give the option of targeting the effect compartment concentration because this reflects pharmacodynamic activity more closely.

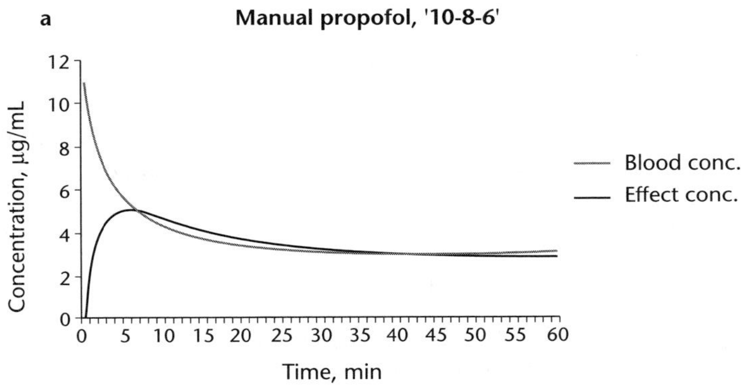

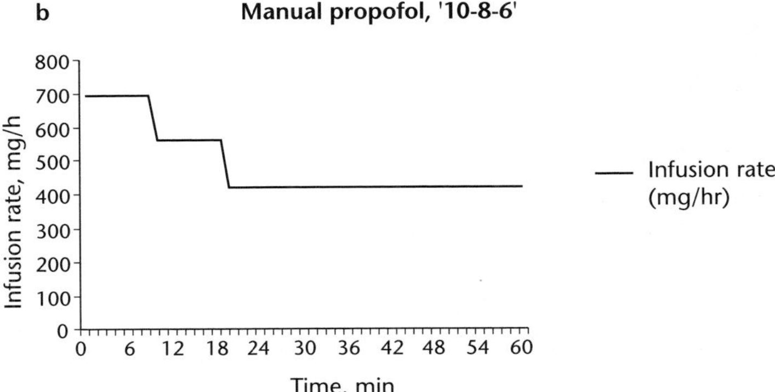

Figure 2.4.3 A. Predicted plasma and effect concentrations using a manual infusion regimen ('10–8–6'). The initial plasma concentrations are high due to a bolus dose, with peak effect compartment concentration of 5 µg/mL. This is commonly compared with TCI propofol to a target of 6 µg/mL. **B.** The corrresponding infusion rates.

Two pharmacokinetic models are available – the original model developed by Marsh et al.[4] and the newer one by Schneider et al.,[5] which uses a different value of k_{eo} and includes an additional age-dependent component. These models therefore differ in the predicted effect compartment concentration during induction and recovery. The Schneider model gives a more rapid rise in effect compartment concentration during induction (Fig. 2.4.4).

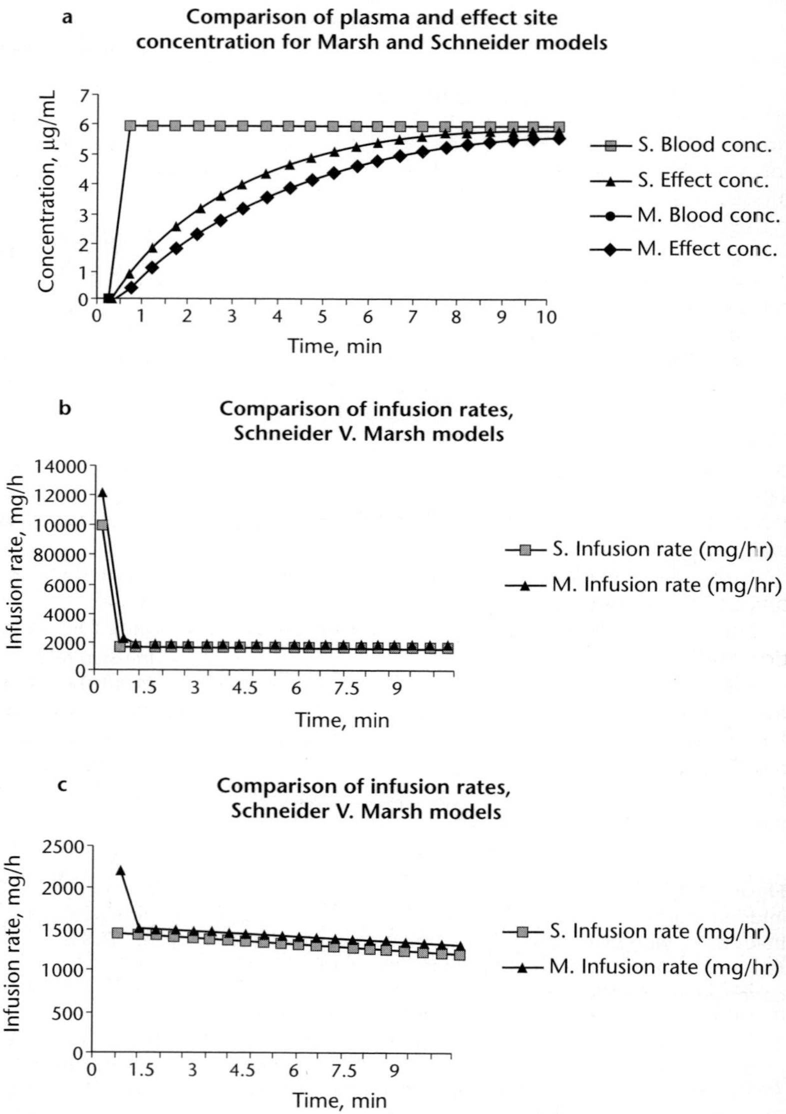

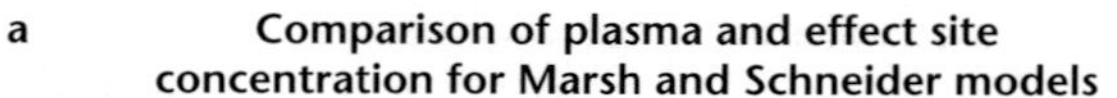

Figure 2.4.4 A. Comparison of the Marsh and Schneider models for predicted rise in plasma and effect compartment concentration for the first 10 minutes during a TCI of propofol to 6 μg/mL. The Marsh model predicts a slower rise of effect compartment concentration because the effect compartment half-life ($t^{1/2}k_{eo}$) is longer (2.6 min), than in the Schneider model ($t^{1/2}k_{eo}$ 1.8 min). **B.** Comparison of the Marsh and Schneider model infusion rates. These are similar, but the Marsh model has a slightly faster initial infusion rate. **C.** Comparison of the Marsh and Schneider model infusion rates. The Schneider model requires a slightly lower infusion rate over the entire 10-minute period of induction

Two microprocessors with different algorithms calculate targeted concentrations. One acts as a monitor to check the accuracy of the control processor, which in turn determines the pump motor speed and rate of infusion. Performance therefore depends not only on the pharmacokinetic model, but also on the algorithms used and the mechanics of the pump, syringe and infusion line.

The performance of such devices has been compared with actual plasma concentrations. There is a positive bias of about 16% (i.e. plasma concentrations tend to be a higher than calculated). Delivery must be within 5% to meet device regulations.

The Diprifusor TCI pumps also require prefilled syringes of 1% or 2% propofol that are magnetically tagged using a radiofrequency technology known as Programmed Magnetic Resonance. The magnetic tag acts as a 'signature' that can distinguish different concentrations of propofol and, once recognised, will be erased once the almost empty signal is received. This is designed as a safety feature to prevent reuse of syringes because refilling with propofol increases friction within the syringe and can alter delivery performance.

A suitable plasma target level for induction depends on premedication, opioid dose at induction, type of surgery, lean body mass and age.

The elderly need a lower target concentration than the young for induction and maintenance.

For a young day-case patient, without opioids, without intubation and for body surface surgery of short duration, a target of 6 μg/mL is suitable. For a premedicated patient requiring intracranial surgery also using a remifentanil infusion, this may be reduced to 3 μg/mL. The maintenance level is usually 4–6 μg/mL without opioids, but reduces to 2–3 μg/mL when using a remifentanil infusion.

TIVA using propofol is associated with a lower incidence of postoperative nausea and vomiting than volatile agent anaesthesia. The rapid awakening is particularly useful in day surgery, and also for neurosurgery where early neurological assessment is required. Long periods of anaesthesia using manually controlled infusion pumps, as opposed to TCI, can lead to longer wake-up times. Recovery cannot be hastened, unlike a volatile technique where agents may be removed by ventilation.

Many anaesthetists are concerned that awareness during TIVA may be greater than for inhalation anaesthesia, although a common time for awareness is during the transition from induction agent to volatile, when intubation takes place. The end-tidal volatile agent concentration needed for adequate anaesthesia shows similar variation between patients to that for plasma levels of propofol measured during TIVA. But there is no similar indirect measure of plasma propofol concentration. End-tidal volatile concentration is measured, so is a surrogate for (indirect measure of) plasma concentration of volatile, but the TCI pump for propofol gives the calculated plasma concentration of propofol according to the pharmacokinetic model. There is therefore a big difference in the confidence anaesthetists attribute to a measured against a calculated value for a plasma concentration. However, there is still a wide individual variation between end-tidal and actual plasma concentration of volatile agent. Monitoring depth of anaesthesia has therefore taken on a greater significance with the rise in popularity of TIVA.

Of the currently available monitors, bispectral analysis (BIS) is probably the most valuable.

Remifentanil

TCI remifentanil devices are available, with a pharmacokinetic model derived by Minto et al.[6] which target both plasma and effect compartment concentration. Unlike with propofol, age is an essential parameter. Effect site concentrations are achieved more rapidly than with propofol (Fig. 2.4.5).

For patients over 70 years of age the infusion rate needs to be reduced to one-third of that for a fit young patient. Typical manually controlled remifentanil infusion rates are 2–2.5 μg/kg/min for induction and 1–2 μg/kg/min for maintenance, adjusted in anticipation of variation in surgical stimulation.

For TCI remifentanil, target levels are 4–10 ng/L depending on the nature of surgery. Offset of action is rapid and almost constant despite prolonged infusion because remifentanil has an almost constant and short CSHT of 3.5 minutes. This means remifentanil can be continued to the end of surgery, after propofol has been discontinued.

Provision of adequate postoperative analgesia is essential because the analgesic effects of remifentanil will dissipate soon after discontinuing the infusion. This may be provided by 5–10 mg morphine intravenously or intramuscularly about 20 minutes before the completion of surgery.

Advantages of propofol TIVA

Advantages of propofol TIVA are:

- predictable and extremely clear-headed awakening, which is especially useful after neurosurgery;
- rapid emergence, especially when used with remifentanil;
- reduced incidence of nausea and vomiting compared to volatile anaesthesia;
- reduced release of scavenged anaesthetic gases into the atmosphere;
- safe in patients susceptible to malignant hyperpyrexia;
- paralysis not always required when used with remifentanil, avoiding reversal agents;

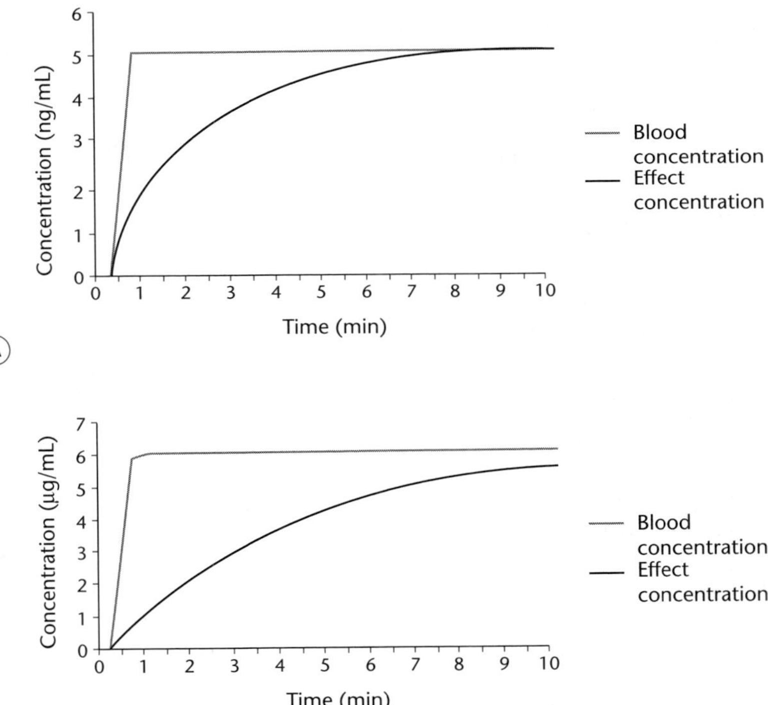

Figure 2.4.5 A. Rate of rise of effect compartment concentration for remifentanil. Remifentanil reaches an effect compartment concentration of 90% of the targeted plasma concentration within 4 minutes. **B.** Rate of rise of effect compartment concentration for propofol. Propofol takes just under 9 minutes to reach an effect compartment concentration of 90% of the targeted plasma concentration (Marsh model).

- can be used when an anaesthetised patient needs to be transferred (e.g. between radiology and theatres).

Disadvantages of propofol TIVA

Disadvantages of propofol TIVA are:

- propofol is more expensive than volatiles used in low-flow systems;
- it needs electrical power and infusion devices;

- it requires experience to run smoothly;
- there is a risk of awareness if intravenous access is not maintained (e.g. disconnection, blockage, dislodgement) – the infusion site must be visible at all times;
- there is no direct monitoring of plasma concentration, unlike end-tidal concentration of volatile agents – BIS or similar monitoring may be desirable to reduce the possibility of awareness.

SEDATION TECHNIQUES

Conscious sedation is a term used to describe a variety of techniques used to enable therapeutic and diagnostic procedures to be carried out without recourse to general anaesthesia. It is of particular importance in children, in the accident and emergency department and for imaging, dental and endoscopic procedures.[7]

Premedication with or without intermittent bolus doses of intravenous anaesthetic agents can be used for short periods of sedation. The dose required is subanaesthetic and depends on the selected combination of agents.

Low-dose TCI propofol, setting a target of 1–1.5 μg/mL, is appropriate for sedation and is particularly useful in conjunction with a regional anaesthetic technique.

Infusions of ketamine have been used successfully in children during dressing changes for burns, when analgesia requirements would otherwise be high.

Patient-controlled sedation, analagous to patient-controlled analgesia, is another technique of interest. Protocols exist for different drugs, doses and lockout times.

Sedation in intensive care

Sedation in intensive care usually consists of a combination of agents tailored to the needs of individual patients and their underlying disease processes. In critically ill patients, changes in pharmacokinetics, protein binding and metabolism lead to much more variable plasma levels as well as responses. Tolerance can also become a problem, particularly in very long-term illness.

Commonly encountered drug combinations are morphine with midazolam for long periods, and propofol with alfentanil for shorter periods. Renal failure can prolong the effects of morphine due to accumulation of the active 6-glucuronide metabolite.

Thiopental is unsuitable for long-term sedation because of accumulation, except in status epilepticus and the management of intractable increases in intracranial pressure.

Etomidate is not licensed in the UK for infusion because of adrenal suppression.

References

1. Beattie D, Jenkins T, McCullough H, et al. The in vivo activity of THRX-918661, a novel, pharmacokinetically-responsive sedative/hypnotic agent. Anaesthesia 2003; 59:100–102.
2. Spelina KR, Coates DP, Monk CR, et al. Dose requirements of propofol by infusion during nitrous oxide anaesthesia in man. I: Patients premedicated with morphine sulphate. Br J Anaesth 1986; 58:1080–1084.
3. Gray JM, Kenny GNC. Development of the technology for 'Diprifusor' TCI systems. Anaesthesia 1998; 53:22–27.
4. Marsh B, White M, Morton N, Kenny GN. Pharmacokinetic model driven infusion of propofol in children. Br J Anaesth 1991; 67:41–48.
5. Schneider T, Minto C, Schaefer S, et al. The influence of age on propofol pharmacodynamics. Anesthesiology 2000; 90:1502–1516.
6. Minto CF, Schneider TW, Egan TD, et al. Influence of age and gender on the pharmacokinetics and pharmacodynamics of remifentanil. I. Model development. Anesthesiology 1997; 86:10–23.
7. Flood RG, Krauss B. Procedural sedation and analgesia for children in the emergency department. Emerg Med Clin North Am 2003; 21:121–139.

Further reading

Engbers F. Basic pharmacokinetic principles for intravenous anaesthesia. In: Vuyk J, Schraag S, eds. Advances in modelling and clinical applications of intravenous anaesthesia. Adv Exp Med Biol 2003; 523:3–18.

Villard V. Clinical applications of pharmacokinetic and pharmacodynamic models. In: Vuyk J, Schraag S, eds. Advances in modelling and clinical applications of intravenous anaesthesia. Adv Exp Med Biol 2003; 523:57–70.

CHAPTER **2.5**

MUSCLE RELAXANTS

Neuromuscular blocking drugs provide skeletal muscle relaxation to facilitate tracheal intubation, control mechanical ventilation, and optimise surgical operating conditions. These drugs principally interrupt the transmission of nerve impulses at the neuromuscular junction. This junction is the most thoroughly studied synapse of any type, and although some questions remain unanswered it is a model for our understanding of synaptic transmission.

PHYSIOLOGY OF NEUROMUSCULAR TRANSMISSION

Motor unit

A motor neuron innervates a muscle, dividing into many nerve fibres, each of which supplies one muscle fibre. The combination of a motor neuron and the muscle fibres it innervates is a motor unit. The number of muscle cells per motor unit varies from fewer than ten to several thousand, depending on the function of the muscle. The motor neurons that control skeletal muscle are long cells with bodies in the ventral horn of the spinal cord, and axons that extend to peripheral muscle cells up to 1 metre away. The axons are typically 10–20 μm in diameter and are myelinated.

The synapse is the area of the nerve lying closest to the muscle cell, situated opposite a specialised area of the muscle cell called the endplate (Fig. 2.5.1). The synaptic cleft is only 20 nm wide. A nerve impulse causes the release of acetylcholine into the cleft, activating the postsynaptic receptors and leading to depolarisation and contraction of the muscle fibres.

Motor endplate

The motor endplate is a small specialised area of muscle that is rich in acetylcholine receptors. The surface of the muscle at the endplate is deeply folded, with many ridges and secondary clefts. The ridges have a high concentration of acetylcholine receptors on the crests of their folds. There are 1–10 million receptors at each endplate, with a high density of 10 000–20 000/μm^2.

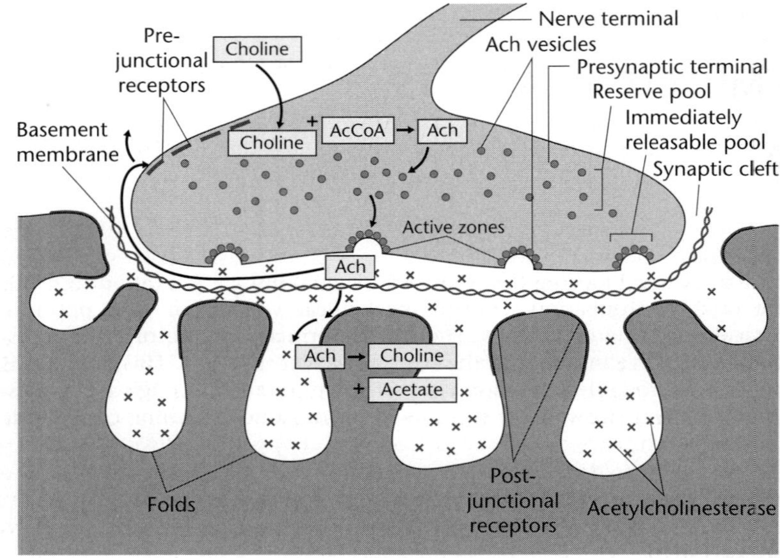

Figure 2.5.1 Synthesis, storage and release of acetylcholine and its interaction with the post-synaptic nicotinic receptor before being broken down by acetylcholinesterase. AcCoA, acetylcoenzyme A. Reproduced from Donati F. Physiology: nerve junction and muscle. In: Harper NJN, Pollard BJ, eds. Muscle relaxants in anaesthesia. London: Edward Arnold; 1995; 1–12.

Acetylcholine synthesis, storage and release

Acetylcholine is synthesised in the presynaptic terminal from the substrates choline and acetate, catalysed by choline acetyltransferase. The majority of the choline is derived from extracellular fluid. Most of this choline comes from the diet although a small amount is synthesised in the liver. About half the choline formed by the breakdown of acetylcholine at the neuromuscular junction is taken up again into the nerve terminals by a carrier-facilitated transport mechanism before being converted back to acetylcholine.

Different pools or vesicles of acetylcholine in the nerve terminal have variable availability for release. About 1% of the vesicles form the immediately releasable store responsible for the maintenance of transmitter release under conditions of low nerve activity. Nearly 80% of acetylcholine is in a reserve pool, released in response to nerve impulses. The remainder is called the stationary store.

Each vesicle contains approximately 12 000 molecules of acetylcholine. Acetylcholine is loaded into the vesicles by an active transport process in the vesicle membrane involving a magnesium-dependent proton-pumping ATPase.

The release of acetylcholine may be spontaneous or in response to a nerve impulse. Random miniature endplate potentials (MEPP) of 0.5–1 mV may be detected by an intracellular electrode in the absence of an axon potential.

When a nerve impulse invades the nerve terminal, calcium channels in the terminal membrane are opened. Calcium enters the nerve terminal and there is a calcium-dependent synchronous release of the contents of from 50 to 100 vesicles.

To enable the contents of the vesicle to be released, the vesicles must be docked at special release sites (active zones) in that part of the terminal where the axonal membrane faces the postjunctional acetylcholine receptors. These are the vesicles from the immediately releasable store. Once the vesicle contents have been discharged, they are rapidly refilled from the reserve store. The reserve vesicles are anchored to actin fibrils in the cytoskeleton by vesicular proteins called synapsins. Some of the calcium ions that enter the axoplasm on arrival of the nerve impulse bind to calmodulin, which then activates an enzyme, protein kinase 2. Protein kinase 2 phosphorylates synapsin, which dissociates from the vesicle allowing it to move forward to the release site. The docking of the vesicle and subsequent discharge of the vesicular contents involves several other proteins.

Acetylcholine release and receptor stimulation in response to a nerve action potential is far greater than that required to elicit a single muscle fibre contraction. This large safety margin means that up to 70–80% of receptors can be occupied by a non-depolarising muscle relaxant before surgical relaxation develops. Conversely, reversal can be clinically adequate even though many receptors are still blocked.

Acetylcholine receptors

Acetylcholine receptors in the postjunctional membrane of the motor endplate are of the nicotinic type. They are made up of five protein subunits, designated α, β, γ, δ and ε joined to form a channel that penetrates through and projects on each side of the membrane. The subunits have different molecular weights and properties. All receptors contain two α-subunits and one δ-, β- and ε-subunit. In the fetus, γ replaces ε.

The protein subunits are assembled like barrel staves into cylindrical receptors. Each receptor has a central funnel-shaped core, which is an ion channel 4 nm in diameter at the entrance, narrowing to less than 0.7 nm within the membrane. The receptor is 11 nm in length and extends 2 nm into the cytoplasm of the muscle cell.

When acetylcholine receptors bind to the pentameric complex, they induce a conformational change in the proteins of the α-subunits which opens the channel. Potassium ions leak from the inside of the cell to the outside, but this movement is minor compared to the movement of sodium ions from the outside to the inside.

The inside of the cell has a resting membrane potential of –80 mV with respect to the outside. Sodium ions are attracted to the inside of the cell, which induces depolarisation. Once a threshold of –50 mV is reached, voltage-gated sodium channels on the sarcolemma are opened and allow the flow of sodium ions into the muscle. This increases the rate of depolarisation, forming an action potential that passes around the whole sarcolemma, causing muscle contraction.

Only 6–25% of acetylcholine normally released is required to reach the threshold potential. The activated acetylcholine receptor stays open for 1 ms. This receptor also acts as a switch, which is closed until the acetylcholine binds to the two α binding sites. The receptor then snaps open and passes current. When the acetylcholine leaves, the channel shuts and the current ceases.

Acetylcholinesterase

Acetylcholine molecules that do not react with a receptor or are released from the binding site are destroyed almost immediately by acetylcholinesterase in the junctional cleft. This protein enzyme is secreted from the muscle, but remains attached to it by thin stalks of collagen attached to the basement membrane. Acetylcholine is destroyed in less than 1 ms after it has been released.

Other acetylcholine receptors

As well as the postjunctional receptors described above, there are also prejunctional and extrajunctional acetylcholine receptors.

Prejunctional receptors

Prejunctional receptors are nicotinic receptors that control an ion channel specific for sodium, which is essential for the synthesis and mobilisation of acetylcholine. They contain protein subunits and are blocked by D-tubocurarine, resulting in 'fade' and exhaustion. They are also blocked by aminoglycosides and polymyxin antibiotics.

Extrajunctional receptors

Extrajunctional receptors tend to be concentrated around the endplate, where they mix with postjunctional receptors, but may also be found anywhere on the muscle membrane. The adult ε unit is replaced by the fetal γ unit.

Extrajunctional receptors are not found in normal active muscle, but appear very rapidly after injury or whenever muscle activity has ended. They can appear within 18 hours of injury and an altered response to neuromuscular blocking drugs can be detected within 24 hours of the insult.

There is a difference in the response to depolarising and non-depolarising muscle relaxants when large numbers of extrajunctional receptors are present. Resistance to non-depolarising relaxants develops, yet there is an increased sensitivity to depolarising relaxants such as suxamethonium. In its most extreme form the increased sensitivity to suxamethonium results in a lethal hyperkalaemic response. Suxamethonium depolarises both postjunctional and extrajunctional receptors with an exaggerated efflux of intracellular potassium resulting in hyperkalaemia. The longer opening time of the ion channel on the extrajunctional receptor also results in a larger efflux of ions from each receptor.

Physical channel blockade

Many different drugs, apart from muscle relaxants, are capable of blocking ion channels at the neuromuscular junction and preventing depolarisation. This blockade can occur in two modes – blocked when open and blocked when closed.

Physical block by a molecule of an open channel (by cationic drugs only) relies on the channel being open in the first place, and the development of this is proportional to the frequency of channel opening. Provided its molecular size is small enough and concentration high enough, any drug may enter and occlude open ion channels. This mechanism may explain the synergy that occurs with certain drugs such as local anaesthetics, antibiotics and other muscle relaxants. In addition, the difficulty in antagonising profound neuromuscular blockade may be due to open channel block by the muscle relaxant itself.

Tricyclic drugs and naloxone may cause physical blockade of a closed channel by impeding interaction of acetylcholine with the receptor.

CHARACTERISTICS OF MUSCLE RELAXANTS

Muscle relaxants used in anaesthesia can be classified as:

- non-depolarising agents (tachycurares);
- depolarising agents (leptocurares).

Under certain circumstances depolarising agents can exert a non-depolarising effect, the so-called phase 2 block described below. Muscle relaxation can also be produced centrally by deep general anaesthesia or peripherally by nerve block.

Mechanisms of neuromuscular block

Cholinergic agonists (such as suxamethonium) and antagonists (such as vecuronium and atracurium) compete at the α-subunit binding site on the nicotinic receptor.

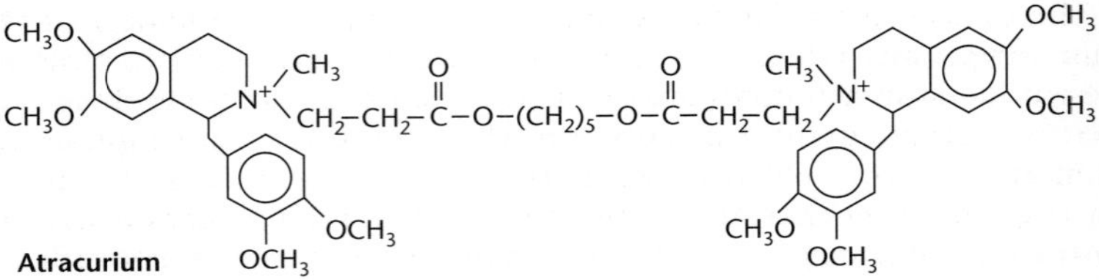

Atracurium

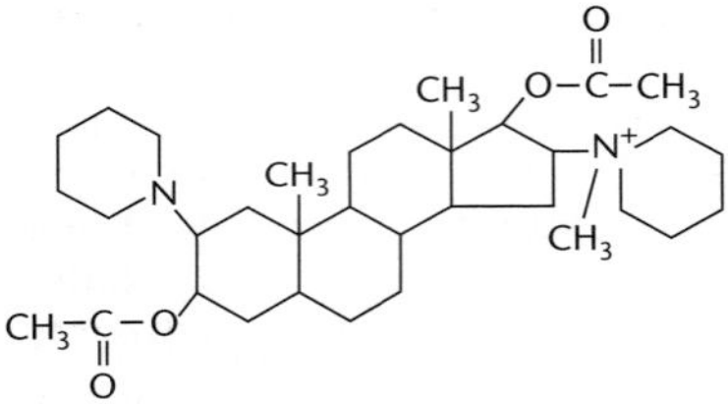

Vecuronium

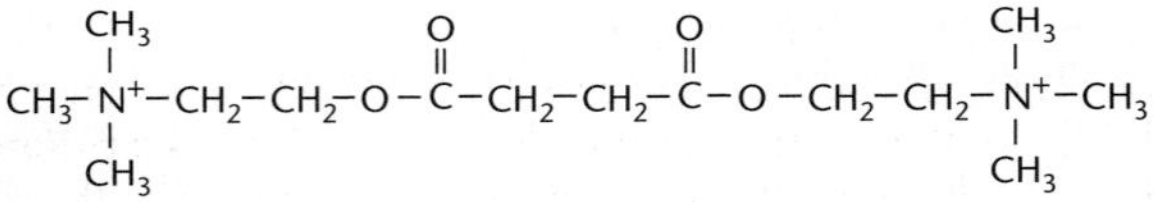

Suxamethonium

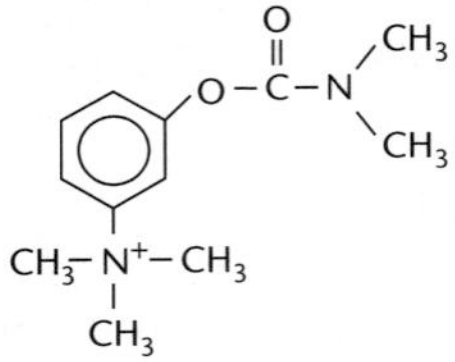

Neostigmine

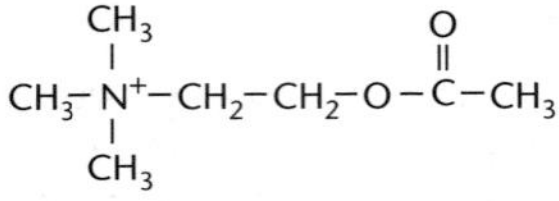

Acetylcholine

Figure 2.5.2 Chemical structures of atracurium, vecuronium, suxamethonium, neostigmine and acetylcholine.

Neuromuscular blocking drugs are positively charged quaternary ammonium compounds (Fig. 2.5.2). The positive charge combines with the α-subunit in the same way as the quaternary nitrogen radical of acetylcholine.

All currently available blocking drugs contain one or more quaternary ammonium groups, which are separated by a lipophilic bridging structure of varying length. The lipophilic bridge may be a major determinant of potency.

With a depolarising or non-competitive block, the drug occupies the α-subunits of a receptor binding site to produce depolarisation, and remains attached for longer than acetylcholine, rendering the receptor insensitive to further stimulation.

With a non-depolarising or competitive block, the drug competes with acetylcholine to occupy the receptor-binding site but does not produce any initial stimulation or depolarisation.

Depolarising (non-competitive) neuromuscular block

The only depolarising drug now available in the UK is suxamethonium chloride (succinylcholine). It is comparable to two molecules of acetylcholine linked together. If the two quaternary ammonium radicals of suxamethonium interact with two α-subunits of a receptor they open the ion channel in the same way as acetylcholine.

Because suxamethonium is not metabolised by acetylcholinesterase in the synaptic cleft, depolarisation of the endplate continues for longer than with acetylcholine, inactivating the voltage-gated sodium channels in the muscle membrane, which are immediately adjacent to the motor endplate. A zone is created around the endplate through which impulses temporarily cannot pass, preventing further action potentials. The muscle becomes flaccid and repolarisation does not occur. Recovery only occurs as the drug diffuses away from the receptor down a concentration gradient as the plasma level falls.

Desensitisation block

Prolonged exposure of the neuromuscular junction to agonists (acetylcholine or depolarising drugs) leads to receptor desensitisation. This may represent a safety mechanism that prevents overexcitation. The membrane potential may return almost to its resting level despite the continued presence of the agonist, yet neuromuscular transmission remains blocked. The exact mechanism of desensitisation block is not fully understood.

Phase 2 block

High doses of suxamethonium (between 3 and 17 mg/kg) generate a phenomenon known as phase 2 block (previously called dual block), when a short-lived depolarising block changes into a non-depolarising block, characterised by fade of the train of four (TOF, see page 196), tetanic fade, and post-tetanic facilitation. It may be reversed by low doses of anticholinesterase.

Possible mechanisms of phase 2 block include postjunctional receptor desensitisation, postjunctional ion channel block or presynaptic receptor blockade inhibiting acetylcholine synthesis or release.

Features of depolarising neuromuscular blocking drugs

Depolarising neuromuscular blocking drugs have the following features:

- they cause muscle fasciculation (but not in myasthenic humans and some other species), and extraocular muscles exhibit a tonic response;
- the sodium channels are blocked open, the muscle is unresponsive to other mechanical or electrical stimuli, and repolarisation does not happen until phase 2 block develops, when the resting membrane potential returns to –80 mV;
- there is fast dissociation at receptors;
- the block is not reversed by neostigmine or other anticholinesterases;
- in partial paralysis there is depression of muscle twitch, no 'fade' and no post-tetanic facilitation;
- they are potentiated by isoflurane, respiratory alkalosis, hypothermia and magnesium;
- they are antagonised by acidosis and non-depolarising relaxants;
- repeated or continuous use leads to phase 2 block.

Non-depolarising (competitive) neuromuscular block

Non-depolarising drugs do not alter the structural conformation of the acetylcholine receptor, but prevent depolarisation by combining reversibly with one or both of the α-subunits, preventing access by acetylcholine and opening of the ion channel. This results in a lower endplate potential, which does not reach the threshold necessary to fire off a propagating action potential. This is a dynamic situation with the various molecules repeatedly combining and being released from the receptor. The outcome (i.e. neuromuscular transmission or block) depends on the relative concentrations of acetylcholine and the blocking drug, and their relative affinities for the postsynaptic nicotinic receptor: 70–80% of receptors have to be occupied by a non-depolarising drug before the response to nerve stimulation is affected. Thus during recovery from a non-depolarising block, even when respiratory force and vital capacity are normal and head lift is sustainable for 5 seconds, 70% of the postsynaptic receptors may still be occupied by the drug.

The phenomena of fade and post-tetanic facilitation are thought to be due to block of the prejunctional nicotinic receptor. The blocking drug is thought to inhibit the positive acetylcholine feedback, which stimulates acetylcholine synthesis and mobilisation in the presynaptic nerve endings.

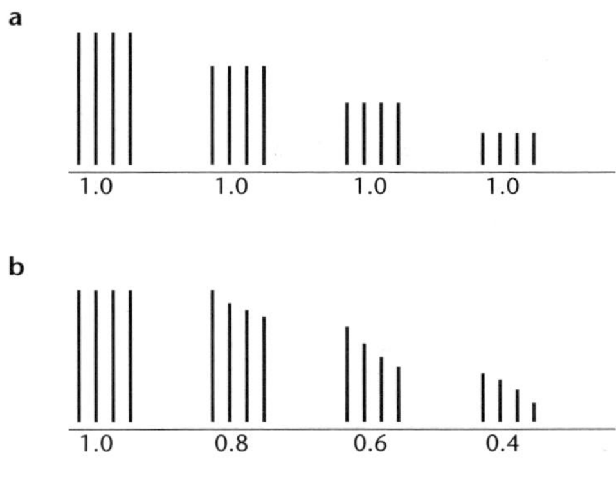

Figure 2.5.3 Representation of train of four (TOF) responses to a depolarising (A) and a non-depolarising (B) relaxant. Note there is no fade with the depolarising relaxant (T_4/T_1 ratio remains at 1.0) and progressive fade with the non-depolarising relaxant (T_4/T_1 ratio decreases to 0.4) as blockade develops.

Features of non-depolarising neuromuscular blocking drugs

Non-depolarising neuromuscular blocking drugs have the following features:

- no muscle fasciculation;
- they are mostly hydrophilic mono- or bisquaternary salts with interonium distances of 0.7–1.4 nm;
- they have a relatively slow onset (1–5 min) and slow dissociation at receptors;
- they are reversed by anticholinesterases;
- the relaxed muscle remains responsive to other mechanical and electrical stimuli;
- in partial paralysis there is depression of muscle twitch, 'fade' and post-tetanic facilitation, followed by exhaustion (Fig. 2.5.3, see also p. 196);
- the effects are reduced by suxamethonium (but not in myasthenics);
- they are potentiated by volatile agents, acidosis, magnesium and hypokalaemia;
- mild cooling antagonises their effects, but further cooling below about 33°C potentiates them.

Pharmacokinetics

The concentration of drug at the receptor (biophase) is in equilibrium with the plasma concentration, which in turn depends on the dose administered and its individual pharmacokinetic behaviour. A relationship therefore exists between plasma concentration and the degree of paralysis, and the time course of action of non-depolarising muscle relaxants is a reflection of the plasma concentration–elimination curve. Pharmacokinetic variables can be calculated from this curve (Table 2.5.1).

As a result of the positively charged quaternary ammonium groups all muscle relaxants are highly water soluble, relatively insoluble in fat and confined to the extracellular fluid. They are poorly absorbed from the gut and their onset is delayed when administered intramuscularly.

Protein binding of muscle relaxants varies between 30 and 85%, and is influenced by changes in protein concentration in disease and protein binding of other drugs. This influences the volume of distribution, metabolism and excretion of the relaxants.

For most muscle relaxants a two-compartment model is suitable and thus two half-lives can be determined: the distribution half-life ($t\frac{1}{2}\alpha$) and the elimination half-life ($t\frac{1}{2}\beta$). The volume of distribution is limited owing to high water solubility.

Drug	Vd_{ss} (L/kg)	Clearance (mL/kg/min)	Excretion	
			Urinary (%)	Biliary (%)
Atracurium	0.09	6.6	10	–
Cisatracurium	0.15	4.5–5.7	15	–
Doxacurium	0.22	2.7	25–30	–
Mivacurium	0.2–0.27	55	<10	–
Gallamine	0.2	1.3	95	<1
Pancuronium	0.24	1.8	40	10
Pipecuronium	0.35	3.0	38	2
Rocuronium	0.21	2.9	9	54
D-Tubocurarine	0.30	2.3	45	–
Vecuronium	0.20	5.3	15	40

Table 2.5.1 Pharmacokinetic data of muscle relaxants

Volume of distribution and clearance can be markedly affected by hepatic and renal disease, and cardiovascular disturbances.

Reduction in cardiac output usually leads to slower and lesser distribution, with lengthening of $t^1\!/_2\alpha$, slower onset of action, and eventually a stronger effect.

In hypovolaemia the volume of distribution is smaller and peak concentration higher, with a stronger clinical drug effect.

In patients with oedema the volume of distribution increases and plasma concentrations are lower, with a weaker clinical effect.

Renal function

Many relaxants are strongly dependent on renal excretion for their elimination. Only suxamethonium, mivacurium, atracurium and cisatracurium are independent of renal function.

Plasma cholinesterase activity is frequently decreased in renal failure, prolonging the effects of suxamethonium and mivacurium.

Changes in renal function have a significant impact on clearance and elimination, but minimal effect on volume of distribution and $t^1\!/_2\alpha$.

Liver function

In comparison with renal function, liver function is a modest determinant of the pharmacokinetics of muscle relaxants.

Decreased liver perfusion (e.g. in shock) results in a lower clearance and prolongation of paralysis.

Increased extraction ratio (e.g. enzyme induction) leads to increased metabolism and a shorter effect for some relaxants.

Decreased protein binding in hypoproteinaemia can increase liver extraction (if not already maximal) and shorten the duration of action.

Cirrhosis may increase the volume of distribution and cause an apparent resistance to many non-depolarising muscle relaxants.

Plasma cholinesterase levels may be depressed in hepatic failure, prolonging the effects of suxamethonium and mivacurium.

Age

Neonates and infants have a decreased plasma clearance, prolonged elimination and prolonged paralysis. In addition the initial volume of distribution is increased, leading to a relative resistance to relaxants.

The elderly usually have a decrease in total body water, lean body mass and protein binding, resulting in an altered volume of distribution and plasma clearance of most relaxants. Increased sensitivity and prolonged effects are seen. A decrease in renal function and renal blood flow contributes to a decreased clearance with a more prolonged effect of muscle relaxants.

Pharmacodynamics

Muscle relaxants have neither anaesthetic nor analgesic properties. Therapeutic doses produce the following effects in sequence: ptosis, imbalance of extraocular muscles with diplopia (which rarely may last several days), relaxation of muscles of the face, jaw, neck and limbs, and finally relaxation of the abdominal wall and diaphragm.

Respiration

Paralysis of respiratory muscles causes apnoea. The diaphragm is less sensitive than other muscles and is usually the last to be paralysed.

Cardiovascular effects

Hypotension with D-tubocurarine, hypertension with pancuronium, tachycardia with gallamine, rocuronium and pancuronium, and skin flushing and hypotension with atracurium (Table 2.5.2).

Histamine release

D-Tubocurarine is the most likely to cause histamine release and vecuronium is the least likely. True allergy with antibody formation is rare, but more frequent in females and atopic individuals. Often there is no obvious history of previous exposure.

Drug	Histamine release[a]	Ganglionic effects	Vagolytic activity	Sympathetic stimulation
Suxamethonium	+	Stimulation	[b]	0
Atracurium	+	0	0	0
Cisatracurium	0	0	0	0
Doxacurium	0	0	0	0
Mivacurium	+	0	0	0
Gallamine	0	0	++	+
Pancuronium	0	0	+	+
Pipecuronium	0	0	0	0
Rocuronium	0	0	±	0
Tubocurarine	++	Blockade	0	0
Vecuronium	0	0	0	0

[a]Histamine release is dose dependent and less pronounced if drugs are given slowly over 75 s
[b]Suxamethonium may cause bradycardia by muscarinic stimulation at the sinoatrial node

Table 2.5.2 Cardiovascular side-effects of muscle relaxants

CLINICAL USE

Following induction of anaesthesia and intravenous administration of the muscle relaxant, the patient's lungs are gently inflated using a face mask, taking care not to inflate the stomach. Anaesthesia is maintained by inhalation or the intravenous route. Tracheal intubation is possible when the relaxant has taken its full effect after 1–3 minutes.

The following signs suggest the need for more relaxant:

- hiccough due to contraction of the periphery of the diaphragm, abdominal wall tightening, coughing on the tracheal tube, or decreased compliance of the chest wall;
- irregular capnograph pattern;
- as indicated by neuromuscular monitoring.

These should be distinguished from signs of light anaesthesia or inadequate analgesia, such as muscle movement in the limbs, head or neck in response to surgical stimulation, or sympathetic activity (i.e. sweating, raised blood pressure and pulse).

Choice of non-depolarising relaxant

The ideal muscle relaxant would have the following characteristics:

- non-depolarising – most side-effects of suxamethonium are related to its depolarising characteristics;
- rapid onset of action, enabling intubation within 45 seconds of administration so that it may be used in a rapid sequence induction technique;
- predictable duration of action, no accumulation, same elimination rate regardless of dose given, and antagonism by a suitable drug;
- no histamine release – this has classically been a problem associated with the benzylisoquinolinium drugs such as D-tubocurarine or atracurium;
- no vagolytic or ganglion blocking action resulting in cardiovascular side-effects;
- potency – increased potency may give fewer side-effects, but lower potency seems necessary for a rapid onset of action;
- properties unaltered by renal or hepatic dysfunction and metabolites should have no pharmacological action.

The duration of surgery will influence the choice of muscle relaxant:

- ultra-short acting (e.g. suxamethonium);
- short duration (e.g. mivacurium);
- intermediate duration (e.g. atracurium, vecuronium, rocuronium, cisatracurium);

- long duration (e.g. pancuronium, D-tubocurarine, doxacurium, pipecuronium).

  The following relaxants are suggested:

- for rapid sequence induction – suxamethonium, or if this is contraindicated, rocuronium;
- for haemodynamic stability (e.g in hypovolaemia or severe heart disease) – vecuronium;
- in renal or hepatic failure – atracurium, cisatracurium or mivacurium;
- in myasthenia gravis (if relaxants are essential) – initially one-tenth of the normal dose of atracurium and then titrate against response from neuromuscular monitor.

PHARMACOLOGY OF SPECIFIC MUSCLE RELAXANTS

Suxamethonium is the only depolarising neuromuscular blocking drug available in the UK. Non-depolarising blocking drugs can be subdivided into two groups of chemical compounds – the benzylisoquinolinium compounds and the aminosteroids (Table 2.5.3).

Drug	ED_{95} (mg/kg)[a]	Intubating dose (mg/kg)	Onset time (s)[b]	Clinical duration (min)[c]
Suxamethonium	0.3	1.0	60	10
Atracurium	0.23	0.5	110	43
Cisatracurium	0.05	0.15	150	45
Doxacurium	0.025	0.05	250	83
Mivacurium	0.08	0.2	170	16
Gallamine	3.0	3.5	240	80
Pancuronium	0.07	0.1	220	75
Pipecuronium	0.045	0.08	300	95
Rocuronium	0.3	0.6	75	33
D-Tubocurarine	0.5	0.5	220	80
Vecuronium	0.05	0.1	180	33

[a]ED_{95} is the mean dose that depresses twitch height by 95%
[b]Onset time is the time to 95% depression of twitch height following an intubating dose
[c]Clinical duration is time to 25% recovery of twitch height

Table 2.5.3 Pharmacodynamic data of muscle relaxants

Depolarising neuromuscular blocking drugs

SUXAMETHONIUM CHLORIDE

Suxamethonium chloride is the dicholine ester of acetylcholine. It is presented as a clear colourless aqueous solution of pH 3.0–5.0 with a shelf-life of 2 years, and stored at 4°C. Spontaneous hydrolysis occurs in warm or alkaline conditions.

Dose

The dose of suxamethonium is 0.3–1.1 mg/kg as an intravenous. bolus. It is effective within 30 seconds and lasts for several minutes, with complete recovery in 10–12 minutes.

Suxamethonium is rapidly acting by virtue of rapid redistribution to the neuromuscular junction and its depolarising mode of action. Its effect is terminated by diffusion away from the neuromuscular junction followed by rapid redistribution and hydrolysis. Elimination is by hydrolysis by plasma cholinesterase and its elimination half-life is 3.5 minutes.

With suxamethonium, blood pressure increases, and bradycardia occurs, especially in children or after a second dose, when prior administration of atropine is advised. There may be a small increase in intracranial pressure, although rapid control of the airway and $Pa\text{CO}_2$ is of greater importance for brain protection. There is an increase in intraocular pressure. Although gastric pressure is increased, barrier pressure (upper and lower oesophageal sphincter pressure) is maintained, so there is no increased tendency for regurgitation.

Mechanism of action

Suxamethonium acts by stimulation of the acetylcholine receptor and depolarisation. Persistence of the agonist at the receptor prevents repolarisation of the endplate, which is therefore refractory to further stimulation. As the suxamethonium diffuses away from the junctional cleft repolarisation occurs and muscle action potentials are once more possible. The block may be enhanced by anticholinesterases.

Clinical features

Suxamethonium has a rapid onset, with muscle fasciculation as groups of muscle fibres are depolarised. Neuromuscular monitoring shows reduced single twitch height, reduced TOF (see page 196), all of equal amplitude, no tetanic fade and no post-tetanic facilitation.

Abnormalities of suxamethonium metabolism

Plasma cholinesterase seems to have no known physiological purpose. Its half-life is about 7–10 days. Abnormal inherited genetic variants of plasma cholinesterase were first identified by the extent to which the enzyme is inhibited by dibucaine, the percentage inhibition using benzylcholine as substrate being called the dibucaine number. The normal value is 75–85%; heterozygotes for the atypical gene have numbers of about 50% and homozygotes about 30%. Different abnormal genetic variants have also been identified using inhibition by sodium fluoride. Other rarer variants have been identified, such as the 'silent' gene.

The atypical genes are autosomal – 1 in 3000 of the population is homozygous, when hydrolysis proceeds at only 5% per hour and there is 1–2 hours of apnoea after suxamethonium, during which phase 2 block may develop. In the commoner heterozygote (about 1 in 25 of the population), apnoea lasts only 10–20 minutes.

Cholinesterase deficiency may also be acquired, as in liver disease, malnutrition, carcinomatosis (reduced production), pregnancy, uraemia, connective tissue disorders or hypothyroidism. The enzyme is antagonised by anticholinesterases such as neostigmine.

Mivacurium and ester local anaesthetics such as cocaine are also metabolised by plasma cholinesterase. Their actions are prolonged if this enzyme if deficient. Esmolol and remifentanil are unaffected because they are metabolised by other esterases.

Side-effects

Hyperkalaemia

The serum potassium may rise transiently by up to 0.5 mmol/L with suxamethonium, even in the normal patient. This is exaggerated after burns, tetanus and spinal cord injuries, and also in patients with many other neurological and muscular disorders, such as stroke, cerebral palsy and muscular dystrophy. This is due to the proliferation of extrajunctional receptors, which cause a massive outpouring of potassium when stimulated by suxamethonium. It is probably safe to use suxamethonium within 24–48 hours of an acute lesion such as burns or spinal cord injury, but the safe period after injury has not been accurately determined.

Intraocular pressure

Intraocular pressure increases by 7–8 mmHg with suxamethonium, with a maximal effect 2 minutes after administration, and is due to tonic contraction of the extraocular muscles. Suxamethonium may still be used in a perforating eye injury if essential (see Ch. 5.9).

Muscle pains

Muscle pains with suxamethonium are more frequent in women, young to middle-aged adults, and those who are ambulant shortly after surgery. They may be prevented by a small dose of a non-depolarising agent 3 minutes before the suxamethonium, although a larger dose of the latter is then likely to be needed.

Malignant hyperpyrexia

Suxamethonium is one of the drugs most commonly implicated in the development of malignant hyperpyrexia, which has an incidence of 1 in 100 000 general anaesthetics.

Allergy

Suxamethonium causes the highest incidence of anaphylaxis of any muscle relaxant, but much more frequently causes histamine release from mast cells and circulating basophils, resulting in flushing or urticaria.

Dystrophia

Suxamethonium should not be given in dystrophia myotonica because it causes severe muscle rigidity, preventing respiration and intubation.

Non-depolarising blocking drugs

BENZYLISOQUINOLINIUM COMPOUNDS

Atracurium besylate

The dose of atracurium besylate is 0.3–0.6 mg/kg. It has a molecular weight of 1243, the pH of the solution is 3.5, and it is stored at 4°C. Atracurium is distributed throughout the extracellular fluid with no effective crossing of the placenta. The speed of onset, which is 1–2 minutes, and duration of action is dose dependent,20–40 minutes, even in anephric patients.

Atracurium is metabolised by Hofmann degradation and alkaline ester hydrolysis in the plasma and elsewhere in the body. The elimination half-life is 20 minutes.

Hofmann degradation is the spontaneous fragmentation of atracurium at the bond between the quaternary nitrogen and the central chain, which occurs at body temperature and pH, producing the tertiary metabolite laudanosine and a quaternary monoacrylate. Laudanosine has slow renal elimination and crosses the blood–brain barrier. It can cause convulsions in dogs if the plasma concentration is greater than 20 pg/mL, but this has not been of significance in clinical practice. Atracurium is also metabolised by ester hydrolysis, producing a quaternary alcohol and quaternary acid. It is a suitable drug for patients with impaired renal or hepatic function.

The effect of atracurium is prolonged in hypothermia.

Histamine release is observed in up to 40% of patients with doses over 0.5 mg/kg, giving transient hypotension and tachycardia associated with facial and truncal flushing. This effect can be prevented by injecting the drug slowly over 75 seconds, reducing the dose, or prior treatment with 0.1 mg/kg chlorpheniramine and 2 mg/kg cimetidine intravenously.

Cisatracurium besylate

Cisatracurium is the purified form of one of the ten isomers of atracurium. It is stored at 4°C, and is approximately three times more potent than atracurium. The dose is 0.15 mg/kg, and the duration of action is about 30 minutes.

The features of cisatracurium are similar to those of atracurium, except that it does not release histamine within the clinical dose range. It is slightly slower in onset, consistent with the inverse relationship between potency and the speed of onset observed in non-depolarising relaxants.

Cisatracurium is haemodynamically stable, non-cumulative and a suitable agent as an infusion in intensive care. It undergoes Hofmann degradation, but not hydrolysis by plasma esterases. Laudanosine levels are much lower than with atracurium.

Mivacurium chloride

The structure of mivacurium resembles that of both atracurium and doxacurium, but in common with doxacurium the ether oxygen and the carboxyl group are reversed and so do not permit Hofmann degradation. Mivacurium exhibits stereoisomerism, is a geometric isomer, and is presented as a racemic mixture – *trans–trans* (58%), *cis–trans* (36%) and *cis–cis* (6%).

Mivacurium is a short-acting muscle relaxant metabolised by plasma cholinesterase. The dose is up to 0.25 mg/kg. It is ideal for use by continuous intravenous infusion at 0.24–0.48 mg/kg/h. The duration of action is 10–20 minutes (about twice that of suxamethonium and one-half to one-third that of atracurium or vecuronium). Transient decreases in arterial pressure as a result of histamine release may be observed following doses greater than 0.15–0.2 mg/kg.

Although the *trans–trans* and *cis–trans* isomers are hydrolysed by plasma cholinesterase, the *cis–cis* isomer may be metabolised in part by the liver. The block is prolonged by atypical or reduced plasma cholinesterase, as with suxamethonium. Heterozygotes for the atypical enzyme show a prolongation of block by about 10 minutes.

Doxacurium chloride

Doxacurium chloride is the most potent neuromuscular blocking drug currently available. Hence it has a slow onset and very long duration of action. Although it has diester groupings, it does not undergo significant hydrolysis by plasma cholinesterase and is largely eliminated by the kidney with some hepatic excretion unchanged in the bile. The cumulative potential is difficult to ascertain because repeat dosing is rarely needed. Antagonism by anticholinesterase is satisfactory provided considerable spontaneous recovery has already taken place.

The dose of doxacurium chloride is 0.03–0.05 mg/kg, and its duration of action is over 1 hour.

Unlike other benzylisoquinolinium analogues doxacurium has no significant cardiovascular effects or histamine-releasing propensity within the clinical dose range.

D-Tubocurarine chloride

D-Tubocurarine chloride was once the main non-depolarising agent, but is no longer used in the UK. The dose is 0.3–0.5 mg/kg and its duration of action is over 40 minutes. It shows cumulation.

D-Tubocurarine chloride may cause histamine release and blockade of sympathetic ganglia, resulting in significant hypotension. It was formerly used to assist controlled hypotension.

AMINOSTEROIDS

The aminosteroids have a bulky steroidal nucleus which, when bound to the nicotinic receptor at the endplate, competitively impedes the interaction of acetylcholine with the α-subunits.

Vecuronium bromide

Ring D of the steroidal nucleus has a quaternary ammonium similar to that of pancuronium and is probably the area that interacts with the endplate nicotinic receptor. Ring A has been modified by a tertiary nitrogen, giving greater vascular stability and less stability in solution, and encouraging elimination in the bile as well as in the urine. The duration of action of vecuronium bromide is therefore shorter than that of pancuronium.

Vecuronium bromide is eliminated by spontaneous deacetylation and hepatic metabolism. Of the total dose, 10–25% is excreted in urine and the rest in bile. Most is excreted unchanged. Hepatic failure may prolong the clinical effect. Phenytoin and other anticonvulsant therapies reduce the efficacy of vecuronium by enzyme induction. There are three potential metabolites – 3-OH, 17-OH and 3,17-OH. The 3-OH metabolite is the only one found in any significant quantity and it has 50% of the neuromuscular blocking potency of vecuronium. This may cause prolonged block if used by infusion in intensive care.

The dose of vecuronium bromide is 0.1 mg/kg and its onset of action is 1–2 minutes, but this can be shortened by priming with one-tenth of the intubating dose 6 minutes before the main dose. There is minimal vagolytic activity. Vecuronium bromide is the gold standard for haemodynamic stability among muscle relaxants.

Pancuronium bromide

Pancuronium bromide is a long-acting bisquaternary aminosteroid, devoid of hormonal activity. The additional quaternary ammonium group on ring A of the steroidal nucleus enhances vagolytic activity by blocking cardiac muscarinic M_2 receptors and neuronal norepinephrine (noradrenaline) reuptake. It can also cause norepinephrine release.

Pancuronium bromide becomes strongly bound to gamma globulin and moderately bound to albumin. Less than 13% of the dose is unbound and active; 50% is excreted unchanged, of which 80% appears in the urine,

40% is deacetylated in the liver to 3-OH, 17-OH and 3,17-OH derivatives, which are eliminated in the bile. The 3-OH metabolite has some neuromuscular antagonist activity.

The dose of pancuronium bromide is 0.05–0.1 mg/kg, and the initial dose lasts 45–60 minutes. There is no histamine release. It tends to cause tachycardia and hypertension, and is safe in patients susceptible to malignant hyperpyrexia.

Rocuronium bromide

Rocuronium bromide is a monoquaternary aminosteroid. It is a rapid-onset deacetoxy analogue of vecuronium and is slightly vagolytic, resulting in a tachycardia at higher doses (more than 0.6 mg/kg). Rocuronium bromide exhibits predominantly biliary excretion and 10% is excreted in urine, but clearance is decreased in renal failure. The elimination half-life is significantly increased in patients with hepatic disease. The main metabolite,17-deacetyl rocuronium, has weak neuromuscular blocking action.

The dose of rocuronium bromide is 0.6 mg/kg. The onset of an equipotent dose is twice as rapid, but the duration is similar. Although the time to 80% block (for intubation) is more rapid than with any other non-depolarising relaxant, the overall time to 100% block is similar to that for vecuronium. Even at high doses, the onset of block is still slower than for suxamethonium.

Rocuronium bromide is stored at 4°C protected from light.

Pipecuronium bromide

Pipecuronium bromide is a quaternary aminosteroid not available in the UK. It is 25% more potent than pancuronium, but clinically and pharmacodynamically very similar, but without pancuronium's vagolytic side-effects. As 85% is excreted by the kidneys it has a prolonged effect in renal failure; 4% is metabolised by the liver to 3-desacetyl pipecuronium, and only 2% is excreted in the bile. Cumulation may occur, particularly with impaired renal function.

The dose of pipecuronium bromide is 0.05 mg/kg. It has a slow onset – over 3 minutes – and a long duration of 1–2 hours. Like other aminosteroids used clinically, it does not produce histamine.

ANTICHOLINESTERASE DRUGS

Acetylcholinesterase has an esteratic site and an anionic site in close proximity. Physiologically the positively charged quaternary amine of acetylcholine binds to the anionic site, the acetyl ester combines with the esteratic site and the acetylcholine is hydrolysed. Anticholinesterases competitively occupy these sites and prevent acetylcholine access.

Anticholinesterases have a quaternary amine group that is attracted to the anionic site and a carbamyl ester that binds covalently to the serine amino acid of the esteratic site. The quaternary amine group conveys enhanced potency and stability, and results in poor absorption following oral administration with minimal transfer of the drug across the blood–brain barrier. When neostigmine is used for the treatment of myasthenia gravis large oral doses are therefore necessary. Anticholinesterases also have some direct cholinergic agonist activity.

Anticholinesterases have widespread effects subsequent to the increased cholinergic, muscarinic and nicotinic activity. Heart rate, vasomotor tone and blood pressure are reduced. At high doses sympathetic ganglion stimulation may predominate.

Excess acetylcholine causes bronchoconstriction, increase bronchial secretion, increased gastrointestinal tone with severe colic, and increased secretion of saliva, sweat and tears. These problems are prevented by the concomitant use of muscarinic anticholinergic drugs such as atropine or glycopyrronium.

Anticholinesterases can also cause a depolarising neuromuscular blockade when used in excess or in the absence of non-depolarising blockade.

Neuromuscular blockade terminates either by endogenous elimination of the muscle relaxant drug and diffusion of the blocking agent away from the neuromuscular junction, or in the case of the non-depolarising agents the effects can be overcome in part by inhibiting the metabolism of acetylcholine.

In administering anticholinesterase drugs, the clearance of relaxants is not accelerated but the dose–response curve for neuromuscular blockade shifts to the right. The pharmacodynamic recovery is therefore accelerated. This process of reversal is superimposed upon the mechanisms responsible for relaxant clearance.

Neostigmine

Neostigmine binds to the esteratic subsite of acetylcholinesterase with its carbonate group. It is the only anticholinesterase routinely used to reverse neuromuscular blockade in anaesthesia. It can cause a depolarising block in its own right owing to build-up of acetylcholine. Phase 2 block can eventually result. The amount of neostigmine needed to cause paralysis by persistent depolarisation is much greater than that required to antagonise a clinical dose of non-depolarising relaxant.

The dose of neostigmine is 2.5 mg to a maximum of 5 mg, with atropine 1 mg or glycopyrronium 0.5 mg. Its duration of action is 40 minutes.

Neostigmine is eliminated via hydrolysis by the acetylcholinesterase that it antagonises, and by plasma cholinesterase to a quaternary alcohol. Renal excretion accounts for 50% of its clearance. Some hepatic metabolism occurs with biliary excretion.

Edrophonium

Edrophonium has similar actions to neostigmine, but is quicker in onset; however, small doses are rapidly metabolised and are not as longlasting. It is used for the assessment of myasthenia gravis, to distinguish between a myasthenic or a cholinergic crisis.

The dose of edrophonium is 1 mg/kg, repeated if necessary, with atropine or glycopyrronium.

Pyridostigmine

Pyridostigmine is used in the treatment of myasthenia gravis in total daily doses up to 720 mg (sometimes more). Its duration of action is 6 hours.

Physostigmine

Physostigmine is an anticholinesterase derived from the West African calabar bean and has a tertiary amine structure that can cross the blood–brain barrier. It does not adequately antagonise neuromuscular block, but may be used in the treatment of anticholinergic syndrome produced by atropine, hyoscine and other related alkaloids.

NEUROMUSCULAR MONITORING

Monitoring of neuromuscular function involves pulsed electrical stimulation of a peripheral motor nerve, and assessment of the muscular response.

Stimulus

Needle or surface electrodes are located over or close to a peripheral motor nerve. The stimulator pulse should be a square wave with an appropriate amplitude (i.e. low amplitude [0.5–5.0 mA] for needle electrodes and higher amplitude for skin electrodes [10–40 mA]).

The optimal duration of the pulse is 0.2 ms for various patterns of pulses including single, trains of pulses at 1–2 Hz, and tetanic bursts at 50–100 Hz. This provides supramaximal stimulation that ensures maximum recruitment of muscle fibres and provides a baseline control twitch for comparison with that obtained when using muscle relaxants.

Single twitch

A single twitch results from application of a single supramaximal stimulus every 10 seconds. The twitch height falls steadily to zero as the nicotinic postsynaptic receptor occupancy increases from 75 or 80% up to 100%. It has limited application owing to the narrow range of receptor occupancy detected (75–95%) and the requirement for a means of measuring twitch height.

Train of four

Train of four (TOF) stimulation is the application of four successive stimuli, each of which is similar to the single twitch, administered at 2 Hz every 10 seconds. The degree of neuromuscular blockade can be more objectively assessed by calculating the ratio of the fourth (T_4) and the first (T_1) measured twitch heights (T_4/T_1). For adequate respiratory function the T_4/T_1 ratio must be greater than 70%.

Tetanic stimulation

Tetanic stimulation results from application of an electrical current identical to the single twitch, but repeated at a higher frequency, usually 50 Hz, applied for 5 seconds. The frequency of 50 Hz is similar to the stimulation of a voluntary maximal muscle movement. The test is painful and can only be used during anaesthesia.

Tetanic stimulation causes mobilisation of acetylcholine from the reserve pools to the readily available store. The depletion of acetylcholine changes the intensity of the basic response and therefore it is necessary to wait 15–20 minutes before the next tetanic stimulus can be given.

Post-tetanic count

Post-tetanic count (PTC) describes the counting of responses to single twitch stimulation following a tetanic stimulation of 50 Hz for 5 seconds. This method can produce a response at relatively high levels of receptor occupancy, and a PTC less than 5 indicates profound neuromuscular blockade. A PTC greater than 15 is at least equivalent to two twitches of a TOF, and at this level reversal of remaining muscle blockade is possible.

Double burst stimulation

Double burst stimulation was introduced to improve manual assessment of fade. This consists of two tetanic bursts at 50 Hz. Each burst is separated by 750 ms. The user sees two contractions (T1 and T2). The ratio of T2 to T1 is more sensitive in detecting fade than the TOF ratio.

Sensitivities of the different modes of stimulation

The different modes of stimulation have different sensitivities. The amplitude of a single twitch does not start to diminish until about 80% of receptors are occupied by muscle relaxants. For normal neuromuscular transmission, only 20% of receptors of the motor endplate are required. Neuromuscular blockade is not complete until 90–95% of receptors are occupied. This percentage varies from muscle to muscle. Paralysis of the diaphragm does not become apparent until 90–95% of the receptors are blocked. Tetanic stimulation is the most sensitive test. The response to stimulation at 50 Hz starts to diminish when 65% of receptors are occupied.

Assessment of muscular response

A variety of methods providing an indirect measure of contractile force have been employed during neuromuscular stimulation.

Vision and touch

Vision and touch provide a simple and convenient method, but are less accurate than other methods and provide only a gross assessment of muscle response.

Mechanomyography

With mechanomyography the muscle contracts against a preload, generating a tension that is proportional to the force of contraction. This is converted to an electrical signal for measurement. Mechanomyography is more accurate than vision and touch, but does require correct positioning of the transducer, selection of the preload and immobilisation of the hand.

Acceleromyography

In acceleromyography a piezo-electrode wafer is fixed to the distal part of the digit. Acceleration is converted into an electrical signal for measurement. This technique is more objective than vision and touch, but problems with joint positioning make this technique inconvenient and inconsistent.

Electromyography

Electromyography measures muscle activity by recording the magnitude of the evoked compound potentials from either skin or needle electrodes overlying a particular muscle. This technique avoids the mechanical problems of using and calibrating transducers attached to joints, but simple alteration in hand position can alter electrode geometry enough to change the measured response.

Interpretation

A normal response to different stimulation patterns demonstrates different percentages of unoccupied or free receptors (Table 2.5.4). Clinically, depression of at least 95% of a twitch is needed to obtain absence of glottic movements, and depression of at least 90% is desirable for surgery when opening

Normal response to stimulation	Percentage of free receptors
Single twitch	>20–25
Train of four	>25–30
30 Hz tetanic	>30
50 Hz tetanic	>40
100 Hz tetanic	>50
200 Hz tetanic	>60

Table 2.5.4 Different stimulation patterns demonstrate the following percentage of unoccupied or free receptors

and closing the abdominal wall. The respiratory vital capacity will be diminished at more than 25% paralysis, but it is possible to maintain a tidal volume until about 75% paralysis. The most sensitive clinical test to evaluate residual paralysis is the 5-second head lift test.

Full recovery of the diaphragm corresponds with only 25% recovery of the adductor pollicis muscle. A much higher degree of receptor occupation is necessary in the respiratory muscles than in the peripheral muscles to obtain the same intensity of neuromuscular blockade. Monitoring of a peripheral muscle therefore enables the anaesthetist to be confident about normal respiratory muscle function when the twitch height is 100%.

SOME LANDMARKS IN THE HISTORY OF MUSCLE RELAXANTS

- 1516 – Pietro Martire D'Anghera described a South American arrow poison in his book *De Orbo Novo*;
- 1595 – Sir Walter Raleigh mentioned curare in his account of the discovery of Guiana;
- 1811 – Sir Benjamin Brodie described experiments with curare and showed that life could be maintained in curarised animals by artificial respiration. He also suggested its use in tetanus;
- 1812 – Charles Waterton introduced curare to England and extended Brodie's experiments;
- 1851 – Claude Bernarde, using nerve muscle preparations, proved that curare acts on the neuromuscular junction;
- 1851 – AW Hofmann first described a novel non-enzymatic degradation mechanism of quaternary ammonium salts, one of the mechanisms by which atracurium is broken down;
- 1891 – Hypodermic curare issued for use in tetanus by Burroughs, Wellcome and Company;
- 1935 – H King isolated the active principle D-tubocurarine from a sample of crude curare;
- 1940 – Bennett successfully used a curare preparation to modify convulsive shock therapy;
- 1942 – Griffith and Johnson reported the first use of curare in clinical anaesthesia;
- 1948 – H King elucidated the structure of D-tubocurarine;
- 1949 – Use of suxamethonium;
- 1967 – Use of pancuronium;
- 1980 – Use of atracurium and vecuronium;

Further reading

Bowman WC. Pharmacology of neuromuscular function. London: Wright; 1990.

Lee C. Structure, conformation and action of neuromuscular blocking drugs. Br J Anaesth 2001; 87:755–769.

Standaert FG. Neuromuscular physiology and pharmacology. In: Miller RD, ed. Anaesthesia. 5th edn. New York: Churchill Livingstone; 2000:735–751.

Appiah-Ankam J, Hunter JM. Pharmacology of neuromuscular blocking drugs. Br J Anaesth cited in Anaesthesia, Critical Care and Pain 2004; 4:2–7.

CHAPTER **2.6**

AIRWAY MANAGEMENT

Airway management seeks primarily to maintain and protect the airway, to allow unimpeded ventilation and a near zero incidence of aspiration of material into the respiratory tract.

The theory of airway management is relatively straightforward. The patient's airway is instrumented by either:

- a facemask;
- a supraglottic airway such as the laryngeal mask; or
- tracheal intubation.

The airway device is maintained in situ from the start to the finish of anaesthesia.

The practice is much more difficult. Substantial morbidity and mortality arise in this core duty of an anaesthetist.

The central problem is the unfavourable anatomy of the human compared with many animals. There is no continuity by means of dedicated tube from the nares to the trachea or from the mouth to the oesophagus. Instead there is a floppy-walled mixing chamber above the entrance to both trachea and oesophagus. Moreover, the mixing chamber is the crossover point at which the ventilation channel passes from posterior to anterior and the nutrition channel passes the other way, possibly a relic of ancestors dwelling in water but breathing air.

ANATOMY OF THE LARYNX

The larynx is the organ of voice, the sphincter between the pharynx and the trachea. It extends from the root of the tongue to the trachea and lies opposite C3–C6 vertebrae, higher in children and females. It is covered by the depressor muscles of the hyoid bone, the thyroid gland and the cricothyroid muscles, and is composed of the following cartilages, joined together by ligaments – thyroid, cricoid, two arytenoids, two corniculate (Santorini), two cuneiform (Wrisberg) and the epiglottis.

The cavity of the larynx extends from the superior laryngeal aperture to the lower border of the cricoid cartilage. The piriform fossa is a recess on each side, bounded by the aryepiglottic fold medially and the thyroid cartilage and thyrohyoid membrane laterally. Beneath its mucosa lie twigs of the internal laryngeal nerve, which may be blocked by topical local anaesthetic. The depression between the dorsum of the tongue and the epiglottis is divided into two valleculae by the glossoepiglottic fold. The epiglottis is not essential for swallowing, breathing or phonation.

The superior laryngeal aperture is wider in front than behind, and slopes downwards and backwards. It is bounded anteriorly by the epiglottis, laterally by the aryepiglottic folds containing the two small nodules on each side, the cuneiform anteriorly and the corniculate posteriorly, and posteriorly by the arytenoids. This view (Fig. 2.6.1) is seen at laryngoscopy.

The vestibule of the larynx is the superior part of the cavity of the larynx and extends from the aryepiglottic folds to the vestibular (ventricular) folds. Each of the latter is a ridge formed by the vestibular ligament and extends from the angle of the thyroid cartilage anteriorly, backwards along the side cavity of the larynx to the cuneiform cartilage. The vestibular folds are the false cords and the space between them is the rima vestibuli, while a depression on the sidewall of the larynx between the vestibular fold and the vocal folds (false and true cords) is the saccule of the larynx.

The vocal folds (cords) stretch from the thyroid cartilage anteriorly to the arytenoid cartilage of the corresponding side posteriorly. The space between the vocal folds is the glottis. It is bounded in front by the intermembranous part of the vocal folds; behind, by the intercartilaginous part.

The glottis is the narrowest part of the larynx in adults and measures about 2.3 cm from front to back in males, and 1.7 cm in females. In children, the narrowest part is found just below the vocal folds at the cricoid ring. The shape and width of the glottis vary with phonation and respiration and the tone of the muscles controlling it. When these are in spasm, the glottis is obliterated.

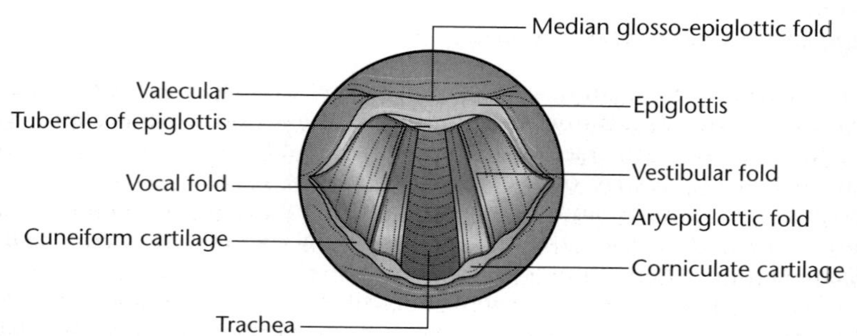

Figure 2.6.1 A laryngoscopic view of the interior of the larynx.

Extrinsic muscles

The extrinsic muscles comprise the suprahyoid group attached to the hyoid (thyrohyoid, mylohyoid, stylohyoid, geniohyoid), the infrahyoid or strap muscles (sternothyroid, omohyoid, sternohyoid) and the inferior constrictor of the pharynx. The first group elevate and the second depress the larynx, whereas the third constricts the pharynx, assisting in deglutition.

Intrinsic muscles

The vocal folds abduct during inspiration and return nearly to the midline on expiration, and on phonation they actually touch. Intrinsic muscles that open and close the glottis are:

- the posterior (open) and lateral cricoarytenoids (close);
- interarytenoid (close).

Intrinsic muscles that control the tension of the cords are:

- the cricothyroids – which tense the cords;
- posterior cricoarytenoids;
- thyroarytenoids – which relax the cords;
- vocales – which relax the cords.

Intrinsic muscles that control the inlet of the larynx are:

- the aryepiglottics;
- thyroepiglottics – in laryngeal spasm both the true and the false cords are adducted.

Nerve supply (from the vagus)

The superior laryngeal branch of the vagus arises near the base of the skull and divides into the internal laryngeal nerve (the sensory supply to both surfaces of the epiglottis and to the larynx down to the vocal cords) and the motor external laryngeal nerve (which supplies the cricothyroid muscle and the inferior constrictor of the pharynx), the division taking place slightly below and anterior to the greater cornu of the hyoid bone.

The external laryngeal nerve may be injured during ligation of the superior thyroid vessels at thyroidectomy, causing temporary huskiness of voice.

The recurrent laryngeal nerve branch of the vagus supplies the remaining intrinsic muscles and is sensory to the mucosa below the cords.

The recurrent laryngeal nerve carries abductor and adductor fibres, but if it is injured abductor, paralysis is greater than adductor paralysis. With bilateral injury there is respiratory difficulty because the cords lie together, and speech is difficult, with valvular obstruction and inspiratory stridor. Complete paralysis of both recurrent nerves inactivates both abductor and adductor muscles, but the tensing action of cricothyroid maintains cords in adduction. Paralysis of one cord may be symptomless, but paralysis of both is serious and may require surgery.

Paralysis of both recurrent and superior laryngeal nerves together (or full muscle relaxation) produces the cadaveric position with the cords relaxed midway between abduction and adduction.

Topical analgesia of the larynx may, by paralysing twigs from the external laryngeal nerves going to the cricothyroids, cause a temporary alteration in both the appearance of the cords and the voice.

All sensory nerve impulses from the larynx reach the nucleus solitarius in the medulla.

Arterial supply

The larynx is supplied by laryngeal branches of the superior and inferior thyroid arteries, which accompany the nerves.

ASSESSMENT OF THE AIRWAY

Preoperative airway evaluation, undertaken in all patients, seeks to determine which airway device is the most appropriate, and whether problems with airway management are likely.

The decision as to whether facemask, laryngeal mask or tracheal intubation is required is based on consideration of the duration and nature of surgery, the requirement for intermittent positive-pressure ventilation (IPPV) and the likelihood of airway soiling.

Prediction of difficult airway management is not always possible because the sensitivity and specificity of the tests are inadequate for the low prevalence of the condition.[1] The prevalence of Cormack and Lehane grade 3 view (epiglottis only) is 1.5% in the general population, and unexpected failed intubation (by direct laryngoscopy) with an experienced anaesthetist is 1 in 2500 in general surgical patients. Plans should always be made for unanticipated difficult facemask ventilation or intubation.

The following findings should be sought routinely.

History

- Any history of previous difficulties with airway management?
- Any past disease or surgery affecting the head, neck or mediastinum?
- Does the current disease affect the head, neck or mediastinum?
- Are there any symptoms of difficulty with breathing, difficulty with swallowing, noisy breathing, alteration of voice or gastric reflux?
- Is there a concurrent medical condition, such as rheumatoid arthritis, obstructive sleep apnoea, acromegaly or longstanding insulin-dependent diabetes mellitus that might indicate an increased likelihood of difficulty?

Examination

- Are there any swellings, scars, burns or indications of radiotherapy to the head, neck or chest?
- Do the tongue, face, jaw, chin and neck look normal in size and proportion?
- Is the patient obese, or does the patient have a beard?
- Are mouth opening and neck mobility normal?
- Are there any caps, crowns, bridges, loose or awkward teeth?
- Is the cricothyroid membrane accessible?

Predictive tests of difficult direct laryngoscopy

- mouth opening less than three fingerbreadths or 5 cm (particularly if <3 cm);
- Mallampati grade 3 or 4 (see Ch. 1.1);
- thyromental distance less than three fingerbreadths or 6 cm;
- jaw slide – inability to protrude lower incisors to reach upper incisors;
- reduction in atlanto-occipital movements.

In some cases, investigations such as chest radiography, magnetic resonance imaging or computed tomography of the airway or a flow–volume loop are needed to fully assess airway pathology.

Difficult airway management may still occur in patients who appear to be quite normal. Some have conditions such as lingual tonsil hyperplasia,[2] a vallecular cyst or unrecognised mediastinal pathology.

MAINTAINING THE AIRWAY

Facemask

To maintain a patent airway in an anaesthetised patient it is usually necessary to displace the mandible anteriorly by holding up the jaw and extending the neck. Either one or two hands are needed to accomplish this. Upper airway obstruction during facemask anaesthesia may be overcome by insertion of an oral or nasal airway. The curved Guedel (US anaesthetist, 1933) oral airway is commonly used, but with caution in those patients with loose or crowned front teeth. Biting on the airway may exert a pressure of 0.25 metric tonne on the teeth, leading to displacement. A nasopharyngeal airway avoids this problem, but may cause bleeding.

When the facemask is applied properly the reservoir bag will fill and empty with spontaneous respiration, and manual inflation to a pressure of approximately 20 cmH_2O will be possible.

Facemask anaesthesia is employed for short procedures when there is no increased risk of aspiration.

Resuscitation of the apnoeic patient by an anaesthetist is usually initially by facemask, although in untrained hands the laryngeal mask is more effective.

Difficult facemask inflation may be defined as inability to maintain oxygen saturations above 90% with 100% inspired oxygen, or to reverse signs of inadequate ventilation.[3] Difficulty may be expected in those patients who have an abnormal facial contour or those presenting with upper airway obstruction. Unexpected failed facemask ventilation is rare.

Some problem with facemask ventilation occurs in about 5% of patients, particularly those with beards, without teeth, with a body mass index (BMI) greater than 26, with a history of snoring or aged over 55 years.[4]

Laryngeal mask airway

The development of the laryngeal mask airway (LMA) series (classic, ProSeal™ and intubating) by Brain (UK anaesthetist) represents the greatest advance in airway management since intubation.

Classic

The classic LMA was introduced in 1988, and over 200 million have been inserted without recorded mortality. It is a cuffed mask designed to be placed in the pharynx, with the tip engaged in the upper oesophageal sphincter and the mask fitting closely over the laryngeal aperture. It is now made in eight sizes: size 1 neonate less than 5 kg, size 1.5 infant 5–10 kg, size 2 child 10–20 kg, size 2.5 child 20–30 kg, size 3 child or small adult 30–50 kg, size 4 adult 50–70 kg, size 5 adult 70–100 kg, size 6 adult over 100 kg. Reinforced or flexible masks are available in which the stem is wire spiralled, floppier and nonkinking.

Before use, the cuff should be deflated and lubricant applied.

After induction of anaesthesia with propofol (which depresses laryngeal reflexes), or the establishment of sufficiently deep inhalational anaesthesia, the classic LMA is introduced blindly into the hypopharynx.

The finger is placed at the junction of the stem and bowl, and the mask is pressed into the curve of the palate and advanced into the pharynx. Over 30 alternative insertion techniques have been described. If the epiglottis is folded downwards by the tip of the mask on insertion, the airway may be obstructed. It is best not inserted immediately after thiopental only because laryngeal reflexes are very active.

The cuff is then inflated. Maximal cuff volumes are 4 mL (size 1), 7 mL (size 1.5), 10 mL (size 2), 14 mL (size 2.5), 20 mL (size 3), 30 mL (size 4), 40 mL (size 5) and 50 mL (size 6). The cuff should not necessarily be inflated to maximum volume. Cuff pressure should not be greater than 60 cmH_2O. The pressure may rise two- to threefold during nitrous oxide anaesthesia.

In one study of 11 000 patients the successful insertion rate (with three attempts) was 99.8%.

The classic LMA forms a seal around the larynx, and allows spontaneous ventilation or gentle IPPV without tracheal intubation. The seal does not always prevent aspiration and the LMA should not be used where there is an increased risk of aspiration of stomach contents. The aspiration rate in selected patients is low, at 1 in 5000–11 000.

IPPV through the classic LMA is common in the UK, but not without debate.[5] Gastric distension may occur if airway pressures exceed about 20 cmH_2O.

A biteblock is useful protection against occlusion during emergence. The mask is best removed when the protective reflexes have fully returned and the patient has started to swallow. Suction is usually not needed.

The LMA provides a relatively secure, hands-free airway in place of a facemask or tracheal intubation for routine anaesthesia in both adults and children. It is valuable in many operations where the airway may present difficulties (e.g. radiotherapy and dental extractions in children). It causes only a small rise in heart rate, blood pressure and intraocular pressure, comparable with those seen after insertion of an oropharyngeal airway. Cricoid pressure is effective with an LMA in place.

The mask can be autoclaved and reused 40 times, but several single-use LMAs are now produced.

The classic LMA has a number of uses:

- as the desired airway conduit;
- where intubation has proved difficult;
- in the 'can't ventilate, can't intubate' scenario;
- as a conduit for smooth emergence;
- as a dedicated airway through which intubation is performed. Five methods of intubation have been described: blind insertion of the tube; blind or fibreoptic insertion of a standard bougie/introducer with subsequent intubation over the bougie; direct fibreoptic placement of the tracheal tube; and fibreoptic placement of an Aintree Catheter with subsequent intubation over the catheter. Fibreoptic guided techniques have success rates >95%. A 6.0 mm tracheal tube passes through a size 3 or 4 LMA, and a 7.0 mm through the size 5.

ProSeal

The ProSeal, introduced in 2001, separates the airway and oesophagus more completely than the classic LMA. Adult sizes are 3 to 5, with smaller sizes in production for children.

The stem consists of two separate tubes, one supplying gases to the bowl and the other passing as a separate duct to the tip of the mask, which overlies the upper oesophageal sphincter. An additional posterior cuff (not present in paediatric sizes) applies the bowl more firmly around the larynx so that inflation pressures of 30 cmH_2O may be applied.

The ProSeal is inserted with a digital technique, the metal introducer, or over a bougie passed through the drainage tube into the oesophagus.[6] The depth of anaesthesia required may be slightly deeper than with the classic LMA. Successful insertion by all techniques is over 98% with three attempts.

When the ProSeal is inserted correctly, a nasogastric tube can be passed through the drainage tube into the stomach in over 98% of cases. There should be no leak through the drainage tube when the mask is positioned correctly.

The ProSeal is being used increasingly in preference to the classic LMA, particularly when IPPV is required, and also instead of tracheal intubation. It has been used successfully in failed rapid sequence induction (RSI).

Other supraglottic airways

More than 15 other supraglottic airway devices have appeared on the market, often with little validation before marketing.[7] Some have performed so poorly that they are already defunct. Comparative trials against the classic or ProSeal laryngeal mask are awaited. The laryngeal tube appears to be one of the best. The Elisha has the particular advantage of being designed to facilitate fibreoptic intubation. They may be classified by the arrangement of the sealing mechanism, as follows:[8]

- cuffed perilaryngeal sealing – classic or single-use LMA, ProSeal, intubating LMA;
- cuffed pharyngeal sealing (no oesophageal sealing) – cuffed oropharyngeal airway (COPA), PAxpress®, Cobra™;
- cuffed pharyngeal and oesophageal sealing – Combitube™, EasyTube™, laryngeal tube, airway management device (AMD), Elisha;
- cuffless – streamlined liner of the pharynx airway (SLIPA™).

Tracheal intubation

Indications

Indications for tracheal intubation are:

- to maintain the airway in the presence of obstruction or laryngeal spasm;
- to protect the airway against aspiration of stomach contents or blood and debris from operations on the head and upper airways;
- for security in head and neck surgery, when the patient is prone or during transfer of an obtunded patient;

- to allow IPPV – if muscle relaxation is needed (e.g. abdominal surgery); in thoracic operations, when suctioning can also be easily carried out; to minimise the dose of volatile agent and allow large doses of narcotics; in infants, where respiration is easily depressed and intubation halves the anatomic dead space; in respiratory failure.

Endotracheal tubes

Endotracheal tubes used to be rubber, coloured red by a preservative. Today virtually all tubes used in the UK are semirigid polyvinyl chloride (PVC) and designed for single use. The size refers to the inside diameter in mm. Other markings include the maker, outside diameter (mm), 'oral' or 'nasal' design, single or multiple use, number of centimetres from the tip, and code of the implantation test (IT).

The toxicity of the PVC is tested by implantation in rabbit muscle (IT, 'implantation tested') or by cell culture.

Red rubber, silicone and PVC are all flammable in concentrations of oxygen and nitrous oxide that are used clinically. Laser-resistant tubes are available.

There are many types of tube for special purposes. A microlaryngeal tube is a 5 mm tube of adult length and cuff size for microlaryngeal surgery. Wire-reinforced silicone rubber tubes resist kinking and are available down to 2.5 mm.

Polar or RAE™ (Ring, Adair, Elwyn) preformed nasal and oral tubes, both north and south facing, are widely used in head and neck surgery.

Double-lumen tubes are used in thoracic anaesthesia.

Inflatable cuffs

Cuffs prevent leakage between the endotracheal tube and the trachea – both leakage of gas outwards during IPPV and of gastric contents, blood and mucus into the lungs. They are available on tubes down to about 3.5 mm. The integrity of the cuff should be tested before use. The tube to the pilot balloon enters the shaft of a nasal tube much nearer its proximal end than for an orotracheal tube. Cuffs are low volume and high pressure, or vice versa. Pressure on the tracheal wall is likely to be less than cuff pressure, but may be nearly equal if the cuff is floppy. Cuff pressure may be monitored and should not exceed 30 cmH_2O (22 mmHg) to prevent ischaemic damage to the tracheal mucosa. It is important that cuffs should not be inflated more than the minimum needed to prevent audible leakage of gas. Overinflation may cause a sore throat, or, at worst, necrosis of the tracheal mucosa. Leakage past low-pressure cuffs has been reported.

Cuff pressure rises substantially if nitrous oxide is used in the anaesthetic gas mixture. Bronchial rupture has been ascribed to rupture of cuffs on double-lumen tubes due to this mechanism. This rise in pressure may be minimised by inflation with normal saline, filling the cuff with anaesthetic gas mixtures, or the use of a pressure-limiting device or a foam-filled cuff.

Laryngoscopes

A wide variety of straight, curved, hinged, flexible and fibreoptic laryngoscope blades, some incorporating prisms and mirrors, have been produced. Most are of historical interest. Those in common current use in the UK will be described briefly.

The Macintosh laryngoscope blade is short, curved and Z-shaped on cross-section and the Magill blade is straight. Each is designed to be inserted into the right side of the patient's mouth, moving the tongue over to the left. There is a blade available for the left side. Adult blades can be used for quite small children, but neonates and babies may require special straight blades. The paraglossal straight blade technique (similar to that used by ENT surgeons) is more difficult to learn but has a higher success rate. Excellent descriptions of the technique accompanied the launch of the Henderson straight blade.[9]

The Polio laryngoscope can be used on patients in tank respirators. Its Macintosh blade makes an angle of approximately 135° with the handle.

The McCoy blade has a hinged tip, actuated by a lever positioned along the length of the handle on the opposite side to the blade. After insertion (with the hand further clockwise round the handle than usual), pressing the lever elevates the hinged tip in the vallecula. It is especially useful in grade 3 intubations, and in combination with cricoid pressure.

The Bullard intubating laryngoscope is a rigid fibrescope and is useful when the neck is immobile and mouth opening restricted.

Technique for direct laryngoscopy and oral intubation

Intubation by direct laryngoscopy is a skill that requires practice over several years before it is mastered. It is usually undertaken in apnoea, with intermittent facemask inflation to avoid hypoxaemia and maintain inhalational anaesthesia. Loose, filled or capped teeth, especially upper incisors, may be protected by a guard. There are five important components, as follows.

Optimal head and neck positioning

Optimal head and neck positioning is obtained by flexion of the neck and extension of the atlanto-occipital joint, usually by means of a small pillow under the occiput. More pillows may be required in obese patients. The head and neck position should be correct before inducing anaesthesia.

Optimal muscle relaxation

Optimal muscle relaxation allows the greatest exposure of the larynx and prevents glottic closure. Muscle relaxants are commonly used. Their effect is easily monitored by nerve stimulation. Reflexes may also be abolished by deep inhalational or intravenous agents, perhaps aided by topical analgesia.

Optimal laryngoscope blade

The curved laryngoscope blade may be the easier to use if the patient has a full set of teeth, and may cause less stretching of the faucial pillars than a straight blade. It is inserted from the right side of the patient's mouth to prevent the tongue blocking the view of the larynx, while watching the blade tip as it is advanced alongside the tongue towards the midline. When the epiglottis is seen, the tip is inserted firmly but not forcibly into the vallecula and used to lift the base of the epiglottis forward to reveal the cords. If the view is poor it is possible to change to a longer, straight or hinged blade.

Optimal external laryngeal manipulation

Backward and lateral pressure on the larynx by the anaesthetist or assistant may help bring the cords into view. It reduces the prevalence of a grade 3 view from 8% to 1.5%. The best manoeuvre is BURP (backwards, upwards, and to the right pressure).

Optimal use of the bougie

The gum elastic bougie (correctly termed an introducer) with Coudé tip is the single most useful aid for difficult direct laryngoscopy. It is introduced into the trachea, sometimes blindly, and used as a guide to railroad a tracheal tube. Indications that it has been successfully placed in the trachea and not the oesophagus are a feeling of tracheal rings, hold-up to advancement at 25 cm as the bougie encounters the carina, and a cough as the carina is stimulated. The laryngoscope should remain in place as the tube is railroaded, and it is often necessary to withdraw the tube slightly and rotate it anticlockwise 90° to avoid the tip of the tube impinging on the right vocal cord. A hollow bougie allows capnography to confirm position before attempting intubation. Single-use plastic bougies are currently inferior to the gum elastic ones owing to differences in memory of the plastic, but this problem will soon be resolved by the use of different plasticisers.

Grading of direct laryngoscopy has been proposed according to the amount of the larynx exposed under optimal conditions. Cormack and Lehane described grades 1 to 4. Grade 1 is the full glottic opening visible, grade 2 is partial glottic opening visible, grade 3 is epiglottis only visible, and grade 4 is when no part of the larynx is visible.

Blind oral intubation is very occasionally necessary when abnormal anatomy precludes the use of a laryngoscope and the nasal route is undesirable, or in animals. An assistant draws the tongue forward while the anaesthetist stands facing the patient on his or her left, passes two fingers of the left hand over the dorsum of the tongue and hooks the epiglottis forwards. The tube, which must be fully curved, is guided by these two fingers into the glottis. Curved introducers may help. Oral airways such as the Berman were designed to facilitate blind oral intubation.

Nasotracheal intubation

Nasal intubation is required when an oral tube will interfere with surgery and may be indicated when oral intubation is difficult. Nasal intubation may be accomplished under vision by oral direct laryngoscopy to guide the tube into the larynx, perhaps using Magill's forceps, or with the intubating fibrescope, or by a blind technique.

Blind nasal intubation

The distance between nares and carina in adults averages 32 cm in men and 27 cm in women. Extreme gentleness should prevail.

Blind nasal intubation is a knack, only acquired by practice. The experienced worker employs tubes of a size, shape and consistency to suit the individual technique, and the steps are as follows:

- the nares should be examined for patency by listening to the patient's breathing with each naris occluded. Nasal polyps should be excluded. The nasal mucosa may be shrunk by 5% cocaine, Moffett's solution or other vasoconstrictor;
- select the largest size of tube that should pass atraumatically through the larger naris: for a man up to 7 mm, for a small woman between 5 and 7 mm. The position of the patient's head depends on the curve of the tube. The greater the curve, the more flexed the head should be. Magill advised the position adopted 'when sniffing the morning air,' the head on a single pillow, with slight extension of the atlanto-occipital joint;
- the anaesthetist may attempt nasal intubation with the patient apnoeic after muscle relaxation, or under deep inhalational anaesthesia. Some find blind intubation easier in the paralysed patient because reflex laryngospasm does not occur;
- the lubricated tube, with its concavity directed to the patient's feet, is inserted into the naris initially upwards for 2–3 cm to clear the inferior turbinate, then directly backwards. Movement of the bevel by rotation of the tube may assist easier passage, both at this stage and when the tube enters the nasopharynx;
- if the patient is breathing spontaneously, the opposite nostril may be occluded so that all breathing is taking place through the tube. The jaw should be slightly elevated to lift the epiglottis from the posterior pharyngeal wall. If the right naris is used the head should be inclined slightly to the right, and vice versa. The anaesthetist should listen carefully to the respiration. The breath sounds conducted through the tube become maximal when its tip is immediately above the glottis. If the tube does not enter the larynx, its direction may be adjusted by rotation of the tube, rotation of the neck or digital movement of the

larynx to meet the advancing tube. Should the tube enter the oesophagus it can be partially withdrawn and its tip directed anteriorly by increased extension of the neck or by using a tube with a larger curvature. Occasionally the tip of the tube impinges on the anterior commissure of the larynx, when it will often enter the larynx if the neck is flexed or a tube of lesser curvature is used. As the tube passes the cords there may be some coughing or breath-holding in the lightly anaesthetised patient, even if muscle relaxants have been used. In the unparalysed patient the tube may enter the trachea during the explosive cough, that may follow spasm of the cords. In the case of failure to intubate through one naris, success may be achieved through the other, or with a tube of different curvature;

- normal free breath sounds at the proximal end of a tube of reasonable length show that it is in the trachea. If the tube is inserted fully and no breath sounds are heard, it is probably in the oesophagus. Capnography should be used to confirm placement.

A prominent arch of the atlas may cause obstruction and perhaps the overlying mucosa to be torn. A small suction catheter may be threaded through the tube and tension kept on it as it is delivered through the mouth, thus displacing the tip of the tube.

Epistaxis, though messy, seldom interferes with the anaesthesia or causes postoperative discomfort. Partial obstruction of a nasotracheal tube by an avulsed piece of turbinate has been described. It may also be compressed by nasal spurs and a deviated septum. Nasal intubation has been followed by bacteraemia in 12% of children and in 17–21% of adults.

General anaesthetic techniques for tracheal intubation

Without muscle relaxation

Intubation is possible under an adequate dose of propofol (up to 3 mg/kg) with alfentanil 10–20 μg/kg or remifentanil 1–2 μg/kg. It is also possible under deep inhalational anaesthesia with spontaneous respiration. Sevoflurane alone is popular in children and adults, and useful where awake intubation is not possible.

With muscle relaxation

Induction followed by suxamethonium 0.5–1.5 mg/kg gives rapid and profound relaxation and helps make intubation quick and atraumatic. Offset of relaxation after a few minutes is a safety factor if intubation fails, although this will not necessarily occur before critical oxygen desaturation. Suxamethonium can also be given intramuscularly (3 mg/kg) or by sublingual injection in an emergency. Non-depolarising relaxants such as vecuronium, mivacurium or atracurium allow intubation about 90 seconds after intravenous administration, during which time gentle facemask ventilation is applied. Rocuronium has a significantly faster onset of action.

Muscle relaxants should not normally be given unless the anaesthetist is confident in his or her ability to ventilate the lungs using a facemask.

Rapid sequence induction (RSI) of anaesthesia

The incidence of perioperative aspiration is 2–3/10 000, only one-third of these at induction. Rapid sequence induction is indicated when there is significant risk of airway soiling from gastro-oesophageal contents (e.g. pregnancy, intestinal obstruction, oesophageal dilatation, inadequate starvation, trauma). It involves preoxygenation, an intravenous induction agent and suxamethonium, with cricoid pressure. A trained assistant, running suction, tilting trolley, selection of tested cuffed endotracheal tubes, laryngoscopes and gum elastic bougie are needed to hand. Cricoid pressure is applied at loss of consciousness and only released when the endotracheal cuff is safely inflated in the trachea. The classic RSI with thiopental and suxamethonium is being challenged by a number of modifications. None has been subjected to proper scientific study.

Other methods[10] to reduce the frequency or seriousness of aspiration include preoperative starvation, nasogastric tube drainage, induced vomiting, non-particulate antacids (30 mL 0.3 M sodium citrate), prokinetic agents (10–20 mg metoclopramide intravenously), proton pump inhibitors (lansoprazole 30 mg) or H_2 receptor antagonists (150–300 mg ranitidine orally or 50 mg intravenously). The aim is to reduce the volume and raise the pH of gastric contents to commonly quoted (but scientifically unproven) 'safe' values of less than 25 mL and greater than 2.5, respectively.

Classic RSI Classic RSI is carried out as follows:

- check assistant, tilting trolley, drugs, suction, airway equipment, machine, monitor;
- take baseline blood pressure, heart rate and oxygen saturation on air;
- preoxygenate for at least 3 minutes tidal volume breathing with tight-fitting facemask, or until the end-tidal oxygen has reached 90%;
- give thiopental 5 mg/kg and suxamethonium 1.5 mg/kg;
- apply cricoid pressure at 30 N, the force to register 3 kg on a weighing machine;
- intubate, inflate cuff and confirm tracheal placement of tube;
- remove cricoid pressure and continue anaesthesia.

Adverse effects of cricoid pressure Cricoid pressure has adverse effects on airway management, which may threaten life. It also appears to reduce lower oesophageal barrier pressure. The adverse effects are related to excessive force. The assistant should know that 30 N is the correct amount and should have practised exerting a 3 kg force on a weighing machine. Forces over 40 N may completely occlude the laryngeal lumen at the level of the cricoid cartilage, particularly in young women. Cricoid pressure may cause difficulty with laryngoscopy and intubation. It may also cause difficulty with facemask inflation of the lungs, insertion of, and intubation through an LMA.

Failed RSI A back-up plan should be formulated before each RSI in case of failed intubation or failed ventilation.[11] The anaesthetist must know whether the patient can be woken and intubated later by an awake technique, or whether the operation is so urgent that the anaesthetic must continue even if intubation fails. The former is more common. A wall flowchart has been produced for this situation at *www.das.uk.com*. It assumes that suxamethonium has been used, and the procedure is as follows:

- announce failed intubation, maintain cricoid pressure;
- call for help and keep the first responder;
- insert a large oral airway and try facemask ventilation with 100% oxygen;
- try four-handed bag mask ventilation using the extra person;
- insert a LMA – release cricoid force temporarily as the LMA is swept into place;
- reapply cricoid force and attempt ventilation;
- release cricoid force and attempt ventilation;
- if ventilation is impossible by any of the above steps, the patient is not waking up and critical hypoxia develops, emergency cricothyrotomy should be initiated.

If a modified RSI with rocuronium has been undertaken, waking up is not an option. The ProSeal may then be best if anaesthesia must be continued.

Confirmation of correct position of a tracheal tube

Trachea (and not oesophagus)?

'When in doubt, take it out'. It is easy to wrongly intubate the oesophagus, no matter how experienced the anaesthetist. This must be recognised immediately. If the clinical state of the patient deteriorates after intubation, or if there is any doubt whatsoever about tube placement, the tube should be removed and the patient ventilated by facemask. A facemask may even be used with the open tube in place if the anaesthetist is unwilling to remove it.

The anaesthetist can only be certain that the tube has been correctly placed in the trachea if:

- it is seen to pass through the cords and is still visible in front of the arytenoids;
- the tracheobronchial tree can be seen when a fibreoptic bronchoscope is passed down the tube.

It is often not possible to use these two gold standard tests. The next best tests are as follows.

Capnography Normal values of CO_2 are present in expired gas and continue for six breaths, which avoids washout of CO_2-containing stomach gas being falsely interpreted. False negatives (i.e. tube in trachea but no CO_2 visible on capnograph) will occur if the capnograph is not attached, the tracheal cuff has not been inflated and there is a large gas leak around the tube, or with cardiac arrest when pulmonary blood flow is absent or low.

Oesophageal detector device The oesophageal detector device uses a self-inflating bulb, which cannot fill with gas if the tube is in the oesophagus. It is effective in normal individuals, gives an immediate response and does not require several positive-pressure breaths to be applied. False negatives may occur in the morbidly obese and in late pregnancy.

Other tests A range of other tests suggest, but do not confirm, tracheal intubation.

- chest movement and auscultation for air entry over the lung fields, and the absence of a gurgle over the epigastrium when the reservoir bag is squeezed;
- feeling of correct lung compliance, refilling of bag in expiration and misting of the tube;
- palpating the tube in the larynx through the mouth or at the front of the neck;
- the use of a lighted stylet down the tube whose light shines through the front of the neck.

Trachea or main bronchus?

The average distance between the central incisors and carina is 27 cm in an adult male and 23 cm in a female. The tip of the tube moves about 4 cm caudad as the neck moves from full extension to full flexion. The following suggest that the tip of the tube is in the trachea, and not in a main bronchus (usually the right):

- bilateral chest movement;
- bilateral equal breath sounds;
- normal compliance;
- carina visualised on fibreoptic endoscopy;
- tip of tube above the carina on chest radiography.

Complications of intubation

Tracheal intubation offers the most secure airway, but intubation by direct laryngoscopy has complications, some of which are fatal.[12]

Direct trauma

Direct trauma to the lips, teeth, gums, eyes, nose, uvula, throat and larynx results in hoarseness, dysphagia, sore throat, etc. Sore throat may also result purely from suxamethonium muscle pain.

Nasal intubation may dislodge nasal polyps, cause epistaxis, damage turbinates, or cause ulceration of turbinates if intubation is prolonged.

Tears in the mucosa of the pharynx, oesophagus, larynx or trachea may result in extensive surgical and mediastinal emphysema and mediastinitis. Retropharyngeal abscess has been reported. Antibiotics and ENT review are required.

A tooth guard may be helpful. If a tooth is knocked out it must be found to prevent it falling into the trachea. If shown to be in a bronchus, it should be removed bronchoscopically. It should be handled only by the crown and placed in saline because reimplantation may be possible.

A haematoma may form in the cords, especially the left, or in the supraglottic region, which may result in dysphonia and dysphagia, but usually clears up in a few days. It bears no constant relationship to the difficulty of intubation.

The arytenoids may dislocate, or more serious damage may be done to the laryngeal muscles and ligaments. Permanent alteration of the voice has been reported in 3% of patients after intubation.

Nerve injuries

Recurrent laryngeal nerve palsy following intubation results in a paralysed cord. This is most commonly due to the surgery, but other possible causes include stretching of nerve if the neck is extended during intubation or extubation, and inflation of the cuff within the larynx. Idiopathic palsy of the recurrent nerve, a transient cranial mononeuropathy, can also occur and has a reasonable chance of good recovery.

The law of F Semon (1849–1921) states that in a disorder of the laryngeal motor nerves, the abductors of the cords are the first and occasionally the only muscles affected. Bilateral cord paralysis, perhaps due to pressure of the inflated cuff on the laminae of the thyroid cartilage and the recurrent nerves, may occur. Increasing airway obstruction results, which requires facemask continuous positive airway pressure (CPAP) or reintubation.

Lingual nerve palsy may occur as a result of compression or stretching in its course from the medial surface of the mandible to the underside of the tongue, especially on the right. The prognosis is good.

Fracture–subluxation of the cervical spine

Fracture–subluxation of the cervical spine is a risk from extension of the atlantoaxial joint in fractures, malformations or abnormal fragility of the cervical spine, as in rheumatoid arthritis or Down's syndrome, where muscle tone has been abolished by relaxants. A cervical collar with in-line fixation may be needed.

Infections

Sinusitis and otitis media may result from nasotracheal intubation. The bronchial tree may also become contaminated, and bacteraemia is associated with nasotracheal intubation.

Tracheal rupture during anaesthesia

Tracheal rupture during anaesthesia may occur in both adults and neonates. It is not necessarily associated with trauma.

Ignition of the tube during laser surgery

See Otorhinolaryngology, Chapter 5.12.

Obstruction of tube

A foreign body, blood clot or mucus plug may obstruct the tube. The cuff may herniate over the end of the tube or internally to occlude the lumen. This was a particular problem with old red rubber tubes. The bevel may impinge on the tracheal wall, allowing inspiration but not expiration. The Murphy (US anaesthetist, 1947) eye is an additional opening opposite the bevel that prevents this.

Acute glottic oedema

Acute glottic oedema rarely follows intubation, especially in a patient with acute laryngitis. This is more serious in children because of the small larynx and loose submucosal tissue in the subglottic region. It presents up to several hours after extubation with hoarseness, cough, choking, restlessness, stridor, and signs of upper airway obstruction (i.e. inspiratory indrawing at the suprasternal notch, epigastrium, intercostal spaces or around the clavicles). Sedation is contraindicated. Humidification and nebulised epinephrine (adrenaline) may be useful. Reintubation with a smaller tube may be needed, or even tracheostomy.

Laryngeal ulceration and granuloma formation

Rarely, a contact ulcer may form in the mucosa over the prominent tip of the vocal process of one or both arytenoids in the posterior third of the rima glottidis, or in the subglottis of children after prolonged intubation. In the trachea, fibrosis, stenosis and tracheomalacia may result. If hoarseness persists for more than 3–4 days after intubation, flexible laryngoscopy should be performed. A contact ulcer will heal if the voice is completely rested. A granuloma may need ENT referral for excision.

Cardiovascular responses

The influence of airway manipulation on heart rate and blood pressure was first documented in 1951.

During light general anaesthesia, irrespective of the type of laryngoscope blade used, direct laryngoscopy and intubation cause afferent vagal stimulation and an efferent sympathoadrenal response. There are increases in heart rate and blood pressure, and intraocular and intracranial pressures. Arrhythmias are common. Hypertensive patients show an exaggerated response. Endorphin release also occurs.

These reflexes are important in patients with coronary artery disease, aneurysms, raised intracranial pressure or open eye surgery. They are less marked under deep general anaesthesia, adequate topical analgesia, and with smooth blind nasal and fibreoptic intubation. These responses may also be minimised by:[13]

- opioids (e.g. fentanyl 2–6 μg/kg, alfentanil 10–30 μg/kg or remifentanil 1–3 μg/kg);
- lidocaine (lignocaine) 1–1.5 mg/kg intravenously;
- induction with propofol;
- esmolol 50–100 μg/kg;
- other hypotensive drugs as premedication or shortly before intubation (e.g. clonidine, an angiotensin-converting enzyme [ACE] inhibitor, verapamil 0.1 mg/kg intravenously, nifedipine 10 mg sublingually, diltiazem 0.2–0.3 mg/kg) orally.

Alternative techniques for tracheal intubation

Fruitless prolonged attempts at intubation are commonly seen when airway-related deaths are analysed. No more than three attempts at direct laryngoscopy should be made. When unsuccessful, an alternative technique should be considered. A wall flowchart for unanticipated difficult direct laryngoscopy is available from *www.das.uk.com.*

Intubating LMA

Devised by Brain in 2001,[14] the intubating LMA consists of a metal handle and curved stem with a 15 mm connector, a cuffed bowl with epiglottic elevator bar, dedicated wire-spiralled tubes (7.0, 7.5, 8.0 mm) with detachable connectors and a stabilising rod for removal of the mask over the inserted tube. The mask is available in sizes 3, 4 and 5 and may be autoclaved 40 times, and the tube ten times. It is latex free.

The mask is inserted by holding the handle low down over the sternum and rotating it into place. Ventilation should be easy. The tube is well lubricated and passed blindly into the stem until a horizontal line on the tube indicates that the tip is engaging the epiglottic elevator bar. Light force advances the tube through into the trachea. This may be blind or under fibreoptic guidance.

Studies indicate that this is the best technique for blind intubation and has been validated in difficult airways.[15] Ventilation via the mask is virtually always possible and successful intubation, allowing three attempts, is possible in 95–100% of patients. The fibreoptic-assisted variant appears to be useful. A new version of the intubating LMA incorporates a camera and screen to view the vocal cords and the tube passing through them, and has just been released. A single-use version is planned.

Fibreoptic intubation

Described by Murphy[16] (anaesthetist, National Hospital, London, UK, 1967) using a flexible choledochoscope, fibreoptic intubation remains the most useful means of nasal or oral intubation in awake or anaesthetised patients with normal or abnormal airway anatomy. The fibrescope is narrow enough to pass easily, its flexible nature means that it conforms to the shape of the airway, its cylindrical shape allows the design of special masks and connectors such that ventilation can be concurrent with endoscopy, and it is a visual technique. The success rate is high and the complication rate low. Fibreoptic intubation through a guide such as the Berman airway or laryngeal mask is promoted as a core skill of an anaesthetist.

The technique requires an expensive (around £10 000) reusable fibrescope with stringent controls for decontamination (special scopes are available if the patient is suspected of variant Creutzfeldt–Jakob disease [vCJD][17]), and an experienced operator, but is essential for modern airway management.[18] Third-generation fibrescopes have a battery attachment and higher-resolution image.

Elective fibreoptic intubation under general anaesthesia

Steps to carry out elective fibreoptic intubation under general anaesthesia are as follows:

- glycopyrronium 0.2 mg intravenously is useful, but not essential, and consider a topical vasoconstrictor before nasal intubation;
- attach and orientate the camera monitor (notch at 12 o'clock), turn on the light, adjust the focus;
- load the selected tube onto the fibrescope;
- induce anaesthesia, maintain with an intravenous or inhalational agent, suppress airway reflexes with deep anaesthesia, muscle relaxants or topical anaesthesia;
- pass the fibrescope through the nose or mouth to the carina, railroad the tube over the fibrescope, confirm the correct position and continue anaesthesia;
- decontaminate the fibrescope, complete the tracking ledger and note the fibrescope details in patient's notes.

Practical tips include the following.

- master manipulation on a model or mannikin before use in patients. Maintain oxygenation by uninterrupted ventilation (and possibly intravenous anaesthesia) until more experienced;
- use an alcohol-impregnated swab on the lens to clear the view;
- remember to load the tube on the fibrescope before insertion. Use a biteblock unless the patient is completely paralysed: a bitten fibrescope is expensive to repair;
- huides such as the Berman (US anaesthetist, 1914–1999) or Williams airway, or a laryngeal mask, make it easier;
- avoid hitting mucosa – it may cover the lens with secretions or cause bleeding;
- ensure continuous vision from the nares or mouth to the carina. If the view is lost withdraw until the structures are recognised;
- chin lift and neck extension are essential in nasal intubation to provide pharyngeal space.

Awake fibreoptic intubation

More correctly termed intubation under conscious sedation, awake fibreoptic intubation is employed when difficult direct laryngoscopy is predicted together with either difficult facemask ventilation or risk of aspiration. It is also used in cervical spine injury, to aid self-positioning of morbidly obese patients, in injuries to the airway, or where the disease process impinges on the airway.

Intubation in the awake patient has been described using various techniques, such as oral or nasal blind, direct laryngoscopy, through an LMA, with the lighted stylet, by the retrograde route, and with a rigid or flexible fibrescope.

When awake flexible fibreoptic intubation is the preferred option, it is carried out as follows:

- the risks and benefits are explained to the patient. Cooperation is needed. Children and intoxicated or neurologically impaired adults may not be suitable. The patient is monitored from arrival and breathes additional oxygen by mask. It is helpful for one anaesthetist to look after the patient and another to perform the intubation;
- glycopyrronium 0.2–0.4 mg intramuscularly or intravenously provides a dry mucosa, and topical anaesthesia acts more quickly and provides more satisfactory analgesia. If the nose is to be used, ephedrine 0.5% or xylometazoline 0.1% nose drops are desirable to shrink the mucosa. The more patent nostril should be determined;

- sedation with opioid and benzodiazepine has a good safety record. Fentanyl 25 μg and midazolam 1 mg increments are given, ensuring the patient maintains breathing and responsiveness. Both agents peak at 5 minutes and it is easy to hurry and give too much sedation. Propofol TCI set initially at 0.6–1.5 μg/mL is increasingly popular. Propofol and remifentanil (manual or TCI) or remifentanil alone may also be used. Opioids certainly improve intubating conditions, but careful monitoring is needed to avoid apnoea;
- topical anaesthesia is with 2–4% lidocaine (lignocaine) initially, supplemented if necessary by 10% to the nose or mouth and pharynx. Inhalation during the spraying will start glottic and tracheal analgesia. Additional laryngeal and tracheal analgesia can be provided by translaryngeal application of 3–4 mL 4% through the cricothyroid membrane or sprayed down the working channel of the fibrescope, perhaps through an epidural catheter. It is usual to limit the dose of lidocaine (lignocaine) to 3 mg/kg when it is injected directly into the airway, but 7–9 mg/kg may be given if much is swallowed.

Lighted stylet

Described initially in 1959, lighted stylets within the lumen of the tracheal tube are placed correctly by the principle of transillumination.[19] The stylet is guided into position by following the spot of light viewed externally. In one early model the distal light bulb became detached and fell into the bronchial tree. The Trachlight is a typical modern version. Reported success rates are very high in anticipated and unanticipated difficult direct laryngoscopy, with mean intubation times of only 20–25 seconds. The bulb of the Trachlight blinks off and on after 30 seconds to remind of continuing apnoea and to reduce the bulb temperature to prevent mucosal burns. It is a popular, simple device for practitioners with sufficient practice.

EXTUBATION

Extubation strategy considers whether the tube is removed in the awake or the anaesthetised state, protection of the airway, and management of complications with facilities for reintubation.

Extubation in routine cases where no problems are envisaged would include suctioning of the pharynx under direct vision, administration of 100% oxygen for at least 3 minutes or until the end-tidal oxygen has reached about 90%, antagonism of any residual neuromuscular blockade, demonstration of satisfactory spontaneous respiration, pressure on the reservoir bag, cuff deflation, tube removal, application of the facemask with 100% oxygen, and confirmation of satisfactory spontaneous respiration before transfer to recovery.

Where there is a risk of aspiration, the patient should be awake (i.e. opening eyes and moving limbs to command), and in the lateral position, possibly head-down as well.

If intubation was difficult, or surgery impinged on the airway, extubation strategy will change to awake extubation, accommodate some testing of airway patency prior to extubation, and may incorporate the introduction of a guide over which reintubation can be undertaken quickly or some means of emergency oxygenation.

Airway patency around the tube can be tested by a simple leak test in which the circuit is pressurised to 20 cmH_2O, the cuff deflated and any leak around the tube evaluated.

A narrow airway exchange catheter can be placed in the tube and left in situ after extubation, providing a means of emergency oxygenation and a guide for reintubation.

Extubation may be deferred unexpectedly at the end of surgery. The usual reasons are hypoxaemia requiring greater than 40% inspired oxygen, core temperature less than 35°C, cardiovascular instability, continued bleeding, retention of surgical packs to be removed later, and continued active resuscitation or developing sepsis.

Common extubation problems are as follows.

Extubation Problems

Residual muscle paralysis

Residual muscle paralysis presents as respiratory insufficiency and possibly laryngospasm. Check neuromuscular function by nerve stimulation and clinical tests before extubation. Treat with 100% oxygen by facemask, additional neostigmine or reintubation. This may be extremely unpleasant for the patient.

Cardiovascular disturbance

Extubation is associated with hypertension and tachycardia, which are prevented by extubation at deep planes of anaesthesia, short-acting opioids or β-blockers such as esmolol. Lidocaine 1 mg/kg intravenously or 60 mg intratracheally is described as beneficial. The tube can be replaced with a laryngeal mask before anaesthesia is terminated.

Hypoxaemia

Hypoxaemia is more common at extubation than at intubation.

Laryngospasm

Laryngospasm at extubation is common and occasionally life-threatening. It only occurs when the patient is partially anaesthetised, and particularly when blood or secretions irritate the glottis. Treat initially by 100% oxygen with facemask and CPAP. Small (10–30 mg) doses of propofol may be helpful but Suxamethonium 15–25 mg may be required in extremis. Other described treatments are with intravenous midazolan 1–2 mg, doxapram 1 mg/kg, nitroglycerin 4 μg/kg or magnesium 15 mg/kg prior to extubation. Larson's manoeuvre is jaw thrust with firm bilateral digital pressure in the posterior part of the temporomandibular joint.

Paradoxical vocal cord movement

Paradoxical vocal cord movement presents with stridor and respiratory difficulty in the early recovery period after awakening. It responds to oxygen by mask, reassurance and midazolam increments, and is more commonly described in women. It is diagnosed by flexible nasendoscopy, when it can be seen that the glottis narrows on inspiration, and is usually self-limiting (in 10–20 minutes).

Pulmonary oedema

Prolonged powerful inspiratory attempts with a closed glottis (as in laryngospasm) may give rise to acute and dramatic pulmonary oedema. Treat by reintubation, ventilation and positive end-expiratory pressure (PEEP). It usually resolves in 4–6 hours.

FAILED VENTILATION

A failed ventilation drill should be activated when it proves difficult to ventilate with a facemask. A suitable flow chart has been produced (*www.das.uk.com*). The breathing circuit, connections and facemask should have been inspected and tested before use to ensure there is no blockage with bits of plastic. The glottic closure reflex, which is active in light planes of anaesthesia without muscle relaxants, will make facemask inflation and intubation impossible.

When mask ventilation is difficult or impossible after induction of anaesthesia, the following steps are recommended:

- optimise facemask ventilation with a large oral airway and four-handed bag–mask ventilation;
- insert a laryngeal mask airway;
- if the glottic closure reflex is active, deepen anaesthesia with an intravenous agent;
- consider rapid direct laryngoscopy and intubation, but do not spend too much time on this;
- undertake emergency cricothyrotomy when the problem is glottic or supraglottic;
- unrecognised anterior mediastinal or tracheal masses may present with 'can't ventilate, can't intubate' – try turning the patient laterally or using a rigid bronchoscope.

EMERGENCY CRICOTHYROTOMY

Emergency cricothyrotomy is a major intervention, with serious complications of its own. It should be used after all efforts to secure the airway by facemask, laryngeal mask or tracheal intubation.

The trigger is the realisation that ventilation is not possible, saturations are falling and the patient will not recover their own airway. The sooner it is commenced, the more favourable the outcome.

Mannikin practice and available equipment are both essential.

Oxygen is delivered via the cricothyroid membrane or upper trachea.

The cricothyroid membrane is convenient, easy to locate, relatively avascular and will accommodate a 6.0 mm tube. The neck needs to be extended.

There are three types of cricothyrotomy – needle or small cannula cricothyrotomy, large purpose-built cannula cricothyrotomy, and surgical cricothyrotomy – which are carried out as outlined below.

Needle or small cannula cricothyrotomy

- Insert a 14 G cannula (in adults, but preferably a specific transtracheal jet ventilation catheter) through the cricothyroid membrane caudad into the trachea, and aspirate air through the cannula to confirm correct placement;
- fix in position, manually or with tape;
- narrow calibre means expiratory flow is impossible and inspiration requires high pressure. Use oxygen at high pressure (2–4 bar) via a Sanders injector;
- watch chest movement during inspiration and expiration to avoid overinflation;
- ensure the upper airway is patent to allow expiration. Possibly insert a LMA;
- no suction of the airway is possible;
- possibility of barotrauma.

Large purpose-built cannula cricothyrotomy

- Minimum 4 mm inner diameter (ID) in adults, preferably 6 mm cuffed;
- cannula over needle (QuickTrach) or Seldinger type (Melker);
- a standard breathing system will provide sufficient pressure for adequate inspiratory flows, though an uncuffed 4 mm tube may be insufficient if the upper airway is open;
- exhalation occurs through cannula;
- capnography possible to confirm correct placement;
- suctioning possible, and cuffed tube provides good airway protection.

Surgical cricothyrotomy

- Stab incision through skin and cricothyroid membrane;
- snlarge incision with handle of scalpel or forceps;

- caudal traction on cricoid cartilage with tracheal hook;
- insert 6.0 mm ID tube.

FOLLOW-UP

The ease of facemask ventilation, laryngeal mask insertion or tracheal intubation should be included on the anaesthetic record. It is common to use the Cormack and Lehane grading of best laryngeal view at direct laryngoscopy. When difficulties with airway management are encountered, follow-up is essential:[20]

- make detailed notes in the anaesthetic record, and an entry in the hospital notes;
- assess the patient to detect and treat morbidity;
- explain the problems to the patient, and advise him or her to inform their next anaesthetist;
- write a letter to the patient, with a copy to the general practitioner, and to any register kept by the anaesthetic department;
- consider advising the patient to register with MedicAlert®.

TRACHEOSTOMY

Tracheostomy may be urgent or elective, and undertaken under local or general anaesthesia.

The tubes may be cuffed or uncuffed and are usually supplied with an inner tube, which may be removed for cleaning. Fenestrated tubes allow gas to pass from the lungs to the glottis, enabling speech. Standard sizes are 4–10, with a size 8 having an outer diameter (OD) 12.0 mm, ID 8.5 mm and length 84 mm.

A standard 15 mm connector is usual except for long-term tracheostomy when the silver or plastic tube may have no connector. A paediatric facemask or laryngeal mask placed over the tracheostomy tube or tracheostome allows initial airway control when no connector is present.

The major indications for performing tracheostomy are:

- relief of upper airway obstruction;
- when prolonged intubation is required;
- to facilitate weaning in intensive care;
- in the management of severe obstructive sleep apnoea;
- to protect the airway when adequate neuromuscular control is absent;
- as part of complex head and neck resection;
- for the removal of foreign bodies.

There are several techniques for insertion of a tracheostomy tube, as outlined below.

Surgical insertion of a tracheostomy tube

The surgeon dissects down to the trachea, opens it and inserts the tracheostomy tube under vision.

Percutaneous insertion of a tracheostomy tube

The operator makes an incision over the trachea and bluntly dissects the pretracheal fascia. A needle is inserted into the tracheal lumen in the midline and a guidewire is inserted into the trachea in the caudad direction.

There are several techniques.[21] In the original Ciaglia technique (1985), dilators of increasing diameter are used until the tracheostomy tube may be placed. A latter, popular modification is the Ciaglia Blue Rhino® (1999) in which a single tapered dilator is used instead of serial dilators. Another technique, once the wire has been placed into the trachea, is to dilate the tracheal wall with guidewire dilating forceps (1990). A more recent design, PercuTwist® (2001),[22] uses a single-step dilator with self-tapping screw to breach the tracheal wall.

A fibrescope placed at glottic level will allow visual confirmation that the guide needle has punctured the trachea in the midline and guide the rest of the procedure. Capnography attached to the guide needle may also be used to confirm tracheal placement.

Percutaneous tracheostomy is also described in difficult airway management.

Serious complications of tracheostomy include tracheal rupture, bleeding and death.

Translaryngeal insertion of a tracheostomy tube

Translaryngeal insertion of a tracheostomy tube is a novel method (1997) in which the needle puncture and wire insertion are cephalad, as in retrograde intubation. The wire is found in the mouth and attached to the tough conical tip of a cuffed tube. The wire is pulled at the neck so that the conical tip passes between the vocal cords and then through the tracheal wall from inside to outside. The conical tip is removed, and the tube is partially withdrawn and then rotated so that the tip passes caudally. Further modifications have been made.[23]

References

1. Yentis SM. Predicting difficult intubation – worthwhile exercise or pointless ritual. Anaesthesia 2002; 57:105–109.

2. Ovassapian A, Glassenberg R, Randel GI, Klock A, Mesnick PS, Klafta JM. The unexpected difficult airway and lingual tonsil hyperplasia. Anesthesiology 2002; 97:124–132.
3. Caplan RA, Benumof JL, Berry FA, et al. A practice guideline for management of the difficult airway. Anesthesiology 1993; 78:597–602.
4. Langeron O, Masso E, Huraux C, et al. Prediction of difficult mask ventilation. Anesthesiology 2000; 92:1229–1236.
5. Sidaras G, Hunter JM. Is it safe to artificially ventilate a paralysed patient through the laryngeal mask? The jury is still out. Br J Anaesth 2001; 86:749–753.
6. Brimacombe J, Keller C, Judd DV. Gum elastic bougie-guided insertion of the ProSeal laryngeal mask airway is superior to the digital and introducer-tool technique. Anesthesiology 2004; 100:25–29.
7. Cook TM. Novel airway devices: spoilt for choice? Anaesthesia 2003; 58:107–110.
8. Miller DM. A proposed classification and scoring system for supraglottic sealing airways: a brief review. Anesth Analg 2004; 99:1553–1559.
9. Henderson JJ. The use of paraglossal straight blade laryngoscopy in difficult tracheal intubation. Anaesthesia 1997; 52:552–560.
10. Ng A, Smith G. Gastroesophageal reflux and aspiration of gastric contents in anesthetic practice. Anesth Analg 2001; 93:494–513.
11. Henderson JJ, Popat MT, Latto IP, Pearce AC. Difficult Airway Society guidelines for management of the unanticipated difficult intubation. Anaesthesia 2004; 59:675–694.
12. Domino KB, Posner KL, Caplan RA, Cheney FW. Airway injury during anesthesia. Anesthesiology 1999; 91:1703–1711.
13. Randell T. Haemodynamic responses to intubation: what more do we have to know? Acta Anaesthesiol Scand 2004; 48:393–395.
14. Brain AI, Verghese C, Addy EV, Kapila A, Brimacombe J. The intubating laryngeal mask airway. A preliminary clinical report of a new means of intubating the trachea. Br J Anaesth 1997; 79:704–709.
15. Ferson DZ, Rosenblatt WH, Johansen MJ, Osborn I, Ovassapian A. Use of the intubating LMA-Fastrach in 254 patients with difficult-to-manage airways. Anesthesiology 2001; 95:1175–1181.
16. Murphy P. A fiberoptic endoscope used for tracheal intubation. Anaesthesia 1967; 22:489–491.
17. Farling P, Popat M, Cooper S. Fibreoptic equipment and variant Creutzfeldt–Jakob disease. Anaesthesia 2003; 58:716–717.
18. Popat M. Practical fibreoptic intubation. Oxford: Butterworth Heinemann; 2001.

19. Davis L, Cook-Sather SD, Schreiner MS. Lighted stylet tracheal intubation: a review. Anesth Analg 2000; 90:745–756.

20. Barron FA, Ball DR, Jefferson P, Norrie J. 'Airway alerts'. How UK anaesthetists organise, document and communicate difficult airway management. Anaesthesia 2003; 58:73–77.

21. Anon JM, Escuela MP, Gomez V, et al. Percutaneous tracheostomy: Ciaglia Blue Rhino versus Griggs' guide wire dilating forceps. A prospective randomized trial. Acta Anaesthesiol Scand 2004; 48:451–456.

22. Sengupta N, Ang KL, Prakash D, Ng V, George SJ. Twenty months' routine use of a new percutaneous tracheostomy set using controlled rotating dilation. Anesth Analg 2004; 99:188–192.

23. Byhahn C, Wilke HJ, Lischke V, Westphal K. Translaryngeal tracheostomy: two modified techniques versus the basic technique – early experience in 75 critically ill adults. Intens Care Med 2000; 26:457–461.

CHAPTER **2.7**

INTRAVASCULAR TECHNIQUES AND BLOOD TRANSFUSION

PERIPHERAL VENOUS CANNULATION

Suitable veins for routine use for peripheral venous cannulation in adults include those on the forearm or dorsum of the hand. Veins in the leg should be avoided if possible.

A cold or frightened patient is likely to have constricted veins that are difficult to cannulate. If this is the case, or if the patient is hypovolaemic, an antecubital fossa or central vein may be preferred.

Prior application of EMLA® cream or tetracaine gel is effective at reducing the pain of venepuncture, especially in children. In infants the external jugular vein, a scalp vein, or one over the ankle or dorsum of the foot is often used.

Complications

Damage to a superficial cutaneous nerve caused by the needle or cannula has been reported after peripheral venous cannulation, and may result in chronic neuropathic pain.

Thrombophlebitis is common if a cannula remains in place for more than a day or two, and it should be removed at the first sign of this developing.

Minor extravasation of fluids is common and does not usually cause harm, but if the solution is irritant or hypertonic (e.g. sodium bicarbonate, calcium, some chemotherapeutic agents) it may cause extensive necrosis of skin, muscle and tendons, with permanent disability.

CENTRAL VENOUS CANNULATION

The commonest approach to a central (i.e. intrathoracic) vein is via the internal jugular vein. The right side is preferred. On the left side, the thoracic duct joins the venous system at the lower end of the left internal jugular vein and can be damaged. Also, a cannula passed from the left internal jugular vein is more likely to pass across into the right internal jugular or subclavian vein.

With the patient tilted head down and the head rotated to the left, the right internal jugular vein is often visible or palpable. The needle punctures the skin midway between the mastoid process and the sternoclavicular joint, and is advanced towards the right nipple to enter the vein. A guidewire is inserted, over which the cannula is then passed.

In 2002 in the UK, the National Institute for Clinical Excellence recommended that two-dimensional imaging ultrasound guidance was the preferred method for internal jugular venous cannulation of adults and children in elective situations.

The subclavian vein is often preferred for long-term use because it is more amenable to subcutaneous tunnelling.

Other approaches that have been used include the axillary, femoral or external jugular veins.

Alternatively, a long catheter may be passed from an antecubital vein, preferably on the medial side of the arm to avoid the pectoral fascia obstructing the passage of the catheter.

The position of the cannula should usually be checked by radiography to ensure its tip lies above the pericardial reflection (i.e. above the level of the carina). This will avoid pericardial tamponade in the rare case where the tip penetrates the wall of the superior vena cava or right atrium. It is also valuable to exclude a pneumothorax.

Complications

Complications of central venous cannulation are air embolism, pneumothorax, damage to other structures in the neck such as the carotid artery, perforation of the vein or right atrium, thromboembolism and infection.

CRYSTALLOIDS AND COLLOIDS

Constituents of some common crystalloid and colloid intravenous fluids are shown in Table 2.7.1 (all are isotonic with plasma).

Gelatins

Gelatins are produced by hydrolysis of collagen. The average molecular weight for both succinylated gelatin 4% and polygeline 3.5% is 30 000. They are widely used for temporary blood volume replacement.

Dextrans

Dextrans are available as dextran 40 and 70 with average molecular weights of 40 000 and 70 000, respectively. Both are available either in 0.9% sodium chloride or in 5% dextrose. Dextran 40 is sometimes used to improve blood flow to ischaemic limbs. Both dextrans have some prophylactic value against

	Na^+ (mmol/L)	K^+ (mmol/L)	Cl^- (mmol/L)	HCO_3^- (mmol/L)	Ca^{++} (mmol/L)
Normal saline (0.9% or 9 g/L)	154	–	154	–	– 0
Hartmann's	131	5	111	29	2
Dextrose (4%) with saline (0.18%)	30	–	30	–	–
Dextrose (5%)	–	–	–	–	–
Succinylated gelatin 4% (Gelofusine®)	154	–	120	–	–
Polygeline 3.5% (Haemaccel®)	145	5.1	145	–	6.25

Table 2.7.1 Constituents of some common crystalloid and colloid intravenous fluids

deep venous thrombosis, but have been replaced for this purpose by heparin preparations. Dextrans interfere with blood grouping and cross-matching.

Starches

Starches are mainly amylopectin etherified with hydroxyethyl groups. Pentastarch is 50% etherified (i.e. 50 hydroxyethyl groups for every 100 glucose units). Tetrastarch and hexastarch are 40% and 60% etherified, respectively. Average molecular weights are generally high (130 000 for tetrastarch; 200 000 for pentastarch and hexastarch). They are usually presented as a 6% solution in normal saline. They are considerably longer lasting as plasma expanders than the gelatins or dextrans.

There is a small but significant incidence of anaphylaxis with all colloids, and this is least common with albumin solutions.

Gastrointestinal fluid losses

For replacement of gastrointestinal fluid losses, it is helpful to compare the figures given above with the approximate volume and electrolyte composition of gut secretions (Table 2.7.2).

	Na^+ (mmol/L)	K^+ (mmol/L)	Cl^- (mmol/L)	HCO_3^- (mmol/L)	Volume (mL/day)
Stomach	30–80	5–15	110–140	*	2000
Pancreas	130	10	60	90	1000–1500
Bile	130	10	100	35	500
Small bowel	130	10	110	30	1500+

* pH is about 1.0

Table 2.7.2 Approximate volume and electrolyte composition of gut secretions

ARTERIAL CANNULATION

Any artery that can be compressed after cannulation may be used for arterial cannulation. The radial artery is normally preferred. Alternative sites are the dorsalis pedis, brachial or femoral arteries. The only sure confirmation of arterial, rather than venous, cannulation is to observe the pulse waveform or to measure a sufficiently high PO_2. It can be misleading to rely only on the colour of the blood. The cannula and any connecting lines should be clearly marked as arterial and kept as separate as possible from intravenous lines, to avoid the possibility of accidental arterial injection of drugs. Extreme care is also taken to avoid entry of air into an artery.

Before radial artery cannulation, some anaesthetists perform Allen's test – press on the radial and ulnar arteries while a fist is made, extend the patient's fingers and release the pressure on the ulnar artery only, when re-flushing of the hand indicates a healthy alternative blood supply to the radial artery. Others consider that the significant incidence of false positives and negatives makes this test misleading and therefore unnecessary.

BLOOD TRANSFUSION

A bloodborne disease, new variant Creutzfeldt–Jakob disease (nvCJD), is now forcing clinicians to re-evaluate their decision to give patients a transfusion.[1] In March 2004 the Minister of Health announced that patients who had received a transfusion since 1980 would not be allowed to donate blood. This has the potential to reduce the donation pool by 6–10%. The government has insisted that hospitals look carefully at their practice, in particular the measures taken to attempt to reduce perioperative transfusion.[2]

It is fundamental to the use of any therapeutic agent to understand its contents and potential physiological effects, both beneficial and harmful. Transfusion of blood and blood products is potentially life saving in acute severe haemorrhage.

Our understanding of the effects of transfusion, the period of blood storage, and when or why to transfuse red cells is still in its infancy. Until such questions are answered we should be cautious with a product used so widely but with so little proven efficacy. It is useful to highlight currently contentious areas of transfusion and blood conservation in the perioperative setting.

Blood and blood products

A transfusion can consist of blood or its related constituents (blood products). Blood is collected from the donor into polyvinyl chloride bags partly prefilled with one of several anticoagulants. It is then subjected to centrifugation, leucodepletion and separation into red blood cells (RBCs) and the haemostatic components. In the UK RBCs are re-suspended in saline, adenine (to preserve cellular ATP stores), mannitol and glucose (to preserve the 2,3-diphosphoglycerate [DPG] as much as possible). They are then stored at 4°C.

Temporal chemical and physical changes result from these mechanical processes and cold storage. These changes are well documented and result clinically in the infusion of hyperkalaemic, acidotic fluids containing RBCs that are much less deformable than normal and sometimes collected in aggregates or clumps. The mark of efficacy of a transfusion is defined by the US Food and Drugs Administration as survival of 70% or more of RBCs 24 hours after a transfusion. By this time, therefore, up to 30 % of the transfused cells may be dead.

Fresh frozen plasma

Fresh frozen plasma (FFP) is separated from whole blood at the time of collection, flash frozen, and the cryoprecipitate withdrawn. A unit of FFP should contain:

- 400 mg of fibrinogen in 200 mL of plasma;
- 1 unit of activity per mL for each clotting factor;
- Na^+ 170 mmol/L; K^+ 4 mmol/L; glucose 22 mmol/L and lactate 3 mmol/L, with a pH between 7.2 and 7.4;
- labile clotting factors V and VIII – may decrease to less than 40% 4 hours after thawing.

UK guidelines for use after thawing may change to allow use up to 24 hours later, provided the plasma has been stored at between 1 and 6°C after thawing.

Solvent detergents and treatment with methylene blue are used as additional measures to reduce viral loads in FFP. All FFP transfused into children born after 1996 should be treated with methylene blue and sourced from the US.

Transfusion-related acute lung injury (TRALI) is increasingly being recognised as a complication of the transfusion of FFP. It occurs if leucoagglutinating specific antibodies are present in donor plasma. If this is the case, the donor is usually a woman who has become immunised against leucocyte antigens during pregnancy.[3]

Cryoprecipitate

Cryoprecipitate is the precipitate of slow-thawing FFP. It contains between 9 and 15 mg/mL of fibrinogen compared to FFP, which contains only 2 mg/mL.

Platelets

Platelets are prepared by centrifugation of whole blood. One pooled unit contains 55×10^9 platelets in 50 mL (normal blood contains this number of platelets in about 200 mL, or 250×10^9/L).

A single unit should raise the platelet count by between 5 and 10×10^9/L.

An apheresis unit, often from a single donor, contains 30×10^{10} platelets and is the equivalent of six pooled platelet units.

Platelets are subject to rapid deterioration during storage, and only 40–60% of platelets are active in any infusion.

Cytokine levels in platelet infusions are higher than for any other blood product and may account for many of their adverse effects. For example, platelet infusions have been associated with a fourfold and sevenfold increase in stroke and death, respectively, after cardiac surgery.[4]

Is blood transfusion necessary?

It is clear from the above discussion that transfusion is not an exact science, and not without risk of considerable complications. Inappropriate transfusion of patients during surgery has often been criticised, but it is of interest to put these patients in the context of all those receiving blood transfusions.

Table 2.7.3, published in 2002, shows that in the north of England just over 50% of all transfused blood is used for medical (i.e. non-surgical) reasons, often with little scientific justification.[5]

Blood is a potentially scarce and expensive resource. Before starting a transfusion in the perioperative setting it is necessary to consider the aim of transfusion and the expected outcome.

For the past 50 years the traditional view of the haematologist was that a transfusion was efficacious if the transfused RBCs had a 24-hour survival rate of over 70%.[6] This is probably not a sensible method of assessment in the surgical patient.

To understand the aim of a perioperative blood transfusion, it is necessary to consider the relationship between oxygen delivery to the tissues (DO_2) and consumption ($\dot{V}O_2$).

	No (% of all transfused; 95% CI) of units ($n = 9774$)	Mean (SD) age (years) of recipients*
Medicine		
All uses	5047 (51.6; 50.6 to 52.7)	64.6 (19.7)
Anaemia	2269 (23.2)	67.1 (17.1)
Haematology	1514 (15.5)	61.2 (20.5)
Gastrointestinal bleed	1054 (10.8)	69.2 (15.5)
Other	148 (1.5)	55.5 (23.0)
Neonatal top-up/ exchange transfusion	62 (0.6)	0
Surgery	3982 (40.7; 39.7 to 41.7)	64.1 (18.2)
Obstetrics and gynaecology		
All uses	612 (6.3; 5.6 to 6.8)	38.7 (18.0)
Gynaecology	307 (3.1)	47.7 (19.5)
Obstetrics	305 (3.1)	29.7 (10.5)
No clinical details	133 (1.4; 1.1 to 1.6)	60.5 (20.14)

*67.2 (20.1) for all transfusions

Table 2.7.3 Indications for red cell transfusion

Oxygen delivery (DO_2) is:

- cardiac output × arterial oxygen content.

Arterial oxygen content depends mainly on the haemoglobin concentration and arterial oxygen saturation.

Oxygen consumption $\dot{V}O_2$ is often calculated by the Fick equation as:

- cardiac output × the arteriovenous oxygen content difference.

The two terms are related by the graph shown in Figure 2.7.1.

It can be seen that, as oxygen delivery is potentially reduced, whether by haemorrhage, myocardial dysfunction or hypoxic hypoxaemia, oxygen consumption is maintained by increasing oxygen extraction. However, as oxygen delivery is reduced further, the critical DO_2 is reached. $\dot{V}O_2$ then moves from being independent of supply to becoming dependent on supply, with resultant ischaemic injury and cell death. The aim of blood transfusion is to ensure that this point is never reached and forms the basis for the term 'transfusion trigger'.

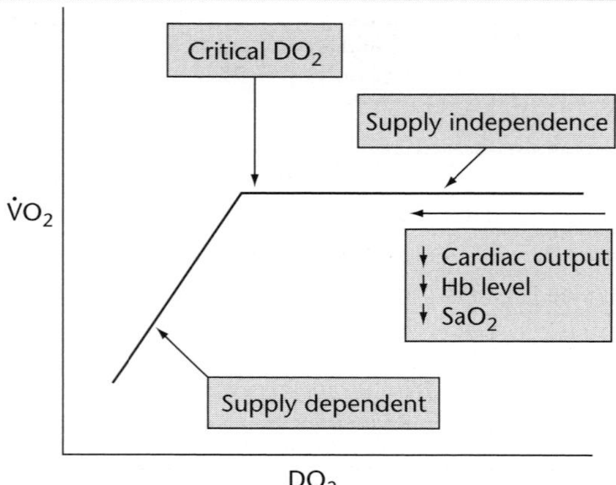

Figure 2.7.1 The relationship between oxygen consumption ($\dot{V}O_2$) and delivery (DO_2). As oxygen delivery to the tissues falls, whether due to reduced cardiac output, haemoglobin concentration or arterial oxygen saturation (SaO_2), $\dot{V}O_2$ is unaltered (i.e. is independent of supply) until delivery reaches a critical value, below which $\dot{V}O_2$ starts to drop (i.e. is dependent on supply).

What is an appropriate transfusion trigger?

What is an appropriate transfusion trigger? This is a difficult question to answer. The main factors that need to be taken into account are:

- how has the patient has become anaemic? Is it due to acute haemorrhage or gradual, well oxygenated haemodilution?
- how old is the patient?
- does the patient have any co-morbidity?

The father of thiopental (Lundy) may be responsible for the often quoted haemoglobin trigger level of 10 g/L. There is no evidence to support this practice.

Young children safely tolerate haemoglobin levels down to 3 g/L during haemodilution for spinal surgery.[7]

An elegant set of experiments has shown that healthy conscious volunteers lose their ability to perform simple tasks at haemoglobin levels as low as 5 g/L.[8]

However, neither of these studies sheds any light on what might be a safe haemoglobin level in the more typical elderly surgical patient with stable angina and peripheral vascular disease who has fallen and requires an emergency hip operation.

The major concern is whether there will be adequate oxygen delivery to the heart. It is well known that the myocardium extracts up to 75% of

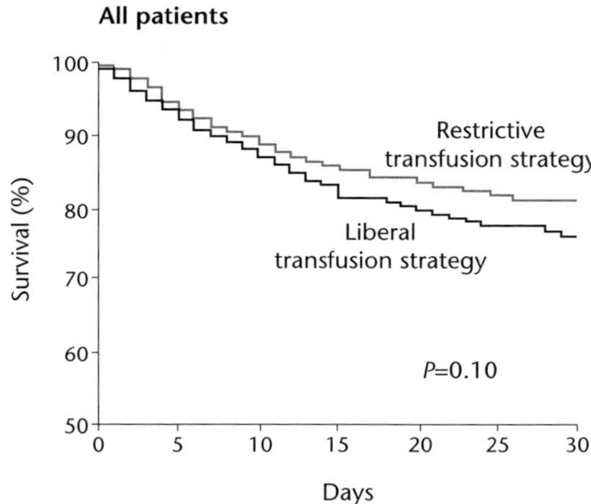

Figure 2.7.2 Improved survival in critically ill patients when the blood transfusion policy is restrictive. From Hebert et al.[9]

the oxygen delivered to it by the coronary arteries. This maximal extraction is unique to the coronary circulation. The delivery of oxygen can only be augmented by increasing blood flow or arterial oxygen content. These facts have led many physicians to assume that anaemia is undesirable in a patient with ischaemic heart disease, and to adopt a liberal transfusion policy. This approach fails to balance the severity of the anaemia with the question of whether there is improvement after transfusion. The evidence is confusing and conflicting. Three studies have attempted to answer this conundrum, one prospective and two retrospective observational studies.

In the first, Hebert et al., in the only prospective randomised study to question the outcome after transfusion, showed that a restrictive transfusion strategy was advantageous compared to a liberal strategy in critically ill patients (patients after heart surgery were excluded).[9] The results are displayed in Figure 2.7.2. They show increased survival with adoption of the more restrictive transfusion policy (i.e. transfusion triggered by a haemoglobin of 7 g/L), compared with the more liberal policy (i.e. transfusion triggered by a haemoglobin of 10 g/L).

This groundbreaking study questioned many of the widely held values of the benefits of transfusion, and led to a further question: Could the transfusion of red cells actually contribute to or cause tissue injury, or did the lower haemoglobin concentration protect against tissue injury? This is still unanswered.

The other two studies looked at patients admitted with acute myocardial infarction. The first, a retrospective review of the Medicare records of 78 974 patients over 65 years of age hospitalised with a primary diagnosis of myocardial infarction, conflicts with Hebert's results.[10] This study can be summarised as:

- anaemia as defined by a haematocrit of less than 39% was present in 50% of patients;
- only 3680 patients (4.7%) received a transfusion;
- if treatment subsequently included a blood transfusion, the 30-day mortality rate was reduced in the cohort of patients who had haematocrits between 33 and 36% on admission.

This is the first and only study to demonstrate that transfusion may be beneficial in patients with acute myocardial infarction. However, it suffers from several major limitations – relatively few patients received transfusion, a significant number of patients with a low haematocrit were deemed not for resuscitation, and there was a lack of statistical adjustments in multivariate analyses.

Despite these biases, an accompanying editorial suggested that all elderly patients whose haematocrit was less than 33% should be transfused following acute myocardial infarction. Such a policy has considerable significance for medical practice in coronary care units.

In contrast, the final study, by Rao and colleagues, demonstrated that the risk of death was 3.94 times higher in patients transfused after acute myocardial infarction than in those who did not receive transfusion.[11] These were prospectively collected data and were analysed in an appropriate manner.

Both animal and human studies of the effects of anaemia on myocardial function show that, in the absence of coronary artery disease, anaemia to levels down to 7 g/L is well tolerated. In animal models with high-grade coronary stenosis, myocardial dysfunction and ischaemia occur earlier and are more pronounced as normovolaemic anaemia reduces the haemoglobin towards 7 g/L.

To transfuse vs to not transfuse

In summary there is now sufficient evidence to assume that transfusion would not be beneficial when the haemoglobin is greater than 10 g/L in the absence of acute blood loss. Anaemia below 8 g/L may be more progressively harmful in patients with ischaemic heart disease. Between 8 and 10 g/L controversy still exists. The individual patient's physiological requirements should be taken into account rather than adopting a slavish adherence to protocols.

Reducing the need for transfusion

How might the incidence of transfusion be reduced in the surgical patient? It would seem reasonable that preoperative screening should exclude the anaemic patient from elective surgery, at least until the anaemia is diagnosed and treated. Having accepted the patient for surgery, the following general factors are important in reducing blood loss in many types of surgery:

- controlling and maintaining body temperature;
- controlling and maintaining a normal $P\text{CO}_2$;
- positioning the patient carefully to aid venous drainage from the site of surgery;
- considering whether a regional anaesthetic technique would help (e.g. central neuraxial blockade);
- controlling blood pressure – avoiding unnecessary hypertension and considering modest hypotension.

There are two principal groups of specific methods to reduce the need for transfusion – mechanical and pharmacological.

Mechanical methods

Mechanical methods to reduce the need for transfusion include acute peroperative normovolaemic haemodilution (APNH) and cell salvage.

Acute peroperative normovolaemic haemodilution

APNH is the withdrawal of a certain amount of blood and its replacement with an equivalent volume of crystalloid or colloid. It is used for surgery associated with major but controlled blood loss. The meta-analysis shown in Figure 2.7.3 demonstrates that APNH significantly reduces the need for blood transfusion in orthopaedic surgery, cardiac surgery and other miscellaneous groups.[12]

It is perhaps not surprising that the efficacy of APNH is improved by withdrawing a greater volume of blood. The odds ratio when this volume was less than 1000 mL was 0.43 (95% CI 0.18–1.02), and when the volume exceeded 1000 mL was 0.16 (95% CI 0.04–0.65).

Cell salvage

An effective approach to reduce the need for transfusion that can be used intra- or postoperatively, and with processed or unprocessed blood, is cell salvage. Processed salvaged blood yields a haematocrit of 50–70% in the transfused mixture, which is reduced to 20% if it is unprocessed.

Unprocessed cell salvage Unprocessed cell salvage is safe and efficacious provided large volumes are not reinfused. Free haemoglobin has a marked left-shifted oxygen dissociation curve and also passes through the glomerular filter. The high free haemoglobin levels in unprocessed salvage blood may therefore lead to acidosis and renal failure.

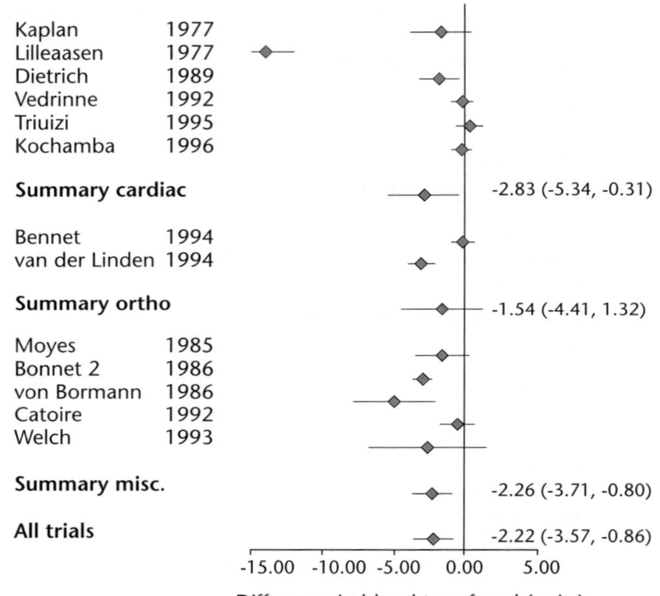

Figure 2.7.3 The number of units of blood transfused in six studies of cardiac surgery, two of orthopaedic surgery, and five of miscellaneous types of surgery (thoracic, ENT, liver and vascular), expressed as the differences with or without acute peroperative normovolaemic haemodilution (APNH). When APNH is used, there is a mean overall reduction in blood transfused of 2.22 units. From Bryson et al.[12]

Processed cell salvage Processed cell salvage yields a quality and quantity of recovered red cells that is dependent on the cell washing. This in turn is dependent on the prime volume of the washing bowl and the rate of washing. For instance, faster wash cycles are likely to lead to a lower haematocrit of the returned red cells in patients with ruptured abdominal aortic aneurysm, whereas recovered red cells from orthopaedic surgery will require larger volumes of wash at lower rates to ensure proper removal of fat and bone debris.

Pharmacological methods

There are two main classes of pharmacological agent used to reduce operative blood loss and the need for blood transfusion. These act in very different ways:

- serine protease inhibitors (e.g. aprotinin) prevent fibrinolysis by direct inhibition of plasmi;

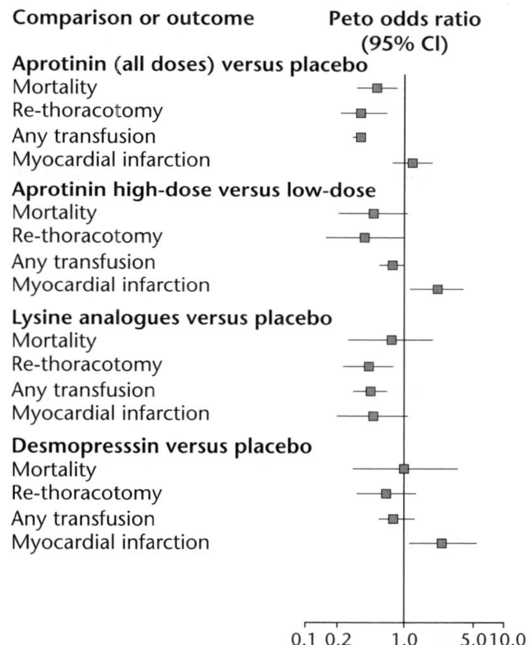

Figure 2.7.4 The odds ratios for various outcomes from a meta-analysis of patients undergoing cardiac surgery. There is a beneficial effect of aprotinin and lysine analogues, but not for desmopressin. From Levi et al.[13]

- lysine analogues (e.g. tranexamic acid, ε-aminocaproic acid) prevent the conversion of plasminogen to plasmin.

In addition, desmopressin has been used for this purpose. It acts by stimulating the release of von Willebrand factor from endothelial cells to promote primary haemostasis.

Both aprotinin and the lysine analogues have been shown to be effective in the meta-analysis of patients undergoing cardiac surgery shown in Figure 2.7.4, with improved mortality rates, need for re-operation, and transfusion requirements.[13] By contrast, desmopressin offered little advantage, and in addition was associated with a 2.4-fold increase in perioperative myocardial infarction.

Aprotinin is considerably more expensive than the lysine analogues. However, it has shown a convincing dose–response curve and greater efficacy in most comparisons. Although the above meta-analysis was in cardiac surgery, aprotinin has also been shown to be effective in preventing blood loss and reducing transfusion requirements in revision or bilateral total hip arthroplasty, although the improvement was less striking. Mean blood loss dropped from 2096 mL to 1498 mL with the use of aprotinin.[14]

References

1. Llewelyn CA, Hewitt PE, Knight RS, et al. Possible transmission of variant Creutzfeldt–Jakob disease by blood transfusion. Lancet 2004; 363:417–421.
2. Department of Health. Better blood transfusion. London: The Stationery Office; 2002.
3. Wallis JP. Transfusion related acute lung injury – under diagnosed and under-reported. Br J Anaesth 2003; 90:573–575.
4. Spiess BD, Royston D, Levy JH, et al. Platelet transfusions during coronary artery bypass graft surgery are associated with serious adverse outcomes. Transfusion 2004; 44:1143–1148.
5. Wells AW, Mounter PJ, Chapman CE, Stainsby D, Wallis JP. Where does blood go? Prospective observational study of red cell transfusion in north England. Br Med J 2002; 325:803.
6. Mollison PL. The life-span of red blood cells. Lect Sci Basis Med 1952; 2:269–286.
7. Fontana JL, Welborn L, Mongan PD, et al. Oxygen consumption and cardiovascular function in children during profound intraoperative normovolemic hemodilution. Anesth Analg 1995; 80:219–225.
8. Weiskopf RB, Viele MK, Feiner J, et al. Human cardiovascular and metabolic response to acute, severe isovolemic anemia. JAMA 1998; 279:217–221.
9. Hebert PC, Wells G, Blajchman MA, et al. A multicenter, randomized, controlled clinical trial of transfusion requirements in critical care. Transfusion Requirements in Critical Care Investigators, Canadian Critical Care Trials Group. N Engl J Med 1999; 340:409–417.
10. Wu WC, Rathore SS, Wang Y, Radford MJ, Krumholz HM. Blood transfusion in elderly patients with acute myocardial infarction. N Engl J Med 2001; 345:1230–1236.
11. Rao SV, Jollis JG, Harrington RA, et al. Relationship of blood transfusion and clinical outcomes in patients with acute coronary syndromes. JAMA 2004; 292:1555–1562.
12. Bryson GL, Laupacis A, Wells GA. Does acute normovolemic hemodilution reduce perioperative allogeneic transfusion? A meta-analysis. The International Study of Perioperative Transfusion. Anesth Analg 1998; 86:9–15.
13. Levi M, Cromheecke ME, de Jonge E, et al. Pharmacological strategies to decrease excessive blood loss in cardiac surgery: a meta-analysis of clinically relevant endpoints. Lancet 1999; 354:1940–1947.

14. Murkin, JM, Shanon NA, Bourne RB, et al. Aprotinin decreases blood loss in patients undergoing revision or bilateral total hip arthroplasty. Anesth Analg 1995; 80:343–348.

CHAPTER **2.8**

ACID–BASE, ELECTROLYTE BALANCE AND NUTRITION

ACID–BASE BALANCE

The pH notation was described by Søren PL Sørensen in 1909, with pH defined as the negative logarithm to the base 10 of the hydrogen ion concentration $[H^+]$. The normal range for arterial blood is 7.36–7.44. However, over the clinical range it is more sensible to use $[H^+]$ directly because the scale is linear and not inverse. For example, from Table 2.8.1 it can be seen that the change in $[H^+]$ from pH 7.4 to 7.2 is not as great as that from 7.2 to 7.0 and that, logically, the acidosis worsens as the $[H^+]$ increases.

Acidosis is a condition that would cause acidaemia (i.e. a higher than normal blood $[H^+]$) if uncorrected, and alkalosis would cause alkalaemia if uncorrected. The pH range compatible with life is about 6.8–7.7, or 160–20 nmol/L of hydrogen ions.

An acid is a chemical that dissociates in aqueous solution to give a hydrogen ion and its conjugate base:

- $\text{Acid} \rightarrow H^+ + \text{Base}^-$

At equilibrium, the law of mass action states that the product of the mass of reactants on one side of the equation must equal that on the other side, where K equals the dissociation constant for the reaction, as follows:

- $K[\text{Acid}] \rightarrow [H^+][\text{Base}^-]$

This is the Henderson equation and can be arranged thus:

- $[H^+] = K \times [\text{Acid}]/[\text{Base}^-]$

Or, using the less than intuitive pH notation that requires the use of negative logarithms:

- $pH = pK + \log[\text{Base}^-]/[\text{Acid}]$

Note that acidity, the $[H^+]$, is determined by the ratio of acid to its conjugate base and not by the absolute value of either.

pH (units)	[H+] nmol/L	Comment
6.6	251	
6.8	158	H^+ concentration of water at 37°C
7.0	100	H^+ concentration of water at 20°C
7.2	63	
7.4	40	H^+ concentration in blood at 37°C
7.6	25	
7.8	16	
8.0	10	

Table 2.8.1 Hydrogen ion concentration from pH 6.6 to 8.0

BUFFER SYSTEMS

Buffers act to minimise the change in pH in the blood that would otherwise occur when acid or alkali is added. There are a number of buffer systems in the blood:

- bicarbonate – the most important;
- haemoglobin – the next most important: reduced haemoglobin is a more effective buffer than oxyhaemoglobin;
- plasma proteins – also act as buffers, but their concentration is only one-third that of haemoglobin;
- phosphate – in low concentrations only.

Bicarbonate buffer system.

Carbonic acid is formed by the hydration of carbon dioxide and exists in a state of equilibrium with hydrogen and bicarbonate ions. The combination of carbon dioxide with water is catalysed by carbonic anhydrase, found in high concentrations in red blood cells, enabling the rapid transfer of carbon dioxide between tissues, blood and alveolar gas.

From:

- $[H^+] = K \times [Acid]/[Base^-]$

Since:

- $CO_2 + H_2O \rightleftharpoons H_2CO_3 \rightleftharpoons H^+ + HCO_3^-$

We can write:

- $[H^+] = K \times [H_2CO_3]/[HCO_3^-]$

When $[H^+]$ is expressed in nmol/L, Pa_{CO_2} in kPa, $[HCO_3^-]$ in mmol/L and α is the solubility coefficient, then $[H_2CO_3]$ is proportional to P_{CO_2} such that:

- $[H^+] = K \times \alpha Pa_{CO_2}/[HCO_3^-]$

Lawrence J Henderson derived this equation and Karl A Hasselbalch expressed it in logarithmic form. In pH notation:

- $pH = pK + \log \dfrac{[HCO_3^-]}{\alpha Pa_{CO_2}}$

In arterial blood $[HCO_3] = 24$ mmol/L, $Pa_{CO_2} = 5.3$ kPa, with a solubility coefficient of 0.225 mmol/L/kPa and pK = 6.1, hence:

- $pH = 6.1 + \log \dfrac{24}{(0.225 \times 5.3)}$
- $pH = 6.1 + \log 20$
- $pH = 6.1 + 1.3$ (i.e. pH = 7.4)

The body tries to compensate for any acid–base disturbance by preserving the ratio of $[HCO_3^-]$ to Pa_{CO_2}, and hence keeps the pH normal.

Pa_{CO_2} is altered by changing alveolar ventilation, and $[HCO_3^-]$ by changing renal bicarbonate handling. Because protein buffers also exist in blood, the change in $[HCO_3^-]$ resulting from a metabolic acidosis or alkalosis is less than expected, and so underestimates the true disturbance.

The potential respiratory acid load from CO_2 produced during oxidative metabolism amounts to some 12 000 mmol/day, and explains the rapid onset of acidosis during episodes of hypoventilation. By comparison, the amount of H^+ produced from lactate, fixed acids and urea production is approximately 3000 mmol/day. The bicarbonate buffer system is the most important because of the ability to excrete CO_2 via the lungs. However, in the long term the kidney must excrete hydrogen ions and regenerate bicarbonate to maintain acid–base balance.

Standard bicarbonate is the bicarbonate concentration in the plasma at 37°C with P_{CO_2} 5.3 kPa and fully oxygenated haemoglobin; it is normally 24 mmol/L.

Buffer base is the sum of all the buffer anions in blood (including the proteins) in mmol/L.

Base excess is a measure of the surplus or deficit of acid needed to titrate the pH of the sample to 7.40 when equilibrated at a Pa_{CO_2} of 5.3 kPa, and is said to reflect the metabolic component of an acid–base disturbance. The normal value is usually taken as 0 to –6 mmol/L. This is the most useful clinical estimate of the metabolic component of any acid–base disturbance, and (like standard bicarbonate) takes account of non-bicarbonate buffers in blood, but not the buffers outside blood.

By convention an acid surplus (base deficit) is referred to as a negative base excess.

Peter A Stewart described in 1983 how the acidity of blood could be related to the strong ion difference (SID), $PaCO_2$ and the total weak acids in the body.[1] SID was originally determined as below, but others have expanded the concept to include other cations (e.g. calcium, magnesium) and other anions (e.g. phosphate, albumin and other proteins etc.).

- SID = (Na^+ + K^+) – (Cl^- + lactate)

In health, the normal value is about 40 mmol/L, for example:

- (140 + 5) – (104 + 1) = 40

The difference between the measured SID and the normal value is equal to the base excess.

As an example, in hyperchloraemic acidosis the measured SID may be:

- (140 + 5) – (114 + 1) = 30

and the base excess would then be (30–40) or –10.

Because all plasma ionic charges must balance any perturbations induced by changes in $PaCO_2$, weak acids or SID must be balanced by changes in [H^+]. Incorporating all the necessary variables requires six complex equations, but the underlying principles appear to hold and help in our understanding of acid–base balance.[2]

For example, in the acidosis seen with infusions of 0.9% saline solution the larger increase in plasma chloride relative to sodium and potassium will reduce the SID and therefore cause a compensatory increase in [H^+]. The hyperchloraemia is accompanied by an equivalent loss of bicarbonate, so it will be a normal anion gap acidosis.

In the next example remember that according to Stewart bicarbonate is a dependent variable. The correction of a metabolic acidosis by sodium bicarbonate is due to the unopposed increase in sodium concentration correcting a reduced SID towards normal and so decreasing the ionisation of water and reducing the [H^+].

ARTERIAL BLOOD GAS ANALYSIS

The proper interpretation of a blood gas sample requires a clinical history and physical examination and it should be reviewed in conjunction with other laboratory investigations. In many cases many of these data will be lacking and one must interpret the initial results with caution and follow trends while other information is being obtained.

The following schema may be helpful; think through each option as you work down the list:

- What is the pH? – normal, acidosis/alkalosis, compensatory changes?
- What is the $PaCO_2$? – normal, high/low, compensated?
- What is the measured bicarbonate or chloride?

- Calculate the anion gap (AG)
- What is the $P\text{aO}_2$? – relate to the fraction of inspired oxygen ($F\text{IO}_2$)

First, look at the pH to see if there is acidaemia or alkalaemia, remembering that a pH may be near normal because of pulmonary or renal compensatory mechanisms.

Next look at the $P\text{aCO}_2$ to see if there is hypoventilation or hyperventilation; are any changes compensatory?

Look at the measured bicarbonate and calculated base excess to assess whether a metabolic alkalosis or acidosis is present; again these may be compensatory.

If a chloride is available, calculate the anion gap:

- $AG = (Na^+ + K^+) - (HCO_3^- + Cl^-)$

This gap is due to the presence of unmeasured anions such as sulphate and ketones, plus phosphate and albumin.

Finally, look at the $P\text{aO}_2$ and interpret this in light of the $F\text{IO}_2$.

Atmospheric pressure is approximately 100 kPa, so 1% is approximately 1 kPa. This would mean that inspiring, say, 40% oxygen from a facemask would lead to an alveolar concentration of at least 30 kPa and a similar value for the $P\text{aO}_2$. If not, there is likely to be hypoventilation, a barrier to alveolar diffusion or a right-to-left shunt.

Problems with blood sampling can lead to erroneous results. Common errors include failure to account for apparatus dead space, excess of heparin or air bubbles in the sample and prolonged delay to analysis.

Metabolic acidosis

Metabolic acidosis results in a negative base excess (i.e. a base deficit) and a low standard bicarbonate.

Causes

Metabolic acidosis may occur due to an excess acid production or administration/ingestion. Further information is obtained from the plasma anion gap, which allows differentiation of the less common normal anion gap acidosis from the more usual high anion gap acidosis.

Normal anion gap acidosis

In normal anion gap acidosis there is decreased plasma bicarbonate but retention of chloride. Causes include:

- failure of renal acidification – renal tubular acidosis, acetazolamide treatment;
- bicarbonate loss from the gut – diarrhoea, small bowel fistulae, ureterosigmoidostomy;

- excessive administration of 0.9% saline;
- hyperkalaemia associated with hypoaldosteronism.

Increased anion gap acidosis

More commonly there is an increased anion gap acidosis due to elevation in the plasma of acids whose anions are not measured. These are usually organic in nature and causes include:

- ketoacidosis – diabetes mellitus, alcoholism, starvation;
- lactic acidosis – poor tissue perfusion, phenformin, severe alkalaemia;
- renal failure – retention of acid metabolites;
- poisoning – salicylates, ethylene glycol, methanol.

These all result in the measured cations (sodium and potassium) exceeding the measured anions (bicarbonate and chloride). The normal anion gap is often quoted as 8–12 mmol/L, but it is useful to correct the anion gap in known hypoalbuminaemia and hypophosphataemia thus:

- AG = 0.2 × albumin (g/L) + 1.5 × phosphate (mmol/L)

Effects

A number of nonspecific effects are difficult to separate from the cause of the metabolic acidosis, including:

- increased respiration (stimulated via the peripheral chemoreceptors);
- palpitations;
- nausea and vomiting;
- hyperkalaemia.

The hyperventilation reduces the $Pa\text{CO}_2$ and this partially compensates for the acidosis.

Treatment

Treatment of metabolic acidosis is mainly of the primary cause. Occasionally, treatment with intravenous sodium bicarbonate is necessary (e.g. following reperfusion).

One common formula for the dose of bicarbonate is:

- (Base excess × weight in kg)/3

Usually, much smaller doses (50 mmol) are given and the effect is monitored by repeat blood gas analysis. An increase in ventilation will be required to excrete the excess carbon dioxide so generated; otherwise this rapidly diffuses into cells and worsens any intracellular acidosis.

The disadvantages of giving bicarbonate in a metabolic acidosis are:

- hyperosmolar load;
- hypernatraemia;

- increased minute ventilation to remove carbon dioxide formed;
- alkalosis produces vasoconstriction;
- left shift of the oxyhaemoglobin dissociation curve, reducing tissue oxygen delivery.

Metabolic alkalosis

Metabolic alkalosis results in a positive base excess and high standard bicarbonate.

Causes

Metabolic alkalosis may occur following:

- loss of acid – pyloric stenosis, vomiting or nasogastric drainage, diuretic-induced hypokalaemia;
- ingestion of large amounts of bicarbonate or its precursors (e.g. citrate drinks, milk–alkali syndrome).

Effects

In metabolic alkalosis the body compensates by hypoventilation and increased renal bicarbonate excretion. The consequences of metabolic alkalosis on organ systems depend on the severity of the alkalaemia and the degree of respiratory compensation and include:

- reduced oxygen delivery due to alkalaemia may be worsened by a compensatory hypoventilation to elevate $Pa\text{CO}_2$;
- arrhythmias;
- muscle weakness;
- renal potassium and magnesium loss that may be symptomatic;
- reduced ionised calcium;
- stimulating of phosphofructokinase, so increasing lactate production.

Treatment

Treatment of metabolic alkalosis is mainly of the primary cause, but potassium and magnesium will need to be replaced. Dilute hydrochloric acid can be given orally or intravenously; acetazolamide may be considered.

Respiratory acidosis

Respiratory acidosis is caused by inadequate alveolar ventilation with a consequent increase in $Pa\text{CO}_2$.

Causes

Hypercarbia is common in anaesthesia and intensive care practice and is usually well tolerated. Common causes of respiratory acidosis include:

- impairment of ventilation due to respiratory depression, obstruction or weakness;
- severe chronic obstructive lung disease;
- asthma;
- accidental administration of carbon dioxide;
- faulty carbon dioxide absorption;
- during apnoea;
- overproduction of carbon dioxide (e.g. severe burns, hyperpyrexia).

Effects

Acute changes produce far more manifestations than chronic carbon dioxide retention, as follows:

- central nervous system – cerebral vasodilatation and increased intracranial pressure; headache occurs. As the $P\text{aCO}_2$ rises towards 25 kPa narcosis deepens into coma, and over 25 kPa there is a profound narcosis and respiratory failure resembling curarisation. If the hypercapnia is chronic the cerebrospinal fluid (CSF) bicarbonate rises, restores the CSF pH, and so sets a new baseline for cerebral vascular resistance;
- autonomic nervous system – sympathetic activation, with a rise of circulating catecholamines and sweating; any parasympathetic activation is overshadowed by the sympathetic effect;
- respiratory system – carbon dioxide stimulates the respiratory centre. There is right shift of the oxyhaemoglobin dissociation curve, the Bohr effect – via an increase in hydrogen ions, which facilitates oxygen release in the tissues;
- cardiovascular system – increased rate and force of contraction, and vasodilatation due to direct effect of carbon dioxide on the blood vessels, increases cardiac output. There is sympathetic stimulation and increased circulating catecholamine; blood pressure often rises. Arrhythmias may occur, particularly during halothane anaesthesia. A direct peripheral effect leads to vasodilatation, with flushed skin and distended veins.

Treatment

Respiratory acidosis is treated by increasing alveolar ventilation plus or minus reducing carbon dioxide production.

Recovery from severe respiratory acidosis may be associated with hypophosphataemia, so this should be monitored carefully.

If the $Pa\text{CO}_2$ is reduced too rapidly after a long period of hypercapnia there may be:

- sudden hypotension;
- a left shift of the haemoglobin dissociation curve;
- a rapid rise in CSF pH leading to cerebral vasoconstriction and convulsions.

Respiratory alkalosis

Respiratory alkalosis is caused by hyperventilation, producing hypocapnia and a rise in pH.

Causes

Excessive mechanical ventilatory support may readily reduce the $Pa\text{CO}_2$ from a normal of 5.3 kPa to half of this value. Other causes of hyperventilation are in response to hypoxia, high altitude, metabolic acidosis or neurological disease (e.g. severe head injury, hyperventilation syndrome).

Effects

Effects of respiratory alkalosis are as follows:

- nervous system – cerebral vasoconstriction and reduced cerebral blood flow, clouding of consciousness and analgesia, voluntary hyperventilation lessens, tetany due to the fall in ionised calcium;
- cardiovascular system – peripheral vasoconstriction, but fall of blood pressure and cardiac output. Coronary vasoconstriction;
- respiratory system – lack of stimulation of the respiratory centre may lead to hypoventilation. Left shift of the haemoglobin dissociation curve;
- fetus – hyperventilation causes a reduction in uteroplacental blood flow that, with the left-shifted haemoglobin dissociation curve, causes a fall in fetal oxygen supply and acidosis.

Treatment

Respiratory alkalosis is treated by a decrease in alveolar ventilation by reducing tidal volume, respiratory rate or both.

ELECTROLYTE BALANCE

SODIUM

Normal serum level is 138–142 mmol/L, and the maintenance requirement is 1.0 mmol/kg. Most sodium is extracellular; normal intracellular concentration is 10 mmol/L.

Hyponatraemia

A relative excess of water to plasma electrolytes is usually noted by the presence of hyponatraemia and a fall in plasma osmolality. The incidence of postoperative hyponatraemia is reported to be approximately 1% and, when severe (Na <110 mmol/L with neurological symptoms), is a medical emergency.[3]

The endocrine stress response to surgery or trauma increases plasma antidiuretic hormone (ADH) and impairs free water excretion (also seen with administration of oxytocin), which leads to an inappropriately high urine osmolality in the face of a low plasma osmolality. Osmolality (normal 280–290 mosmol/L) is calculated as:

- $2 \times [Na^+] + [urea] + [glucose]$

Causes

An assessment of volume status and total body water should be attempted and the urine sodium concentration, and plasma osmolality (calculated and measured), should be determined. An increase in the plasma calculated to measured osmolar gap suggests the presence of unmeasured substances such as alcohol or mannitol. Pseudohyponatraemia may be seen with severe hyperlipidaemia/hyperproteinaemia.

The causes of hyponatraemia in hypovolaemic, euvolaemic and hypervolaemic patients are given in Box 2.8.1.

Effects

The effects of hyponatraemia relate to the speed at which it develops, as well as the absolute degree. Anorexia and vomiting occur first, but then neuropsychiatric effects predominate when sodium is below 125 mmol/L. There is brain swelling with lassitude, apathy, confusion, weakness, and eventually peripheral circulatory failure. In chronic hyponatraemia, compensatory mechanisms such as loss of solutes from the brain lead to a decrease in brain swelling.

Treatment

Rapid correction of hyponatraemia, especially if chronic, may lead to central pontine myelinolysis.

Box 2.8.1

Causes of hyponatraemia in hypovolaemic, euvolaemic and hypervolaemic patients

Hypovolaemic patient

Extrarenal salt loss (urine [Na^+] <20 mmol/L)

Vomiting, diarrhoea, intestinal fistulae

Unrecognised losses in burns, pancreatitis or bowel obstruction

Renal salt loss (urine [Na^+] >20 mmol/L)

Diuretics including osmotic effect

Mineralocorticoid deficiency

Salt-losing nephropathy

Euvolaemic patient (urine [Na^+] >20 mmol/L)

Water excess

Intravenous hypotonic solutions

Primary polydipsia

Fluid absorption during transurethral resection of prostate (TURP) or endometrial surgery

Associated factors

Glucocorticoid deficiency

Syndrome of inappropriate antidiuretic hormone secretion (SIADH)

Hypothyroidism

Drugs (e.g. antipsychotics)

Hypervolaemic patient (urine [Na^+] <20 mmol/L)

Nephrotic syndrome

Cirrhosis

Heart failure

Acute or chronic renal failure

The management of acute severe symptomatic hyponatraemia should be on an intensive care unit to allow careful monitoring and measurement of electrolytes every hour.

In hypovolaemic patients ADH will be high, so first resuscitate with isotonic fluids.

Treatment of hyponatraemia is as follows:

- treat the primary cause;
- stop any implicated drug therapy;
- water restriction;
- for acute symptomatic hyponatraemia, hypertonic saline (1.8%) is given to raise the sodium by 1–2 mmol/L/h;
- loop diuretic to increase free water clearance;
- in chronic and asymptomatic hyponatraemia, the rate of increase should be no more than 1 mmol/L/h.

Hypernatraemia

An assessment of volume status and total body water should be attempted and the urine sodium concentration, and plasma osmolality (calculated and measured), should be determined.[4]

Causes

The causes of hypernatraemia in hypovolaemic, euvolaemic and hypervolaemic patients are given in Box 2.8.2.

Effects

Intense thirst is prominent in hypernatraemia, but there is unlikely to be any oedema. Central nervous system symptoms predominate, with confusion, apathy, hyper-reflexia and eventually coma.

Treatment

As with hyponatraemia, the speed of correction of the high sodium depends on the degree and acuity of the hypernatraemia. Because of the generation of 'idiogenic osmols' in the brain in chronic hypernatraemia there is a high risk of acute brain swelling if the plasma osmolality is decreased too quickly. In hypovolaemic patients, first use isotonic fluids to correct any haemodynamic abnormality. Treatment of hypernatraemia is as follows:

- treat the primary cause – consider desmopressin for diabetes insipidus, and review drug therapy, especially diuretics;
- withhold sodium-containing fluids;
- administer water by the enteral route or hypotonic fluids intravenously;
- furosemide (frusemide) or dialysis may be needed if hypervolaemic;
- the rate of decrease in plasma sodium should be no more than 1 mmol/L/h.

Box 2.8.2

Causes of hypernatraemia in hypovolaemic, euvolaemic and hypervolaemic patients

Hypovolaemic patient

Extrarenal losses of more water than salt (urine [Na^+] <20 mmol/L)

Excessive sweating

Burns, diarrhoea, intestinal fistulae

Renal loss of more water than salt (urine [Na^+] >20 mmol/L)

Diuretics including osmotic effect

Renal disease

Post-obstruction diuresis

Euvolaemic patient

Excess water loss

Diabetes insipidus
- Neurogenic (e.g. head injury)
- Nephrogenic (e.g. congenital or acquired, e.g. severe hypokalaemia)
- Drug induced (e.g. amphotericin B, demeclocycline or lithium)

Hypervolaemic patient (urine [Na^+] >20 mmol/L)

Excess sodium administration

High sodium-containing fluids (e.g. hypertonic saline, sodium bicarbonate)

Inappropriate replacement of daily insensible losses with high-sodium fluids

Inability to excrete sodium

Primary hyperaldosteronism

Cushing's syndrome or high-dose corticosteroid therapy

POTASSIUM

Normal serum potassium level is 3.5–5.0 mmol/L. The maintenance requirement is 1.0 mmol/kg or 5–7 mmol/g nitrogen, with a higher requirement if severely malnourished. Most potassium is intracellular, with about 2% in the extracellular compartment, and only 0.4% in the serum. Normal intracellular concentration is 150 mmol/L.

Hypokalaemia

Causes

Causes of hypokalaemia are:

- inadequate intake, especially when reliant on intravenous therapy;
- excessive loss from the gastrointestinal tract – vomiting, diarrhoea, fistulae etc.;
- excessive loss in the urine – diuretics, aminophylline overdose, renal tubular acidosis etc.;
- hyperadrenal states or intensive steroid therapy;
- catecholamine-induced shift of potassium into cells – e.g. intravenous salbutamol;
- alkalosis – causes potassium to move into cells;
- insulinoma – drives potassium into cells;
- familial periodic paralysis.

Effects

Hypokalaemia results in a clinical picture of lethargy, apathy, anorexia and nausea related to disordered function of the three types of muscle:

- smooth muscle – resulting in constipation, distension and ileus;
- skeletal muscle – resulting in hypotonia, weakness and paralysis;
- cardiac muscle – resulting in hypotension, arrhythmias and cardiac arrest – the ECG shows ST segment depression, lowering, widening or inversion of T waves, prolongation of PR and QT intervals and the appearance of U waves.

  Hypokalaemia increases the risk of digoxin toxicity.

Treatment

Treatment of hypokalaemia is as follows:

- if there are life-threatening arrhythmias, a small slow bolus dose of potassium may be needed, say 5 mmol over 60 seconds with ECG monitoring and repeated as necessary;
- replace the expected deficit, either orally or intravenously; the deficit may well be in the order of 200 mmol or more. Only dilute solutions are given peripherally – no more than 40 mmol/L because of pain and thrombosis;
- the recommended maximum replacement rate is quoted to be 20 mmol/h, but this can be exceeded, if clinically indicated, under close monitoring;

- potassium administration may not increase intracellular potassium concentration in the presence of magnesium deficiency;
- the correction of hypokalaemia with potassium chloride will correct any concurrent metabolic alkalosis;
- in renal tubular acidosis potassium hydroxide will ameliorate the metabolic acidosis;
- surgery may have to be delayed if the serum potassium is below 3.0 mmol/L because of the risk of cardiac arrhythmias, muscle weakness, inability to reverse relaxants, myopathy and renal failure.

Hyperkalaemia

Hyperkalaemia is dangerous, chiefly because of its effects on the heart; acute changes are more dangerous than chronic changes.

Causes

Causes of hyperkalaemia are:

- excessive administration – usually intravenously, but may occur with commercial salt substitutes;
- renal failure;
- administration of suxamethonium – the hyperkalaemia occurs within minutes and may be up to 1.0 mmol/L in normal patients, but is often much higher in patients with trauma and burns, muscle injury or diseases such as myopathies, motor neuron disease, muscular dystrophy, denervation and spinal cord transection and tetanus. The hyperkalaemia may be ameliorated by pre-treatment with a non-depolarizing agent;
- metabolic acidosis, including diabetic ketosis;
- massive blood transfusion – stored blood may contain 25 mmol/L potassium.
- potassium-sparing diuretics, angiotensin-converting enzyme (ACE) inhibitors, angiotensin II blockers and non-steroidal anti-inflammatory drugs (NSAIDs);
- major trauma and rhabdomyolysis;
- hypoaldosteronism;
- hyperkalaemic periodic paralysis.

Effects

Toxic manifestations of hyperkalaemia may occur at concentrations above 7.0 mmol/L, when the ECG shows peaking of the T wave, ST depression, absence of the P wave, widening of the QRS and finally a biphasic QRST. Ventricular fibrillation may supervene.

Treatment

Treatment of hyperkalaemia is as follows:

- stop further administration or precipitating factors;
- calcium 5 mmol intravenously opposes the action of potassium on the heart;
- increase cellular uptake of potassium – glucose and insulin – 25 g of dextrose (50 mL of 50%) plus 5–15 units of insulin as appropriate for the patient, over 15 minutes sodium bicarbonate, 1 mmol/kg, over 15 minutes; β2 agonists by injection (salbutamol 500 μg over 15 minutes) has been described, but should probably be avoided in ischaemic heart disease (large doses by inhalation may also be effective);
- loop diuretic;
- cation exchange resin – give 15 g 6-hourly orally or 30 g as a retention enema;
- dialysis.

CALCIUM

The normal serum level of calcium is 2.1–2.6 mmol/L; the maintenance requirement is 0.2 mmol/kg. Calcium binding to albumin is pH dependent and the ionised level is the active fraction, so it is more appropriate to measure this fraction, which is normally 1.15–1.25 mmol/L.

Hypocalcaemia

Causes

Causes of hypocalcaemia are:

- postoperative hypoparathyroidism;
- alkalosis – usually due to acute hyperventilation;
- acute pancreatitis – associated with fat necrosis;
- acute hyperphosphataemia – tumour lysis syndrome, crush injury;
- transfusion with citrated blood – rarely requires treatment;
- hypoparathyroidism;
- chronic renal failure due to chronic hyperphosphataemia and reduced renal mass.

Effects

The symptoms of hypocalcaemia correlate with the rate and magnitude of the fall in serum calcium. Neuromuscular irritability leads to circumoral and distal paraesthesia, muscle cramps, tetany and seizures. Hypocalcaemia results in a long QT interval.

Treatment

Treatment of hypocalcaemia is as follows:

- the first line is oral or intravenous calcium and correction of any concurrent hypomagnesaemia. Calcium is irritant to veins and can cause tissue damage if extravasation occurs;
- treating any acidosis will cause the ionised calcium to fall further, so defer this until the hypocalcaemia is corrected;
- dialysis against high calcium and bicarbonate dialysate will correct both hypocalcaemia and acidosis;
- further treatment will depend on the underlying cause, but may include vitamin D analogues, phosphate binders and parathyroidectomy.

Note that calcium and bicarbonate solutions must not mix in the giving set.

Hypercalcaemia

Causes

Hypercalcaemia may be genetic or associated with malignancy, primary hyperparathyroidism, secondary hyperparathyroidism associated with chronic renal failure, thiazide diuretics, immobilisation, sarcoid, excessive vitamin D and the milk–alkali syndrome.

Effects

Symptoms of hypercalcaemia correlate with the rate and magnitude of increase in serum calcium. Above 3.0 mmol/L nausea, vomiting, constipation, polyuria and polydipsia are common; peptic ulcers may occur. Higher levels lead to confusion, coma and death. The ECG shows a short QT interval; the toxicity of digoxin is enhanced.

Treatment

Treatment of hypercalcaemia is as follows:

- treat or remove any obvious cause;
- those with symptomatic, moderate or severe hypercalcaemia should be well hydrated;
- consider furosemide (frusemide) to enhance urinary calcium loss (the opposite occurs with thiazide diuretics);
- those with primary hyperparathyroidism may need urgent surgery when stabilised;
- further treatment involves bisphosphonates to reduce bone resorption, although precipitated calcium biphosphate may lead to renal insufficiency;

- in very severe cases calcitonin may be considered;
- corticosteroids may be useful in malignancy or sarcoidosis;
- haemodialysis against a low-calcium dialysate can be used for dialysis-dependent patients.

MAGNESIUM

The normal serum level of magnesium is 0.9–1.1 mmol/L; the maintenance requirement is 0.2 mmol/kg or 1 mmol/g nitrogen.

Hypomagnesaemia

Causes

Causes of hypomagnesaemia are as follows:

- serum magnesium levels frequently fall in ill patients;
- gastrointestinal losses – gastric aspiration, diarrhoea, malabsorption;
- renal losses – vigorous fluid therapy, diuretics, alcohol, aminoglycosides, amphotericin and cisplatin, phosphate depletion.

Effects

Effects of hypomagnesaemia are as follows:

- magnesium is a cofactor in various cellular enzymes – insufficient activation of Na^+K^+ATPase reduces intracellular potassium concentration;
- chronic hypomagnesaemia leads to hypocalcaemia by inhibiting parathyroid hormone;
- neuromuscular – paraesthesia, muscle twitching, tremor, cramps, tetany;
- neuropsychiatric – apathy, depression, hallucinations and coma;
- cardiovascular – arrhythmias, prolonged QT interval, hypertension.

Treatment

Treatment of hypomagnesaemia is routine replacement of 40 mmol/day, preferably by the oral route, although magnesium sulphate is cathartic. Therapeutic infusions may be larger and more rapid, but hypotension may occur because magnesium is a direct-acting vasodilator.

Hypermagnesaemia

Causes

Hypermagnesaemia results from excessive administration, either intravenously or by mouth, especially in those with renal impairment.

Hypermagnesaemia may be associated with a reduced inability to excrete magnesium and calcium via the kidney and a hypokalaemic alkalosis.

High levels of magnesium (1.5 – 4.0 mmol/L) have been used therapeutically in many conditions including pre-eclampsia, cardiac arrhythmias and asthma.

Effects
Above 2 mmol/L hypermagnesaemia causes nausea, flushing and reduced deep tendon reflexes. When levels are over 3 mmol/L there is drowsiness, decreased muscle tone, hypotension and bradycardia. Levels over 5 mmol/L lead to paralysis of voluntary muscle and respiratory depression; eventually there is cardiopulmonary arrest.

Treatment
To treat hypermagnesaemia stop administration of magnesium. In severe cases 5 mmol of intravenous calcium is given as necessary. Haemodialysis may be needed.

PHOSPHATE

The normal serum level of phosphate is 0.9–1.4 mmol/L; the maintenance requirement is 0.3 mmol/kg (less if in renal failure and more if very catabolic).

Hypophosphataemia

A low serum phosphate is common in critically ill patients.

Causes
Causes of hypophosphataemia are:

- poor nutrition – chronic alcoholism, poor feeding in hospital;
- malabsorption – chelating antacids, diarrhoea, vitamin D deficiency;
- uptake of phosphate into cells – β_2-agonists, insulin and alkalosis;
- excessive renal loss – acetazolamide, acidosis, hyperparathyroidism and loss during haemodialysis.

Effects
Hypophosphataemia results in irritability, confusion and eventual metabolic encephalopathy with coma. Muscle weakness may lead to respiratory failure or failure to wean from mechanical ventilation. Dysphagia and ileus may occur. The oxygen dissociation curve shifts to the left, which may hinder offloading of oxygen in the tissues.

Treatment
To treat hypophosphataemia phosphate is best administered orally as effervescent tablets containing 16 mmol. Rapid or large infusions are dangerous,

but in severe cases regimens have been described as high as 20 mmol over 12 hours; it should not be mixed with calcium or magnesium for injection. Phosphate levels should be monitored at least daily.

Hyperphosphataemia

Causes

Causes of hyperphosphataemia are:

- excessive administration – oral or intravenous supplements, vitamin D poisoning;
- increased endogenous load – tumour lysis syndrome, rhabdomyolysis;
- reduced excretion – renal failure, bisphosphonates, magnesium deficiency.

Effects

Hyperphosphataemia results in hypocalcaemia and tetany if the increase is acute. Metastatic calcification occurs if the product of the serum Ca^{2+} and PO_4^- exceeds 70.

Treatment

To treat hyperphosphataemia stop administration and reduce absorption with phosphate-binding salts (not aluminium-based in renal failure).

NUTRITION

NUTRITIONAL REQUIREMENTS

Calorie requirements can be highly variable, but are normally about 30 kcal/kg/day. This can be assessed at the bedside using indirect calorimetry, which determines $\dot{V}O_2$, $\dot{V}CO_2$ and respiratory quotient (RQ).

A number of formulae and tables purport to assess changes in calorific needs under different clinical conditions (e.g. 6% increase per °C temperature rise; Fig. 2.8.1). However, direct measurement is preferable in critically ill patients to avoid the deleterious effects of overfeeding, particularly with carbohydrate.

Overfeeding may lead to:

- increased fat synthesis, with an increased metabolic rate and carbon dioxide production – for the individual with respiratory compromise this is hazardous and may lead to failure to wean from the ventilator;
- fatty deposition in the liver and disturbances in hepatic function;
- impaired neutrophil function;
- elevation in sympathetic nervous activity and increased catecholamine production.

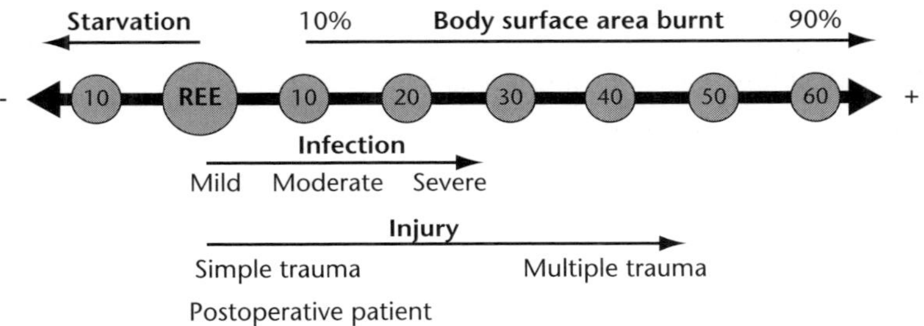

Figure 2.8.1 Nomogram for metabolic rate adjustment. REE, resting energy expenditure.

ASSESSMENT OF NUTRITIONAL STATUS

Malnutrition is common in hospitalised patients and is rarely recognised and then adequately treated; the malnutrition screening tool (MUST) outlined in Box 2.8.3 is recommended.[5]

Box 2.8.3
Malnutrition screening tool (MUST)
History of associated disease (e.g. alcoholism, inflammatory bowel disease)
Dietary history
Present problem (e.g. burns, trauma, sepsis)
Recent severe weight loss; body mass index (BMI) <20 kg/m^2
Signs of malnutrition (e.g. muscle wasting)
Simple measurements of body composition (have limited use in seriously ill patients e.g. due to the presence of oedema) such as: mid-triceps skinfold thickness (indicates fat stores) mid-arm muscle circumference (indicates muscle mass) muscle ultrasound and bioelectrical impedance analysis
Biochemical markers albumin is a poor marker because of its long half-life proteins with a rapid turnover (e.g. transferrin, retinol-binding protein fibronectin) are more appealing — there is normally a turnover of some 100 g of protein per day.
Immunological anergy on skin testing is of limited use

ARTIFICIAL FEEDING

Indications

Indications for artificial feeding include:

- gastrointestinal failure (e.g. paralytic ileus, multiple fistulae or blind loops);
- major surgery, trauma, burns, sepsis;
- preoperative malnutrition;
- some patients with kidney or liver failure;
- chemotherapy resulting in intractable nausea and vomiting;
- coma;
- severe anorexia nervosa.

Aims

Feeding aims to provide:

- calories in the form of carbohydrate and fat because this is optimal for protein anabolism and provision of essential fatty acids;
- protein to provide essential amino acids and nitrogen so reducing muscle breakdown;
- water and electrolytes, phosphate etc.;
- trace elements, vitamins, folate etc.

Daily requirements

Daily requirements vary with the clinical situation, but approximate baseline values are given in the table 2.8.2.

Most feeds have about 1 kcal(4.2 kJ)/mL. Vegetable oils are used as sources of fat, and starch or corn syrup for carbohydrate; alcohol provides 7 kcal/g (29 kJ/g).

Carbohydrate

Body stores of carbohydrate are limited, the average adult having only 5 g of blood glucose and 100 g of liver glycogen. Adequate carbohydrate is needed to allow fat utilisation without ketosis, the minimum for this being 400 kcal (1.7 MJ) of carbohydrate energy per day, although normally at least 50% of the administered calories are from glucose.

Glucose provides 4.0 kcal (17 kJ)/g; 1L of isotonic (5%) solution provides only 200 kcal (840 kJ), so concentrated solutions are needed to give enough calories without overhydration. Twenty-five per cent glucose supplies 250 g glucose and 1000 kcal (4 MJ) per litre. Twenty-five per cent or 50% is commonly used, and these solutions require a central vein.

	Requirement per kg body weight	Requirement for 70 kg man
Water	30–35 mL	2100–2500 mL (lower range in the elderly)
Sodium	1.0 mmol	60–100 mmol
Potassium	1.0 mmol	50–100 mmol
Phosphate	0.3 mmol	25 mmol
Calcium	0.2 mmol	20 mmol
Magnesium	0.2 mmol	12 mmol
Protein	1 g	70 g
Nitrogen	0.15–0.2 g	10–14 g
Carbohydrate	2 g	140 g
Fat	1–2 g	140 g
Calories	30 kcal/125 kJ	2100 kcal/8750 kJ

Table 2.8.2 Daily nutritional requirements

The metabolic response to surgery, sepsis or trauma includes an increase in energy expenditure and impaired glucose tolerance, but insulin does not often need to be given if less than 500 g glucose is given per day. If needed it may be given intravenously by infusion, normally about 1 unit per 4 g glucose infused, to ideally keep the blood sugar normal. There is good evidence of improved outcome from intensive care when blood glucose is kept at 4.4–6.1 mmol/L.[6]

Fat

Fat provides 9.0 kcal (38 kJ)/g. Advantages include iso-osmolarity and neutral pH (it can be given into a peripheral vein). No losses occur in the faeces or urine.

Fat is provided as a 10% or 20% soya oil emulsion, with particle diameters 0.2–1.0 μm, much the same as a chylomicron. The surfactant is egg phospholipid and glycerol is added to make the solution isotonic; 500 mL of 20% emulsion provides 1000 kcal (4.2 MJ). This also provides essential fatty acids.

Excessive milkiness of serum calls for a reduction in fat intake. This is more likely in liver insufficiency, acute pancreatitis, uraemia and septicaemia. Occasional side-effects are shivering, flushing and fever.

Patients on infusions of propofol for sedation may receive a considerable proportion of their daily fat requirements by this route, and this should be considered when planning a parenteral feeding regimen.

Patients with a severe limitation of ventilatory reserve may benefit from a higher percentage of fat as their calorie source because less carbon dioxide is produced than with carbohydrate (RQ 0.71 vs 1.0).

Protein

Protein intake should be 1.2–1.5 g/kg/day (0.2–0.25 g nitrogen/kg/day). Nitrogen excretion in critical illness can exceed 20 g/day, which represents the breakdown of 125 g of protein or 600 g of muscle. This can be estimated from urea and protein loss in the urine and any rise in total body urea plus an estimate of losses from skin and stool. In practice, these calculations are rarely done.

Protein can theoretically supply 4 kcal/g (17 kJ/g), but it is recommended that non-protein calories are provided concurrently to maximise nitrogen uptake.

For enteral feeding standard polymeric solutions are used that do not contain gluten or lactose. These solutions contain long-chain triglycerides and may also contain fibre. Elemental and semi-elemental feeds are also available that contain amino acids or peptides, glucose or oligosaccharides and medium-chain triglycerides.

For parenteral feeding a mixture of essential and non-essential crystalline amino acids is given in the physiological laevo-rotatory form. Solutions with higher proportions of branched-chain amino acids have no real advantage. Most solutions are hyperosmolar and acidic. Some, however, are less so and have been designed for peripheral use, but they are only suitable for short-term use.

Micronutrients

Many micronutrients are conveniently provided by commercial additive preparations, although others are given individually (e.g. vitamin B_{12}) or in much higher doses according to the clinical circumstances (e.g. folate). The B vitamins and vitamins A and C degrade when exposed to light (Table 2.8.3).

Enteral feeding

Contraindications to enteral feeding include severe gut pathology (e.g. generalised peritonitis, ischaemia and severe shock), but in general enteral feeding is the preferred route if the gut is functioning at all because it is less costly, more effective and less hazardous than intravenous nutrition. Also, gut integrity and function are enhanced.

Some nutrients, such as glutamine, short-chain fatty acids and polyunsaturated fatty acids, may be trophic to the gut and be of particular benefit

Nutrient	Parenteral daily requirement
Pyridoxine (B6)	4–6 mg
Riboflavine (B2)	3–8 mg
Thiamine (B1)	3–20 mg
Biotin	60 μg
Folate	0.2–0.4 mg
Niacin	40 mg
Pantothenic acid	10–20 mg
Vitamin A	1–2.5 mg
Vitamin B_{12}	5–15 μg
Vitamin C	100 mg
Vitamin D	5 μg
Vitamin E	10 mg
Vitamin K	1.0 μg/kg
Chromium	0.2–0.4 μmol
Copper	20 μmol
Fluoride	50 μmol
Iodine	1 μmol
Iron	20–70 μmol
Manganese	5–10 μmol
Molybdenum	0.2–1.2 μmol
Selenium	0.25–0.5 μmol
Zinc	100 μmol

Table 2.8.3 Parenteral daily requirements of vitamins and minerals

to septic patients. Glutamine is central to protein synthesis and the function of enterocytes and the immune system. During critical illness glutamine becomes a conditionally essential amino acid and the demand has to be met by skeletal muscle breakdown. There is now good evidence in a number of critical illnesses that glutamine supplementation, especially parenterally, improves outcome.[7] There is some evidence that the newer immunomodulating feeds, particularly those containing ω-3 fatty acids are beneficial, for example in acute respiratory distress syndrome (ARDS), but further work is needed.[8]

Confirmation that a tube is in the stomach is achieved using a pH indicator/paper strips covering the appropriate range; do not use blue litmus paper.

For longer-term feeding small-bore feeding tubes are placed in the stomach or duodenum. These need a wire stylet insertion, but are less traumatic and better tolerated, although blockage is more common. Aspiration is difficult through such small-lumen tubes, so to rule out misplacement into the lungs their position must be checked by radiography or endoscopy.

Percutaneous gastrostomy and jejunostomy tubes may also be used postoperatively and for longer-term feeding.

Numerous protocols are available for starting and maintaining enteral feeding. Feeding continuously at a constant rate over 24 hours makes glycaemic control easier. There is growing evidence that early nutrition, even after major colorectal surgery, enhances recovery.[9]

A number of complications may arise during enteral feeding:

- tube related – trauma and ulceration of the nose, pharynx and gut mucosa; sinusitis (if nasal); misplacement in the lungs; regurgitation and aspiration (reflux can be reduced by nursing the patient head up): aim for 45°;
- gastrointestinal – change of gut flora, vomiting, regurgitation, large residue on aspiration of the nasogastric tube, and diarrhoea; diarrhoea is common and may have a number of causes (e.g. antibiotics, lactose intolerance or high osmolality feed) and loperamide or codeine phosphate can be useful;
- metabolic – water and electrolyte abnormalities, hyperglycaemia, deficiencies of essential nutrients.

Parenteral feeding

Intravenous nutrition is used when full feeding via the gut is not possible, and so may be as total parenteral nutrition (TPN) or to supplement enteral feeds. In some conditions where parenteral nutrition was formerly used extensively (e.g. acute pancreatitis), the evidence now suggests that enteral feeding is better.[10]

The aim with TPN is to maintain nutrition until the gut failure is corrected, so it is usually started when prolonged feeding difficulties are expected (e.g. major abdominal surgery).

A central venous catheter is necessary for most parenteral solutions, except those designed for peripheral veins using a fine-bore silicone catheter.

Catheters must be inserted under aseptic conditions and scrupulous care is needed in use (e.g. stopcocks should not be used). Ideally, the line should be tunnelled and not used for other infusions or blood sampling, but if a multi-lumen catheter is used, one lumen should be reserved exclusively for parenteral nutrition.

Best practice is to have the desired mixture made up aseptically in pharmacy, presented in a 'big-bag' and infused over 24 hours with a controlled volumetric pump. The electrolyte composition can be varied, within limits, by the pharmacy.

Total parenteral nutrition is best managed by a dedicated multidisciplinary team and can be successfully carried out at home. Complications may occur related to catheter insertion and use (e.g. pneumothorax, haemorrhage, infection, thrombophlebitis etc.).

Other complications can be minimised by adequate biochemical monitoring and include the following:

- glucose related – hyperglycaemia, ketoacidosis, hypercapnia;
- amino acid metabolism – patients in acute renal failure will have to be dialysed or have haemofiltration more frequently due to prerenal uraemia. Hyperchloraemic metabolic acidosis;
- fats – sicker patients are less able to metabolise fat; fatty liver and cholestasis may occur. Essential fatty acid deficiency may occur with predominantly glucose-based feeds;
- water and electrolytes – circulatory overload, electrolyte imbalance (e.g. hypophosphataemia, pseudohyponatraemia);
- vitamin and trace element deficiencies – thiamine, vitamin K, vitamin B_{12}, folate, zinc and copper deficiency should be considered and rectified.

References

1. Stewart PA. Modern quantitative acid–base chemistry. Can J Physiol Pharmacol 1983; 61:1444–1461.
2. Morfei J. Stewart's strong ion difference approach to acid–base analysis. Respir Care 1999; 44:45–52.
3. Androgue HJ, Madias NE. Hyponatremia. N Engl J Med 2000; 342:1581–1589.
4. Androgue HJ, Madias NE. Hypernatremia. N Engl J Med 2000; 342:1493–1499.
5. Elia M. Nutrition in acute care. Clin Med 2004; 4:405–407.
6. Van den Berghe G, Wouters P, Weekers F, et al. Intensive insulin therapy in the critically ill patients. N Engl J Med 2001; 345:1359–1367
7. D'Souza R, Powell-Tuck J. Glutamine supplements in the critically ill. J Roy Soc Med 2004; 97:425–427.
8. Stechmiller JK, Childress B, Porter T. Arginine immunonutrition in critically ill patients: a clinical dilemma. Am J Crit Care 2004; 13:17–23.
9. Soop M, Carlso GL, Hopkinson J, et al. Randomized clinical trial of the effects of immediate enteral nutrition on metabolic responses to major colorectal surgery in an enhanced recovery protocol. Br J Surg 2004; 91:1138–1145.

10. Marik PE, Zaloga GP. Meta-analysis of parenteral nutrition versus enteral nutrition in patients with acute pancreatitis. Br Med J 2004; 328:1407.

Further reading

Arieff AI. Electrolyte disturbance. In: Webb AR, Shapiro MJ, Singer M, Suter PM, eds. Oxford textbook of intensive care. Oxford: Oxford University Press; 1999:552–572.

CHAPTER **2.9**

RESUSCITATION

Resuscitation is an art as old as mankind itself. More recently, it has evolved into a science, which has led to the development of evidence-based resuscitation guidelines.

The current guidelines were developed by the International Liaison Committee on Resuscitation (ILCOR), of which the Resuscitation Council (UK) is a member, and were published in 2000.

Successful resuscitation relies on a chain of survival that begins with calling for help, progresses to basic life support (BLS) and early defibrillation, and concludes with the provision of advanced life support (ALS). Delivery of this chain of survival is equally important for cardiac arrest both outside and inside hospital.

ADULT RESUSCITATION

Basic life support

Basic life support[1] must be initiated immediately, and when performed correctly will double the survival from cardiac arrest outside hospital. It follows the sequence of ABC – opening the Airway, supporting Breathing and assisting the Circulation (Fig. 2.9.1).

A precordial thump is only indicated for witnessed arrest, when it may be able to deliver early cardioversion of ventricular fibrillation (VF) or ventricular tachycardia (VT).

With the increasing availability and simplicity of use of automated external defibrillators, defibrillation is now considered as part of BLS.

Most adult cardiac arrests are secondary to shockable arrhythmias, primarily VF and VT. Every minute's delay in defibrillation increases the mortality rate by 7–10%.

The public access defibrillation schemes in the UK aim to place defibrillators in public areas (e.g. airports, shopping centres) to enable early defibrillation before the arrival of the emergency services.

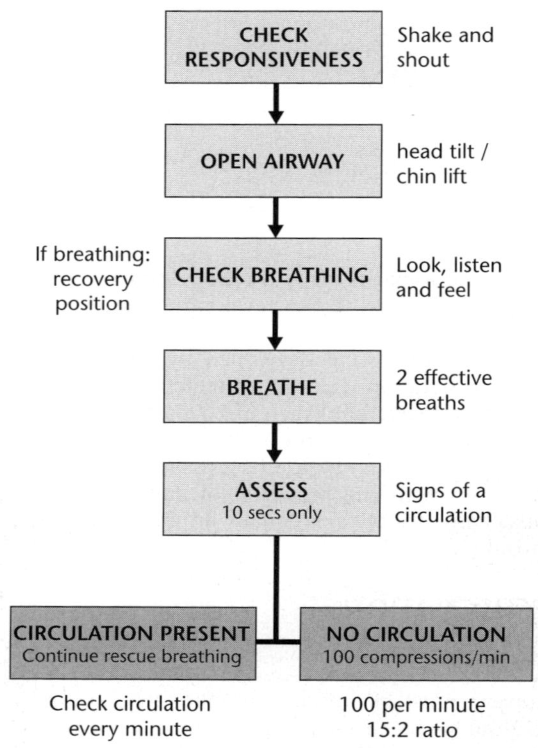

Figure 2.9.1 Algorithm showing adult basic life support. Reproduced from algorithms published in the 2000 Resuscitation Guidelines (available on www.resus.org.uk) with permission from the Resuscitation Council UK.

Advanced life support

Advanced life support[2] secures the airway and supports the circulation with pharmacological adjuncts, aiming to restore sinus rhythm and a spontaneous cardiac output. The ALS algorithm is shown in Figure 2.9.2. The treatment pathways follow the routes of VF/VT or non-VF/VT (i.e. asystole or pulseless electrical activity).

The gold standard in terms of airway management is endotracheal intubation. This secures the airway from aspiration, allows ventilation while

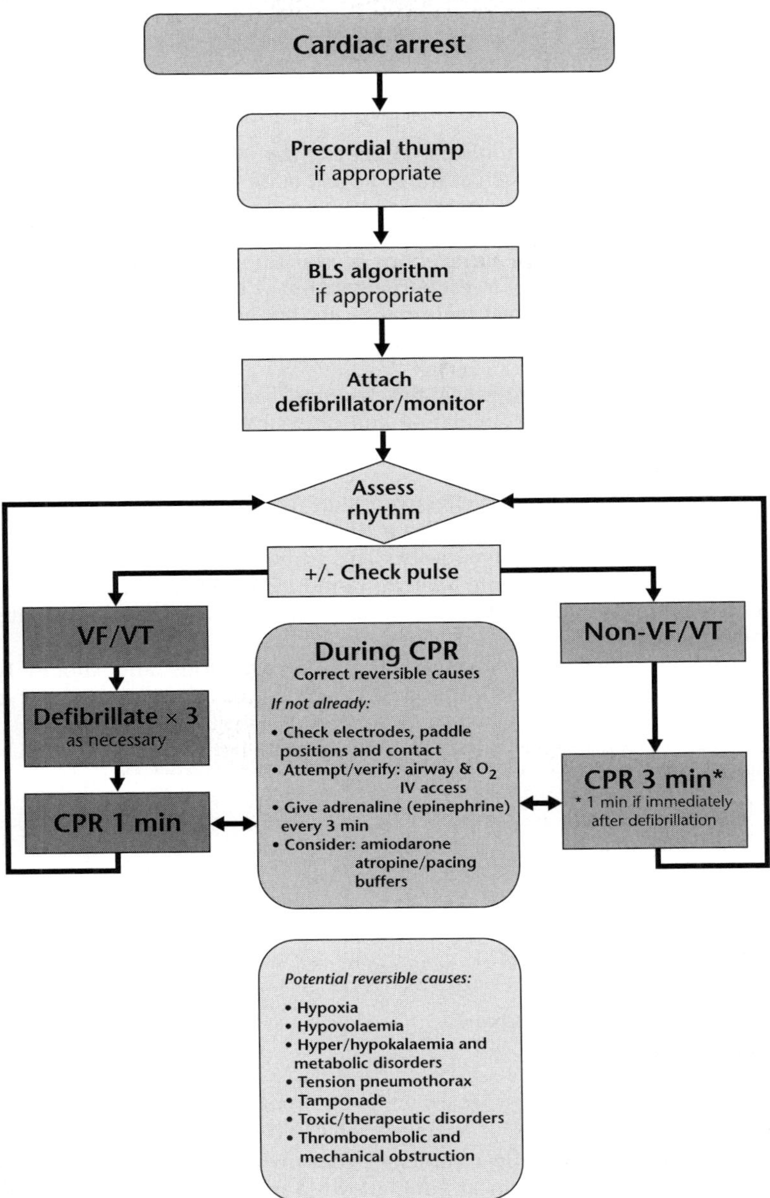

Figure 2.9.2 Algorithm showing adult advanced life support. CPR, cardiopulmonary resuscitation; VF, ventricular fibrillation; VT, ventricular tachycardia. Reproduced from algorithms published in the 2000 Resuscitation Guidelines (available on www.resus.org.uk) with permission from the Resuscitation Council UK.

chest compression is performed, and enables delivery of drugs via the endotracheal tube.

In situations where those first attending the patient are not skilled in intubation, alternatives such as the laryngeal mask airway have been shown to be effective in delivering early ventilation and are easy to insert after relatively little training.

Early establishment of intravenous access is necessary for the administration of drugs according to the ALS algorithm. A large forearm vein or the external jugular vein is ideal for initial access, but both require a saline infusion to flush the drugs through to the central circulation. Central venous access is optimal.

Administration of drugs via the endotracheal tube is a poor route, delivers little drug to the circulation and causes hypoxia.

The intraosseous needle is a suitable device for drug delivery and is now available for adults.

The evidence base for the effectiveness of ALS drugs is limited.

The initial drug indicated for both VF/VT and non-VF/VT is adrenaline (epinephrine) 1 mg intravenously. This should be administered with caution as excessive doses are liable to re-induce VT/VF after the establishment of sinus rhythm. Epinephrine should be administered every 3 minutes when indicated.

Atropine 3 mg intravenously will block vagal tone and should be administered following the initial dose of epinephrine for patients in asystole.

Causes of pulseless electrical activity should be actively sought and treated, and include:

- hypoxia;
- hypovolaemia;
- hyper/hypokalaemia;
- hypothermia;
- tension pneumothorax;
- tamponade;
- toxic/therapeutic disturbance;
- thromboembolism.

DEFIBRILLATION

Defibrillation aims to deliver sufficient transmyocardial current to depolarise a critical mass of myocardium, allowing restoration of synchronised electrical activity.

Inadequate energy fails to defibrillate, but excessive energy causes myocardial damage and risks the resumption of fibrillation.

Defibrillation of supraventricular arrhythmias should be synchronised to avoid delivering a shock on the T wave of the ECG, which may induce VF.

Defibrillation can be performed using either paddles or self-adhesive pads. Either should be placed with the sternal pad to the right of the sternum below the clavicle and the apical pad in line with the nipple in the left mid-axillary line.

Firm force of at least 8 kg should be applied to manual paddles during defibrillation.

The monophasic defibrillation waveform has been superseded by a biphasic waveform which has a positive, followed by a negative phase, delivered over approximately 10 ms (Fig. 2.9.3).

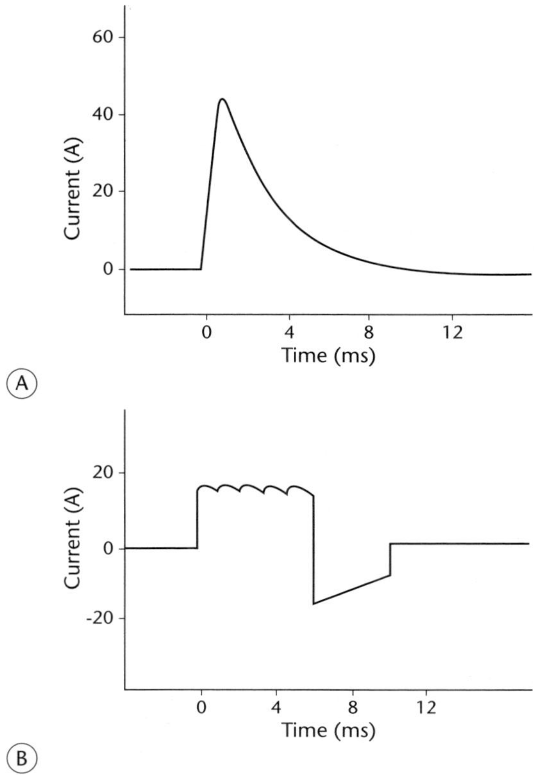

Figure 2.9.3 Current versus time profiles for (A) older monophasic, and (B) newer biphasic defibrillators.

Biphasic waveforms are more effective than monophasic waveforms for any given energy level, more likely to achieve cardioversion and cause less myocardial injury.

Monophasic defibrillators use a sequence of 200 J, 200 J, 360 J; the optimal sequence for biphasic defibrillators has not been established, but 150 J is considered at least as effective as 200 J monophasic.

Defibrillation may result in the ECG showing 'asystole' immediately following a shock and actually masking continuing VF, particularly when using gel pads.

Standard ECG leads should be used to examine the ECG and exclude spurious asystole.

Amiodarone has replaced lidocaine (lignocaine) as the drug of choice for refractory VF/VT. Current guidelines recommend amiodarone 300 mg intravenously if the patient remains in VF/VT after the first three shocks.

OTHER THERAPY

Future changes to resuscitation guidelines are likely to recommend that thrombolysis should be considered for adult cardiac arrest patients when the presumed etiology would be an indication for thrombolysis if there was no cardiac arrest (e.g. acute myocardial infarction or pulmonary embolus). Cardiopulmonary resuscitation (CPR) is not a contraindication to thrombolytic therapy.

In the critically ill adult survivor of cardiac arrest who requires mechanical ventilation after return of spontaneous circulation, strict control of blood glucose with insulin may be beneficial to outcome.

There is good evidence that patients with a spontaneous circulation who remain comatose after cardiac arrest benefit from active cooling to 32–34°C for 12–24 hours. This is now recommended treatment.[3]

RESUSCITATION DURING PREGNANCY

The main causes of cardiovascular collapse during pregnancy are amniotic fluid embolus, pulmonary embolus, eclampsia, congestive cardiomyopathy, drug toxicity (e.g. hypermagnesaemia, total spinal anaesthetic) and haemorrhage:

- below 25 weeks of gestation, treatment is as for a non-pregnant adult;
- above 25 weeks of gestation, a wedge is required to tilt the body to the left to relieve aortocaval compression, which would otherwise impede venous return;
- above 32 weeks of gestation, the extent of aortocaval compression precludes effective CPR and immediate caesarean section is indicated while CPR is continued.

In the third trimester, the mediastinum is pushed cranially by the gravid uterus and external chest compressions should be performed higher on the sternum than usual.

PAEDIATRIC RESUSCITATION

This section refers to children under 8 years old.

Unlike adults, in whom cardiac arrest is usually due to ischaemic heart disease, paediatric arrests are usually secondary to hypoxia. Resuscitation of patients in this age group therefore emphasises the importance of securing the airway and delivering high-concentration oxygen as a priority in the resuscitation sequence.

Basic life support[4]

The algorithm for paediatric BLS is shown in Figure 2.9.4 and, as with adults, follows the ABC sequence. The 15:2 compression ventilation ratio recommended for adults is replaced by a 5:1 ratio.

Choking is more common in infants than adults. Conscious infants should be encouraged to cough. Never perform a finger sweep that may impact the foreign body further. Unconscious infants should be given five back blows in the prone position, alternating with five chest thrusts. In children, abdominal thrusts replace chest thrusts (when they are less likely to damage abdominal viscera) after the second round of back blows. Subsequently, back blows are alternated with chest thrusts/abdominal thrusts until the airway is cleared.

Advanced life support[5]

The algorithm for paediatric ALS is shown in Figure 2.9.5.

The airway must be secured early in the resuscitation sequence. Endotracheal intubation with an uncuffed tube is recommended in infants and young children. The following formula is useful in estimating the appropriate endotracheal tube internal diameter:

- Internal diameter (mm) = (age in years/4) + 4

If endotracheal intubation is difficult, BLS must not be interrupted for long and it is vital to re-oxygenate the child at short intervals. Once the airway is secured, high-flow oxygen (>15 L/min) must be delivered to ensure inspired oxygen concentrations over 90%.

Having secured the airway, breathing must be assessed. It is particularly important to exclude a tension pneumothorax in both trauma patients and those with acute asthma. In the latter, a high index of suspicion must be maintained for a bilateral tension pneumothorax. If there is any doubt, decompress the chest once the child is intubated.

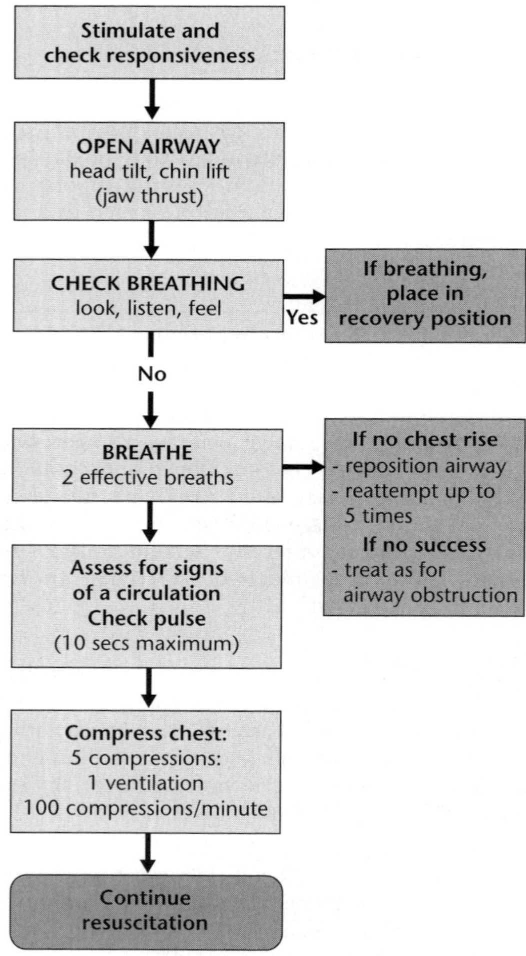

Figure 2.9.4 Algorithm showing paediatric basic life support. Reproduced from algorithms published in the 2000 Resuscitation Guidelines (available on www.resus.org.uk) with permission from the Resuscitation Council UK.

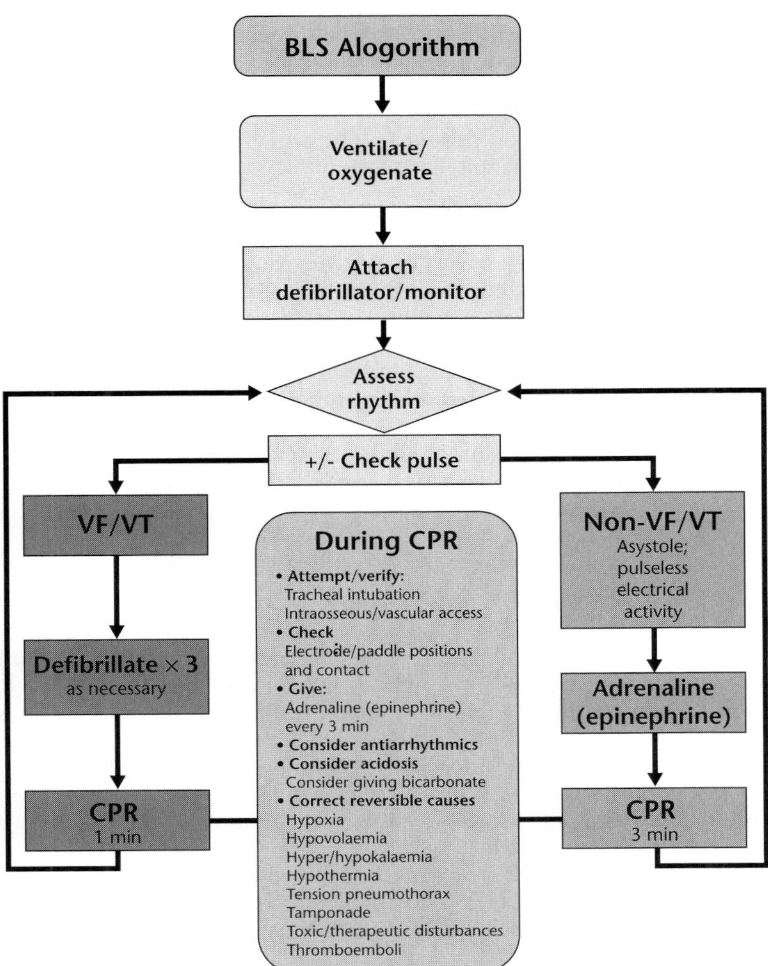

Figure 2.9.5 Algorithm showing paediatric advanced life support. Reproduced from algorithms published in the 2000 Resuscitation Guidelines (available on www.resus.org.uk) with permission from the Resuscitation Council UK.

Management of the circulation requires early establishment of intravenous access for resuscitation drugs and fluid.

Intravenous access is particularly difficult in infants, and if venous access has not been gained within 90 seconds, the intraosseous route should be attempted. Resuscitation drugs and fluids can be given safely via this route and marrow aspirate used to estimate haemoglobin, electrolytes, venous pH and blood group.

Drug doses are based on patient weight, which in infants and children can be estimated from the following formula:

- Weight (kg) = (age + 4) × 2

An annotated tape measure (Broselow tape) or a length–weight–age nomogram (Oakley chart) both give specific drug doses according to the length or weight of the child and reduce the chances of error.

The initial drug for all arrhythmias is epinephrine 10 μg/kg intravenously. If subsequent doses are required, 100 μg/kg can be considered if arterial blood pressure monitoring has been established. Atropine 20 μg/kg intravenously is only indicated as a treatment for bradycardia once any hypoxia has been reversed.

Ventricular fibrillation in children is uncommon. If present, the following diagnoses should be actively excluded:

- tricyclic overdose;
- hypothermia;
- hyperkalaemia;
- congenital heart disease.

Energy levels of 2, 2 and 4 J/kg are recommended for paediatric defibrillation for both monophasic and biphasic waveforms.

Bicarbonate is ideally given titrated against arterial blood gases, Although acidosis is known to depress myocardial contractility, reduce tissue oxygen delivery and increase susceptibility to VF, there is no good evidence that correction of pH improves the outcome of CPR. When given without knowledge of acid–base status after prolonged arrest a dose of 1 mmol/kg is recommended.

When circulatory collapse results from hypovolaemia (e.g. blood loss, acute gastroenteritis) or sepsis and fluid resuscitation is required, give a 20 mL/kg bolus of crystalloid. Repeat three times and then give 10 mL/kg of blood if shock persists.

Hypoglycaemia is common in infants and blood sugar should be checked and treated appropriately.

ETHICAL ASPECTS OF RESUSCITATION

Ethical aspects of resuscitation have recently been addressed in a joint statement from the British Medical Association and Resuscitation Council.[6] They stress that literature on CPR should be available to patients, who should be involved in decision-making, and these decisions should be reviewed regularly. In emergencies, CPR should be performed unless:

- the patient has refused CPR;
- the patient is in the terminal phase of an illness;
- the burdens of treatment outweigh the benefits.

References

1. Part 3: adult basic life support. European Resuscitation Council. Resuscitation 2000; 46:29–71.
2. Part 6: advanced cardiovascular life support. Section 7: algorithm approach to ACLS. 7C: a guide to the international ACLS algorithms. European Resuscitation Council. Resuscitation 2000; 46:169–184.
3. Nolan JP, Morley PT, Hoek TL, Hickey, RW. Therapeutic hypothermia after cardiac arrest. An advisory statement by the Advanced Life Support Task Force of the International Committee on Resuscitation. Resuscitation 2003; 57:231–235.
4. Part 9: pediatric basic life support. European Resuscitation Council. Resuscitation 2000; 46:301–341.
5. Part 10: pediatric advanced life support. European Resuscitation Council. Resuscitation 2000; 46:343–399.
6. Decisions relating to cardiopulmonary resuscitation: a joint statement from the British Medical Association, the Resuscitation Council (UK) and the Royal College of Nursing. J Med Ethics 2002; 27:310–316.

Further reading

Colquhoun MC, Handley AJ, Evans TR, eds. ABC of Resuscitation. London: BMJ Publishing Group; 2004.

Detailed guidelines for adult and paediatric resuscitation can be found on the website of the Resuscitation Council (UK) at www.resus.org.uk.

Section 3

Care of the patient after surgery

CHAPTER **3.1**

CARE IN THE RECOVERY AREA

THE POSTOPERATIVE RECOVERY WARD

Location

Common sense dictates that the recovery ward should occupy a central area within the operating suite, as far as possible equidistant from all the theatres, but with separate access for patients to and from the wards. As well as minimising transfer times this also means that recovery staff will have more ready access to expert anaesthetic help should it be required.

Ideally the recovery area should also be located close to the critical care units. Typically these comprise the intensive therapy unit (ITU) and high-dependency unit (HDU), but may also include the specific step-down post-operative critical care units (POCCU) that now exist in some hospitals.[1] These different units will admit, as appropriate, patients who are too sick or too unstable to be cared for safely on the general ward, who require invasive monitoring, or who require the organ and ventilatory support offered by full intensive care. They may also be appropriate for those for whom specialised pain regimens have been prescribed, such as those delivered by patient-controlled epidural analgesia (PCEA) devices with which ward staff may not be familiar. This generalisation will not apply to all hospitals, many of whose general nursing staff may well have received specific training in some of these areas.

Design

Some recent recommendations from the NHS Agency of the Department of Health (in the UK) assert that the ratio of beds to operating theatres should be not less than two, and that a suite of eight theatres should have a total floor space of 164 m^2.[2,3] Some flexibility is necessary: a patient entering recovery after prolonged major surgery requires much more space and equipment, including if necessary the ability to maintain or resume intermittent positive-pressure ventilation (IPPV), than say a young fit adult who has undergone knee arthroscopy as a day case.

The recovery bays should be matched for purpose. There should be curtains or screens to allow privacy, and where possible there should be separation of the sexes. This is rarely done, although it is commonplace to have a designated area for children. Such an area should be decorated appropriately and should allow access to parents who wish to be reunited with their children rather than waiting until they return to the ward.

It is clear that any design should incorporate adequate storage, a dirty utility area, washing facilities, adequate provision of electrical outlets and desk space for clerical tasks.

Each bay should have pipeline outlets for oxygen, air and suction.

It is increasingly common for each bay to require a computer terminal.

In design terms what may be less immediately obvious is the importance of ensuring adequate air exchange, because exhaled anaesthetic gases in a busy recovery will otherwise accumulate in the working area.

Equipment

Potential post-anaesthetic and surgical problems mean that there must be immediate access to the same drugs and equipment, both standard and emergency, as are available in the anaesthetic room and operating theatre.

Such equipment must therefore include airway adjuncts such as oropharyngeal and nasopharyngeal airways, laryngoscopes and a range of tracheal tubes. There should also be readily available an effective (and familiar) cricothyroidotomy puncture device with a means of attachment, after insertion, to the fresh gas supply.

A breathing system (circuit) must be present in every bay. Typically this is a Mapleson C system, which although convenient does require a high gas flow of two to three times minute volume to avoid rebreathing. Some units prefer to use self-inflating bags, particularly during resuscitation, although these tend to be less popular with anaesthetists.

Capnography should be available to confirm correct tracheal tube placement.

Powerful and effective suction must be present in every bay, together with a range of suction catheters. There should also be provision for the emergency insertion of a chest drain should an acute or tension pneumothorax make it necessary. Intravenous cannulae and fluids should be available for immediate fluid resuscitation. A defibrillator must also be present in the recovery area.

It would clearly be impractical to have all this equipment at each bed space, but it is useful to contain it within a cart that can be mobilised along with other resuscitation equipment. Trolleys that can be rapidly tipped head-down should be standard. There must also be sufficient room round the bed or trolley to allow whatever resuscitative or emergency manoeuvres may be necessary.

Monitoring

The sophistication of the monitoring that is used depends on the complexity of the case.

After major surgery the anaesthetist may wish to continue the invasive monitoring that was established in theatre, and so depending on the surgical case mix there should be this facility in at least one bay.

More straightforward cases may be monitored simply with intermittent noninvasive blood pressure measurements, intermittent tympanic infrared temperature measurements, electrocardiographic monitoring (ECG) and pulse oximetry. In most recovery units this would be considered to be the minimum for all patients.

Staffing

There should be sufficient trained staff to allow continuous one-to-one care of every patient passing through the recovery unit. An anaesthetist must also be immediately available. Ideally this would be a named individual with responsibilities only to the patients in recovery, but at the least they should be supernumerary to requirements in the operating theatre.

The particular skills of the staff will vary according to the case mix of the surgical unit, but their core skills should include basic airway management, immediate life support, and the ability to assess accurately a patient's cardiac, respiratory and volaemic status.

Whether or not staff feel competent to manage patients in whom a laryngeal mask or tracheal tube remains in place depends usually on local policies and training. The laryngeal mask airway is a forgiving device and much of its inherent safety lies in the fact that patients will tolerate it as consciousness returns and after airway reflexes are restored. The same is not true of a tracheal tube. Yet although the uneventful removal of an endotracheal tube can be more difficult to achieve, there is no reason why this task cannot also be undertaken by properly trained recovery personnel, given appropriate anaesthetic supervision and support.

Part of the satisfaction of working in the recovery area is being able to provide total care, albeit for a short period of time, and so staff should also be trained to administer intravenous drugs, and in particular opiate analgesics. Ideally they should in addition be allowed by local protocols to set up and initiate patient-controlled analgesia (PCA) and PCEA devices.

TRANSFER TO RECOVERY

The imperative to maintain surgical throughput means that the anaesthetist rarely has the luxury of transferring a patient who is fully conscious and whose protective reflexes are intact. More commonly the patient is in the inherently unstable state of emergence from anaesthesia. Transfer from the operating theatre to the recovery area should therefore be as swift as possible, but with supplemental oxygen provided as a routine.

HANDOVER

It is standard practice for a member of the theatre team to convey operative information such as details of the surgical procedure and the presence of any drains or other devices. The anaesthetist, who should have accompanied the patient to recovery, should supplement this with a brief verbal summary detailing any other relevant information. In a simple case this is at the least a professional courtesy to the individual to whom continuing care is being delegated, but in less straightforward cases such information may be crucial to the quality of that care. The handover should therefore include any intraoperative surgical or anaesthetic complications or interventions that might influence recovery, as well as any pre-existing medical condition that may be of significance. Such conditions might include not only diseases such as asthma, hypertension or coronary ischaemia, but also mild dementia or excessive preoperative anxiety.

Recovery staff should also be warned what to expect in relation to any chronic or acute cardiac arrhythmia (such as atrial fibrillation).

The anaesthetist should ensure that the anaesthetic record is legible and that prescriptions for fluid therapy, oxygen therapy, analgesia and antiemesis are clear and comprehensive.

RECOVERY

The plan for recovery from anaesthesia should in effect begin at the stage of the preoperative assessment, because even though the effects of anaesthesia on the major systems are usually only temporary, they are nevertheless almost uniformly deleterious.

Cardiovascular function may often worsen, renal function may be compromised, CNS function is by definition impaired and respiratory function can only deteriorate.

These changes are not surprising because the list of anaesthetic 'poisons' is long. A patient undergoing emergency laparotomy may receive as many as ten different drugs in total, and even non-anaesthetic agents may have significant contributory effects. Aminoglycoside antibiotics, for example, may potentiate neuromuscular blockade.

At the preoperative assessment therefore, the anaesthetist should be planning a technique that will mitigate these effects in any given patient and will facilitate rapid and safe recovery from anaesthesia. There do remain, however, a large number of potential complications that can still occur, such careful anaesthetic planning notwithstanding.

PROBLEMS ENCOUNTERED IN THE IMMEDIATE POSTOPERATIVE PERIOD

There are a number of ways of viewing the various clinical problems that may occur in recovery.

One is to apply the typical Airway, Breathing, Circulation, Disability (ABCD) algorithm and to list the critical events with which each may be associated.

A different, and arguably more practical, method of dealing with these events is to incorporate the ABCD algorithm within a problem-based approach, because recovery staff will ask an anaesthetist to review a patient not because they have 'upper airways obstruction' or 'cardiogenic shock', but because they have low oxygen saturations or are hypotensive (Box 3.1.1). What follows, therefore, is an account of the presentations of important problems that may require the urgent attention of an anaesthetist during the immediate postoperative period.

Low oxygen saturation

Airway

Upper airway obstruction

Falling oxygen saturations may reflect the fact that the airway is obstructed, either partially or totally. There are no exceptions to the rule that noisy breathing is always partially obstructed breathing.

Obstruction may occur at any part of the respiratory tract.

Upper airway obstruction may be due to common and well-recognised causes such as the position of the tongue, persistent loss of tone in the pha-

Box 3.1.1
Common problems in recovery
Low oxygen saturation
Hypotension
Hypertension
Delayed awakening
Confusion and agitation
Pain
Nausea
Temperature disturbance
Shivering
High, low or irregular pulse

ryngeal muscles and inappropriate positioning of the neck and jaw. It may also be due to foreign bodies in the oropharynx (such as a pack that has not been removed) or to blood clot or debris. These latter causes are all likely to be difficulties associated with intraoral and maxillofacial surgery.

A more general and common problem is laryngeal spasm, in which there is reflex closure of the vocal cords, precipitated often by stimulation during a light stage of anaesthesia. Traditional wisdom has it that if the anaesthetist is able to obtain a good seal with a facemask delivering 100% oxygen then laryngeal spasm will always eventually 'break'. Most anaesthetists prefer not to put this wisdom to the test, and tend to treat the complication earlier.

Definitive management of laryngeal spasm comprises tracheal intubation following a full dose of neuromuscular blocking agent, but laryngeal spasm may also respond to a small dose of suxamethonium (10 mg in an adult), to a subhypnotic bolus dose of propofol, to low-dose midazolam (0.5–1.0 mg increments), to doxapram (in a dose of 1 mg/kg) and (historically) to the administration of 5% carbon dioxide.

The patient will desaturate at a rate proportional to the oxygen that remains within the functional residual capacity, which in an adult is about 2000–2500 mL. The basal requirement for oxygen is around 250 mL/min, and so if a patient has been breathing 50% oxygen the alveolar oxygen reserve of 1000–1250 mL will be exhausted within 5 minutes.

If upper airway obstruction is total then there will be pronounced ventilatory efforts, but the airway will be silent. These extreme respiratory efforts, particularly if the patient is young and fit, can generate negative intrathoracic pressures as great as –100 cmH_2O. This is more than sufficient to cause negative-pressure pulmonary oedema. Onset can be rapid (within a few minutes) or delayed (up to 2–3 hours) and will usually resolve within 12–24 hours. Treatment meanwhile is supportive with oxygen therapy, continuous positive airways pressure (CPAP), and occasionally IPPV.

Lower airway obstruction

Bronchoconstriction in the lower airways may occur in patients with a history of asthma, in individuals who are atopic, and de novo in response to airway irritants, to the presence of inhaled gastric contents and as part of an allergic drug response. Wheeze is often transient, but if it persists to the detriment of gas exchange it can be treated with nebulised β-sympathomimetics (such as salbutamol, 2.5–5.0 mg) or with intravenous salbutamol (4 μg/kg slowly) or aminophylline (5 mg/kg over 20 minutes).

Breathing

Apnoea

A patient may be apnoeic because of drug-induced respiratory depression. Opiates are the most potent agents in this respect, but most anaesthetic agents, including nitrous oxide, also depress respiration and may exert a synergistic effect. Oxygen desaturation may occur relatively late in this situation.

If the airway remains patent ambient gas is drawn into the lungs by mass movement down the trachea. If room air is the ambient gas then hypoxia will occur almost as swiftly as it does in obstructed apnoea. If, however, the ambient gas is 100% oxygen then (in theory) it will take about 100 minutes before hypoxia supervenes.

Other causes of apnoea include residual neuromuscular paralysis, and hypocapnia associated with mechanical hyperventilation. Rarely, in the worst scenario of all, patients may fail to breathe because of an intracranial catastrophe.

Hypopnoea (hypoventilation)

Hypoventilation results in the failure of the patient to generate minute ventilation sufficient to supply tissue oxygen needs. This may be due to drug-induced respiratory depression and residual neuromuscular block, although inadequate ventilation may also be associated with poor pain control. Under all these circumstances low oxygen saturation may return to normal if the patient is given supplemental oxygen. It is vital to realise, however, that should the cause be left untreated the high inspired oxygen concentration has no influence on carbon dioxide elimination and so it may actually mask respiratory failure.

As a corollary it is important also to be aware that an oxygen saturation of 95% in the presence of high inspired oxygen concentrations is not in fact normal, but is low.

Patients who remain partly paralysed by the effects of residual neuromuscular blocking agents may exhibit characteristic jerky and athetoid movements, which are instantly recognisable to anaesthetists trained before the widespread use of atracurium, but which happily are much less familiar to the newer generation of specialists. The diagnosis is supported if a patient has weak grip strength or is unable to support the head lifted off the pillow for 5 seconds. It is preferable to make the diagnosis clinically because the painful alternative is to use a peripheral nerve stimulator. The best means of demonstrating residual block is tetanic stimulation (which is more sensitive than double burst or train-of-four stimulation.) This requires stimuli of 50 or 100 Hz for 5 seconds, but should not be used in the conscious patient, who may be aware of marked lingering discomfort even if the stimulus has been applied during anaesthesia.

Circulation

Low oxygen saturation may also reflect impaired cardiac output (CO), which is the product of heart rate (HR) and stroke volume (SV). From this relationship several possible causes can be inferred. The effects of a pronounced bradycardia are obvious, while an abnormally high heart rate may compromise diastolic filling and coronary artery perfusion times. The commonest cause of decreased stroke volume is hypovolaemia, but acute left ventricular dysfunction may also be seen in the recovery room. Hypotension will be an associated sign.

Hypotension

Hypotension has numerous causes, and although the immediate reason may be very obvious, such as excessive blood loss via a wound drain, it is better to follow a systematic diagnostic path that is based on first physiological principles. This may lead to a quicker diagnosis in a difficult case, and may help unravel situations in which causation is multifactorial.

The prime determinants of systemic blood pressure are CO (SV × HR) and systemic vascular resistance (SVR). A main determinant of SV is venous return. This will decrease if there is actual hypovolaemia, following blood and/or fluid loss, or when there is effective hypovolaemia, with insufficient volume effectively to fill the capacity of the venous system.

A patient undergoing surgery in the lithotomy position under subarachnoid (spinal) anaesthesia, for example, will maintain adequate venous return to the heart until the legs are laid flat and blood pools in the expanded venous compartment.

Effective hypovolaemia may be associated with neuraxial (and hence sympathetic) block, with peripheral vasodilatation due to pyrexia or sepsis, and with severe drug reactions.

Stroke volume may also be diminished by myocardial depression, injury and ischaemia.

The influence of extremes of heart rate is outlined above. Primary causes of bradycardia include vagal reflexes, due for example to visceral distension, and the persistent effects of preoperative cardiac medication (such as β-adrenoceptor blockers).

A decrease in SVR is associated with most anaesthetic agents, and their effects may persist into the recovery period. Other influences on SVR include pyrexia, hypercapnia and sepsis.

In respect of hypotension however, it is important to remember that pressure is not the same as flow. An inflated arterial tourniquet cuff has a high internal pressure, but no flow. As long as the patient's brain is receiving oxygenated blood (as manifest by normal cerebration) the absolute blood pressure is of little importance. It is the patient who should be treated and not the numbers.

Hypertension

Hypertension occurs less frequently in recovery than hypotension, and its most common cause is likely to be unrelieved pain. It can be due to distension of viscera, particularly of the urinary bladder, and it may also be associated with pre-existing essential hypertension. Rarely it may be a rebound phenomenon secondary to the preoperative withdrawal of anti-hypertensive drugs (typically clonidine and β-adrenoceptor blockers). Volume overload can be a contributory factor, as can hypercapnia and the perioperative use of ketamine.

Severe postoperative hypertension may be associated with coronary ischaemia, particularly if it is accompanied by a tachycardia, and so it should be treated. In addition to managing the cause it may be necessary to prescribe a glyceryl trinitrate patch (5–10 mg). Sublingual nifedipine (5 mg) may also be effective.

Delayed awakening

The most common cause of delayed awakening is persistent central nervous system (CNS) depression by anaesthetic and analgesic drugs. The clinical context may suggest that this is the case, and if opiates or benzodiazepines are implicated then their effects can be reversed by the cautious intravenous administration respectively of naloxone (1–3 μg/kg) or flumazenil (3 μg/kg stat, followed by 1.5 μg/kg at 60-second intervals).

As discussed above, high inspired oxygen concentrations may disguise the fact that a patient is retaining carbon dioxide. In non-habituated patients carbon dioxide narcosis will supervene at a $Pa\text{CO}_2$ of around 12 kPa.

Persistent coma may rarely be due to a hypoxic or ischaemic insult during surgery and anaesthesia. A number of metabolic derangements may also be responsible. The most important of these is hypoglycaemia, not because it is especially common, but because diagnosis and treatment are so simple. Other abnormalities include the hyponatraemia associated with the irrigation of large volumes of glycine-containing solutions during transurethral procedures, and rare endocrine disorders such as undiagnosed myxoedema coma associated with hypothyroidism.

If a patient has received a neuraxial or major plexus block in addition to a general anaesthetic then consideration must be given to the possibility of extensive central spread. Interscalene block, for example, can be complicated by total spinal anaesthesia.

Confusion and agitation

Confusion, agitation, disorientation and aggression may complicate immediate postanaesthetic recovery, and such psychological upsets may be relatively common in elderly patients. That should not stop the anaesthetist seeking a cause, the most important of which is hypoxaemia (which can be both cause and effect).

Confusion may be a nonspecific manifestation of persistent anaesthetic drug actions, but may follow as a direct adverse effect of an agent such as racemic ketamine. It can also be a sign of an alcohol withdrawal syndrome.

More commonly it results from the residual hypnotic effects of drugs, which may prevent a patient being able to communicate effectively that they are in pain or have urinary retention. Other causes of immediate postoperative confusion include pyrexia and sepsis as well as hyponatraemia and hypoglycaemia, as above.

In some patients, usually the elderly, such mental changes may persist for some days or longer, as postoperative cognitive deficit. It is an oversimplification to assume that this is related wholly to intermittent failures of cerebral oxygenation. It may be associated with pre-existing mental infirmity in which dementias and mild confusional states are exaggerated by the effects of anaesthetic drugs on memory processing. It is also associated with procedures in which there is a risk of embolism, such as joint replacement surgery and carotid endarterectomy.

Pain

Pain is a routine problem. One obstacle to its rapid remedy can be the initial attitude of the anaesthetist concerned. There is a tendency among some anaesthetists to react to the statement that one of their patients is in pain as if it were a personal criticism of their anaesthetic technique. It usually is not, of course, but reflects rather the reality that the severity of postoperative pain is not always easy to predict. The recovery area provides a very safe environment in which to manage acute pain properly, and there should be no arbitrary limit on the dose of opiate that can be given. Pain scoring need not be complex. A simple scale (0 = pain free, 1 = mild, 2 = moderate, 3 = severe, 4 = very severe) should be sufficient to grade the response to analgesic drugs. The anxiety that may increase the patient's perception of pain can often be treated effectively by small doses of anxiolytic (intravenous midazolam, 0.5–1.0 mg). A patient should be discharged from recovery only when they themselves are satisfied that their pain is tolerable.

Nausea

Immediate postoperative nausea (PON) is also common, probably affecting more than 15% of all patients. It is multifactorial, with the vomiting centre receiving afferents from the cerebral cortex, the viscera and the chemoreceptor trigger zone, and so the prescription of an antiemetic has become almost routine. This reflex administration should be preceded at least by an attempt to identify the most likely cause. An antiemetic should not be the first-line treatment for nausea and vomiting caused by hypoxia, hypotension or pain.

If there is no obvious cause amenable to treatment and the PON is due to predisposition, the nature of the surgery or drugs then there is a range of agents available that act at different sites. These include those with antihistaminic and antimuscarinic actions, such as cyclizine (dose 50 mg intramuscularly), serotonin (5-HT_3) antagonists such as ondansetron (dose 4 mg orally, intramuscularly or intravenously), and dopamine D_2-antagonists such as prochlorperazine (dose 6.25–12.5 mg intramuscularly). Intractable postoperative nausea with or without vomiting may need treatment with combinations of these agents together with other antiemetic adjuncts such as dexamethasone (8 mg intravenously).

Temperature disturbance

A high temperature always excites the brief suspicion that it may herald of malignant hyperpyrexia, but the diagnosis needs to be considered only to be dismissed, because it almost certainly will not be. More probable causes include sepsis, transfusion reactions and reactions to medication. The overefficient use of a warm air blanket perioperatively can also lead to a rise in core temperature. The use of anticholinergic drugs in the presence of any of these factors may cause pyrexia by preventing effective heat loss through the inhibition of sweating.

A fall in core temperature is more common, especially in the elderly and the very young, and is associated with factors such as intraoperative exposure, prolonged surgery and the intravenous infusion of cool fluids.

Shivering

Shivering that is not associated with a drop in body temperature may accompany the use (particularly) of volatile anaesthetic agents. Not only is it a distressing symptom, but by increasing metabolic oxygen consumption by 300–500% it may also impose an unacceptably high metabolic burden on susceptible individuals (such as those with ischaemic coronary or cerebrovascular disease). The shivering may be aborted by a small dose of pethidine (25 mg intravenously); clonidine (1 μg/kg) may also be effective. High-flow oxygen should be given continuously.

High, low or irregular pulse

Sinus tachycardia is a response to unrelieved pain, hypoxia, hypercapnia and hypovolaemia. It may also be caused by sympathomimetic drugs and by agents with anticholinergic actions.

Sinus bradycardia at worst may be a pre-agonal rhythm due to hypoxia; more usual causes include treatment with β-adrenoceptor antagonists, overdose of neostigmine, vagal stimulation and the higher vagal tone that may accompany physical fitness.

Bradycardia needs treating only if it is causing symptoms.

Any tachyarrhythmia that is accompanied by loss of cardiac output needs urgent treatment, if necessary by DC cardioversion (usually synchronised, unless the rate is so fast that the defibrillator cannot identify the R wave on the ECG).

First-line pharmacological treatment of supraventricular tachycardia (SVT) is with adenosine (3 mg intravenously initially, increasing to 12 mg). Amiodarone (5 mg/kg, in glucose 5%) is useful both for SVT and for ventricular arrhythmias.

The irregularly irregular rhythm of atrial fibrillation (AF) is typically chronic. Acute AF may be provoked by relatively trivial stimuli, but is also associated with sepsis.

PAEDIATRIC RECOVERY

The same principles that govern the care of adults following anaesthesia also apply to children, but there are some important additional aspects. The smaller paediatric airway may be more vulnerable to the complications already described in adults, and the higher metabolic rate and enhanced oxygen consumption in children mean that airway or breathing problems will lead to a more rapid fall in oxygen saturation. The smaller the child the more pronounced these factors become, and this applies also to the maintenance of body temperature.

Postoperative distress in children can be difficult to interpret. It may be due to pain, which should be managed just as energetically as it is in adults, but it may also be due to disorientation, hunger or separation (from parent, dummy or other comforter). This means that it is important that children should be cared for by recovery staff who, as well as being trained in the general aspects of paediatric postoperative care, are experienced enough to be familiar with these particular considerations.

PROTOCOLS AND DISCHARGE CRITERIA

Various scoring systems have been described, based on physical signs, but none holds universal currency. Their main advantage lies in the fact that they encourage a systematic approach to patient assessment before discharge from the recovery area.

The criteria are neither complex nor ambiguous. Patients must be able to maintain their airway unassisted and protective reflexes should be intact. Respiratory and cardiovascular indices should be within the anticipated range for that particular patient. Patients should be able to demonstrate recovery from neuromuscular blockade by sustaining a head lift off the pillow for at least 5 seconds, and symptoms such as pain and nausea should be under control to the patient's own satisfaction.

In routine practice much of the care during the immediate period of postoperative recovery is delegated to recovery room staff. It remains good professional practice for the anaesthetist to leave the theatre and recovery suite only when the patient is awake and comfortable, with airway reflexes restored, and with a circulation that is stable. If the anaesthetist wishes to delegate discharge to the ward to another individual, he or she is free so to do, but must not lose sight of the uncomfortable reality that the final legal responsibility for ensuring that patients are safe when they leave the recovery area is going to be theirs.

References

1. Jones AG, Harper SJ. 'Ventilating in recovery' – the way forward: intensive therapy or postoperative critical care? Br J Anaesth 2002; 88:473–474.
2. Immediate postanaesthetic recovery. Association of Anaesthetists of Great Britain and Ireland. September 2002.
3. Health Building Note 26. Operating Department. London: HMSO; 1991.

CHAPTER **3.2**

ACUTE PAIN MANAGEMENT

There are many causes of acute pain other than postoperative, including trauma, infection, cancer and medical conditions (such as sickle cell crisis and rheumatic disease). Post-surgical pain may be severe, persistent, and become chronic.[1–4] Effective management of acute pain requires a multidisciplinary, evidence-based approach.[5]

PATHOPHYSIOLOGY OF ACUTE PAIN

Tissue damage and inflammation

Noxious stimuli sufficient to cause tissue damage are associated with the release of numerous inflammatory mediators,[6,7] which may be directly algogenic or enhance the algogenic effects of other stimuli.

Chemical mediators of inflammation exert their effect on membrane ion channels of nociceptive neurons either by direct coupling to membrane receptors for specific substances (hydrogen ion, adenosine triphosphate, serotonin [5-HT_3]) or, more commonly, by an indirect action mediated by intracellular second messengers (bradykinin, cytokines, prostanoids, histamine H_1, serotonin [5-HT_1]). Some mediators act on other parts of the neuron to control the expression of receptor proteins and ion channels or to control the release of mediators by other cells.

In addition, many inflammatory cells express receptors for neuropeptides that are released from peripheral nerve terminals (substance P, calcitonin gene-related peptide [CGRP]).[6,8]

Important mediators involved in inflammatory hyperalgesia include bradykinin, cytokines and eicosanoids.

Inflammatory mediators

Bradykinin

Bradykinin is a potent algogenic agent that also sensitises nociceptors to the action of other algogens, increases vascular permeability and enhances leucocyte chemotaxis.

Bradykinin receptor activation releases prostaglandins from sympathetic fibres as well as from other tissues.

Binding sites for bradykinin are found on sensory nerve fibres and in the dorsal horn.

Catecholamines

Catecholamines have been implicated in nociception at the spinal cord level, the effect being mediated by α_2-adrenoreceptors.

Cytokines

Cytokines are regulatory peptides produced in all cells. They have pleiotropic actions; anti-inflammatory cytokines and growth factors contribute to inflammatory hyperalgesia. Thus tumour necrosis factor-α release is stimulated by bradykinin; this stimulates the production of interleukin (IL)-1β and IL-6, which induce hyperalgesia via the production of cyclo-oxygenase products. The effect of IL-8 is mediated via sympathetic nerve fibres.

Histamine

Histamine released from damaged cells and mast cells in response to substance P and nerve growth factor causes activation of nociceptors, vasodilatation and oedema.

Serotonin

Serotonin released by platelets is directly algogenic and enhances the nociceptive effect of bradykinin on sensory nerves.

Protons

Inflammatory exudates tend to be acidic and there is evidence that protons at the site of tissue damage enhance the action of algogenic substances as well as exciting neurons directly.

Prostaglandins

Tissue damage releases phospholipids from cell membranes, which are broken down by phospholipase to form arachidonic acid.

Cyclo-oxygenase-catalysed oxidation of arachidonic acid results in the production of cyclic prostaglandins.

Two forms of the cyclo-oxygenase enzyme (COX-1 and COX-2) have been characterised. COX-1 is a constitutive member of normal cells and is important in platelet function, gastric mucus production, regulation of renal haemodynamics and electrolyte balance. COX-2, the inducible form of the enzyme, is the major isozyme associated with inflammation.

Prostaglandins sensitise nociceptors to the action of other algogenic substances and to mechanical stimuli.

Leukotrienes, the lipoxygenase products of arachidonic acid metabolism, may also have algogenic properties.

Pain signalling and modulation

Information signalling acute injury is transmitted along fast conduction velocity (20 m/s) myelinated A-δ fibres (sharp first pain) and slow conduction velocity (0.5–2.0 m/s) unmyelinated C fibres (dull second pain).

These first-order neurons synapse with second-order neurons in the dorsal horn of the spinal cord. A-δ fibres terminate mainly in lamina I, while C fibres terminate in lamina II. After acute tissue injury there is increased release of neuropeptides such as substance P, and excitatory amino acids such as glutamate, in the dorsal horn.

Projection of nociceptive information to the thalamus is conducted up the spinothalamic tracts.

Synapse of second-order with third-order neurons in the ventral portion of the thalamus results in onward transmission of the nociceptive impulse to the sensory cortex, where it is ultimately perceived as pain.

Endogenous opioid modulation

Endogenous opioid peptides are found in high density in areas of the central nervous system (CNS) involved in nociception.

Three groups of endogenous opioids (enkephalins, β-endorphins and dynorphins) have been identified.

Endogenous opioids modulate nociception by binding to specific receptors. There are several types of opioid receptor (μ1 and μ2, κ, δ, ε and σ), each mediating a spectrum of pharmacological effects. Activation of the μ-receptor is largely responsible for supraspinal analgesia, whereas activation of the κ- and δ-receptors results in spinal analgesia. Recently opioid receptors have been reclassified as OP1 (δ), OP2 (κ) and OP3 (μ).[9] Opioids also act peripherally to block the release of inflammatory mediators, but this action is only manifest in injury and inflammation.

Endogenous non-opioid modulation

Inhibition by a descending monoaminergic pathway may modulate pain traffic at the spinal level. Peripheral chemical sensitisation of the receptor transduction mechanism is, however, independent of central connections.

Hyperalgesia

Tissue damage induces a state of hyperalgesia (increased response to a given stimulus intensity).

Primary hyperalgesia

Primary hyperalgesia occurs within the area of injury and is due to sensitisation of primary afferent neurons by inflammatory mediators.[10]

Secondary (mechanical) hyperalgesia

Secondary (mechanical) hyperalgesia develops in the surrounding uninjured tissue and is thought to be due to activation of the *N*-methyl-D-aspartate (NMDA) receptor (a subtype of the glutamate receptor) in the dorsal horn of the spinal cord – the phenomenon of 'wind-up'.[10]

ACUTE POSTOPERATIVE PAIN

Pain measurement

Knowledge of the incidence and severity of postoperative pain is essential for the establishment of effective pain treatment programmes.

Acute pain is commonly assessed using single-dimension pain scales (behavioural, verbal and numerical rating scales, and visual analogue scale [VAS]) as opposed to multidimensional scales (McGill pain questionnaire). Clinically verbal rating scales (VRS) tend to be preferred to the VAS for the measurement of acute postoperative pain because of their perceived greater ease of use.

Pain scoring

The simplest subjective measure is to ask the patient whether or not he or she feels any pain. Greater sensitivity is obtained if ordered categories are used to grade the pain, but the maximum number of grades a patient can define is limited. A simple VRS with which a patient is asked to describe the amount of pain that he or she feels according to an arbitrary scale is:

- none;
- mild/slight;
- moderate;
- severe;
- very severe/intolerable.

Sedation scores must also be recorded.

Incidence of postoperative pain

Between one-third and one-half of all surgical patients experience significant postoperative pain. The incidence and severity of acute surgical pain depend on:

- site of operation;
- age;
- sex;
- premedication;
- anaesthetic agents;

- psychological factors;
- diurnal factors.

Adverse effects of uncontrolled postoperative pain

Adverse sequelae of uncontrolled postoperative pain include delayed postoperative recovery, increased postoperative morbidity, delayed return of normal physiological functions, restriction of mobility with risk of thromboembolism, and heightened catecholamine response leading to increased oxygen consumption.

Uncontrolled pain is recognised as the primary cause of pulmonary dysfunction after surgery, with reduced sputum clearance, atelectasis, regional underventilation, perfusion inequality, shunting of venous blood and reduced functional residual capacity all contributing to hypoxia.

DRUGS USED IN ACUTE POSTOPERATIVE PAIN MANAGEMENT

Non-steroidal anti-inflammatory drugs

Non-steroidal anti-inflammatory drugs (NSAIDs) may be sufficiently effective as sole analgesics after minor to intermediate surgery. They are also useful after major surgery, when their opioid-sparing effect (≈30%) will help contribute towards a reduction in overall side-effects. They may usefully be combined with paracetamol. NSAIDs can be classified on the basis of their chemical structure (Table 3.2.1).

NSAIDs have widespread actions, including:

- exerting a direct analgesic effect on higher centres;
- modifying the nociceptive responses caused by bradykinin;
- reducing platelet adhesivenesss;
- causing hypothrombinaemia in large doses;
- lowering body temperature in pyrexia (low dose);
- lowering blood sugar (low dose; reverse effect at high dose);
- causing acid–base imbalance and acidosis (rarely).

Inhibition of prostaglandin biosynthesis is considered to be the main mechanism of analgesic action of NSAIDs. However, some NSAIDs also exhibit significant prostaglandin-independent mechanism(s) of action, which augments analgesia.

COX-selective NSAIDs

Traditional NSAIDs block both COX-1 and COX-2, whereas the COX-2 inhibitors (Coxibs) selectively block COX-2.

Chemical classification	NSAID
Acetic acids	
Indoleacetic acids	Acemetacin, indomethacin, sulindac
Naphthylacetic acid	Nabumetone
Phenylacetic acids	Aceclofenac, diclofenac
Pyrroleacetic acids	Ketorolac, tolmetin
Coxibs	Celecoxib, etoricoxib, valdecoxib
Fenamates	Mefenamic acid
Oxicams	Piroxicam, tenoxicam, meloxicam
Propionic acids	
Phenyl proprionic acids	Ibuprofen, fenbufen, fenoprofen, flurbiprofen, ketoprofen, tiaprofenic acid
Naphthyl proprionic acids	Naproxen
Pyrazolones	Azapropazone, phenylbutazone
Salicylic acids	
Acetylated	Aspirin
Non-acetylated	Diflunisal, salicyl salicylate
Others	Licofelone, paracetamol (acetaminophen)

Table 3.2.1 Chemical classification of NSAIDs

The Coxibs were expected to be associated with a reduction in adverse reactions mediated through COX-1 compared to conventional nonselective NSAIDs and a longer duration of action than traditional NSAIDs. However, COX-2 inhibitors contribute to an increased risk of adverse thromboembolic events.

The renal adverse effects of COX-2 inhibitors are similar to those of conventional NSAIDs.

There is some evidence that aspirin-induced asthma may not be precipitated by COX-2 inhibitors. Currently there is a limited number of COX-2 selective NSAIDs (Table 3.2.2), including a parenteral formulation of one of them.

Enantioselective NSAIDS

Ketorolac and all of the profen group of NSAIDs are formulated as racemic mixtures. There may be benefits to using the *S*-enantiomer as opposed to racemic mixtures because stereoselectivity is exhibited in pharmacokinetics, and COX inhibition is also enantioselective. Thus single-isomer NSAIDs exhibit greater peak and faster time to peak plasma concentration than racemic preparations.

COX-1:COX-2 ratio >1	Intermediate COX-1:COX-2 ratio = 1	COX-1:COX-2 ratio <1
Celecoxib	Diclofenac	Aspirin
Etodolac	Ketoprofen	Indomethacin
Etoricoxib	Naproxen	Ibuprofen
Meloxicam		Piroxicam
Valdecoxib (Parecoxib)		

Table 3.2.2 COX selectivity of current NSAIDs

Routes of administration of NSAIDs

Many NSAIDs are available in a range of formulations, including oral, sublingual, rectal and topical. Parenteral preparations of aspirin, diclofenac, indomethacin, ketoprofen, ketorolac, piroxicam and tenoxicam are available

Pharmacokinetics

NSAIDs are rapidly absorbed from the gastrointestinal tract and the speed of absorption is increased using arginine salts.

NSAIDs are highly protein bound (>90%), and are metabolised in the liver. Some are given as inactive 'prodrugs', which are converted to active drugs in the liver (e.g. sulindac, fenbufen).

Glucuronic acid conjugation is followed by the excretion of inactive metabolites in the urine. The rate of elimination is reduced in the elderly and in those with renal impairment.

Adverse effects

NSAIDs have a number of adverse effects affecting the gastrointestinal, respiratory, renal and haematological systems. They should be used with caution in the elderly. Clinical guidelines for their safe use in the perioperative period have been produced.[11]

Gastrointestinal system

NSAIDs may cause gastrointestinal perforation, ulceration and bleeding with diarrhoea and faecal blood loss. They may worsen ulcerative colitis. Risk factors include:

- female gender;
- increasing age;
- cigarette smoking;
- history of alcohol excess;
- history of peptic ulceration;
- the particular NSAID used.

The risk of NSAID-induced gastropathy can be reduced by co-prescription of cytoprotective drugs such as the synthetic prostaglandin E_1 analogue misoprostol or a histamine H_2 receptor antagonist (less effective). An alternative approach is to use NSAIDs devoid of gastroduodenal toxicity, such as selective inhibitors of the COX-2 enzyme and enantioselective NSAIDs.

Respiratory system

The prevalence of sensitivity to NSAIDs in adult asthmatics is 21%. The mechanism of the reaction is unclear.

Renal system

Long-term use of NSAIDs can cause sodium and water retention, which may exacerbate hypertension or even induce cardiac failure. NSAIDs should be avoided when there is evidence of fluid retention or renal impairment and in patients who are hypovolaemic or in circulatory arrest.

Haematological system

Traditional NSAIDs impair platelet function and blood clotting may be altered. The use of some NSAIDs with anticoagulant therapy and low-dose heparin may be contraindicated postoperatively. In contrast, coxibs may have a procoagulant effect. Blood dyscrasias are rare (except with phenylbutazone).

NSAIDs for postoperative pain management

NSAIDs can provide effective postoperative pain relief after many different types of operation. The number of patients who need to receive the active drug for one patient to achieve at least 50% relief of pain (number needed to treat; NNT) is a measure of analgesic efficacy. Most effective analgesics, including many NSAIDs, have low NNT values (Table 3.2.3).

Dexketoprofen

Dexketoprofen, the *S*+-enantiomer of ketoprofen, is a good analgesic with rapid onset and a favourable safety profile. The dose is 75 mg/day.

Diclofenac

Diclofenac is versatile and can be given orally, intramuscularly, intravenously or rectally during or after the operation. Intramuscular diclofenac should be avoided because it may be very painful for a long time. A combination oral preparation of diclofenac with misoprostol is available. The dose is 150 mg/day by any route.

Etoricoxib

Etoricoxib is currently the most selective COX-2 inhibitor. The median time to onset of analgesia is 10–20 minutes. The dose is 60–90 mg once daily.

Analgesic agent	NNT (95% CI)
Diclofenac 100 mg	1.9 (1.6, 2.2)
Paracetamol 1000 mg/codeine 60 mg	2.2 (1.7, 2.9)
Diclofenac 50 mg	2.3 (2.0, 2.7)
Naproxen 440 mg	2.3 (2.0, 2.9)
Ibuprofen 400 mg	2.4 (2.3, 2.6)
Ibuprofen 200 mg	2.7 (2.5, 3.1)
Piroxicam 20 mg	2.7 (2.1, 3.8)
Pethidine 100 mg (intramuscular)	2.9 (2.3, 3.9)
Morphine 10 mg (intramuscular)	2.9 (2.6, 3.6)
Ketorolac 30 mg (intramuscular)	3.4 (2.5, 4.9)
Paracetamol 1000 mg	3.8 (3.4, 4.4)
Aspirin 600/650 mg	4.6 (3.9, 5.5)
Tramadol 100 mg	4.8 (3.8, 6.1)
Codeine 60 mg	16.7 (11.0, 48.0)

Table 3.2.3 Number of patients who need to receive the active drug for one patient to achieve at least 50% relief of pain (NNT) for some commonly used analgesic agents

Indomethacin

Indomethacin can be given orally as well as intravenously and rectally. The dose is 150–200 mg/day.

Ketorolac

Ketorolac is structurally related to zomepirac and tolmetin. It provides analgesia equivalent to opioids in single-dose studies but may adversely affect renal function. Peak plasma concentrations are achieved within 30–60 minutes after oral and parenteral administration.

In excess of 99% of ketorolac is plasma protein bound.

Ketorolac is metabolised in the liver, conjugated and excreted by the kidneys.

Dose and duration of ketorolac should be reduced in the elderly. It can be used as continuous intravenous infusion and in PCA. The dose is 10–30 mg intravenously or intramuscularly

Meloxicam

Meloxicam is a COX-2 selective NSAID, but probably no better than other NSAIDs with respect to adverse gastrointestinal events. The dose is 7.5–15 mg/day

Parecoxib

Parecoxib is a water-soluble prodrug that is rapidly hydrolysed to valdecoxib following injection. The prodrug has no inherent pharmacological activity. Analgesic efficacy is similar to that of ketorolac. The median time to onset of analgesia is 10–20 minutes. It exhibits fewer gastrointestinal side-effects than ketorolac. The dose is 40 mg intravenously

Piroxicam

Piroxicam has a very long half-life, hence dosing is 'once daily'. Dispersible (sublingual) tablets are available. The dose is 10–20 mg once daily.

Other non-opioid analgesic drugs

Paracetamol

Paracetamol is an active metabolite of phenacetin. It is analgesic and antipyretic, but not anti-inflammatory. It does not cause gastric irritation and is relatively nontoxic in therapeutic doses, but 5 g may be enough to cause centrilobular hepatic necrosis.

The efficacy of single-dose paracetamol as a postoperative analgesic has been confirmed by various studies.[12] The mechanism of action remains unclear because paracetamol has no known endogenous binding sites and does not significantly inhibit peripheral cyclo-oxygenase activity. There is increasing evidence of a central antinociceptive effect, and potential mechanisms include inhibition of a CNS COX-2, inhibition of a putative central cyclo-oxygenase 'COX-3' that is selectively susceptible to paracetamol, and modulation of inhibitory descending serotinergic pathways.

Paracetamol is therefore an effective postoperative analgesic, with potency slightly less than that of a standard dose of morphine or the NSAIDs.[12,13]

An intravenous preparation and reports of the analgesic and anti-inflammatory properties and safety advantages of a nitric oxide (NO)-releasing form may be significant advances in the use of paracetamol.

The dose of paracetamol is 10–15 mg/kg orally or rectally. The maximum dose is 60 mg/kg/day

Opioid analgesic drugs

Opiates are very effective as postoperative analgesics and are the main drugs used for the treatment of moderate to severe pain. Doses have to be titrated for each patient, because of considerable interpatient variation in requirements. In adults, age is a better determinant of dose than weight.

Opiates influence the emotional aspects of pain, such as anxiety and fear, as well as reducing the actual pain threshold, so making intolerable pain tolerable. They act on specific opioid receptors in the brain and spinal cord. The piperidine ring structure is essential for opioid activity.

Opiates can be arranged depending on their affinities for endorphin receptors, ranging from pure agonists, through partial agonists and partial antagonists to pure antagonists. Some (e.g. morphine) are more active at the supraspinal μ- receptor, whereas others (e.g. nalbuphine) are more active at spinal δ- and κ-receptors.

Opiate analgesia can be potentiated by pretreatment with oral clonidine, a partial α_2-adrenoceptor agonist, at a dose of 50–150 μg orally, intravenously, intramuscularly or epidurally. In contrast, naloxone antagonises opioid analgesia as well as most side-effects (Table 3.2.4).

Actions of opioids

Central nervous system

Opioids:

- depress – awareness, anxiety, pain sensation, respiration;
- stimulate – vomiting centre, secretion of antidiuretic hormone, Edinger–Westphal nucleus (causing small pupils), hallucinations (rarely).

Smooth muscle

Opioids:

- depress – vascular tone, peristalsis;
- stimulate – bronchoconstriction, bowel sphincters, biliary sphincter, fallopian spasm, arrectores pilorum.

Psychological and physical addiction

Patients may develop both tolerance (tachyphylaxis) and dependence (or addiction). In addicts, withdrawal results in agitation, severe abdominal cramps, diarrhoea and lacrimation (so called ‘cold turkey’). It is relieved by further doses of morphine or methadone.

Other

Opioids:

- stimulate – secretion of catecholamines;
- depress – metabolism;
- release – histamine;
- induce – vagally mediated bradycardia (short-acting opioids).

Agonists	Mixed agonist/antagonist	Antagonist
Phenanthrene alkaloids of opium		
Codeine		Methylnaltrexone
Morphine		
Papaveretum		
Thebaine	Buprenorphine	
Semisynthetic alkaloids		
Diamorphine		
Dihydrocodeine		
Dihydromorphinone		
Oxycodone		
Oxymorphone	Nalbuphine	Naloxone
Synthetic agents		
Morphinans		
Levorphanol	Butorphanol	
	Dezocine	
Benzomorphinans	Meptazinol	
	Pentazocine	
Phenylpiperidine derivatives		
Alfentanil		
Fentanyl		
Pethidine		
Phenoperidine		
Remifentanil		
Sufentanil		
Tramadol		
Diphenylheptane derivatives		
Dipipanone		
Dextromoramide		
Methadone		
Piritramide		
Propoxyphene		

Table 3.2.4 Opioid drugs

Routes of administration of opioids

Oral

Oral opioids can give good analgesia and should be used in preference to parenteral injection when possible. There are several oral formulations of oral morphine – morphine in solution and immediate-release and controlled-release tablets. Peak plasma concentrations occur within 1 hour of morphine in solution and immediate-release tablets, with analgesia lasting 4 hours. Controlled-release tablets produce delayed peak plasma concentrations and longlasting analgesia (12 h MST Continus®; 24 h MXL®). The potency ratio of oral:parenteral morphine is 1:6 for acute pain, but 1:2 to 1:3 for non-acute pain. An antiemetic may be needed.

Oral oxycodone is an effective analgesic and is available in immediate-release (Oxynorm® 5–10 mg 4-hourly) and sustained-release (Oxycontin® 12-hourly) preparations. Oxycontin may have a more rapid onset than other sustained-release opioid preparations.

Rectal

Morphine suppositories have similar bioavailability and duration to oral morphine. The potency ratio to oral morphine is 1:1.

Parenteral

Traditionally opioids have been given intramuscularly or subcutaneously. Neonates, infants, the elderly and the unfit are more susceptible to respiratory depression. Children and young adults are often quite resistant.

Continuous intravenous infusions of opioid analgesic can be given until pain is relieved, and then the dose titrated against the pain. Infusions of fentanyl efficiently relieve postoperative pain. Opioid infusions are not necessarily followed by either psychological dependence or physical sequelae. Intravenous PCA gives good pain relief at a lower dosage than intramuscular injection.

Postoperative pain relief can be provided by a continuous subcutaneous infusion. A simple infusion regimen for subcutaneous morphine is 0.8 mg/kg/24 h. Continuous subcutaneous pethidine infusion (2 mg/h) has also proved successful, but carries the associated risk of norpethidine toxicity. A bolus facility for extra pain (dressings, turning) or to regain pain control is useful.

Opioid requirements of patients receiving high doses of corticosteroids are less than normal for the control of postoperative pain.

Transdermal

The high lipophilicity of fentanyl makes it ideal for transdermal delivery. Fentanyl patches provide sustained delivery of 25–100 μg/h, and although these are not recommended for routine acute pain management, they can be of use for patients who have high or prolonged opioid requirements.

Recently an 'on-demand' iontophoretic fentanyl skin patch has been introduced, and is the subject of much clinical research.

Extradural

Lipophilic opioids are no more potent by this route than when given systemically, unless they are mixed with local analgesics.

Adverse effects

Opioids have a number of adverse effects affecting the gastrointestinal, respiratory and cardiovascular systems. Adverse gastrointestinal effects include nausea and vomiting in up to 50% of patients. Respiratory depression and hypotension may be troublesome[14]. Bradycardia can also occur with short-acting opiates.

Opioids have a relatively slow onset of analgesia. Intravenous remifentanil and alfentanil are fastest (1–2 minutes), whereas fentanyl may take 15–20 minutes to produce analgesia; unfortunately, respiratory depression has a faster onset. However, because of the considerable variation of individual response (up to tenfold) it is difficult to predict the correct dose.

In susceptible individuals addiction may be a problem, and tachyphylaxis and occasional hallucinations may occur with prolonged administration.

Opioid agonists

Naturally occurring alkaloids of opium

Morphine

Morphine (Morpheus, Greek God of dreams, son of Somnos, God of sleep) has been in use for over 2000 years and is still the best available analgesic. It was first used by Theophrastus in the third century BC.

Opium comes from the dried latex of unripe capsules of the poppy head (*Papaver somniferum*). Morphine is one of over 25 alkaloids (alkaloid = like alkali) contained in opium, but only morphine, codeine and papaverine have wide clinical use. The concentration of morphine in opium is 9–17%. Morphine was isolated from opium in 1806, its chemical structure determined in 1925 and synthesised in 1952. Morphine salts are not destroyed by boiling.

Morphine is a good analgesic and a poor relaxer of smooth muscle. (Papaverine is a poor analgesic but a good relaxant of smooth muscle.) There is large interpatient variability with morphine.

Pharmacodynamics

Central nervous system Morphine is analgesic, sedative, anxiolytic, euphoric, addictive, a respiratory depressant, and causes nausea and vomiting. It is more effective against dull, continuous, visceral, than against sharp, intermittent pain. Very rarely, restlessness and delirium follow its injection and dysphoria follows. Intracranial pressure increases because of the raised $Pa\text{CO}_2$.

Effect on the eye Morphine causes miosis by a central action, via the oculomotor nerve, stimulating the Edinger–Westphal nucleus. Atropine can counteract this miosis. Intraocular tension is reduced in both normal and glaucomatous eyes.

Cardiovascular system With morphine, there is mild vasodilation in clinical doses, and sometimes bradycardia. Patients in shock should be given morphine intravenously so that it does not accumulate unabsorbed in the ischaemic tissues only to produce a massive effect when absorption occurs with improvement in the circulation. Only small doses are needed.

Respiratory system With morphine, the response of the respiratory centre to $Pa\text{CO}_2$ is diminished, with 50% depression of the $Pa\text{CO}_2$ response curve at plasma levels of 100 μg/L (postoperative analgesia occurs at 12–25 μg/L). Respiratory rate, rather than tidal volume, is decreased. Arterial and alveolar $Pa\text{CO}_2$ are not usually raised much.

Respiratory depression is difficult to define or measure clinically, and the respiratory rate is often used, by default. However, sedation scores are a better indicator of morphine toxicity.

Breathing may become periodic (Cheyne–Stokes) or irregular.

Bronchoconstriction can occur and is worse in asthmatic patients.

Maximal respiratory depression comes on 30 minutes after intramuscular injection, and sooner after intravenous injection. Morphine also depresses the cough reflex.

Gastrointestinal tract Morphine constricts the sphincters of the gut and reduces peristalsis – more so when given intramuscularly than when given orally. Constipation is a significant adverse effect of prolonged morphine administration.

Nausea and vomiting are due to central stimulation. This is seen most strongly with the allied drug apomorphine. Vomiting after morphine depends partly on the movements of the body and the position of the patient; it sensitises the vomiting centre to vestibular movements. Early ambulation after morphine will cause more nausea than quiet bed rest. Antiemetics can control this nausea, some more effectively than others. About one-third of postoperative patients feel sick after opioids, females much more so than males.

Morphine contracts the sphincter of Oddi, raising the pressure in the bile ducts, which rarely causes severe pain. Atropine does not fully antagonise this action, but glyceryl trinitrate, nalorphine, levallorphan, epinephrine (adrenaline), aminophylline and amyl nitrite do.

Genitourinary tract The tone and peristalsis of the ureters and other smooth muscle (e.g. of the hollow viscera, bladder sphincter, fallopian tubes etc.), are increased with morphine, an action antagonised by atropine.

The tone of the vesical sphincter is increased and may hinder micturition – a common postoperative problem. Urinary output is decreased owing to stimulation of secretion of antidiuretic hormone. There is little relaxation of the uterus during labour. Morphine crosses the placental barrier and depresses fetal respiration.

Endocrine system The posterior pituitary and adrenal medulla are stimulated by morphine, so antidiuretic hormone and blood catecholamine levels increase. Blood sugar may rise.

Other Morphine sometimes causes itching, especially of the nose. It may occasionally cause anaphylactoid and allergic reactions, ranging from slight syncope due to histamine release to anaphylactic shock. Morphine is useful in the management of paroxysmal nocturnal dyspnoea (cardiac asthma). Sweating may be stimulated.

Pharmacokinetics

Routes of administration of morphine are many – oral, buccal, intramuscular, intravenous, subcutaneous, rectal, transcutaneous and intra-articular.

Morphine has a p*K*a of 7.9, is poorly lipid soluble, is 40% bound to plasma albumin (30% in neonates), and exhibits triexponential elimination kinetics. The elimination half-life varies with age – neonate 629 minutes, infant 233 minutes, child 120 minutes, adult 180 minutes.

Oral morphine undergoes significant first-pass metabolism. Biotransformation is by conjugation with glucuronic acid in the liver, followed by excretion in the bile and by the kidneys. Both active (morphine-6-glucuronide [M6G]) and inactive (morphine-3-glucuronide [M3G]) metabolites depend on the kidneys for excretion. Deficient renal excretion may cause accumulation and respiratory depression.

Morphine appears in breast milk, saliva and sweat. Special care is necessary in infants under 6 months of age, elderly or debilitated patients, and in patients with a raised $Pa\text{CO}_2$, suprarenal insufficiency, myasthenia, myotonia, hypothyroidism, asthma, raised intracranial pressure, respiratory depression, hepatic failure, renal failure, acute alcoholism and diverticulitis and in labour.

The dose of morphine is 0.15 mg/kg intramuscularly, although in adults age rather than weight is a better determinant of dose; 0.03 mg/kg intravenously (0.1–1 mg/kg intravenously prevents the 'stress response'); infusion rate 0.03 mg/kg/h, (5–15 μg/kg/h in neonates) (Table 3.2.5).

Onset of analgesia with morphine is 3–10 min (intravenously) and 10–20 minutes (intramuscularly). The duration is 3–4 hours.

Age (years)	Dose (mg)
20–39	7.5–12.5
40–59	5–10
60–69	2.5–7.5
70–85	2.5–5.0
>85	2–3

Table 3.2.5 Adult dosing regimen for intramuscular morphine

Papaverine

Papaverine was isolated from opium in 1848. It does not suppress intestinal peristalsis, and relieves spasm in arteries. It has almost no central effects. The dose is up to 30 mg intravenously or intra-arterially (very slowly), and 120–250 mg orally.

Codeine phosphate

The name is from the Greek name for poppy-head. Its structure is methyl morphine, and together with morphine and papaverine forms the chief alkaloidal derivative of opium. It was isolated in 1832.

Codeine is classed as a weak opioid, and metabolic conversion to morphine accounts for most of the analgesic effect. The enzyme responsible for this conversion, cytochrome isoenzyme P450 (CYP) 2D6, is lacking in 10% of the Caucasian population. The major metabolic pathway is conversion to codeine-6-glucuronide, which like codeine has little opioid agonist activity and is excreted by the kidneys. The analgesic effect is one-tenth that of morphine. Compound preparations of codeine and paracetamol have considerable analgesic effect. Codeine phosphate may release histamine in children.

Codeine undergoes very little first-pass metabolism, hence the oral route is effective. It should never be given intravenously

The dose of codeine phosphate is 15–50 mg as an analgesic, antitussive and antidiarrhoeal agent.

Semi-synthetic alkaloids of opium

Diamorphine hydrochloride

Diamorphine hydrochloride (heroin) is the diacetyl ester of morphine. It is a prodrug and is hydrolysed to 6-monoacetyl morphine and morphine. It is a drug of addiction, because of the euphoria it creates, and was introduced into medicine in 1898. In the US and in Australia its use is proscribed. It should be freshly prepared from powder.

Diamorphine hydrochloride depresses the respiratory centre and the cough reflex more than morphine and is twice as efficient as an analgesic.

Diamorphine 5 mg has a faster onset of activity and fewer emetic sequelae than morphine 10 mg. It is an excellent postoperative analgesic, although its effect does not last as long as that of morphine.

In coronary occlusion, 5 mg intravenously cause little cardiovascular depression or vomiting if given slowly.

Diamorphine hydrochloride is useful by mouth in the treatment of chronic pain in doses up to 30 mg and as an epidural opioid.

Excretion of diamorphine hydrochloride is chiefly by the kidneys after conversion to morphine in the body.

The dose of diamorphine hydrochloride is 2.5–5 mg intravenously or intramuscularly. The onset of action is 5 minutes intravenously and 10 minutes intramuscularly.

Dihydrocodeine tartrate

Dihydrocodeine tartrate is a semisynthetic derivative of codeine with inherent analgesic activity. It is metabolised to dihydromorphine, and is an analgesic, constipator and antitussive. It may cause nausea, dysphoria and vertigo, and it releases histamine.

The dose of dihydrocodeine tartrate is 0.5 mg/kg, orally, intramuscularly or intravenously.

Oxycodone

Oxycodone is a potent opioid agonist that is very useful for the treatment of even severe pain. It produces predictable and reliable analgesia after oral administration because of its higher, and less variable, bioavailability than morphine (50–75%). Intravenous oxycodone produces similar analgesia to the same doses of morphine, and can be given by PCA. It is metabolised in the liver to noroxycodone and oxymorphone (the latter is weakly active).

The dose of oxycodone is 5–10 mg 2–3-hourly (immediate release).

Hydromorphone

Hydromorphone is five times as potent as morphine, from which it is derived. It has a similar efficacy and side-effect profile to morphine, and is metabolised to hydromorphone-3-glucuronide, which is dependent on renal excretion.

The dose of hydromorphone is 8 mg daily in divided doses.

Synthetic alkaloids of opium

Pethidine (meperidine) hydrochloride

Pethidine (meperidine) hydrochloride is the hydrochloride of the ethyl ester of 1-methyl-4-phenyl-piperidine-4-carboxylic acid.

Pethidine use is diminishing because of multiple disadvantages, of which the accumulation of norpethidine is the most significant. Norpethidine toxicity is associated with a variety of neuroexcitatory effects, ranging from nervousness to convulsions.

In clinical practice there is no evidence that pethidine is better than morphine for the relief of renal or biliary colic.

Pharmacodynamics

Analgesia Pethidine relieves most types of pain, especially those associated with plain muscle spasm. It depresses the respiratory centre and cough reflex, and is also a local analgesic. It has no effect on the ciliary body or iris. It raises the cerebrospinal fluid pressure and can cause addiction.

Smooth muscle Pethidine has a direct papaverine-like effect on the smooth muscle of the bronchioles, intestine, ureters and arteries. It will often relieve bronchospasm. Vasodilation may be unwelcome in trauma patients and uncontrolled hypertensives.

Cholinergic effects Pethidine has an atropine-like effect on cholinergic nerve endings.

Histamine release Pethidine may release histamine from tissues.

Side-effects Side-effects of pethidine include sweating, hypotension, vertigo and limb tingling.

Postoperative nausea is similar to that following morphine, but comes on earlier. It is worse after intravenous than after intramuscular injection.

Like morphine, pethidine may cause hypotension if the head of the patient is raised, or with sudden movement. Because of its circulatory depressant effects it is probably not the ideal drug for the relief of pain in myocardial infarction.

Norpethidine can produce nervousness, tremors, twitches, myoclonus and seizures.

Phenobarbital enhances the production of toxic metabolites of pethidine. These two drugs should not be given together.

Precautions The administration of pethidine to patients receiving monoamine oxidase inhibitors may cause severe reactions and even death. There is restlessness, hypertension, convulsions and coma, with absent tendon jerks and an extensor plantar response; hypotension may also be seen. The reaction is said to be due to serotonin reuptake inhibition.

Pharmacokinetics

The routes of administration of pethidine are the same as for morphine. Oral bioavailability is 45–75% and 64% is bound to plasma protein.

Pethidine is metabolised at the rate of 17%/h. The biological half-life is 3–4 hours in man, and 80% is hydrolysed in liver. About 5–10% is excreted unchanged by the kidneys. One metabolite, norpethidine, may cause convulsions or hallucinations if pethidine is given in large doses, for prolonged periods or with monoamine oxidase inhibitors. Patients in renal failure are at increased risk of norpethidine toxicity.

The dose of pethidine is 0.5 mg/kg intravenously and 1.5 mg/kg intramuscularly. Its onset of action is 2–5 minutes, and its duration 2 hours.

Fentanyl

Fentanyl, a 4-anilidopiperidine compound, is a pure opioid agonist with a high affinity for the μ-receptor. It is 75–125 times more potent than morphine as an analgesic. Unlike morphine it has high lipid solubility and as a result is rapidly and extensively distributed in the tissues. Its metabolites are inactive and hence it is useful in patients with renal disease.

Fentanyl is usually used for PCA, with a 5–10-minute lockout interval.

Because of its high lipid solubility fentanyl can also be administered ransdermally, but the fixed delivery rate of the patches is a major disadvantage in postoperative pain control.

The dose of fentanyl is a 10–20 μg intravenous bolus using PCA, and from 25 up to 100 μg/h using a transdermal patch.

Tramadol

Tramadol is a synthetic 4-phenyl-piperidine analogue of codeine. It has a weak central action on opioid receptors and also acts on descending monoaminergic pathways, and thus is commonly referred to as an atypical centrally acting analgesic. The M1 metabolite shows higher affinity for opioid receptors than the parent drug.

The risk of respiratory depression is significantly lower with tramadol than with other opioids given at equianalgesic doses. Tramadol also causes less constipation. However, nausea and vomiting are common side-effects.

The half life of tramadol is 5 hours after oral dosing, and its potency is comparable to that of pethidine. It can be given orally, rectally, intravenously or intramuscularly. The dose is 100 mg orally or intravenously to a maximum of 250 mg. Its duration is 3–6 hours after 100 mg orally.

Methadone hydrochloride

Methadone hydrochloride is a powerful analgesic. It causes less sedation and has a more prolonged action than morphine (half life 40–90 hours, increasing with subsequent doses). It exhibits high oral bioavailability. Absorption from fatty sites (e.g. subcutaneous and epidural) is very slow.

Methadone has been used to wean addicts from morphine and for chronic pain. It is used for the maintenance treatment of patients with an opioid addiction because of the high oral bioavailability (60–95%), high opioid potency and sustained effect. The use of methadone for acute pain management is limited by the long unpredictable duration of action. Careful dosage titration is required to avoid accumulation and adverse effects.

The dose of methadone is 0.1 mg/kg intramuscularly or 0.05 mg/kg intravenously. The onset of action is 1 minute (intravenously) and 5 minutes (intramuscularly).

Dextropropoxyphene

Dextropropoxyphene is the only one of the four isomers of propoxyphene to have analgesic activity. It undergoes extensive first-pass metabolism.

Dextropropoxyphene may cause dependence and, if taken with alcohol, respiratory depression. It is commonly combined with paracetamol – co-proxamol contains dextropropoxyphene 32.5 mg and paracetamol 550 mg. Overdose will result in liver toxicity and respiratory depression.

Dextromoramide acid tartrate

Dextromoramide acid tartrate is a morphine-like analgesic but twice as potent. It is relatively non-soporific, and can be given by mouth. The dose is a 5 mg tablet or 5–10 mg by intramuscular injection.

Mixed agonist/antagonists and partial antagonists of opium

Buprenorphine

Buprenorphine is a powerful, long-acting synthetic thebaine derivative with partial agonist properties. Its duration of action is up to 10 hours. A single dose may therefore last throughout the night, which is important in postoperative analgesia. Buprenorphine may accentuate urinary obstruction. A dose of 0.3 mg relieves the pain of ureteric colic. Buprenophine has altered pharmacokinetics in patients with renal impairment.

Buprenorphine is only partly reversed by naloxone, but because of its partial agonist properties, respiratory depression shows a 'ceiling effect' and apnoea, or even a respiratory rate below 4/min, is very unlikely to occur. Buprenorphine is associated with a particularly high incidence of emesis, especially in mobilising patients.

Routes of administration of buprenorphine are sublingual, intramuscular, intravenous and epidural. The dose is 0.2–1 mg.

Butorphanol

Butorphanol is a synthetic morphinan derivative and potent opioid agonist/antagonist.

Butorphanol undergoes significant hepatic first-pass metabolism after oral dosing, with only 5–17% bioavailability. It is extensively metabolised in the liver by hydroxylation, and only 5–10% is excreted unchanged by the kidney after a single intravenous dose. Respiratory depression is dose related, the ceiling being reached with a 2 mg dose. It can be given transnasally.

The dose of butorphanol is 1–2 mg intramuscularly.

Pentazocine

Pentazocine is an opioid agonist/antagonist analgesic derived from benzmorphinan. It is an agonist at κ/σ-receptors and a very weak opioid antagonist (1/50th the activity of nalorphine).

Respiratory depression with pentazocine is dose related, but has a ceiling effect. Pentazocine is non-addictive and not euphoric. It raises rather than lowers blood pressure and the dextroisomer has a positive inotropic effect on the myocardium (α-receptor stimulation). It does not influence pupil size or intraocular tension, and crosses the placental barrier less easily than pethidine. Hallucinations may follow its use, but may be controlled by diazepam.

Nalbuphine hydrochloride

Nalbuphine hydrochloride is a partial κ-receptor agonist and μ-receptor antagonist. It undergoes extensive first-pass metabolism with oral bioavailability of only 10%.

Nalbuphine hydrochloride has been used for perioperative analgesia. It has less effect on delay of coordinated bowel motility than morphine, and is not likely to cause bronchoconstriction in asthmatics.

The dose of nalbuphine hydrochloride is 10–20 mg.

Meptazinol

Meptazinol is an opioid agonist/antagonist with partial agonist activity at the μ1 receptor and some cholinergic activity. It has a shorter duration of action than morphine, and is used for perioperative analgesia.

The dose of meptazinol is 200 mg orally and 75–100 mg intramuscularly.

Opiate antagonists

Specific antagonism to opioids was first described in 1915. Antagonists are usually the *n*-allyl derivatives of opiate analgesics. The more potent the narcotic, the smaller the dose of its allyl derivative necessary to antagonise opioid-induced respiratory depression. They have high receptor affinity and low receptor activity. They do not lead to addiction. They may cause signs of withdrawal in narcotic addicts. The probable mode of action is competition at receptor sites on cell surfaces. Antagonists counteract the analgesia produced by morphine, pethidine and oxymorphone.

Naloxone

Naloxone *is* *n*-allyl noroxymorphone, derived from oxymorphone. It was first synthesised in 1972. It also antagonises the respiratory depression caused by pentazocine and dextropropoxyphene.

The short duration of effect of naloxone (1 hour) may be less than that of the opiate it is designed to antagonise, so repeat dosage or an infusion may be necessary. It relaxes spasm of the sphincter of Oddi induced by opiate analgesics. With careful titration of dosage, analgesia is not reversed.

Naloxone can be used in the treatment of opiate-induced respiratory depression and in midwifery to reverse fetal respiratory depression due to opiates.

Naloxone reverses respiratory depression, but not the analgesia of intrathecal morphine.

Naloxone may raise blood pressure in septic shock, suggesting that endorphins may contribute to this hypotension, and can cause acute pulmonary oedema in previously fit patients. It has caused arrhythmia and even sudden death, and can be given intramuscularly for a more prolonged effect.

Pharmacokinetics The half-life of naloxone is 20 minutes. It is metabolised in the liver.

The dose of naloxone is 0.1–0.4 mg intravenously, repeated as required (0.01 mg/kg in neonates).

Methylnaltrexone

Methylnaltrexolone is epoxymorphinan. It has a very long half-life, and its main use is as an aid in maintaining abstinence in opioid withdrawal. It has been suggested that with careful titration of dosage, analgesia is not reversed.

Opioid overdose

Opioid overdose causes coma, respiratory depression, hypoxia, acidosis and muscle compression (from deep sedation), all leading to rhabdomyolysis and acute renal failure. Pulmonary oedema (non-cardiogenic), cerebral oedema, convulsions and aspiration pneumonia also occur. Treatment is by immediate reversal with naloxone and by organ support.

Controlled drugs and drug dependence

There are legal requirements relating to the prescription of controlled drugs (CDs). In the UK Misuse of Drugs Regulations 1985 divide drugs into five schedules, whereas the Misuse of Drugs Act 1971 divides drugs into three classes according to their harmfulness when misused.

Most opiates are CDs and as such subject to full controlled drug requirements relating to prescription, safe custody and the need to keep a register. There are a few notable exceptions, such as pentazocine and oral (but not parenteral, codeine, which are subject to special prescription but not safe custody requirements.

MANAGING ACUTE PAIN

Methods of pain relief

It is important to identify and if possible remove the cause of pain (e.g. distended bladder). Thereafter treatment may be by pharmacological (analgesics and regional blocks) or non-pharmacological (e.g. hypnosis, acupuncture) methods.

In general terms, acute pain is best treated by a multimodal approach, using drug combinations to enhance analgesia and minimise side-effects. Paracetamol is the fundamental component, to which NSAIDs (or COX-2 inhibitors) are added in the absence of contraindications, with opioid therapy completing the combination. Other analgesic therapies, including regional blockade, adjuvant agents and non-pharmacological techniques, are valuable additions to this simple approach.[5,15]

Pharmacological techniques

Pharmacotherapy includes the use of simple analgesics either as single or combination preparations, and opioid analgesics, often administered using PCA.

Combination preparations include aspirin–paracetamol, codeine–paracetamol, ibuprofen–codeine and tramadol–paracetamol.

Caffeine, which has been shown to have adjuvant analgesic activity when combined with simple oral analgesics, may be added to simple analgesics. A dose of more than 65 mg is needed. In a large meta-analysis of over 10 000 patients, analgesia from paracetamol or paracetamol-and-aspirin with caffeine 65 mg added was approximately 1.4 times more potent than without added caffeine.

Patient-controlled analgesia

Patient-controlled analgesia (PCA) refers to the on-demand, intermittent self-administration of analgesic drugs by a patient. PCA is predominantly used to deliver opioid analgesics, but other classes of drugs can be administered in this way. Any opiate can be used. The traditional route of drug delivery has been intravenous (IV-PCA), but subcutaneous (SC-PCA) and epidural (PCEA) routes can also be used. The recent development of an iontophoretic patient-controlled fentanyl skin patch may be of considerable significance. The quality of analgesia is normally good, and allows for wide interpatient variation. The basic variables of PCA are:

- demand (bolus) dose;
- lockout interval (length of the time between patient demands);
- background infusion rate (if used);
- hourly or 4-hourly limit.

The use of background infusion in adults is controversial, tending to increase sedation and other side-effects without improving analgesia, but is more often used in children.

Most PCA infusers incorporate sophisticated pump technology with a lockable syringe compartment to prevent tampering (non-disposable).

Compact ambulatory devices are a further refinement. Alternatively, lightweight disposable infusers that combine an elastomeric pressure mechanism (a cylinder containing the analgesic drug within an elastic balloon) with a non-electronic non-programmable wristwatch control device are available

A one-way Y-connector enables use with intravenous infusions. Antireflux valves are recommended to prevent reflux delivery of drug into gravity-fed infusion tubing in the event of an occlusion. However, these valves may store a large bolus of drug or impede the intravenous infusion.

Preoperative counselling in the use of PCA is helpful.

Opiates administered by PCA are associated with less severe falls in oxygen saturation than when given as intermittent intramuscular boluses.

Pain control, respiration and sedation should be monitored.

PCEA with lipophilic opioids may be improved by the addition of local analgesics.

Patients express high satisfaction with PCA. The advantages include not having to bother nurses, rapid pain relief, self-control of their own pain, exact titration of dose and lack of intramuscular injections.

Some patients worry about overdose, addiction, lack of personal contact with nurses and machine dysfunction.

PCA is also useful in children over 5 years of age, in obstetrics and in acute medical diseases (e.g. sickle cell crisis and malignant pain). Parent-controlled analgesia, nurse-controlled and spouse-controlled analgesia have all been described.

Drawbacks of PCA include:

- problems with patient selection/education;
- opioid side-effects, especially respiratory depression (rare 0.019%) and excessive sedation; also nausea, vomiting, itching, ileus and hallucinations;
- complex equipment leading to programming errors – equipment malfunction occurs in 5% of cases;
- underutilisation, overutilisation and syphoning.

Regional blockade with local anaesthetic infusions

Local anaesthetic infusions avoid the side-effects of the opioids, can be applied to an area of the body no larger than the source of pain, and can give supremely good analgesia. Prolonged action is possible with the insertion of microcatheters to the site of the block, and top-ups or infusion of local analgesic. Extra vigilance is needed when epidural opioids have been given.

Blockade of pain afferents by regional techniques (e.g. postoperative high extradural analgesia, intercostal and paravertebral nerve block, axillary and femoral sheath catheters and subcutaneous bupivacaine after herniorrhaphy).

Ketamine infusion

A low-dose (5–15 mg/h) continuous (intravenous or subcutaneous) infusion of ketamine has been successfully used to treat postoperative pain, even in the absence of any neuropathic component (see below). The main adverse effect is hallucination.

Inhalational analgesia

Entonox can be used for dressing changes. When using this technique the potential haematological and neurological adverse effects of repeated nitrous oxide exposure, disrupting vitamin B_{12} metabolism and methionine synthesis, should be considered.

Non-pharmacological techniques

A number of non-pharmacological interventions can be used for pain relief, including:

- transcutaneous electrostimulation;
- acupuncture;
- psychological techniques;
- cryoanalgesia of intercostal nerves (no longer used because of the high incidence of dysaesthesia).

ACUTE NEUROPATHIC PAIN

Neuropathic pain can develop after surgery and must be diagnosed promptly and managed correctly to ensure the best outcome for the patient and avoid chronicity.[1,2,3,4] The diagnosis of neuropathic pain can be obtained from the presenting features of burning, stinging or shooting pain, increasing despite apparent tissue healing, with a relative lack of response to doses of opioids used in the postoperative period (this does not imply that neuropathic pain is unresponsive to opioids), and some or all of the features of allodynia, hyperaesthesia and dysaesthesia.[5]

Long-term therapy comprises either an anticonvulsant or a tricyclic antidepressant, but in the early postoperative period when patients cannot take oral medications the angioneuropathic effects of systemic low-dose lidocaine (lignocaine) or ketamine can be employed. A reasonable approach to control postoperative neuropathic pain would be initially to use a continuous subcutaneous infusion of either lidocaine (lignocaine) (1–1.5 mg/kg/h) or ketamine (5–15 mg/h), followed by oral anticonvulsant or tricyclic antidepressant maintenance therapy.[16]

ACUTE PAIN MANAGEMENT

An 'Acute Pain Service' can teach, encourage and oversee the delivery of analgesia. It involves surgeons, physicians, pharmacists, physiotherapists, anaesthetists and nurses working in a concerted manner to reduce pain, facilitate rehabilitation and improve outcome for the patient.

The relief of postoperative pain can be badly managed, simply by neglect. Failure can occur at the point of writing prescriptions and at the point of delivery of analgesia by nurses. Experience with 'pain teams' has heightened awareness of this, but the risk is that the whole of the pain (and fluid and other) management of the hospital may be transferred by default to the team by those surgeons and nurses who previously looked after it. Thus, pain team activity may need to be mainly advisory in continuing effective analgesia and developing even more efficient methods by nurses, surgeons etc. Invaluable roles of the pain team include education of patients and staff about pain relief techniques, introduction of treatment protocols based on scientific evidence, regular audit of efficacy and safety of techniques used, and provision of a consultation service for difficult pain management cases.

References

1. Cousins MJ, Power I. Acute and postoperative pain. In: Wall PD, Melzack R, eds. Textbook of pain, 4th edn. London: Churchill Livingstone, 1999.
2. Cousins MJ, Power I. Acute and postoperative pain. In: Melzack R, Wall PD, eds. Handbook of pain management. London: Churchill Livingstone; 2003:13–30.
3. Cousins MJ, Power I, Smith G. Pain – a persistent problem. Reg Anesth Pain Med 2000; 25:6–21.
4. Perkins FM, Kehlet H. Chronic pain as an outcome of surgery – review of predictive factors. Anesthesiology 2000; 93:1123–1133.
5. National Health and Medical Research Council. Acute pain management: scientific evidence. Canberra, Australia: National Health and Medical Research Council; 1999.
6. Dray A. Inflammatory mediators of pain. Br J Anaesth 1995; 75:125–131.
7. Dray A, Bevan S. Inflammation and hyperalgesia: highlighting the team effort. Trends Pharmacol Sci 1993; 14:287–290.
8. Rang HP, Bevan C, Dray A. Chemical activation of nociceptive peripheral neurons. Br Med Bull 1991; 47:534–548.
9. Lambert DG. Recent advances in opioid pharmacology. Br J Anaesth 1998; 81:1–2.
10. Rice ASC. Recent developments in the pathophysiology of acute pain. Acute Pain 1998; 1:27–36.

11. Guidelines for use of non-steroidal anti-inflammatory drugs in the perioperative period. London: Royal College of Anaesthetists; 1998.
12. Barden JEJ, Moore A, McQuay H. Single dose oral paracetamol (acetaminophen) for postoperative pain (Cochrane Review). The Cochrane Library. Chichester, UK: John Wiley & Sons Ltd; 2004.
13. Kehlet H, Werner MU. Role of paracetamol in acute pain management. Drugs 2003; 63:15–22.
14. Cashman JN, Dolin SJ. Respiratory and haemodynamic effects of acute postoperative pain management: evidence from published data. Br J Anaesth 2004; 93:212–223.
15. Commission on the Provision of Surgical Services Royal College of Surgeons and College of Anaesthetists. London: 1990.
16. Wilson JA, Colvin LA, Power I. Audit and the evidence base of anaesthesia: acute neuropathic pain after surgery. Bull Roy Coll Anaesth 2002; 15:739–742.

Further reading

Breivik H. Post-operative pain management. Baillière's clinical anaesthesiology. Vol. 9. No. 3. London: Baillière Tindall; 1995.

Ferrante FM, VadeBoncouer TR, eds. Postoperative pain management. New York: Churchill Livingstone; 1993.

Cousins MJ, Power I. Acute and postoperative pain. In: Melzack R, Wall PD, eds. Handbook of pain management. London: Churchill Livingstone; 2003:13–30.

CHAPTER 3.3

COMPLICATIONS OF ANAESTHESIA

Death due to anaesthesia alone is very rare, but complications of anaesthesia are not uncommon. Patients often come to harm when several problems combine to result in adverse outcome;[1] minimising and treating complications is an important aspect of patient safety. Awareness of the risks of anaesthesia and surgery plays a major part in deciding the proposed anaesthetic technique for an individual patient.

This chapter is laid out by system and by diagnosis. In clinical practice the initial presentation of problems is often confusing and the diagnosis is not always immediately obvious. The immediate management of all acute complications must follow an orderly Airway, Breathing and Circulation approach.

RESPIRATORY COMPLICATIONS

Hypoxaemia is best detected by a pulse oximeter or measurement of blood gases. Cyanosis is a late sign, particularly if the patient is anaemic. Furthermore, hypoxaemia is a late sign of hypoventilation if the patient is breathing additional oxygen.

Upper airway obstruction

Upper airway obstruction is diagnosed by:

- excessive abdominal movement and paradoxical movement of the chest wall (see-saw movement) and use of accessory muscles of inspiration;
- noisy breathing, especially inspiration (stridor), unless obstruction is complete when no sound is heard;
- progressive hypercapnia and hypoxaemia;
- during anaesthesia, reduced or absent movement of the reservoir bag, high airway pressure during intermittent positive-pressure ventilation (IPPV) and an absent or diminished capnograph trace.

Extreme negative intrathoracic pressures generated by upper airway obstruction may result in acute pulmonary oedema, which can be mistaken for aspiration.

Causes and management

Equipment faults

Causes include equipment faults such as misplacement, kinking or obstruction of a tracheal tube or connector. There have been several recent reports of connectors becoming blocked by small items of equipment such as caps for intravenous tubing. These should be stored separately.

Less common faults are absence of gas flow to the patient owing to empty cylinders, blockage within the machine itself and sticking valves.

Seeing a tracheal tube pass through the cords, auscultation and capnography confirm that a tube is correctly placed in the trachea.

If an apparatus fault is suspected it may be useful to remove all the anaesthetic apparatus, including the tracheal tube, and ventilate the lungs with a self-inflating bag while checking the apparatus.

Obstruction above the glottis

The lips and cheeks can fall back, especially in edentulous patients, and this is easily corrected by the use of an oro- or nasopharyngeal airway.

The tongue is held away from the posterior pharyngeal wall by the tone in the genioglossus muscles. The activity of these muscles is abolished by anaesthesia, and the tongue falls against the posterior pharyngeal wall ('swallowing the tongue'). It is remedied by extending the head at the atlanto-occipital joint (chin lift) and lifting the jaw up and forwards (jaw thrust), or by placing the patient in the lateral position. An oropharyngeal airway, laryngeal mask airway or even tracheal intubation may be needed.

Foreign bodies such as swabs, dislodged teeth, saliva, vomitus or blood must be removed, usually by suction or Magill's forceps. Very rarely, dislocation of the epiglottis or cysts or tumours of the epiglottis are encountered.

Obstruction at the glottis

Laryngeal spasm may result from intense surgical stimulation such as dilatation of the cervix or anus under insufficient anaesthesia. Briefly stopping surgical stimulation and giving oxygen while anaesthesia is deepened with either an intravenous or a volatile agent may be necessary. Occasionally intubation will be necessary to gain control of the airway. This is a powerful reason always to have suxamethonium readily available.

Incomplete reversal of muscle relaxants prevents cord abduction.

Impaction of the epiglottis into the larynx can be corrected under direct vision with a laryngoscope. Foreign bodies (see above).

'Can't ventilate, can't intubate'

Very rarely it may be impossible to ventilate an apnoeic patient or to pass a tracheal tube or other airway device. In these circumstances a 'can't ventilate, can't intubate'[2] protocol should be followed. This involves needle cricothyroidotomy with a narrow needle connected to a jet ventilator, or a surgical cricothyroidotomy. Commercially available cricothyroidotomy sets with an internal diameter greater than 4 mm can be connected directly to an anaesthetic circuit.

Lower airway obstruction

Lower airway obstruction (bronchospasm) is caused by:

- asthma;
- surgical stimulation, or airway stimulation such as intubation under light anaesthesia, or carinal stimulation by a tracheal tube that is too far down – all airway complications are commoner in smokers, and have also been shown to be commoner in children who are passive smokers at home;[3]
- drug reaction (see p. 356);
- aspiration;
- respiratory infection;
- pulmonary oedema;
- tension pneumothorax.

The underlying cause must be treated. Severe bronchospasm can be treated by increasing the inspired oxygen concentration while deepening anaesthesia. If drugs are required, use sympathomimetics such as inhaled salbutamol or intravenous aminophylline.

Atelectasis and infection

Atelectasis is collapse of dependent areas of the lung, and can be complicated by infection. It is caused by inadequate coughing due to pain, residual neuromuscular block or sedatives. The impairment of mucociliary transport in the lungs after inhalation of cold, dry gas mixtures may also play a part. It is most common after upper abdominal operations, and in obese patients, smokers, and those with pre-existing lung disease.

Atelectasis is diagnosed by:

- rapid breathing (30–60/min), with use of accessory muscles of respiration;
- tachycardia;
- hypoxaemia;
- restricted chest movements, quiet breath sounds, decreased resonance;
- radiographic shadows similar to those in bronchopneumonia.

Elevation of a hemidiaphragm is very common after upper abdominal operations, even in the absence of clinical signs.

Ventilation–perfusion mismatching causes hypoxia after general anaesthesia, even when respiratory function is normal. It is influenced by the site of operation, smoking, age, the presence of cardiorespiratory disease and obesity, and is readily treated by oxygen administration, which may have to be continued for some days.

When problems are anticipated, continuous epidural block or another regional technique is helpful. Arrange physiotherapy with appropriate use of analgesics. Prescribe antibiotics if infection is suspected.

Sleep apnoea

Sleep apnoea[4] is due to either airway obstruction or central respiratory depression (Ondine's curse). Obstructive sleep apnoea is much more common than central sleep apnoea. It is most common in the obese and those with airway abnormalities, including children with large adenoids and tonsils. If severe it can produce pulmonary hypertension.

Preoperative management

Those who are susceptible to sleep apnoea include those with a preoperative history of sleep apnoea, often with daytime sleepiness, and the obese snoring patient. Assess the airway carefully because difficult intubation is common. If previously undiagnosed refer for assessment of oxygen saturations at night and possible correction with nasal continuous positive airway pressure (CPAP).

Management during anaesthesia

Use regional techniques if at all possible, and avoid opiates and long-acting relaxants.

Postoperative management

Extubate with the patient wide awake and sitting up. Use regional techniques for analgesia. For a patient with significant sleep apnoea undergoing major surgery, there is a strong case for monitoring the oxygen saturation or blood gases in a high-dependency unit for several days, giving oxygen continuously, and considering the use of CPAP.

Pulmonary barotrauma and pneumothorax

Barotrauma[5] can occur if the alveoli are overinflated (perhaps better thought of as 'volutrauma'), especially if the lungs are at risk because of disease (especially emphysema) or trauma. The alveolar capillary membrane is disrupted and air enters the interstitial space, producing subcutaneous surgical emphysema, closed pneumothorax which is likely to develop into a tension pneumothorax, pneumomediastinum or gross hyperinflation of the lungs. Mediastinal emphysema shows on radiography as a small air space running parallel to the border of the heart. Management is by insertion of a chest drain.

Open pneumothorax can occur when the pleura is accidentally opened during operations such as cervical sympathectomy, rib resection and nephrectomy. The lungs should be inflated to expel air as the hole is closed. Pneumothorax can also occur as a complication of anaesthetic techniques such as intercostal and brachial plexus blocks or central venous line insertion.

CARDIOVASCULAR COMPLICATIONS

Myocardial ischaemia and infarction

See Chapter 1.2 for factors that predispose to cardiac risk during and after surgery. Myocardial ischaemia can be thought of as an imbalance between myocardial oxygen supply and demand.

Factors affecting oxygen supply are:

- coronary perfusion pressure – the difference between pressure in the aorta and that in the ventricles during diastole;
- oxygen content of arterial blood;
- coronary vascular resistance, especially the presence of atheroma;
- tachycardia, because this shortens diastole, when most coronary flow occurs.

Factors affecting oxygen demand are:

- heart rate;
- ventricular pressure during systole (afterload, can be taken as mean arterial pressure) and diastole (preload, taken as central venous pressure [CVP] or pulmonary artery [PA] wedge pressure);
- contractility, the amount of work done for a given pre- and afterload;
- muscle mass (e.g. left ventricular hypertrophy);
- episodes of ischaemia can occur in the absence of major haemodynamic change due to coronary artery spasm, microthrombosis, or coronary steal syndrome.

The aim is to consider the above factors and avoid changes that may precipitate ischaemia.

Tachycardia produces both a decrease in oxygen supply and an increase in demand.

Hypertension can cause an increase in demand that exceeds the reserve.

Hypotension is particularly dangerous in patients who have had coronary artery grafting or recent angioplasty because of the risk of graft or stent thrombosis.

The major sign of intraoperative ischaemia is a fall in the ST segment on the ECG. Newer monitors display ST segment trends. Arrhythmias may also occur.

There continues to be considerable interest in the use of perioperative β-blockade. A systematic review[6] suggests benefit in high-risk patients undergoing major non-cardiac surgery.

Hypotension

Hypotension may be due to a low cardiac output, a low peripheral vascular resistance or both. It is difficult to give a precise value for systolic pressure that requires treatment. The lower limit of cerebral autoregulation is at a mean pressure of 60 mmHg, but many patients have intercurrent disease, which may make this blood pressure dangerous. A pragmatic approach is to aim to keep the blood pressure within 20% of the patient's normal value. ST depression and ectopic beats suggest poor myocardial perfusion. In conscious patients undergoing regional anaesthesia, nausea and reduced consciousness are symptoms of hypotension.

Common causes of hypotension are as follows:

- hypovolaemia due to haemorrhage is the most serious and readily correctable cause of hypotension. Blood pressure may not fall in a fit young person until more than 30% of the circulating volume has been lost.[7] Blood loss may be concealed or difficult to measure;
- other causes of hypovolaemia, such as trauma, burns, dehydration and metabolic causes, are often obvious;
- mild drops in cardiac output and peripheral resistance are common owing to the effects of anaesthetic drugs, notably induction agents and inhalation agents, and often require no treatment. Blood pressure can drop precipitously in the elderly on induction of anaesthesia unless care is taken with dose and speed of administration of induction agents;
- intradural or extradural administration of local anaesthetics causes vasodilatation by sympathetic blockade, with a secondary reduction in cardiac output due to reduced venous return. High blocks, above T4, can also block the sympathetic nerve supply to the heart, reducing contractility and preventing reflex tachycardia. In obstetric patients the combination of aortocaval compression by the uterus coupled with neuraxial blockade can cause profound hypotension;
- in patients with cardiac disease, hypotension from any cause can reduce myocardial perfusion, leading to a drop in cardiac output and a further fall in blood pressure.

Hypertension in the immediate postoperative period

Possible causes of hypertension in the immediate postoperative period are:

- pain or full bladder (common);
- hypercapnia;

- confusion after anaesthesia, especially in the elderly;
- vasoconstriction after cardiopulmonary bypass and other vascular surgery;
- thyroid crisis (rare);
- unsuspected phaeochromocytoma (very rare).

The risks are mainly of extra myocardial oxygen demand. There is often an associated tachycardia, which will also impair coronary perfusion. These two factors may lead to myocardial ischaemia and even infarction. A history of hypertension should be taken into consideration when assessing postoperative blood pressure.

If an obvious cause cannot be treated, it may be useful to administer a vasodilator drug such as hydralazine 10 mg intravenously or nifedipine 10 mg sublingually with full monitoring and facilities to correct hypotension.

Cardiac arrhythmias

When trying to ascertain the cause of an arrhythmia, apart from intrinsic cardiac disease, it is useful to think in terms of the 'four Hs and four Ts' taught in advanced life support as causes of pulseless electrical activity at a cardiac arrest (see Ch. 2.9):

- hypoxia;
- hypovolaemia;
- hypo/hyperkalaemia;
- hypothermia;
- tension pneumothorax;
- tamponade
- toxic/therapeutic disturbance (including metabolic disorders);
- thromboembolism (including mechanical obstruction).

In anaesthetic practice hypoxia, hypovolaemia and electrolyte disturbances are the most commonly encountered, often in the context of a patient with existing cardiac disease. Often the only treatment required is correction of the precipitating factor. However, some situations may require more specific treatments, as follows:

- ventricular fibrillation and pulseless ventricular tachycardia require chest compression and rapid defibrillation (200–200–360 J). In the context of anaesthesia there is often a precipitating cause that also requires attention;
- ventricular tachycardia not only impairs cardiac output, but may proceed to ventricular fibrillation. If there are signs of haemodynamic decompensation treatment is with synchronised defibrillation

(100–200–360 J). If there are no signs of decompensation, amiodarone or lidocaine (lignocaine) are the initial treatments. Once again it is important to check for a precipitating cause;

- ssupraventricular tachycardia usually occurs in patients who have a history of paroxysmal tachycardia. Initially treat with vagal manoeuvres such as carotid sinus massage and adenosine (but take care with adenosine in Wolff–Parkinson–White syndrome). If there are signs of decompensation synchronised defibrillation (100–200–360 J) may be required. If there is no decompensation verapamil, esmolol, amiodarone or digoxin may be used;
- atrial fibrillation requires synchronised defibrillation (100–200–360 J) if there are signs of decompensation. If there is no decompensation, amiodarone or digoxin are the most commonly used drugs to control the ventricular rate;
- sinus tachycardia usually responds to correction of the common underlying causes: pain, light anaesthesia and hypovolaemia. If necessary a small dose of a β-blocker such as 1–2 mg metoprolol can be used;
- sinus or nodal bradycardia can be treated by a small dose of an anticholinergic agent such as atropine or glycopyrrolate;
- atrial ectopics and occasional ventricular ectopics are usually benign and require no specific treatment other than correction of any reversible cause.

Stroke

Stroke has an incidence of approximately 0.2% after general surgery in patients without known cerebrovascular disease.[8] It occurs typically from 2 to 10 days postoperatively. The choice of anaesthetic agent is probably of little importance. The causes are sometimes uncertain, but include:

- emboli when in atrial fibrillation;
- thrombosis due to hypotension;
- the hypercoagulable state that occurs after surgery;
- obstruction to a vertebral artery when the neck is rotated.

Air or gas embolism

If gas enters the venous circulation it accumulates in the right side of the heart and pulmonary artery. Since gas is compressible, blood is no longer ejected from the heart and cardiovascular collapse occurs. The volume of gas required is of the order of 0.5–1 mL/kg. If the gas enters the arterial side of the circulation through a potential right-to-left shunt such as a patent foramen ovale, paradoxical embolism occurs, which usually obstructs coronary or cerebral arteries.

Surgical causes

Air can enter the circulation if the site of operation is above the heart and atmospheric pressure exceeds the pressure in an open blood vessel (e.g. in operations involving veins in the neck, thorax, breast and pelvis (especially if the patient is tilted); operations on the brain and spinal cord in the sitting position, or operations on the heart). Carbon dioxide may enter the circulation during laparoscopy.

Anaesthetic causes

Air accidentally entering the circulation during intravenous techniques.

Diagnosis:

- an abrupt fall of the end-tidal carbon dioxide – usually the first sign, and precedes clinical signs;
- a hissing sound in the wound if air enters the veins in any quantity;
- a loud continuous precordial murmur, the so-called 'mill-wheel' murmur.

Clinical signs become evident only after a significant amount of gas has entered the circulation. There may be sudden cyanosis, hypotension, engorged neck veins, tachycardia, irregular gasping respiration, and cardiac arrest.

In situations where there is a significant risk (e.g. neurosurgical operations in the sitting position), a Doppler probe on the praecordium has been used as a sensitive early detector, although the output may be obscured by diathermy at the time of highest risk.

Treatment is as follows:

- prevent further entrance of air into the circulation by compressing veins to raise venous pressure. Tilt the patient so that the entry site is below the heart. Flood the wound with saline;
- place the patient on his or her left side so that bubbles are kept away from the pulmonary artery;
- give 100% oxygen and stop administration of nitrous oxide, which is much more soluble in blood than nitrogen and so will diffuse into the gas bubbles and increase their size.;
- if a CVP catheter is in place, aspirate directly from the right heart. If no CVP catheter is in place attempt to insert one while normal resuscitative procedures continue.

Thromboembolism

Thrombosis in the veins of the calf is common, but only likely to result in pulmonary embolism (PE) when it extends into the iliofemoral veins or if it originates in pelvic veins. Deep venous thrombosis (DVT) usually starts before, during or very soon after operation.

A PE most commonly occurs postoperatively, but can occur during an operation by the detachment of a venous clot in the leg following the application of an Esmarch bandage or a change in the patient's position. Postoperatively there is reduced fibrinolytic activity and increased platelet adhesiveness.

Regional techniques such as central neuraxial blockade improve blood flow and reduce the incidence of DVT, although it is not certain whether this results in a reduction in mortality due to pulmonary embolism.

Non-thrombotic emboli can occur from a fat embolus, a renal tumour or amniotic fluid in obstetric patients.

Risk factors are described in more detail in Chapter 1.1. In summary they are:

- age over 40 years;
- a previous history of DVT;
- immobilisation;
- oral contraceptives containing oestrogen;
- cancer;
- certain operations, including pelvic surgery, hip surgery and varicose veins;
- factor V Leiden mutation and similar conditions.

Presentation

The classic presentation of PE is the sudden onset of chest pain during the second postoperative week. In practice, symptoms of PE are very varied, and include unexplained fever, faintness, dyspnoea, substernal discomfort, pleural pain, haemoptysis and collapse. The onset may coincide with getting up or straining at stool.

Signs of DVT in the calf are those of inflammation – pain, especially on dorsiflexion of the foot (Homan's sign), tenderness, redness and swelling.

Signs of PE include tachycardia, hypotension, cyanosis, raised CVP, gallop rhythm, pleural rub and signs of consolidation.

ECG changes in PE are common, but are usually not specific (e.g. sinus tachycardia and ST segment changes). The major value of the ECG is to exclude other conditions such as myocardial infarction. Signs of right heart strain (S wave in lead I, Q-wave and T-wave inversion in lead III – S1, Q3, T_3) only occur with a massive PE.

The chest radiograph is usually normal, but may show linear shadows, effusion or pulmonary oligaemia if the embolus is large.

Arterial blood gases typically show hypoxaemia with a normal or low $P\text{CO}_2$ due to hyperventilation.

Because clinical symptoms, signs and basic investigations are not specific, other tests are sometimes performed. A ventilation–perfusion scan was the commonest method of imaging, but its place has been taken by multislice spiral computed tomography scanning.

Plasma D-dimer enzyme-linked immunosorbent assay (ELISA) detects fibrinolysis. This can be raised in other states such as chest infection and is difficult to interpret after recent surgery. Echocardiography can detect thrombus in the right side of the heart and pulmonary arteries.

Pulmonary angiography is seldom used because it is expensive, invasive, and carries a small mortality rate.

Treatment

Heparin is given as an intravenous loading dose of 5000 units followed by an infusion. Its main action is by binding to antithrombin III, the naturally occurring inhibitor of the coagulation cascade. Heparin binding accelerates the rate of action of antithrombin III and therefore inhibits fibrin formation. The activated partial thromboplastin time (APTT) should be checked after 6 hours and the infusion adjusted to maintain an APTT ratio of 2–2.5 times normal.

Low molecular weight heparin may be give in a full treatment dose of 1.5 mg/kg daily.

Warfarin takes several days to achieve its full effect and heparin is therefore continued for several days until the international normalised ratio (INR) is 2–3 times normal.

Thrombolysis is controversial. There is little evidence that it improves mortality and it carries a risk of haemorrhage, especially after recent surgery, including intracranial bleeding.

Pulmonary embolectomy can only be used with cardiopulmonary bypass and its application is very limited.

Prevention

Hospitals should have local guidelines to prevent PE (see Ch. 1.1 for risk assessment, Chapter 4.3 for a fuller discussion on central neuraxial blockade and anticoagulation, and Chapter 5.11 for the special problems of orthopaedic surgery). In general, preventive measures include:

- early ambulation;
- prevention of hypovolaemia by adequate fluid therapy;
- elevation of the legs during operation;
- intermittent pneumatic calf compression, replacing the normal muscle pump;
- elastic support stockings;
- a heel cushion on the operating table, preventing pressure on calf veins;
- stopping oral contraceptives that contain oestrogen 4 weeks before major surgery or surgery to the legs;

- heparinoids such as danaparoid and hirudins such as lepirudin for patients who develop thrombocytopenia in association with heparin;
- aspirin 75 mg daily;
- low-dose subcutaneous heparin;
- low-dose heparin and elastic support stockings (commonly used).

The rationale for low-dose heparin is that only small amounts of heparin are required to inhibit the clotting cascade in its early stages before coagulation is established.

Low molecular weight heparins are particularly used in orthopaedic surgery and have a long duration of action, so they only need to be given once daily. Extradural and intradural blocks should only be given 12 hours after the last prophylactic heparin injection because of the risk of haematoma and paraplegia. A convenient organisational approach to minimising this risk is to ensure that only low molecular weight heparins are used and that all injections are given in the evening.

NEUROLOGICAL COMPLICATIONS

Abnormal muscle movements and convulsions

Several types of abnormal muscular action may occur during anaesthesia:

- clonus, usually occurring in light anaesthesia and disappearing when anaesthesia is deepened;
- severe myoclonus (wrongly called shivering) after volatile agents – may be mistaken for a convulsion;
- involuntary muscle movements – occur with some induction agents (e.g. etomidate);
- true convulsions – can occur due to hypoxia, hypoglycaemia or local anaesthetic toxicity;
- increased activity on the EEG and epileptiform seizures were reported with the little-used agents enflurane and methohexital;
- propofol has been associated with convulsions, which can be delayed for hours or even days after anaesthesia;
- epilepsy;
- eclampsia.

Delayed recovery from anaesthesia

Delayed recovery from anaesthesia may be caused by:

- sedative drugs taken preoperatively;

- disturbances resulting from surgery (e.g. septicaemia, haemorrhage, fat embolism, air embolism, operative trauma in neurosurgery);
- disturbances resulting from anaesthesia (e.g. hypercapnia, hypoxic episode, electrolyte and acid–base disturbances, fainting (especially in the dental chair), induced hypotension, hypothermia);
- drugs used during operation in relative overdose (e.g. phenothiazines, opioids, thiopental, volatile agents);
- diseases (e.g. stroke, myocardial infarction, myxoedema, hypopituitarism, hypoglycaemia, hyperglycaemic coma, adrenal deficiency, uraemia, liver failure, undiagnosed brain tumour – all very rare).

Acute dystonic reactions

Dopamine is involved in the pathways controlling movement. By mechanisms that remain poorly understood drugs affecting dopamine, such as phenothiazines, butyrophenone derivatives such as haloperidol (droperidol was withdrawn in the UK because of concerns about cardiac toxicity of the oral formulation) and metoclopramide, can cause a variety of acute dystonic movement disorders. Akathisia is an uncontrolled restlessness; oculogyric crisis is a spectrum of blepharospasm, periorbital twitches and protracted staring episodes with a characteristic upward deviation of the eyes. These are more common in the young, especially girls and young women, and the elderly.

These conditions are not very common and their onset may be delayed. The key is recognising the reaction and withdrawing the offending drug. For acute dystonic states antimuscarinic drugs such as benzatropine (benztropine) 1–2 mg intravenously or procyclidine 5–10 mg intravenously are useful. Otherwise the reaction subsides within 24 hours of stopping the responsible drug.

Awareness during general anaesthesia

Awareness during anaesthesia is a spectrum which ranges from full consciousness of the surroundings, through awareness of pain, auditory awareness, subconscious awareness, to unconsciousness with some movement to strong stimuli:

- in conscious awareness without amnesia, pain is felt and conversations are overheard and remembered. Meaningful sounds are more easily remembered afterwards. Incidence of awareness with pain is about 1 in 10 000 elective general anaesthetics, but it is more common to have awareness without memory of pain.;
- conscious awareness with amnesia can be detected by the isolated arm technique. There is obedience to spoken commands during surgery, but this is not remembered as amnesia appears to develop very early as anaesthesia deepens;

- in subconscious awareness there may be purposeful limb movements but no response to spoken command. This is not usually remembered afterwards, but may be uncovered later by hypnosis (implicit memory). The extent to which subconscious awareness matters is not known.

Patients much more commonly remember sounds and other sensations during emergence from anaesthesia, whether in theatre or in recovery, and may mistakenly assume they occurred during surgery. If a patient complains of operative awareness some time later, listen, establish the facts, do not disbelieve what the patient says, and arrange suitable psychological counselling. It may be helpful to have a witness to your conversation. Make full notes.

The causes of awareness are:

- pharmacodynamic variability between patients;
- faulty technique (including one relying only on oxygen, nitrous oxide and opioids);
- faulty equipment (empty vaporiser, oxygen flush on, failure of nitrous oxide supply);
- justified administration of very light anaesthesia in a very sick patient.

Auditory awareness is the most common clinically, closely followed by awareness of intubation, when the intravenous induction agent is wearing off, yet before an adequate amount of inhalation agent has been taken up. Incautious derogatory comments are more likely to be registered and remembered.

Detection of awareness

Clinical detection

Look for movement and phonation in the unparalysed patient. In the paralysed patient look for sweating, reactive pupils, hypertension, tachycardia and lacrimation. These show a fairly poor correlation with purposeful responses to surgery, and the connection between cortical and autonomic function in a conscious patient is not well maintained during adequate anaesthesia. Changes in pulse rate and blood pressure are an unreliable guide to awareness. The 'isolated arm technique'[9] enables an otherwise paralysed patient to respond by squeezing the anaesthetist's hand if awareness develops. This has been useful in research, but not in routine clinical practice.

Electroencephalogram

See Chapter 2.2 for more detail. The raw EEG is transformed by Fourier analysis into a spectrum of power as a function of frequency. The median power frequency is reduced to 5 Hz by anaesthesia. Spectral edge frequency also shows reductions, but cannot accurately predict depth of anaesthesia.

The bispectral index (BIS) is probably the most promising index derived from the EEG.[10] This monitor displays a dimensionless number between 0 (deep unconsciousness) and 100 (wide awake). It has been used with some success during inhalation and during intravenous propofol anaesthesia. A BIS value of 40–60 indicates depth sufficient for surgical anaesthesia.

Evoked potentials

Evoked potentials may be auditory, visual or somatosensory. These show changes related to depth of anaesthesia, but are difficult to interpret reliably. They are affected differently by different anaesthetics. Auditory evoked potentials have shown most promise. Volatile agents affect the amplitudes and especially the latencies of the responses, but intravenous agents and opiates do so much less.[11]

Other techniques

Respiratory sinus arrhythmia diminishes with increasing depth of intravenous or inhalation anaesthesia, but the variability of response is great.

Frontalis electromyography shows a reduction of tonic activity with deepening anaesthesia, but has proved too unreliable for routine use.

Lower oesophageal contractions decrease in rate and pressure from several times a minute during consciousness to zero at about 2 minimum alveolar concentrations (MAC) of volatile anaesthesia, but are an unreliable sign of awareness.

Complications resulting from posture

Supine position

Pressure on and stretching of nerves of the arm, particularly the ulnar nerve at the elbow, must be avoided. The elbow should be padded and the forearm supinated, which provides more protection for the ulnar nerve. Legs should be flat on the table and not crossed. The Achilles tendon must not rest on the unpadded edge of the table. A soft pad, raising heels from the table, avoids pressure on the calf veins, and may lessen the incidence of DVT.

Backache is not infrequent after operations performed in the supine position in patients with lumbar lordosis. It can often be prevented by the use of an inflatable wedge as a lumbar support.

Changes of position of the head and neck

A patient with a decreased cardiac output or cerebrovascular disease is at risk of reduced cerebral blood flow if changes in position alter the relationships of the vertebral arteries to surrounding bony structures. This is possible on rotation of the head or hyperextension of the neck at the atlanto-occipital joint. This can be assessed preoperatively, when full neck extension may result in a faint. Patients with cervical pathology may have nerve symptoms following immobilisation from any cause, including surgery.

Trendelenburg position

The Trendelenburg is a head-down position and is generally well tolerated in anaesthetised patients breathing spontaneously. However, in obese patients or those with an abdominal mass, pressure on the diaphragm may reduce lung volumes considerably, and IPPV may be preferred. Cyanosis occurs in the face and neck of plethoric patients in this position owing to venous stasis, even with adequate ventilation. There is an increased risk of regurgitation.

To prevent pull on the brachial plexus, if the arm has to be abducted it should not be to greater than a right-angle, the elbow slightly flexed and pronated, and the head turned slightly to the side of the arm. The arm should not drop down below the plane of the body. It should not be necessary to use shoulder braces to support the patient.

The increase in CVP will cause a fall in cerebral perfusion, particularly if the patient is hypotensive. Prolonged head-down tilt can cause cerebral oedema and retinal detachment.

Prone position

A special mattress should be used so that pressure is completely removed from the abdomen and inferior vena cava (IVC) and breathing is not unduly interfered with. This prevents the extradural veins becoming unduly distended.

A cuffed, armoured tracheal tube may be wise to secure the airway, although some experienced anaesthetists use a laryngeal mask airway (or even a facemask) with success.

Skeletal injury readily occurs when turning the unconscious patient. Particular care should be taken when moving the arms that a shoulder is not dislocated.

Corneal abrasions are a particular risk. The eyes should be carefully protected with pads. Retinal arterial occlusion and blindness from pressure on the eye have been reported.

Lithotomy position

When putting a patient in the lithotomy position, both legs should be moved together to avoid strain on the pelvic ligaments. If the patient is arranged so that the anterior superior iliac spines are on a level with the break in the table, he or she will be in a good lithotomy position when the legs are supported on the stirrups. The knee should be outside any metal supports, to avoid pressure on the lateral popliteal nerves. If the hips are very flexed, sciatic nerve stretch may occur. Compartment syndrome has occurred after prolonged surgery (see Ch. 5.5 for more detail).

Lateral position

The lateral position impairs spontaneous respiration, especially if a bridge is also used. In the lateral position with an anaesthetised patient breathing spontaneously, more ventilation goes to the upper lung while more blood flow goes to the lower lung, thus causing ventilation–perfusion mismatch and impaired gas exchange. This is made worse by IPPV.

Care should be taken with the position of the arms to prevent nerve compression.

Moving the patient

The reflexes that maintain blood pressure are greatly reduced in an anaesthetised patient, who therefore reacts adversely to minor changes in body posture. This is particularly true if the patient is also hypovolaemic or under central neuraxial blockade. All movements should be smooth and gradual.

Nerve palsies

Nerve palsies are more common in patients with existing risk factors such as diabetes mellitus or multiple sclerosis, and in longer operations (more than 30 minutes). Nerves may be stretched or compressed as a result of positions that would be uncomfortable if the patient was conscious. Tourniquets can also cause problems if excessive pressure is applied over a nerve trunk. The cuff should be adequately wide and padded. The pressure for upper limb ischaemia need only exceed arterial blood pressure by 50 mmHg, and for the lower limb by 100 mmHg.

Patients with established or suspected damage should be referred to a neurologist for conduction studies to establish the site and degree of damage.

Nerves may be damaged as follows:

- aupraorbital nerve – can be compressed by the connector to a tracheal tube, causing forehead numbness;
- facial nerve – compressed between fingers and ascending ramus of mandible when holding a facemask, causing facial paralysis;
- brachial plexus – particularly at risk from stretching or compression in the Trendelenburg position, but also whenever an arm is abducted. The deltoid, biceps and brachialis are the muscles most commonly affected;
- radial nerve – stretched if the arm is allowed to sag over the side of the table or compressed by the use of a vertical screen support, causing wrist drop;
- ulnar nerve – damaged if the elbow is allowed to fall over the sharp edge of the table so that the nerve is compressed against the medial epicondyle of the humerus. If the elbow is extended, it is best to supinate the forearm to provide more protection to the nerve. Injury causes hypothenar weakness, and later 'claw hand'. It is a relatively common injury (1 in 2700), but can occur even if positioning appears to be perfect. Abnormalities of nerve conduction are often found in the other arm;

- median nerve – may be damaged as a result of intravenous injections in the antecubital fossa, from direct needle trauma or extravasation, causing an inability to oppose the thumb and little finger;
- pudendal nerve – can be compressed against a poorly padded perineal post during hip surgery with traction to the legs, so that the nerve is pressed against the ischial tuberosity, causing loss of perineal sensation and faecal incontinence;
- femoral nerve – use of a self-retaining retractor during lower abdominal surgery can result in loss of flexion of the hip and loss of extension of the knee with loss of sensation over the anterior thigh and anteromedial aspect of the calf;
- sciatic nerve – often damaged by intramuscular injections not given in the recommended upper and outer quadrant of the buttock. It may also be damaged in emaciated patients lying on a hard table with the opposite buttock elevated, as for hip surgery. Injury results in paralysis of the hamstrings and all the muscles below the knee, and sensory loss below the knee;
- saphenous nerve – compression between a lithotomy pole and the medial malleolus of the tibia when the leg is suspended lateral to the pole causes sensory loss along the medial border of the foot;
- lateral popliteal nerve – this is the most frequently damaged nerve in the lower limb – it can be compressed between the head of the fibula and a badly placed lithotomy pole, resulting in foot drop.

OTHER COMPLICATIONS OF ANAESTHESIA

Vomiting, regurgitation and aspiration

Vomiting and regurgitation involve the movement of gastric contents into the pharynx. Aspiration is the movement of those contents from the pharynx into the lungs.

Vomiting

Vomiting is an active reflex whose physiological function is the removal of toxins from the upper gastrointestinal tract, as follows:

- sensors are mechano- and chemoreceptors in the gut, including mechanoreceptors in the pharynx, and receptors in the chemoreceptor trigger zone (CTZ) in the area postrema in the caudal part of the fourth ventricle. The CTZ is outside the blood–brain barrier and has many different receptors – muscarinic, histamine, serotonin (5-HT), dopaminergic, μ, α_1 and α_2. There are also sensors in the vestibular system whose protective function is not clear;

- central coordination – through the vomiting centre, several discrete areas of the brainstem integrate respiratory, cardiovascular, somatic and autonomic nervous control;
- efferents produce an early wave of nausea, sympathetic activity and parasympathetic activity, including salivation. The proximal stomach then relaxes, and retrograde giant contraction waves move small bowel contents back into the stomach. Ejection is the movement of gastric contents into the pharynx and out of the mouth. During this phase there is apnoea and closure of the cords to protect the airway.

Vomiting can occur in very light anaesthesia, especially if the base of the tongue or pharynx is stimulated by an airway. Although the glottis closes during the expulsive phase, it soon relaxes, so that some aspiration of stomach contents into the bronchial tree is almost bound to happen in the supine patient if consciousness is impaired.

Regurgitation

Regurgitation is passive movement of gastric contents into the pharynx under the force of gravity. In the upright position a pressure of 40 cmH_2O is required to move gastric contents into the pharynx. When lying flat regurgitation is normally prevented by the barrier pressure between the stomach and lower oesophagus produced by the cardiac sphincter. This is a functional rather than discrete anatomical area at the gastro-oesophageal junction. Therefore regurgitation is made more likely by:

- anaesthesia, which itself reduces the barrier pressure;
- atropine, hyoscine or glycopyrronium;
- head-down position;
- increased gastric pressure (e.g. pregnancy, full stomach or bowel obstruction, gas from facemask ventilation, high intra-abdominal pressure during laparoscopy);
- incompetence of the cardiac sphincter (e.g. hiatus hernia, presence of a nasogastric tube).

Aspiration

Consequences

Food particles can physically block airways. Acid with a volume of greater than 25 mL and a pH below 2.5 is traditionally quoted as sufficient to cause lung damage. Acute chemical trauma to bronchial and alveolar epithelia results in acute exudative pneumonitis or Mendelson's syndrome.[12] Soon after aspiration the patient develops cyanosis, dyspnoea, bronchospasm, hypotension and tachycardia. There are crackles and wheezes in the lungs, and a characteristic radiographic appearance of irregular mottled densities. In severe cases acute pulmonary oedema causes rapid death.

Infection may develop and can be primary (although gastric contents are normally sterile) or secondary to lung injury. Foreign material gravitates into the dependent apex of the lower lobe (usually the right) with the patient lying supine, and into the dependent upper lobe with the patient on their side. These are the commonest sites of abscess formation. Clinical onset may be mild, after a latent period of 2–10 days, simulating early bronchopneumonia. The earliest radiographic sign is a patch of consolidation, and later a fluid level may be seen. An abscess is treated by postural drainage and antibiotics.

If aspiration occurs, the patient should be tilted head-down, turned on to one side and given oxygen and pharyngeal and tracheal suction. Bronchoscopy may be needed, and supportive treatment such as bronchodilators and physiotherapy. Corticosteroids are no longer given because they may increase the risk of secondary infection.

Prevention

There is no foolproof method of prevention, but the following are well-established practices:

- use a regional block technique, and allow the patient to remain awake with full protective reflexes. If general anaesthesia is needed, perform a fibreoptic awake intubation under topical airway analgesia. In any event, avoid heavy preoperative sedation, which may result in aspiration on the ward before or after operation;
- ensure an empty stomach by adequate preoperative starvation. Typically patients are fasted for 6 hours for solids and 3 hours for clear fluids. If a nasogastric tube is in place, use it to remove liquid from the stomach, but this will not remove solids. Metoclopramide 10 mg is prokinetic and may hasten gastric emptying;
- inhibit secretion of gastric acid by giving H_2 antagonists, such as ranitidine 150 mg orally the night before and on the morning of operation. Residual acidity can be neutralised by antacids, typically sodium citrate (15–30 mL of 0.33 M solution) immediately preoperatively. Efficacy may be improved by turning the patient to promote mixing;
- rapid sequence induction of anaesthesia – adequate pre-oxygenation (100% for at least 3 minutes), intravenous induction agent in a predetermined dose, followed by suxamethonium 1.0–1.5 mg/kg. If suxamethonium is contraindicated, rocuronium is an alternative. Cricoid pressure is used to prevent regurgitation by occluding the oesophagus between the cricoid cartilage and the sixth cervical vertebra, as recommended by Sellick.[13] It should be applied as the patient loses consciousness, using the tips of the first two fingers and thumb of an assistant to apply pressure on the cricoid cartilage. The

pressure required is 30 N (about 3 kg weight). It may be necessary to place the other hand behind the neck to steady it. This method must not be used during active vomiting because it may lead to oesophageal rupture. Cricoid pressure should ensure that the onset of unconsciousness, full muscular relaxation and the application of firm cricoid pressure occur simultaneously. It should not be released until the position of the tracheal tube has been confirmed and the cuff inflated;

- extubate when awake, with the patient in the lateral position, perhaps head-down, and leave in that position until airway reflexes have fully returned.

Postoperative nausea and vomiting

The overall incidence of postoperative nausea and vomiting (PONV) is usually quoted to be of the order of 25–30%, but this is an underestimate for some patient groups, such as those undergoing major gynaecological surgery. As well as being profoundly disliked by patients, vomiting may also harm skin flaps, the abdominal wall or other areas recently operated on, as well as raising the intraocular and intracranial pressure.

Causes

PONV may be central (from causes acting on the brainstem and higher centres), peripheral (from causes acting on the gut), or vestibular. It can be influenced by the following:

- patient factors – some patients are prone to PONV – those who suffer from travel sickness, women more than men, and the young (especially children) more than the old. Other important factors include suggestion and the example of surrounding patients. Smokers seem to suffer less PONV;
- anaesthetic factors – barbiturates, opioids, inhalation agents, nitrous oxide and hypoxia are all important contributors. Poor airway management and filling the stomach with gas make the situation worse;
- surgical factors – vomiting is more frequent after prolonged operations and after gynaecological, abdominal, eye, ear, throat and neurosurgery.

Treatment and prevention

Treatment and prevention include preventing the above factors, using regional techniques when possible, and using propofol rather than barbiturates. Consider antiemetics. Acupuncture may also be useful and is inexpensive, easy, and carries few hazards. The P6 (pericardium 6) acupuncture point is in the forearm, three fingerbreadths proximal to the proximal wrist crease, between the tendons of the palmaris longus and the flexor carpi radialis.

Many acute pain teams now use protocols to decide on the antiemetics for a given patient, use some drugs prophylactically and others for 'rescue' or treatment if PONV occurs. These protocols often involve scoring the patient's risk of PONV, for example using gender, smoking history, history of motion sickness or PONV, and the need for postoperative opioids.[14] When using combinations of drugs it is sensible to choose from different groups. The following groups are commonly used:

- phenothiazines – these act as dopamine antagonists in the chemoreceptor trigger zone (e.g. prochlorperazine 12.5 mg intramuscularly). They can cause acute dystonic reactions;
- antihistamines – cyclizine 50 mg intramuscularly; this can also be given slowly intravenously, but causes tachycardia and a slight drop in blood pressure;
- dopamine antagonists – metoclopramide 10 mg acts both centrally and peripherally. It speeds gastric emptying time and increases the tone of the lower oesophageal sphincter. It may cause acute dystonic reactions. Domperidone 30 mg rectally crosses the blood–brain barrier very slowly and so does not usually cause neurological or psychological side-effects;
- butyrophenone derivatives – droperidol is no longer available in the UK. Haloperidol is used in palliative care. It has a specific effect on the chemoreceptor trigger zone and may cause acute dystonic reactions;
- anticholinergic drugs – hyoscine 0.4 mg inhibits the muscarinic activity of acetylcholine on the gut and may also have a central action;
- serotonin (5-HT_3) antagonists – ondansetron 4–8 mg intramuscularly or intravenously at induction of anaesthesia or 16 mg orally 1 hour before anaesthesia is useful for high-risk patients. It is effective and potentiates other antiemetics. It is widely used in chemotherapy and radiotherapy but may be less effective in opioid-related PONV. It is relatively free of side-effects but expensive. Several alternative 5-HT_3 antagonists are available;
- corticosteroids– dexamethasone 4–8 mg is widely used.

Malignant hyperthermia

Malignant hyperthermia (MH) is a genetically determined condition (autosomal dominant) in which trigger agents, typically suxamethonium or volatile agents, cause an abnormal rise in intracellular calcium.

Suxamethonium is thought to cause a brief, marked rise in intracellular calcium and its effects are predominantly related to muscle damage (i.e. myoglobinuria and renal failure).

Inhalation agents cause a more sustained rise and their effects are predominantly metabolic owing to the effect of calcium on enzymes of the glycolytic pathway, with hypercapnia, hypoxia, hyperkalaemia and acidosis.

Many patients will be exposed to both types of trigger in the same anaesthetic. For unknown reasons patients do not necessarily react on every exposure to a trigger agent, so previous uneventful anaesthetics with suxamethonium and inhalation agents do not exclude MH.

Malignant hyperthermia is potentially fatal, and despite its name, the rise in temperature is a relatively late clinical sign.

Malignant hyperthermia is genetically heterogenous. Many patients have a genetically determined defect in the ryanodine receptor in the sarcoplasmic reticulum that opens to permit the outpouring of calcium into the cytoplasm, but the defect is not known in all patients. The incidence is about 1 in 15 000 patients.

If the condition is allowed to run its course unchecked it may ultimately lead to damage to mitochondria and the sarcolemma and become irreversible. The improvement in prognosis over the past decades is due to awareness of the condition, early detection by improved monitoring (particularly capnography) and early treatment, both with dantrolene and also with aggressive general supportive measures. The mortality rate in the UK from established MH is currently about 4%.

Presentation

Malignant hyperthermia presents with:

- masseter muscle spasm (see below);
- tachycardia and arrhythmias;
- rise in end-tidal carbon dioxide (often the first sign);
- tachypnoea if breathing spontaneously;
- unexpected changes in blood pressure;
- fall in oxygen saturation and cyanosis;
- rising temperature (late).

Repeated blood gases will show increasing hypoxaemia, rising $P\text{CO}_2$, increasing acidosis and rising serum potassium. Creatine kinase levels are an indicator of the degree of muscle damage. Disseminated intravascular coagulation can occur, usually late.

Treatment

Specific

Specific treatment is dantrolene 1 mg/kg intravenously, repeated as necessary every 5 minutes until the $P\text{CO}_2$ has started to fall, up to a cumulative maximum of 10 mg/kg. Dantrolene is difficult to dissolve and it is wise to assign one person just to this task.

Supportive

Stop the operation if possible. If it is not possible to stop the operation discontinue the use of volatile agents and continue with total intravenous anaesthesia. Cool the patient using ice packs to the axillae and groins, and chilled intravenous saline. Gastric, rectal and bladder lavage with iced saline have also been used. Give further dantrolene as required.

Admit the patient to intensive care, monitor and treat changes in pH (using sodium bicarbonate), potassium (with intravenous insulin and dextrose) and oxygen. Monitor renal function and use fluids to promote a diuresis to prevent myoglobin-induced renal failure. Dantrolene contains 3 g of mannitol per 20 mg ampoule. Monitor the clotting status.

Further treatment

Refer the patient to a MH unit for further investigation by muscle biopsy and in-vitro testing of susceptibility, in which fresh muscle is tested for contracture on exposure to halothane or caffeine. Family members will also need to be investigated.

Management if MH susceptibility is known or suspected

If MH susceptibility is known or suspected:

- avoid trigger agents (suxamethonium and all volatile agents);
- use total intravenous anaesthesia or regional anaesthesia;
- remove the vaporisers from the anaesthetic machine, flush with oxygen for 30 minutes to remove any traces of volatile agent, and use new anaesthetic tubing;
- monitor body temperature;
- have access to a supply of dantrolene – prophylactic treatment is not indicated.

Masseter muscle spasm

If a patient develops severe spasm after suxamethonium, lasting several minutes such that it is very difficult to open the mouth to intubate, there is a significant (about 20–30%) possibility that they may have a susceptibility to MH. Whether to stop the operation or not is a clinical judgement based on whether other signs of MH manifest themselves and the clinical urgency of the operation. It may be wise to avoid volatile agents and instead use total intravenous anaesthesia. Patients should be closely observed and their blood gases and creatine kinase checked. If there is sufficient clinical suspicion they should be referred to an MH unit for muscle biopsy and in-vitro testing.

Stress response

Surgery and trauma induces a neurohumoral 'stress response' with increased levels of catecholamines, antidiuretic hormone and gluco- and mineralocorticoids. This response can be blocked by the use of high-dose opioids and adequate extradural analgesia, but the benefits of doing so remain uncertain. More importantly, the stress response leads to water and, to a lesser extent, sodium retention, and a tendency to hyperglycaemia. This needs to be taken into account when considering postoperative fluid balance.

Accidental hypothermia

Hypothermia is defined as a core temperature of less than 36°C. Body temperature should be monitored during major or lengthy surgery. Heat loss may be prevented by increasing the environmental temperature, keeping the patient covered, the use of active warming blankets and mattresses, warming intravenous fluids, and warming and humidifying inspired gases.

Heat may be lost during anaesthesia by:

- radiation – the most important route of heat loss, and can account for up to 50% of loss; it is increased by uncovering parts of the body, low ambient temperature and the vasodilatation caused by many anaesthetic agents;
- convection – increased by frequent air changes in the operating theatre;
- conduction – due to cold inspired gases and intravenous fluids;
- evaporation – due to dry inspired gases and evaporation of sweat or body fluids.

In anaesthetised patients body temperature falls rapidly. Heat production falls and shivering and normal behavioural mechanisms to conserve heat are totally lost. Vasodilatation tends to occur, hypothalamic temperature regulatory centres are depressed, and in particular neonates and elderly patients cannot raise their metabolic rate to counteract heat loss. Long operations inevitably increase heat loss. Accidental hypothermia can also be secondary to conditions such as hypothyroidism, hypopituitarism, adrenal failure, drug overdose, near drowning, exposure, immobility and coma.

Physiological effects

Metabolism

Oxygen consumption is reduced by 6–7% for each 1°C drop in temperature. Liver and kidney function is depressed during hypothermia, so drugs must be given in small amounts. Renal blood flow, glomerular filtration and selective reabsorption are diminished. Below 30°C the kidney cannot concentrate urine. Glucose utilisation is depressed, and continued glucose administration may result in hyperglycaemia. Metabolism of substances such heparin, lactic acid and citrate is inhibited. Immune depression may lead to infection.

Cardiovascular system

Arrhythmias can occur at temperatures below 30°C, and spontaneous ventricular fibrillation below 28°C. There is a progressive bradycardia and fall in cardiac output and blood pressure. Stroke volume is little affected and coronary blood flow is well maintained. ECG changes include lengthening of the QRS complex, prolongation of the PR interval, elevation of the ST segment, T-wave depression and the appearance of a J wave (a small positive wave on the downstroke of the S which may appear at about 30°C). Blood viscosity is increased. Blood clotting is impaired, and the platelet count drops rapidly.

Respiratory system

The oxyhaemoglobin dissociation curve is shifted to the left so that liberation of oxygen to the tissues is hindered. More dissolved oxygen is carried in the plasma. Breathing is depressed.

Central nervous system

There is a reduction in cerebral blood flow, brain volume and intracranial pressure. Consciousness is usually lost between 28°C and 30°C. The MAC of volatile agents is reduced.

Acid–base balance

Respiratory acidosis occurs in spontaneously breathing patients because of hypoventilation. Metabolic acidosis occurs due to increased formation of lactic acid with the inadequate circulation, and decreased breakdown in the liver. Impaired renal function prevents correction of acidosis. Measurement of pH and $P\text{CO}_2$ are carried out at 37°C, so must be corrected for lower temperatures by entry of body temperature into the blood gas analyser. Base excess measurements require no temperature correction.

Electrolytes

There may be a rise in serum potassium. The cold heart is more sensitive to potassium, so small changes are of significance.

Neuromuscular block

Neuromuscular block is potentiated by hypothermia.

Adverse drug reactions during anaesthesia

Non-allergic reactions may be caused by:

- relative overdose (i.e. the known effects of a drug to a greater degree than anticipated in a susceptible patient, such as hypotension in an elderly patient after intravenous induction);
- intolerance of known side-effects (e.g. pruritus or nausea with opioids);

- rare but recognised side-effects (e.g. triggering of porphyria by barbiturates);
- wrong drug or diluent. This may be human error or systems error (e.g. drugs with similar packaging, ampoules replaced in the wrong box);
- drug interactions, either pharmaceutical, pharmacokinetic or pharmacodynamic – the common interactions are pharmacodynamic, relating to the effects of two drugs on the same body system (e.g. intravenous induction agents and volatile anaesthetics both decrease blood pressure).

Anaphylactic and anaphylactoid reactions

Clinically anaphylactic and anaphylactoid reactions manifest themselves identically and the management is identical.[15] They have a final common pathway – release of potent inflammatory mediators from mast cells. The distinction lies in the cellular mechanisms.

Anaphylactic reactions are a type I hypersensitivity reaction involving cross-linking of IgE antigen-specific antibodies causing degranulation of mast cells to release powerful mediators, including histamine, prostaglandins, leukotrienes and platelet-activating factor.

An anaphylactoid reaction is when the drug precipitates the release of these mediators directly without the involvement of IgE.

The incidence of anaphylactic and anaphylactoid reactions is of the order of 1 in 10 000 anaesthetics. The drugs responsible are most commonly neuromuscular blocking agents, latex and antibiotics, and less commonly colloids, induction agents and opioids. Anaphylactic reactions to local anaesthetics are very rare, and to inhalation agents unknown.

There is no reliable screening test for allergy to particular drugs, and therefore no method of predicting anaphylaxis in any particular patient.

Presentation

Reactions to intravenous drugs normally occur within minutes of exposure, even though the dose given may have been very small.

Latex allergy typically occurs 30–40 minutes after exposure. The commonest presentation of any reaction is cardiovascular collapse with some combination of bronchospasm and skin changes. However, cardiovascular collapse is the only feature in 10% of patients, and hypotension which is resistant to treatment should therefore arouse the suspicion of anaphylaxis. The severity of the reaction may be worse in patients with a reduced endogenous catecholamine response – those with asthma, those taking β-blockers and those with extra- or intradural blockade.

Immediate management

Immediate management of anaphylactic and anaphylactoid reactions is as follows:

- withdraw all likely responsible drugs and stop anaesthesia and surgery if possible;
- administer oxygen and ensure airway patency;
- elevate the legs if possible. Get help;
- give intravenous epinephrine (adrenaline) in a bolus dose of 50–100 μg (1 μg/kg), which can be repeated as needed up to 1 mg. Never give undiluted epinephrine (adrenaline) (1 in 1000) intravenously;
- rapidly infuse intravenous crystalloid or colloid (unless colloid is suspected as the cause), at least 2 L. Up to 25% of plasma volume may have been lost;
- consider the need for IPPV and further drug therapy: bronchodilators (aminophylline 250 mg slowly or salbutamol 250–500 μg), antihistamines (chlorphenamine [chlorpheniramine] 10–20 mg), corticosteroids (hydrocortisone 100–500 mg) and bicarbonate if there is an acidosis;
- beware of extubation if laryngeal oedema is present;
- epinephrine (adrenaline) is the mainstay of treatment. If intravenous access is not available, it may also be given intramuscularly (0.5–1.0 mg, or 0.5–1.0 mL of 1 in 1000), or intratracheal (10 mL of 1 in 10 000). The dose should be titrated against the response. Note that it may need to be continued by intravenous infusion after the immediate crisis.

Further management

Tryptase is released by mast cells and the concentration rises after anaphylactic and anaphylactoid reactions. A rise confirms the nature of the event, but not the causative agent. Take 10 mL blood samples in plain glass tubes immediately after the reaction, 1 hour later and 6–24 hours later. Separate serum and store at 4°C if the sample can be analysed within 48 hours or at –20°C if there may be a delay.

Refer the patient to an allergist at a regional allergy centre for skin prick tests to identify the causative agent. Specific IgE antibodies can be measured for a few drugs (suxamethonium and latex).

Write full clinical notes, and send a yellow card adverse drug reaction notification to the Committee on Safety of Medicines.

Explain the situation to the patient, and encourage him or her to carry a warning card and Medic-Alert bracelet.

Communicate the plan and any conclusions to the patient and their GP, and suggest safe drug combinations for future anaesthesia.

Prevention

There is no evidence to support the common practice of giving a small test dose before the main dose of an antibiotic. It is more sensible to separate the administration of antibiotics from the anaesthetic agents by several minutes. There is also no evidence to support the prophylactic use of antihistamines or corticosteroids.

A patient known to be sensitive to latex should be first on the operating list (latex particles persist in the air) and all equipment in contact with the patient must be latex free. This will include gloves, airways, tubes, breathing circuits, monitoring apparatus, and intravenous equipment.[16] Most modern equipment is latex free.

ELECTRICAL HAZARDS

Electrocution

Skin has a high resistance unless wet (hence the need for gel pads with defibrillators). The interior of the body is a relatively good conductor, particularly nerve and muscle.

A passage of several mA of electricity through the body may cause arrhythmias, skin and tissue damage including burns, and gross muscle contractions. The extent and type of damage depends on the path through the body, the duration and the current frequency. The frequency of the mains supply in the UK (50 Hz) is particularly likely to provoke ventricular fibrillation.

The basis of safety is to prevent the patient becoming part of an electrical circuit, achieved by either earthing equipment (class I), double insulating it (class II) or using batteries as the power supply. In addition, isolating transformers in the patient circuit protect against electrocution via earth. Microshock can be produced by electrolyte solutions in catheters near the heart when very small currents (50 μA) can cause arrhythmias. Any equipment used near the heart has to be designed to avoid this.

Surgical diathermy

Surgical diathermy uses a radiofrequency (about 3 MHz) alternating current (used continuously for cutting, and in 20 ms bursts at a lower frequency for coagulation) with the patient forming part of the circuit. This high frequency allows the use of the heating effect of electricity without affecting excitable tissue.

Diathermy has the potential to cause explosions or interfere with monitors and cardiac pacemakers. Poor contact of the earth plate with skin may cause burns. A broken earth plate lead may cause the patient to earth themselves to part of the operating table and thus acquire a burn. A sparking earth plate lead may ignite a spirit-based skin preparation. Unintended use, when the active electrode is touching the wrong part of the patient, or a surgeon or assistant may also cause a burn.

Bipolar diathermy, where the current just passes from one blade of a forceps to the other, is of limited power, but interferes least with monitors and pacemakers.

Fires and explosions

Fire or explosions require oxygen, fuel and an ignition source. Oxygen is in atmospheric air and anaesthetic pipelines and cylinders. Nitrous oxide also supports combustion and at high temperatures breaks down to liberate oxygen. Flammable anaesthetic agents are now of historical interest only.

Flammable substances include:

- alcohol-based skin preparation solutions, which can pool in skin creases and under drapes;
- paper surgical drapes;
- intestinal gases such as hydrogen and methane, which may be ignited by diathermy;
- hydrogen produced by diathermy applied to the bladder;
- tracheal tubes, ignited by diathermy in the mouth.

Sources of ignition include:

- heat from hot surfaces, wires or diathermy;
- electric current, either in normal use such as diathermy or monitors, or sparks from electric motors and switches, short circuits;
- static electricity produced by non-conductive materials such as artificial fibres, especially in a dry atmosphere;
- lasers in or near the airway – may ignite vapours or plastic equipment;
- spontaneous (e.g. when a rapid pressure rise heats up a gas, any oil or grease in contact with nitrous oxide or oxygen may ignite when a cylinder is opened) – lubricants must never be used, and cylinder valves opened slowly.

OPHTHALMOLOGICAL COMPLICATIONS

Corneal abrasions

Corneal abrasions are the most common ophthalmological complication of anaesthesia.[17] During anaesthesia protective reflexes are lost and tear production and tear film stability are reduced, which can lead to corneal epithelial drying. Chemical injury can result from any antiseptic except povidone–iodine 10% in aqueous solution. Antiseptic solutions not only damage the corneal epithelium, but if they contain detergents they can penetrate and cause damage to the iris, ciliary body, lens and blood vessels.

Direct trauma to the eye can occur at any time in the perioperative period from poorly fitting facemasks, watches, oximeter probes, staff or the patient's own fingers and surgical drapes. Prevention is by taping the eyelids closed and vigilance, particularly when the patient is moved. For longer operations some anaesthetists use occlusive dressings or instill viscous ointments or gels.

Ischaemic optic neuropathy

Blood flow to the eye, as for any organ, is determined by the perfusion pressure and resistance. The retinal circulation autoregulates to maintain flow across a range of pressures; however, flow to the posterior part of the optic nerve is not autoregulated and is therefore more vulnerable to ischaemia. Ischaemia can be caused by reduced perfusion pressure from low arterial pressure, elevated venous or intraocular pressure, or increased resistance to flow as seen in diabetes mellitus, hypertension and atherosclerosis.

High-risk procedures are bilateral radical neck dissection, spinal surgery and cardiopulmonary bypass. The risk in radical neck dissection is due to the disruption of venous plexuses and the rise in venous pressure. The prone position for spinal surgery elevates venous pressure, a degree of hypotension is often used to control bleeding from epidural veins, and there may be direct pressure on the eye. Eye pads should be used in the prone position.

Ischaemic optic neuropathy presents as painless visual loss after anaesthesia and surgery. The patient needs to be referred urgently to an ophthalmologist. The aims are to reduce optic nerve oedema with corticosteroids and diuretics and to maintain normal oxygenation by management of blood pressure and haemoglobin. The prospects of recovery are poor.

Central retinal artery occlusion

Central retinal artery occlusion is often caused by emboli and can occur together with ischaemic optic neuropathy. It presents with a painless visual defect, which may improve if treated promptly by an ophthalmologist.

TURP syndrome

Transient blindness can follow absorption of the inhibitory neurotransmitter glycine when used as an irrigant during transurethral resection of prostate (TURP) (see Ch. 5.16).

MINOR SEQUELAE

Minor sequelae are often the cause of considerable discomfort to the patient. They include trauma to lips, gums and teeth, sore throat, pharyngeal or laryngeal abrasions, superficial thrombophlebitis or simple bruising following intravenous injections, backache following supine or lithotomy position, nausea, and an occipital bald spot following pressure during prolonged surgery. Following minor surgery these can cause significant distress.

HAZARDS TO HOSPITAL STAFF

Pollution

Exposure to high levels of anaesthetic gases and vapours causes drowsiness. There has also been concern about the effects of chronic low-level exposure.

Nitrous oxide is teratogenic in experimental animals, and known to affect DNA synthesis through inhibition of methionine synthetase. The current consensus view is there is no significant risk to long-term health from chronic low levels of exposure. Even so, regulations exist in many countries to limit pollution by anaesthetic agents in the atmosphere of operating rooms, in the UK through COSHH (Control of Substances Hazardous to Health). Maximal suggested levels in different countries range from 2 to 50 ppm for volatile agents, and from 25 to 100 ppm for nitrous oxide. These values may be difficult to achieve in areas such as recovery, or if there are substantial leaks in breathing circuits.

Measures to reduce pollution include:

- adequate ventilation of operating theatres;
- disposal of waste gases to outside air – for active scavenging an appropriate device is essential to prevent negative pressure being transmitted to the patient circuit;
- the use of low-flow breathing circuits;
- use of total intravenous anaesthesia (TIVA) or regional analgesia combined with intravenous sedation if needed;
- careful filling of vaporisers with anti-spill devices at a time when few staff are present.

Radiation

X-rays are electromagnetic radiation produced when a beam of electrodes is accelerated from a cathode to strike an anode, and are used for imaging and in the treatment of cancer.

Unstable isotopes decay into different elements by nuclear fission. During this decay different sorts of radiation may be produced: α particles consisting of a helium nucleus (two protons and two neutrons), β particles (electrons), and γ-radiation (high-energy electromagnetic radiation, of shorter wavelength than X-rays). Radioactive isotopes are used in cancer treatment and γ-ray-emitting isotopes such as technetium-99m are used in imaging techniques.

All ionising radiation can cause tissue damage and chromosomal changes, and it is important to minimise the dose. Most protection comes from having safe procedures for safe handling of isotopes and arrangements to contain spillage.

For anaesthetists the hazard most commonly encountered is X-rays, particularly from image intensifiers in theatres. The intensity of X-rays declines as the square of distance from the source – staying well back is therefore a good starting point. Lead coats, impervious to X-rays, must be worn by all staff.

Magnetic resonance imaging

Magnetic resonance imaging does not produce ionising radiation, but presents hazards associated with the intense magnetic field, acoustic noise and difficulties in scavenging anaesthetic gases.[18] In particular ferromagnetic objects can become dangerous projectiles within the delimited area where the magnetic field strength exceeds 0.5 mT. Safety is ensured by only allowing unsupervised access to trained, authorised personnel.

Bloodborne viruses

Bloodborne viruses represent a potential hazard to staff. However, immune compromised patients are at great risk from infections and must be treated in the same way as other patients with immune deficiency.

Hepatitis A and E

Hepatitis A and E are commonly transmitted by the faecal–oral route. After an incubation period of a few weeks there is a prodromal illness, which leads to hepatocellular jaundice and resolves without chronic damage. There is a very small risk of infection with hepatitis A after transfusion, if the donor was in a viraemic phase.

Hepatitis B

Hepatitis B is a much more serious condition. Following infection there is usually an acute illness and 5–10% of patients will go on to develop a carrier state characterised by the presence of hepatitis B surface antigen in the circulation. The long-term consequences include chronic active hepatitis, cirrhosis and primary liver cancer. The presence of the 'e' antigen in blood is a marker of high levels of virus and increased risk of transmission. In the UK the prevalence of the carrier state is about 0.1%. The risk of infection after a needlestick injury is one in three for individuals who have not been immunised.

Hepatitis C

Hepatitis C virus was responsible for most non-A, non-B post-transfusion hepatitis. Blood is now screened for hepatitis C antibodies and the risk from transfusion is very low. Of those infected 40–85% will go on to develop chronic liver disease. The carrier state has a worldwide prevalence of about 1%, but less in the UK. The risk of infection after a needlestick injury is one in 30.

Human immunodeficiency virus

Patients with human immunodeficiency virus (HIV) may be completely well and unaware they carry the virus. The other end of the spectrum is full-blown acquired immune deficiency syndrome (AIDS) with immunocompromise and encephalopathy. The virus is delicate, easily destroyed, and has low infectivity. It can be transmitted by blood (needle-sharing drug users and haemophiliacs have been particular victims), sexual contact and transplacentally. Amniotic fluid, pericardial fluid and peritoneal fluid are also considered as carrying a risk of transmission, whereas faeces, nasal secretions, sputum, saliva, sweat, urine and vomit are not thought to present a risk for transmission. The risk of seroconversion following a needlestick injury is one in 300.

Prevention

Most patients with transmissible bloodborne viruses are asymptomatic and may not know they are carrying the infection. Screening all patients presenting for surgery is impractical, and even if carried out only for patients considered high risk would miss large numbers of patients and carry difficult ethical problems. The sensible solution is to regard all contact with patients as carrying a degree of risk and adopt universal precautions. In particular, every effort must be made to avoid needlestick injuries to oneself and others and observe the following:

- wear gloves during induction of anaesthesia and while inserting vascular cannulae, setting up infusions, and inserting and removing airways and tubes;
- where substantial spillage of blood is possible, wear a plastic apron, mask and eye protection;
- dispose of all needles directly into a sharps box. Never resheath needles;
- cover cuts and abrasions that might come into contact with body fluids;
- the hospital or theatre suite should have infection control policies and procedures in place for cleaning and sterilising equipment and the theatre environment;
- all medical staff should be immunised against hepatitis B;
- if a needlestick injury occurs, the puncture or wound should be encouraged to bleed by squeezing the area, then thoroughly washed with soap and water. Splashes into the eye should be washed immediately with sterile eye wash or clean water;

- all hospitals should have procedures in place for any victim of a sharps injury to receive prompt consultation with an appropriately trained physician to discuss further measures. These may include the use of antiviral drugs – the side-effects of some of these drugs make compliance difficult.

Back injury

Heavy lifting can predispose to mechanical low back pain and can even precipitate a prolapsed intervertebral disc. Hospitals should have policies and training in place for manual handling. Where possible aids (such as a 'Pat-slide') should be used to move patients.

References

1. Reason J. Human error: models and management. Br Med J 2000; 320:768–770.
2. Difficult Airway Society: Failed intubation and failed ventilation protocol. 2004. Online at http://www.das.uk.com/guidelines/cvci.html.
3. Skolnick ET, Vomvolakis MA, Buck KA, et al. Exposure to environmental tobacco smoke and the risk of adverse respiratory events in children receiving general anesthesia. Anesthesiology 1998; 88:1144–1153.
4. Loadsman JA, Hillman DR. Anaesthesia and sleep apnoea. Br J Anaesth 2001; 86:254–266.
5. Whitehead T, Slutsky AS. The pulmonary physician in critical care 7: ventilator induced lung injury. Thorax 2002; 57:635–642.
6. Auerbach AD, Goldman L. Beta blockers and reduction of cardiac events in non-cardiac surgery. JAMA 2002; 287:1435–1444.
7. American College of Surgeons Committee on Trauma. Advanced trauma life support manual for physicians. 7th edn. Chicago: ACS; 2003.
8. Kam PCA, Calcroft RM. Perioperative stroke in general surgical patients. Anaesthesia 1997; 52:879–883.
9. Tunstall ME. Detecting wakefulness during general anaesthesia for caesarian section. Br Med J 1977; 1:1321.
10. Johansen JW, Sebel PS. Development and clinical application of the electroencephalographic bispectrum monitoring. Anesthesiology 2000; 93:1336–1344.
11. Tooley MA, Stapleton CL Greenslade GL, Prys-Roberts C. The auditory evoked response during propofol and alfentanil anaesthesia. Br J Anaesth 2004; 92:25–32.
12. Mendelson CL. The aspiration of stomach contents into the lungs during obstetric anesthesia. Am J Obstet Gynecol 1946; 52:191.

13. Sellick BA. Cricoid pressure to control regurgitation of stomach contents during induction of anaesthesia Lancet 1961; 2:404–406.
14. Apfel CC, Creim CA, Haubitz I, et al. A risk score to predict the probability of postoperative vomiting in adults. Acta Anaesthesiol Scand 1998; 42:495–501.
15. Association of Anaesthetists of Great Britain and Ireland. Suspected anaphylactic reactions associated with anaesthesia – 3. London: AAGBI; 2003.
16. Dakin MJ, Yentis SM. Latex allergy: a strategy for management. Anaesthesia 1998; 53:774–781.
17. White E, Crosse MM. The aetiology and prevention of perioperative corneal abrasions. Anaesthesia 1998; 53:157–161.
18. Association of Anaesthetists of Great Britain and Ireland. Provision of anaesthetic services in magnetic resonance units. London: AAGBI; 2002.

Section 4

Regional anaesthesia

CHAPTER **4.1**

LOCAL ANAESTHETIC AGENTS

GENERAL CONSIDERATIONS

Local anaesthetics (LA) are drugs that reversibly block nerve conduction by blocking sodium and potassium ion channels in the nerve membrane. Increases in local anaesthetic concentration progressively inhibit the transmission of autonomic, sensory and motor impulses, resulting in sympathetic blockade, analgesia and anaesthesia.

The first local anaesthetic introduced into medical practice was cocaine, a naturally occurring ester of benzoic acid that is present in large amounts in the leaves of *Eythrwylon coca*, a tree growing in the Andes mountains. In 1850, an Austrian, von Scherzer, brought a sufficient quantum of coca leaves to Europe to permit the isolation of cocaine.

After discussions about the properties of cocaine with Sigmund Freud, in 1884 Koller performed the first clinical operation under local anaesthesia, by administration of cocaine on the eye. The use of cocaine for local and regional anaesthesia rapidly spread throughout Europe and America.

Halsted recognised the ability of injected cocaine to interrupt nerve conduction, leading to the introduction of peripheral nerve block and subarachnoid block (spinal) anaesthesia.

Awareness of the serious adverse effects of cocaine, including psychological dependence, led to the synthesis of another ester, procaine, introduced by Einhorn in 1905.

The first amide local anaesthetic, lidocaine (lignocaine), was synthesised by Lofgren in 1943 and remains the standard against which all other local anaesthetics are still compared.

Common to all local anaesthetics is their propensity for toxicity. With local anaesthetics, the relative difference between therapeutic plasma concentrations and life-threatening plasma concentrations is small compared to many other drugs. If given in sufficiently high dose, local anaesthetics may block excitable tissue such as brain and myocardium, leading to convulsions, cardiac arrest and death.

Clinical application of local anaesthetics for peripheral infiltration, nerve block or neuraxial block requires an understanding of nerve anatomy and physiology and the molecular site of action of local anaesthetics.

Nerve anatomy and physiology

Nerves allow long-distance conduction of electrical signals from the centra nervous system (CNS) to the periphery without loss of information Myelinated nerves are protected by the myelin sheath, which acts as ar insulator. Nerves consist of a cell body and an axon, which ends as a presy naptic terminal. The space between a presynaptic terminal and the cel body of another neuron is termed the synaptic cleft, across which pass neu rotransmitters such as acetylcholine or norepinephrine (noradrenaline).

Nerve fibres are classified as A, B and C according to their velocity of con duction.[1] A and B fibres are myelinated, whereas C fibres are unmyelinated

The largest A fibres are subdivided into alpha (α), beta (β), gamma (γ) anc delta (δ). Aα fibres supply skeletal muscle; Aβ fibres transmit tactile sen sation; Aγ fibres supply skeletal muscle spindles; and Aδ fibres transmi stabbing, acute pain.

Type C fibres transmit dull, aching pain from skin and viscera.

Within the myelinated A and B fibres are interruptions of the myelir sheath called nodes of Ranvier. Action potentials, carried distally down th nerve, pass from node to node rather than continuously down the nerve as in unmyelinated C fibres.

Two or three adjacent nodes must be affected to prevent conduction corresponding to a 6–10 mm segment of nerve fibre. Conduction betweer successive nodes allows higher transmission velocity and conservation o energy because fewer ions move across the nerve membrane.

At rest, an electrical potential of –70 mV exists on the outside of the nerv membrane. Impulse generation down a nerve alters membrane potential b rapid movement of sodium inwards and potassium outwards through dedi cated ion channels. Once the membrane potential rises to –55 mV an actior potential is generated which spikes to +40 mV – a change of over 100 mV Reversal of ion movement repolarises the nerve back to its resting state.

Molecular site of action

The structure of the nerve membrane is that of a bimolecular framework o phospholipid molecules associated with a globular protein channel pro truding through the lipid bilayer. The globular protein is a sodium or potas sium ion channel, which allows fast transmission of information betweer the intracellular and extracellular tissues.

Cryoelectron microscopy and image reconstruction have recently reveale the three-dimensional structure of the sodium channel (Fig. 4.1.1).[2,3] Viewe parallel to the membrane surface, the sodium-channel protein is bell-shape with four transmembrane domains arrayed symmetrically around a centra pore that splits into four passages that communicate between the intra- an extracellular spaces.[4]

The four homologous domains (I–IV) contain six transmembrane α-helice (S1–S6) and an inactivating particle connecting domains III and IV. Th

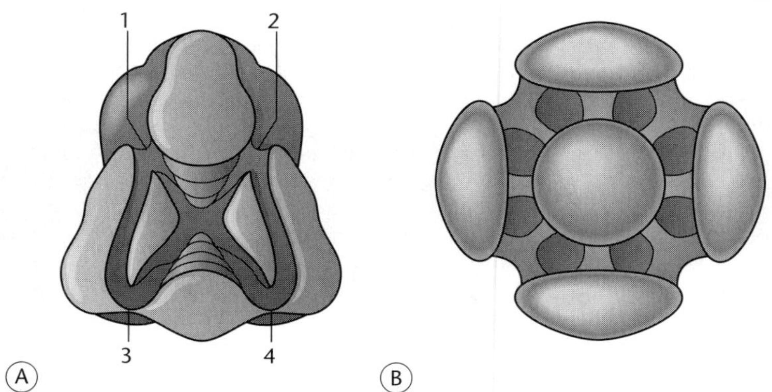

Figure 4.1.1 Three-dimensional representation of sodium channel. **A.** 1 & 2, central ion conducting pores. 3 & 4, gating pores, containing the S4 segments. **B.** View from below showing conducting pores.

S5 and S6 segments and the short loops between them form the pore (Fig. 4.1.2). The fourth helix (S4) has positively charged arginine or lysine residues at every third position and is regarded as the 'voltage-sensitive' region of the sodium channel. Parts of the local anaesthetic (LA) binding site are located in the pore-lining transmembrane segments 6 of domains I, III and IV (DI-S6, D3-S6, D4-S6). Residues L1280 in D3-S6 and N434 in DI-S6 interact directly with local anaesthetics and face each other in the ion-conducting pore.[5]

Three major conformational states of the sodium channel exist (i.e. resting, open, and inactivated).

In the resting state, the membrane potential is negative inside because of the presence of large concentrations of sodium ions outside the cell and a relatively large concentration of potassium ions inside the cell. The S4 segments are in the 'down' position, making the channel non-conductive. Outward movement and spiral rotation of the S4 segments through special, narrow-waisted pores in each domain, moves positive gating charges across the membrane's electric field and opens the ion channel.

Subsequent channel inactivation involves the closure of a hydrophobic inactivation gate or motif called IFMT (isoleucine, phenylalanine, methionine, threonine) between domains III and IV. The gate has little affinity for the mouth of the channel when all S4 segments are down. When they are in the up position, the affinity of the inactivating particle for the mouth increases and it docks in, inducing inactivation.

In contrast to voltage-gated sodium channels, potassium channels are a diverse family of membrane proteins with many subtypes, although their distribution in nerve cells is still not clear. They fulfil a number of roles in

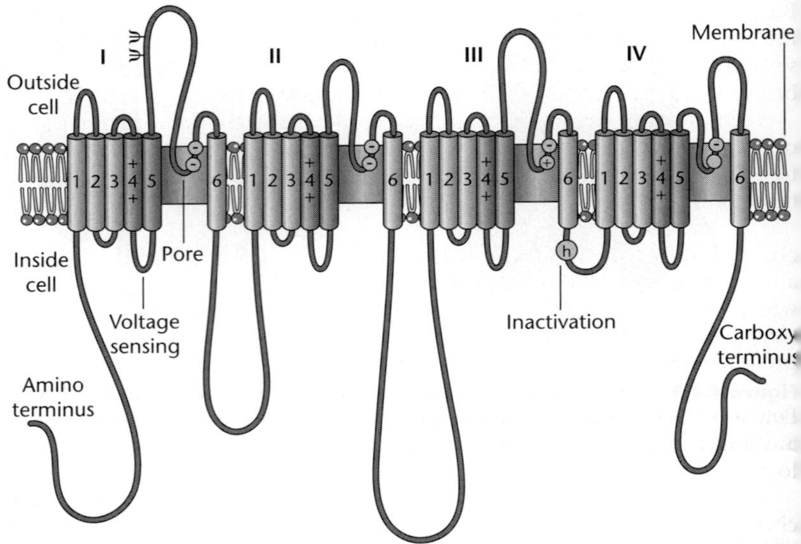

Figure 4.1.2 Schematic representation of sodium ion channel with domains I–IV and segments 1–6. Inactivation gate represented by 'h'.

peripheral nerves, such as establishing the resting membrane potential and accomplishing repolarisation.

Potassium channels[6] are configured to allow only potassium ions to pass through the cell membrane. Unlike sodium channels, the potassium channel only contains the equivalent of one domain that folds over. The pore presents a wide, nonpolar intracellular opening, and narrows on the extracellular side. This region of the pore acts as a 'selectivity filter' by allowing only the passage of potassium ions in single file across the cell membrane. As with sodium channels, the S4 transmembrane segment is the voltage sensor and the inactivation gate 'swings in', binds to the S4–S5 loop and blocks the channel.

Local anaesthetic mode of action

Local anaesthetics reversibly inhibit peripheral nerve conduction by blocking voltage-gated sodium and potassium channels on the internal nerve cell membrane. As the concentration of local anaesthetic increases the height of the action potential is reduced, the firing threshold is elevated, the spread of impulse conduction is slowed and the refractory period lengthened. Finally, nerve conduction is completely blocked

Binding to receptors is achieved by the ionised moiety of the anaesthetic molecule in a reversible and concentration-dependent manner. The binding sites of local anaesthetics at sodium receptors on domain IV, loop S6 have been recently discovered by molecular cloning studies.

The affinity of the sodium receptor for local anaesthetics is higher in the open or inactivated states than in the resting state. Binding of anaesthetics to open sodium channels increases with the frequency of nerve depolarisation and is described as use-dependent or phasic block.

Local anaesthetics that bind with more affinity to open or inactivated channels or that dissociate more slowly (such as bupivacaine) will generate a more potent block than local anaesthetics such as lidocaine (lignocaine), which dissociates four times faster. Consequently, bupivacaine accumulation during diastole is likely to delay recovery of cardiac sodium channels, prolong conduction and cause re-entry-induced arrhythmias.

Potassium channel blockade further enhances local anaesthetic blockade.[7] Potassium block broadens the action potential and encourages the open and inactivated sodium channel states, thereby enhancing the binding of local anaesthetic.

Electrophysiological differences exist between the nerve and heart ion channels.

Nerves undergo a very brief depolarisation owing to rapid flux of sodium ions and neural blockade, probably of resting state sodium channels at a potential of –70 to –80 mV, and need relatively high concentrations of bupivacaine for blockade.

In contrast, cardiac depolarisation lasts 200–400 ms, owing to an initial sodium flux followed by a longer-lasting influx of calcium that prolongs the duration of the action potential and produces a characteristic long plateau phase. As a result, blockade is produced by much lower drug concentrations binding frequently to more available and higher-affinity inactivated sodium channels. Thus, the heart is more susceptible to ion channel blockade from local anaesthetics than are peripheral nerves.

The minimum concentration (Cm) is the concentration of local anaesthetic that prevents transmission of electrical impulses. The Cm represents the balance between channel-bound and channel-released local anaesthetic such that the net sodium current is decreased below the firing threshold level. Each local anaesthetic has its own Cm.

Peripheral nerve fibres are differentially sensitive to local anaesthetics.[1] The principle that the smaller the fibre diameter the greater its blockade holds among the myelinated axons. The most susceptible are the Aγ spindle efferents and the Aδ nociceptive fibres. With myelinated fibres the length of exposed nerve and the number of nodes of Ranvier it contains are important. Preganglionic sympathetic nervous system B fibres are also easily blocked with low concentrations of local anaesthetics. However, the non-myelinated C fibres are generally less susceptible to block than the myelinated axons and, among themselves, the slowest and smallest conducting C fibres are the least sensitive.[1]

Differential sensitivity to local anaesthetics manifests clinically in two ways.

First, block height is higher according to the modality of testing – sympathetic > temperature (cold) > pain (pinprick) > proprioception (light touch with cotton wool).

Second, during operations under epidural anaesthesia, patients may experience paraesthesia to skin incision (Aδ) and motor block (Aγ), but still experience unpleasant pain (unmyelinated visceral C fibres) and sensation of movement (Aβ).

To minimise unpleasant sensations, studies have recommended that adequate anaesthesia for caesarean section should equate to a block height of at least T5 to light touch. Increased sensitivity to local anaesthetics is also found in pregnancy.

Recent evidence has highlighted the many diverse actions of local anaesthetics. Not only do they block sodium and potassium ion channels, but they also interact with G-coupled receptor proteins, muscarinic receptors and endothelial nitric oxide.

Attachment of local anaesthetics to G-coupled receptor proteins linked to lysophosphatilic acid[8,9] (LPA) attenuates neutrophil,[8] macrophage and monocyte function.

Lidocaine (lignocaine) has reduced surface expression of adhesion molecules on polymorphonucleocytes (PMN), reduced priming of PMN by cytokines, and reduced chemotaxis, lysozyme release and free radical production.

Epidural anaesthesia has been shown to preserve lymphocyte function after surgery by reducing natural killer cells and preserving B-cells and T-helper cells.[10] Effects on lymphocytes are protein lipase C- and protein kinase C-dependent and Gq-mediated. As yet, however, these interesting discoveries have not translated to clinical studies of the effect of local anaesthetics on the local inflammatory response to surgery.

Structure of local anaesthetics

Local anaesthetic drugs are water-soluble salts of lipid-soluble alkaloids. Each molecule is composed of a lipophilic aromatic ring connected to a hydrophilic amide by an intermediate chain (Fig. 4.1.3).

The lipophilic, aromatic ring aids the molecule's penetration through the perineurium and nerve cell membrane, where dissociation occurs into the ionic and the non-ionic forms of the tertiary amine.

Two types of intermediate chain exist – ester (–C–) and amide (–NCH–). Examples of esters are cocaine, procaine, chloroprocaine and tetracaine (amethocaine) and examples of amides are lidocaine (lignocaine), prilocaine, mepivacaine, etidocaine, bupivacaine, ropivacaine and levobupivacaine.

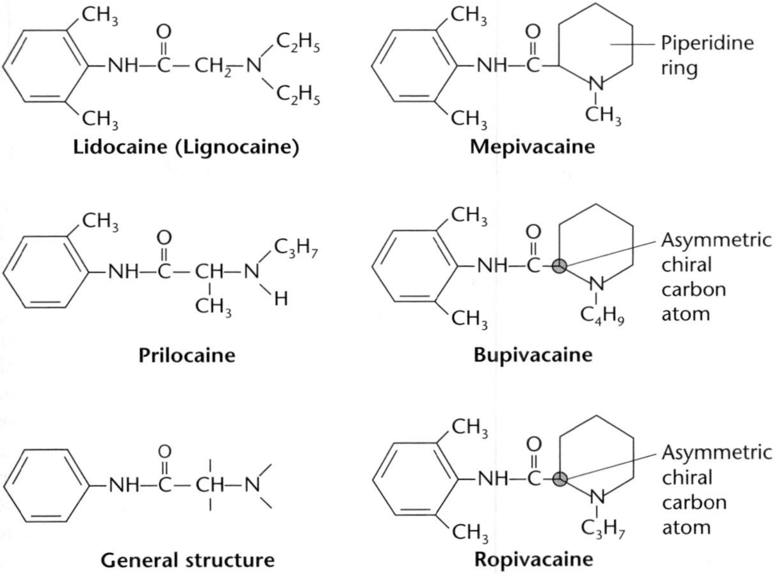

Lidocaine (Lignocaine)

Mepivacaine

Piperidine ring

Prilocaine

Bupivacaine

Asymmetric chiral carbon atom

General structure

Ropivacaine

Asymmetric chiral carbon atom

Figure 4.1.3 Structure of commonly used local anaesthetics.

Modification of the chemical structure of local anaesthetics alters the pharmacologic effect. For example, increasing the length of carbon chains attached to either the aromatic ring, amide linkage or the tertiary amine results in a molecule with a higher lipid solubility, potency and increased duration of action.

Replacement of the tertiary amine by a piperidine ring increases lipid solubility and duration of action; the addition of a butyl group in place of the amine on the benzene ring of procaine results in tetracaine (amethocaine); the addition of an ethyl group to lidocaine (lignocaine) on the α carbon of the amide link creates etidocaine; and the addition of a propyl group or butyl group to the amine end of mepivacaine results in ropivacaine or bupivacaine, respectively.

The greater the number of carbons and branching the greater the potency (and toxicity) up to three to four carbons. After this, the activity drops off, since the analogues are too lipid soluble.

Halogenation of the aromatic ring of procaine creates chlorprocaine, an ester with faster hydrolysis and shorter duration of action.

Bupivacaine exists in two forms called enantiomers, which are mirror images of each other. Although structurally identical, enantiomers can

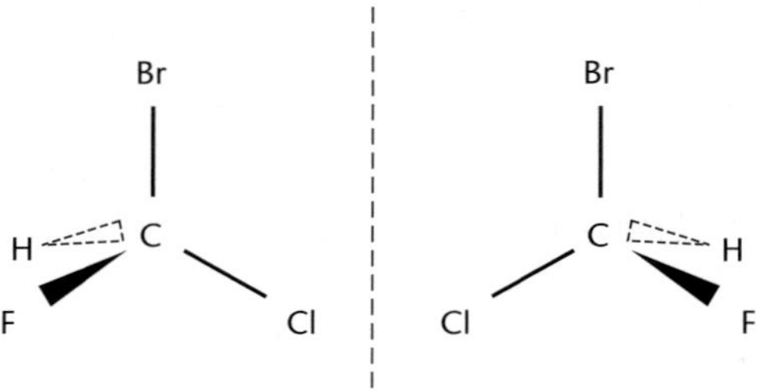

Figure 4.1.4 Schematic example of a chiral molecule.

exhibit pharmacodynamic and pharmacokinetic differences which manifest clinically as differences in potency or in side-effects. The discovery, 30 years ago, of a stereoselective blockade of cardiac sodium channels by the enantiomers of bupivacaine and advances in chiral chemistry created two new local anaesthetics – ropivacaine and levobupivacaine.

A chiral molecule has no internal plane of symmetry and is non-superimposable on its mirror image (Fig. 4.1.4). Even after rotating one of the molecules it remains different from its partner in the same way a right hand will not fit properly into a left-handed glove.

Enantiomers can be classified according to their ability to rotate the plane of polarised light through a polarimeter. This is described as optical activity. Right-handed or clockwise rotation is called dextrorotatory, 'D' or '+' and left-handed or counterclockwise rotation is called levorotatory, 'L', or '–'. A solution that contains a mixture of the two optical isomers will not change the plane of polarised light, because the effects of the two isomers cancel each other out.

The *S* and *R* descriptors are based on the configuration of the four asymmetrical groups around the central carbon atom (Fig. 4.1.5). An accurate description is determined by the following sequence rules:

- put the lowest priority towards the back by rotating the molecule;
- look at the direction of highest to lowest – if clockwise, then *R* (rectus), otherwise it is *S* (sinister).

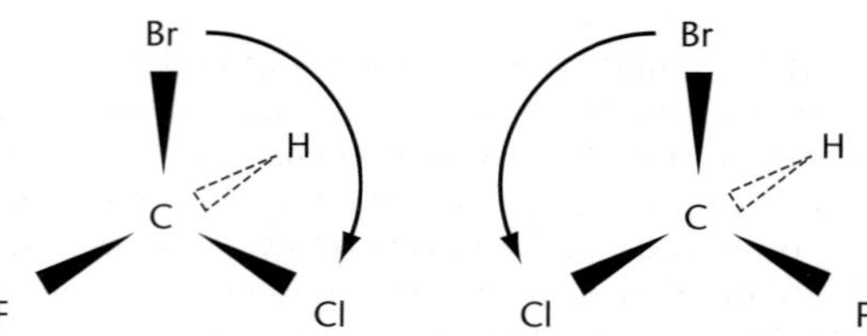

Figure 4.1.5 Sequence rules for chiral molecules.

Chirality	Spatial arrangement of atoms, non-superimposable on each other
Isomer	A molecular entity with the same atomic composition but different stereochemical formulae and hence different physical or chemical properties
Stereoisomers	Isomers that possess identical constitution, but which differ in the arrangement of their atoms in space
Enantiomers	One of a pair of molecular entities which are mirror images of each other and non-superimposable
Racemate	An equimolar mixture of a pair of enantiomers

Table 4.1.1 Chiral terminology

Bupivacaine exists in two forms called enantiomers, which are mirror images of each other. Although structurally identical, *stereoisomers* can exhibit pharmacodynamic and pharmacokinetic differences which manifest clinically as differences in potency or in side-effects. The discovery, 30 years ago, of a stereoselective blockade of cardiac sodium channels by the enantiomers of bupivacaine and advances in chiral chemistry created two new local anaesthetics – ropivacaine and levobupivacaine. Definitions of chiral terminology are given in Table 4.1.1.

For the purposes of this chapter *S*, L and levo (bupivacaine) and *R*, D and dextro (bupivacaine) are considered the same and are interchangeable.

In-vitro studies[11–15] have shown that both ropivacaine and levobupivacaine are less likely to dwell on myocardial sodium channels, have much less potency at potassium channels and are less likely to impair myocardial electrical conduction and contractility than bupivacaine. In-vivo animal studies[16–18] have shown increased convulsive, arrhythmogenic and lethality thresholds and improved resuscitation from cardiac arrest.[19] In a study comparing the effects of intracoronary injection of local anaesthetic in anaesthetised pigs,[20] ropivacaine induced the least QRS and QT widening, but there was no difference in the lethal dose between levobupivacaine and ropivacaine. Resuscitation of dogs after local anaesthetic-induced cardiovascular collapse[21] was better with ropivacaine (90% success) > levobupivacaine (70%) > bupivacaine (50%). The unbound plasma concentrations at collapse were larger for ropivacaine than for bupivacaine after resuscitation.

Human volunteer studies[22] have shown less decrement in myocardial contractility using thoracic bioimpedance monitoring and less propensity to arrhythmias. Acute tolerance of intravenous infusion of 10 mg/min of bupivacaine, ropivacaine[23,24] and levobupivacaine has been studied in five crossover, randomised, double-blind studies in volunteers previously acquainted with the CNS effects of lidocaine (lignocaine). Changes in conductivity and myocardial contractility were monitored using ECG (PR interval,

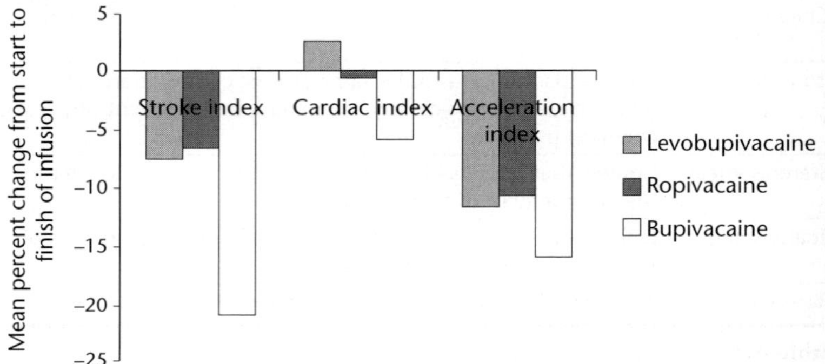

Figure 4.1.6 Mean cardiac indices during intravenous infusion of local anaesthetic. Results for levobupivacaine and ropivacaine taken from Stewart et al.[26] and for bupivacaine taken from Bardsley et al.[25]

QRS duration, QTc (time-corrected QT interval), QTd (QT dispersoin, i.e. difference between longest and shortest QT intervals)), echocardiography or thoracic bioimpedance. Bupivacaine impaired myocardial contractility, extended QRS duration and was less likely to be tolerated than ropivacaine. Using thoracic bioimpedance, levobupivacaine had significantly less effect on stroke index, acceleration index and ejection fraction.[25] In a further study of 22 volunteers, those who received over 75 mg of drug had significantly less QTc dispersion with levobupivacaine. Comparison of intravenous levobupivacaine and ropivacaine in volunteers[26] has shown no difference in cardiovascular parameters but fewer CNS symptoms in patients with levobupivacaine (Fig. 4.1.6).

Pharmacological properties of local anaesthetics

Speed of onset, duration, potency, speed of offset and motor sensory separation determine the clinical efficacy of local anaesthetics. Structurally, the benzene ring restricts the movement of the amide (hydrophilic) group to an axis perpendicular to that of the aromatic ring, helping direct it towards the sodium receptor. Substitutions on the ring or the tertiary amine portion of the local anaesthetic molecule alter p*K*a, lipid solubility and protein binding, determining respectively the speed of onset, potency and duration of action.

pKa

To pass through lipid-soluble membranes then attach to ion receptors on the internal nerve membrane, a drug is required to be both ionised and non-ionised.

The dissociation of local anaesthetics into their ionised and non-ionised modalities is determined by the pH of the solution in which they are dissolved. The pH at which the ionised and non-ionised form of a compound is present in equal amounts is defined as the p*K*a. For bases, such as local anaesthetics, the higher the p*K*a, the greater the ionised fraction in solution.

As diffusion across the nerve sheath and nerve membrane is related to the degree of non-ionised drug, local anaesthetics with low p*K*a have a fast onset of action and local anaesthetics with a high p*K*a have a slow onset of action. For example, lidocaine (lignocaine) (p*K*a 7.6) has a fast onset in comparison with bupivacaine (p*K*a 8.1), because at pH 7.4, 35 % of lidocaine (lignocaine) exists in the non-ionised base form compared to only 20% of bupivacaine.

Molecular weight

Molecular weight has an influence on the rate of nerve membrane and transdural transfer. The smaller the molecular weight the more rapid the transfer.

Lipid solubility

The lipid solubility of local anaesthetics is expressed as the partition coefficient, which is defined as the ratio of concentrations when local anaesthetic is dissolved in a mixture of a lipid and aqueous solvents. Thus, lipid solubility may also contribute to onset of action because local anaesthetics must diffuse through lipid-soluble membranes to reach their site of action.

Protein binding

Protein binding influences the duration of action of local anaesthesia, reflecting attachment to protein components of the nerve membrane. Protein binding parallels lipid solubility.

In plasma, amide local anaesthetics bind predominantly to α-acid glycoprotein (AAG), a high-affinity limited-capacity protein, and albumin, a low-affinity large-capacity protein. Thus, the free fraction or bioavailability of local anaesthetics is determined by the availablity of plasma proteins: the greater the AAG, the greater the binding of local anaesthetic and the lower the free plasma local concentrations. However, many patients have falls in plasma proteins after surgery, major trauma or malignancy. In these circumstances, the free plasma fraction of local anaesthetic would be expected to rise and increase the likelihood of toxic side-effects. Fortunately, after surgery, trauma or malignancy, AAG levels increase significantly and protect patients receiving local anaesthetic epidural or perineural infusions from anaesthetic toxicity by attenuating rises in the free fraction of local anaesthetics.

In the critically ill, however, hypoxia, hypercarbia and acidaemia all decrease protein binding, increasing free fraction and the risk of toxicity.

Neonates and children under 6 months of age have less protein binding of local anaesthetics.

Vasoactivity

Intrinsic vasodilator activity influences in-vivo potency and duration of action. For example, the enhanced vasodilatatory action of lidocaine (lignocaine) compared to that of bupivacaine results in greater vascular absorption and a shorter duration of action.

The newer local anaesthetics have less intrinsic vasoactivity than bupivacaine in the ratio: bupivacaine > levobupivacaine > ropivacaine.[27] All demonstrate a biphasic vasoactive response when measured in the forearm skin of human volunteers,[28] with vasodilatation at anaesthetic concentrations greater than or equal to 0.25% and vasoconstriction at less than 0.25%. Addition of epinephrine (adrenaline) (1 in 200 000 to 1 in 800 000) increases vasoconstriction. The cause of local anaesthetic vasodilatation is partially nitric oxide release.

Pharmacokinetics

Absorption

The site of injection, dosage, rate of injection, use of epinephrine (adrenaline), and the pharmacological characteristics of the drug influence the absorption of local anaesthetic from its site of injection into the systemic circulation. The order of peak plasma concentration after a single dose is intrapleural > intercostal[29] > lumbar epidural > brachial plexus > subcutaneous > sciatic > femoral.

All amides show a biphasic absorption pattern, with an initial rapid phase followed by a slow phase.

Following rapid entry of local anaesthetics into the venous circulation, pulmonary extraction limits the concentration of drug that reaches the systemic circulation for distribution to the coronary and cerebral circulations. For bupivacaine, this first-pass pulmonary extraction is dose dependent, suggesting that the uptake process rapidly becomes saturated. For lidocaine (lignocaine), 40% is removed by the lung during a single passage in pigs. The lungs act as a buffer, reducing the arterial plasma concentrations of local anaesthetic after inadvertent intravenous injection.

Distribution

The plasma concentration of local anaesthetic is determined by the relative rate of tissue distribution and clearance of the drug (Table 4.1.2). Tissue distribution is in proportion to the tissue:blood partition coefficient of the local anaesthetic and the mass and perfusion of the tissue.

The age, cardiovascular status and hepatic function of patients influence tissue blood flow.

Amide local anaesthetics are more widely distributed in tissues than ester local anaesthetics following systemic absorption.

	Molecular weight	pK_a	Protein binding (%)	Partition coefficient (lipid solubility)	Vd_{ss} (L)	$t_{1/2}$ (min)	Clearance (L/min)	Onset	Duration
Procaine	236	8.9	6	0.02	–	–	–	Fast	Short
Chloroprocaine	271	8.7	–	0.14	–	–	–	Fast	Short
Tetracaine (amethocaine)	264	8.5	76	4.1	–	–	–	Slow	Long
Prilocaine	220	7.9	55	0.9	–	–	33.8	Fast	Short
Etidocaine	276	7.7	94	141	1.9	156	17.4	Moderate	Long
Lidocaine (lignocaine)	234	7.9	64	2.9	1.3	96	12.6	Fast	Short
Mepivacaine	246	7.6	78	0.8	1.2	114	11.1	Fast	Short
Bupivacaine	288	8.1	95	28	1.0	210	8.3	Moderate	Long
Ropivacaine	274	8.1	94	8.7	0.8	111	10.3	Moderate	Long
Levobupivacaine	288	8.1	95.5	–	0.8	157	4.6	Moderate	Long

Table 4.1.2 Physicochemical characteristics of local anesthetics[30] Vd_{ss}, volume of distribution-steady state

Metabolism

Ester and amide local anaesthetics differ concerning metabolism and allergic potential.

The aminoesters are rapidly hydrolysed in plasma by pseudocholinesterase to the metabolite para-aminobenzoic acid (PABA), which is responsible for allergic reactions. Plasma half-life varies from less than 1 minute (chloroprocaine) to 8 minutes (tetracaine [amethocaine]) and is prolonged in the presence of atypical cholinesterase.

In contrast, enzymes in the liver degrade amides more slowly. The initial step is conversion of the amide base to aminocarboxylic acid and a cyclic aniline derivative. Complete metabolism usually involves additional steps, such as hydroxylation of the aniline moiety and *N*-dealkylation of the aminocarboxylic acid. As they are not metabolised to PABA, allergic reactions with these agents are extremely rare. Metabolism of amides is dependent on hepatic blood flow, decreasing with age, hypovolaemia and congestive heart failure. Drug interactions very few. Metabolism of amides may be reduced by potent inhibitors of cytochrome P450 isoenzymes. For example, CYP1A2 is inhibited by fluvoxamine and CYP3A4 by ketoconazole.

Cumulation and systemic toxicity of amides are more likely with prolonged infusions in elderly, sick patients, although the relative increase in AAG offers some protection.

Clearance

Clearance values and elimination half-times for amide local anaesthetics probably represent mainly hepatic metabolism because renal excretion of unchanged drug is minimal. Cumulation of metabolites may occur in renal failure. The rate of metabolism is fastest to slowest in the order prilocaine > lidocaine (lignocaine) = mepivacaine > bupivacaine = etidocaine. Poor water solubility of local anaesthetics limits renal excretion of unchanged drug. In heart failure, distribution and clearance of local anaesthetics are reduced.

Placental transfer

Protein binding determines the rate and degree of diffusion of local anaesthetics across the placenta. Bupivacaine, which is highly protein bound (about 95%), has an umbilical vein/maternal arterial ratio of 0.3 compared to lidocaine (lignocaine), which is less bound to protein (about 70%) and has a ratio of 0.52 to 0.71.

Ester local anaesthetics, because of their rapid hydrolysis, are not available to cross the placenta in significant amounts.

Acidosis in the fetus, as occurs during prolonged labour, can result in accumulation of local anaesthetic in the fetus by ion trapping.

Clinical preparation of local anaesthetics

Local anaesthetics are poorly soluble in water and therefore presented as stable hydrochloride salts with pH from 5 to 6. Alkaline pH destabilises local anaesthetics.

Local anaesthetics may also be administered as a carbonated solution (pH 6.5). Carbonated lidocaine (lignocaine) has a faster onset of action and a greater intensity of blockade than do hydrochloride solutions. Carbon dioxide diffuses into tissues, reducing pH and stimulating the conversion of local anaesthetic amide to the more active ammonium ion. An acidic tissue environment, such as occurs with infection, has the opposite effect to carbonation. Acidosis hinders the ionisation and efficacy of local anaesthetics.

Improving clinical efficacy

Epinephrine (adrenaline), in concentrations of 1 in 200 000 or 1 in 400 000 is sometimes added to local anaesthetics to reduce vascular absorption and potential local anaesthetic toxicity.[31] Preparation of 1 in 200 000 epinephrine (adrenaline) involves dilution of 0.1 mL of 1 in 1000 (0.1 mg) epinephrine (adrenaline) or 1 mL of 1 in 10 000 (0.1 mg) epinephrine (adrenaline) to a 20 mL volume of local anaesthetic; 1 in 400 000 dilutions are made with half the above doses of epinephrine (adrenaline).

Epinephrine (adrenaline)-containing solutions contain a reducing agent, sodium metabisulphite, to prevent oxidation of the epinephrine (adrenaline). In addition, a small amount of preservative and fungicide may be added.

The vasoactive effect of epinephrine (adrenaline) is greater with the more lipid-soluble amides. For example, the recommended dose of plain lidocaine (lignocaine) is 3 mg/kg but increases to 7 mg/kg with the addition of epinephrine (adrenaline). However, the addition of epinephrine (adrenaline) to bupivacaine increases the recommended dose from 2.5 mg/kg to 3 mg/kg.

Carbonated local anaesthetics are sometimes used to improve onset of the block. Free base is liberated quickly owing to rapid buffering and liberation of carbon dioxide, which diffuses across cell membranes. Thus the analgesic base is brought closer to nerve tissue more rapidly and in higher concentration, resulting in a more widespread and more intensive block.

Toxicity

CNS toxicity

CNS toxicity manifests initially as circumoral numbness, metallic taste, tinnitus, lightheadedness and dizziness followed by confusion, slurred speech and then convulsions. Increasing plasma levels lead to respiratory arrest.

Treatment consists of oxygen and intravenous injection of propofol to control convulsions. There is increasing evidence that lipid-based solutions reduce plasma levels of local anaesthetics.

Cardiovascular toxicity

Cardiovascular toxicity manifests as initial excitatory symptoms such as tachycardia and high blood pressure followed by myocardial suppression, peripheral vasodilatation, hypotension, bradycardia, conduction abnormalities, ventricular arrhythmias such as torsades de pointes, and finally cardiac arrest.

The treatment is give oxygen, intubate, ventilate, give intravenous fluids, epinephrine (adrenaline) and cardiac massage if necessary. Resuscitation after the longer-acting drugs bupivacaine and etidocaine may be difficult and lengthy.

Inadvertent intravascular injection of local anaesthetics, or frank overdosage and systemic absorption from the site of injection, can block sodium, potassium and calcium channels within conducting tissue such as in the CNS and cardiovascular system. Cardiovascular collapse, without prodromal CNS symptoms, in six pregnant women following inadvertent intravascular injection of bupivacaine or etidocaine was reported by Albright[32] in 1979.

At a meeting of the Food and Drugs Administration (FDA) in 1983, 53 cases of cardiac toxicity with bupivacaine were reported, 39 after epidural injection and 14 with other regional techniques. Twenty-seven patients received 0.75% bupivacaine. In all, 31 deaths were recorded (24 in pregnancy), three patients had a partial recovery and 19 made a full recovery. The medical response to these deaths was twofold. First, bupivacaine was highlighted as a potentially toxic drug (black boxed) and the 0.75% preparation was withdrawn from use in pregnant patients. Second, and most importantly, profound changes in anaesthetic practice occurred, such as slow incremental dosing and the use of test doses.

Incidence of toxicity

Changes in anaesthetic practice have undoubtedly reduced mortality rates, but have failed to eliminate toxicity.

A survey[33] of 25 697 patients undergoing brachial plexus, caudal or epidural block between 1985 and 1992 was the first to show that clinical toxicity was still a problem. The incidence of toxicity for each intervention was caudal (69/10 000), brachial plexus (20/10 000), epidural (1/10 000). Fortunately, no patient required epinephrine (adrenaline).

A larger survey[34] of 103 730 patients receiving regional anaesthesia, including 30 413 epidural anaesthetics and 21 278 peripheral nerve blocks, identified 23 patients with toxicity (Table 4.1.3), although none suffered a cardiac arrest. Convulsions are seven times more likely after limb block

	Neurological injury	Seizure	Cardiac arrest	Death
Spinal	24 (5.9)	0 (0)	26 (6.4)	6 (1.5)
Epidural	6 (2.0)	4 (1.3)	3 (1.0)	0 (0)
Peripheral block	4 (1.9)	16 (7.5)	3 (1.4)	1 (0.5)
Intravenous regional analgesia (IVRA)	0 (0)	3 (2.7)	0 (0)	0 (0)
Total	34 (3.3)	23 (2.2)	32 (3.1)	7 (0.9)

Table 4.1.3 Morbidity and mortality due to local anaesthetics (from Auroy et al.[34]). Number (rate per 10,000 local anaesthetic blocks).

(1 in 1400) than epidural block (1 in 10 000). Increased toxicity with limb blocks may be attributed to the proximity of nerve plexuses to major vessels and the need for high doses of local anaesthetics.

Of increasing concern is the toxicity of lidocaine (lignocaine) during ambulatory tumescent liposuction. Doses of lidocaine (lignocaine) up to 45–50 mg/kg have been administered for pain relief during plastic surgery. A typical regimen consists of 500–1000 mg lidocaine (lignocaine), 0.25–1 mg epinephrine (adrenaline) and 12.5 mmol sodium bicarbonate added to 1 L of crystalloid.

Two recent surveys have highlighted the problem. In the first, 95 deaths were identified from 496 245 lipoplasties (1 in 5224), and in the second, Rao et al.[35] identified five deaths in 48 527 patients in New York between 1993 and 1998 (1 in 9705). Three patients died due to hypotension and bradycardia, one patient died of fluid overload, and one died of deep venous thrombosis of calf veins with pulmonary thromboembolism.

The new local anaesthetics levobupivacaine and ropivacaine are undoubtedly safer than bupivacaine, but case reports of convulsions[36–39] and cardiac arrest[40,41] are emerging. In the clinical evaluation programmes for both ropivacaine and levobupivacaine, intravascular injection occurred with an incidence of approximately 1:500 to 1:600, despite all the procedures being undertaken in a controlled, elective setting by experts.[22]

The reasons for continuing toxicity are manifold: more limb operations are being conducted under regional anaesthesia, the new drugs are not sensitive enough as a test dose[42] compared to lidocaine (lignocaine), and there are increasing case reports of toxicity after administering dosages of local anaesthetics over twice the recommended limits (Table 4.1.4).

It must also be remembered that the mode of action of local anaesthetics is also the mode of toxicity – blockade of sodium and potassium ion channels – and that inadvertent intravascular injection can and will occur.

	Plain	With adrenaline (epinephrine)	Over 24 h
2-Chloroprocaine	800 mg	1000 mg	
Prilocaine	600 mg	600 mg	
Lidocaine (lignocaine)	300 mg	500 mg	
Mepivacaine	400 mg	500 mg	
Bupivacaine	175 mg	225 mg	400 mg
Levobupivacaine	150 mg		400 mg
Ropivacaine	225 mg		800 mg

Table 4.1.4 Maximum doses of local anaesthetics (from Tucker et al.[43]).

If given intravenously, in high enough doses, all local anaesthetics can have perilous consequences. The new drugs are safer – not safe – and clinical vigilance will always be necessary

Allergic reactions

Allergy reactions are rare and may take the form of bronchospasm, urticaria or angioneurotic oedema. They are well documented in association with the use of ester-linked agents, including contact dermatitis in personnel handling procaine. Allergy to amide-linked agents is extremely rare, but has been reported. Allergic reactions may be due to methylparaben, which is sometimes used in commercial preparations of local analgesic solutions as a stabilising agent.

Treatment of allergy reactions is with oxygen, injections of epinephrine (adrenaline) and hydrocortisone.

Reactions to vasoconstrictor drugs include pallor, anxiety, palpitations, tachycardia, hypertension and tachypnoea and may respond to a β-blocker. Care should be taken in patients receiving monoamine oxidase inhibitors or tricyclic antidepressants.

Children

In children, the above adult doses do not apply, but the dose can be calculated on a 'dose for weight' basis (e.g. the maximum dose for a 7 kg child would be one-tenth of the adult dose).

DRUGS USED IN LOCAL ANALGESIA

Cocaine

Cocaine is a naturally occurring plant extract. It is a derivative of the nitrogenous base ecgonine and an ester of benzoic acid. The alkaloid was isolated in 1855 and synthesised in 1924.

Cocaine was first used in surgery (of the cornea) in 1884. It is easily decomposed by heat sterilisation. Cocaine is soluble in water and alcohol and is an excellent surface analgesic and vasoconstrictor, 4% being a suitable strength. It is often toxic when injected.

Cocaine is also a dangerous drug of addiction. Its duration of effect is 20–30 minutes. Solutions should be protected from the light and the p*K*a is 8.7.

In the cortex, cocaine causes excitement and restlessness and mental powers are increased. There is euphoria, agitation, decreased sleep, anxiety, hyperexcitability, psychosis, paranoia, suicidal tendency, violence and confusion.

As cocaine is a powerful vasoconstrictor, epinephrine (adrenaline) added to it is not only unnecessary, but also increases the risks of cardiac arrhythmia and ventricular fibrillation. The two drugs should not be used together.

Cocaine inhibits monoamine oxidase and is not destroyed by cholinesterase.

Small doses of cocaine increase the pulse rate, raise the blood pressure and potentiate the effects of epinephrine (adrenaline) on capillaries (dilatation or constriction). Arrhythmias may occur, but can be reversed by β-blockade. Cutaneous vasoconstriction prevents heat loss. Hypertension and vasospasm may lead to vascular accidents.

Mydriasis occurs with cocaine, perhaps owing to sympathetic stimulation. There is blanching of the conjunctiva from vasoconstriction, clouding of the corneal epithelium and, rarely, ulceration, together with excellent analgesia. Cocaine is used as a 1% solution for analgesia. Eserine counteracts the mydriatic effect of cocaine and atropine increases it. Cocaine is now rarely used in ophthalmology.

There is some evidence that stronger solutions are absorbed less readily than weaker solutions, owing to the increased vasoconstriction they produce. In nose and throat surgery cocaine is used in 1% to 20% solution.

Cocaine can be employed usefully as a spray to vasoconstrict nasal mucosa before nasal intubation.

Cocaine is detoxified in the liver, one metabolite being ecognine, a CNS stimulant. About 10% is excreted by the kidneys unchanged. A safe dose of cocaine for surface analgesia is 2 mL of 4% solution.

Procaine

Procaine is *p*-amino-benzoyl-diethyl amino-ethanol hydrochloride and has a p*K*a of 8.9. It was the standard local analgesic agent until the advent of lidocaine (lignocaine). It was first synthesised in 1899.

For infiltration the strength of procaine used is 0.25–1% and for nerve block 1–2%.

Less than 5% of procaine is excreted unchanged in the urine. It is hydrolysed by serum cholinesterase to diethyl amino-ethanol and *p*-aminobenzoic acid is formed. Biotransformation requires absorption into the bloodstream because neural tissue and cerebrospinal fluid lack esterases.

Analgesia with procaine lasts 45–90 minutes when epinephrine (adrenaline) is added.

Procaine is relatively nontoxic. It has been recommended as the agent of choice for patients with a history of malignant hyperpyrexia. A concentration of 5% may be necessary for successful extradural block.

Chloroprocaine

Chloroprocaine has been in use in the US since 1952. It has a rapid onset of effect, but analgesia may disappear suddenly. Addition of a chlorine atom to the benzene ring of procaine to form chloroprocaine increases threefold the rate of hydrolysis by plasma cholinesterase. Rapid hydrolysis makes it relatively nontoxic and it is not easily transferred across the placenta. Its effect lasts about 45 minutes.

Chloroprocaine is used as a 2 or 3% solution and has a p*K*a of 8.7.

Maternal and neonatal plasma cholinesterase activity may be decreased up to 40% at term, but minimal placental passage of chloroprocaine confirms that even this reduced activity is adequate to hydrolyse most of the chloroprocaine absorbed from the maternal epidural space.[44]

The initial dose of chloroprocaine for an obstetric extradural block is 8–10 mL, which can be followed by bupivacaine or ropivacaine.

Chloroprocaine is the most acid of local analgesic agents commonly used (3% solution has a pH of 3.3). Paraplegia has been reported following its use, particularly after intradural injection, for which it is not recommended. This may be due to sodium metabisulphite in the commercial solution.

Tetracaine (amethocaine)

Tetracaine (amethocaine) was first synthesised in 1928. Like cocaine, it may cause cardiac asystole or ventricular fibrillation. It is used for topical and corneal analgesia in 0.5% solution. The solution should be protected from light. For infiltration the usual strength is 1:2000 to 1:4000, preferably with epinephrine (adrenaline). Up to 200 mL of 1:2000 solution with epinephrine (adrenaline) can safely be used for infiltration analgesia.

Tetracaine (amethocaine) is hydrolysed completely by serum cholinesterase but four times more slowly than procaine. None is found in bile or urine. It is used for intradural block.

The maximum dose of tetracaine (amethocaine) is 100 mg or 1.5 mg/kg of body weight. Large doses are unwise and the maximum for surface analgesia should be 8 mL of 0.5% solution in two or three divided doses, with an interval of 5 minutes between each dose. A lozenge containing

60 mg tetracaine (amethocaine) is available. Absorption from the bronchial tree, when analgesia for bronchoscopy is being induced, is almost as rapid as that following intravenous injection. A 4% gel is available for topical analgesia in children. Onset of cutaneous analgesia is rapid (≈30 minutes).

Tetracaine (amethocaine)'s effect lasts longer than that of procaine and lidocaine (lignocaine), roughly 1.5–3 hours. The onset of analgesia is slow. For intradural block, 0.5–1% solution may be used; for extradural block 0.25–0.5% with epinephrine (adrenaline). The addition of epinephrine (adrenaline) greatly reduces its toxicity, toxic signs being similar in appearance and treatment to those of cocaine.

Tetracaine (amethocaine) undergoes hydrolysis by plasma cholinesterase, but the rate is slower than for procaine, and renal elimination. Poor water solubility of local anaesthetics limits renal excretion of unchanged drug to usually less than 5% of the injected dose. Acidification of the urine facilitates renal elimination of the nonionised local anaesthetic fraction by converting it to the more water-soluble ionised fraction.

Lidocaine (lignocaine)

Lidocaine (lignocaine) is the most commonly used local analgesic agent. It is a tertiary amide and was first synthesised in 1943 in Sweden. It was first used by Gordh in 1948. Solutions are:

- 0.5% for infiltration, with epinephrine (adrenaline) 1:200 000 to 1:400 000;
- 4% for topical analgesia, in surgery of throat, larynx, pharynx etc.;
- for nerve block and extradural block 1.5–2% with epinephrine (adrenaline);
- for corneal analgesia 4% – this causes no mydriasis, vasoconstriction or cycloplegia;
- for urethral analgesia 1–2% in jelly;
- for tracheal tubes 5% as an ointment.

It is less toxic than bupivacaine, but cardiovascular and CNS symptoms of poisoning may occur.

The metabolism of lidocaine (lignocaine) is extensive, such that clearance of this local anaesthetic from the plasma parallels hepatic blood. The principal pathway of metabolism of lidocaine (lignocaine) is oxidative dealkylation in the liver to monoethylglycinexylidide, followed by hydrolysis of this metabolite to xylidide. Monoethylglycinexylidide has about 80% of the activity of lidocaine (lignocaine) for protecting against cardiac arrhythmias in an animal model. Xylidide has only about 10% of the cardiac antiarrhythmic activity of lidocaine (lignocaine). In humans, about 75% of xylidide is excreted in the urine as 4-hydroxy-2,6-dimethylaniline.

Accumulation of metabolites of lidocaine (lignocaine) is predictable in the presence of renal failure.

The metabolism and volume of distribution of lidocaine (lignocaine) are decreased in patients with cardiac failure and cirrhosis of the liver. In these patients, the plasma concentration of lidocaine (lignocaine) produced by a continuous intravenous infusion, as used to suppress cardiac arrhythmias, may be unexpectedly elevated, introducing an increased risk of systemic toxicity.

The clearance of lidocaine (lignocaine) is reduced in the presence of propranolol, with an increased risk of toxicity. As in the case of prilocaine, the metabolism of lidocaine (lignocaine) can give rise to the formation of methaemoglobin. It has a cerebral effect, causing drowsiness and amnesia. It is metabolised by oxidases and amidases from microsomes in the liver, but this is retarded in chronic liver disease.

It is excreted renally, hastened when the urine is acid.

Duration of effect of the 1% solution of lidocaine (lignocaine) is 1 hour; with epinephrine (adrenaline) it is 1.5–2 hours. The onset is rapid.

Lidocaine (lignocaine) has been given intravenously in 40 mg doses at 5-minute intervals, to potentiate the analgesia of the thiopental–gas–oxygen–relaxant combination, and also intramuscularly in 250 mg doses in 2% solution. Lidocaine has also been used in the treatment of status epilepticus, and because of its cell membrane-stabilising effect on cardiac tissue for ventricular arrhythmias, by intravenous injection.

The elimination half-time of lidocaine (lignocaine) is increased more than fivefold in patients with liver dysfunction compared to normal patients. Decreased hepatic metabolism of lidocaine (lignocaine) should also be anticipated when patients are anaesthetised with volatile anaesthetics. Likewise, drugs such as propranolol and norepinephrine (noradrenaline) may decrease hepatic blood flow and subsequent metabolism of lidocaine (lignocaine).

Mepivacaine

Mepivacaine was synthesised and first used in 1956. Its structure and pharmacologic properties resemble those of lidocaine (lignocaine), but its duration of action is somewhat longer. In contrast to lidocaine (lignocaine), mepivacaine lacks vasodilator activity. It is resistant to acid and alkaline hydrolysis. The p*K*a is 7.8 and 70% of the drug becomes protein bound (greater than in the case of lidocaine [lignocaine], but less than with bupivacaine). Most of the drug is metabolised in the liver and some has been recovered from the urine (increased by acidification). Unlike lidocaine (lignocaine), it is not metabolised by neonates; it is eliminated via the kidneys.

Mepivacaine is claimed to be a little less toxic than lidocaine (lignocaine) and its local analgesic effects last rather longer. When injected into the extradural space of patients in labour it passes rather rapidly into the fetal circulation, where it may cause harm. It would appear to have few advantages over lidocaine (lignocaine). A dose of 400 mg should not be exceeded (about 5 mg/kg body weight). Recommended doses for are extradural analgesia 15 mL of 2% or 20 mL of 1.5% solution and for intradural block 1–2 mL of 4% solution. It has anti-arrhythmic properties. The onset may be speeded by alkalinisation.

Bupivacaine

Bupivacaine is an aminoamide local anaesthetic. It is a member of the homologous series of *n*-alkyl substituted pipecholyl xylidines first synthesised by Ekenstam in 1957, and was used clinically in 1963. Debutylation of bupivacaine results in the production of a xylidide metabolite.[45] This metabolite undergoes further breakdown.

Bupivacaine causes more sensory than motor block. It is not recommended for intravenous regional analgesia because leakage past the tourniquet into the bloodstream may cause toxic or even fatal complications. The duration of effect is between 5 and 16 hours – it is one of the longest-acting local analgesics known. This may be more related to binding to nerve tissue than to its overall retention in the body. A small percentage of a given dose of bupivacaine is excreted unchanged in the urine. The remainder is metabolised in the liver. The *N*-dealkylated metabolite, pipecolxylidine, is found in the urine.

The maximal dose of bupivacaine is 2.5 mg/kg body weight (30–35 mL of 0.5% solution) and the strength used is 0.125–0.75% with or without epinephrine (adrenaline) 1:200 000 or 1:400 000; epinephrine (adrenaline) does not greatly prolong its effect, but reduces its toxicity.

Etidocaine

Etidocaine is a long-acting local anaesthetic which was first described in 1972. The onset of action is rapid and the duration of action is long (comparable to bupivacaine or ropivacaine). It is very lipid soluble and almost completely protein bound; its metabolic pathways are not yet determined. Less than 1% of etidocaine is excreted unchanged in the urine. It is probably retained in the body longer than other local analgesic drugs. It is less toxic than bupivacaine but more toxic than lidocaine (lignocaine), and is associated with motor block.

Etidocaine has been used in extradural block, but in obstetric analgesia has the disadvantage that motor block is readily produced. It has been used in 0.25 and 0.5% concentrations. The former may give inadequate analgesia, the latter inappropriate motor block. Concentrations of up to 15%

have been used with success in extradural block for surgical operations. The maximal dose is 4 mg/kg.

Etidocaine is a useful topical analgesic, similar to bupivacaine or ropivacaine and stronger than lidocaine (lignocaine).

Prilocaine

Prilocaine is a secondary amide and was first used clinically in 1959. It is less toxic than lidocaine (lignocaine), and metabolised in lung and kidneys as well as liver, and so has high clearance. Prilocaine is metabolised to ortho-toludine, which is an oxidising compound that converts haemoglobin to methaemoglobin. When the dose of prilocaine exceeds 600 mg there may be sufficient methaemoglobin present for the patient to appear cyanotic, and oxygen-carrying capacity is reduced. There is an associated shift of the oxygen dissociation curve of the remaining haemoglobin, which hinders oxygen liberation at tissue level. Methaemoglobin crosses the placenta. Methaemoglobinaemia is readily reversed by the intravenous administration of methylene blue 1–2 mg/kg, injected over 5 minutes. This therapeutic effect, however, is short-lived because methylene blue may be cleared before conversion of all the methaemoglobin to haemoglobin. A maximal safe dose is 600 mg.

Prilocaine is most useful when high dosage and strong concentration are required of a local analgesic drug, as when injection is into vascular areas (e.g. pudendal block and blocks about the face and neck), and for Bier's intravenous local analgesia in 0.5% solution, for which it is most suitable. For topical analgesia 10 mL of 4% solution is reasonable.

Prilocaine is no longer commercially available in the UK and parts of Europe.

Cinchocaine

Cinchocaine hydrochloride was first synthesised in 1925. It was used for many years for spinal analgesia (intradural), and also for infiltration and surface analgesia, but is no longer commercially available in the UK.

Ropivacaine

Ropivacaine[46] is a single *S*-enantiomer drug rather than a racemic mixture (as is bupivacaine), that is structurally similar to bupivacaine but with a propyl side chain replacing the butyl group. The smaller side chain contributes less lipid solubility, less toxicity and an increased separation of sensory and motor blockade compared to bupivacaine. Has differential effect on motor and sensory nerves at low concentrations. Most studies have found that onset and duration of sensory block in epidural analgesia are similar to those of bupivacaine, whereas motor block is slower in onset, shorter in duration and less intense with ropivacaine. In animal studies ropivacaine is less cardiodepressant, less arrhythmogenic and less toxic to the CNS than bupivacaine. These findings have been confirmed in human volunteers. The greater lipid solubility of bupivacaine compared to ropivacaine may explain the greater peak plasma concentration and the shorter half-life of ropivacaine. Plasma clearance is similar for both drugs. Peak blood levels are unaffected by the addition of epinephrine (adrenaline).

Ropivacaine has been used in many techniques (labour, hip replacement and varicose vein surgery) with good results. A dose of 225 mg should not be exceeded (about 3 mg/kg body weight).

Levobupivacaine

Levobupivacaine,[22] an enantiomer of bupivacaine, shares the same molecular structure as bupivacaine. The altered spatial arrangement of both levobupivacaine and bupivacaine accounts for differences in their pharmacokinetic and pharmacodynamic profiles, manifesting clinically as differences in efficacy and side-effects such as motor block. The physicochemical properties of levobupivacaine and ropivacaine are compared in Table 4.1.2 to those of bupivacaine and other commonly used local anaesthetics.

FUTURE LOCAL ANAESTHETICS

Slow-release formulations of bupivacaine

Prolonged excellent postoperative analgesia can be achieved by continuous or repeated administration of slow-release formulations of bupivacaine via indwelling catheters for regional, epidural or spinal anaesthesia. However, complications associated with catheterisation are not uncommon and include leakage, intravascular injection, catheter migration and infection.

Long-acting anaesthetic placed accurately has the potential to provide longlasting pain relief and eliminate technical problems and possibly to prevent or reverse hyperalgesia.[47] Strategies in the search for prolonged postoperative analgesic have focused on drug delivery systems for slow release of local anaesthetics held in liposomes and microspheres.

Liposomes are amphipathic lipid molecules with a polar head and two hydrophobic hydrocarbon tails which form lipid bilayers not unlike a cell membrane when suspended in an aqueous solution. Liposomal function is dictated by size, structure and composition. Possession of both aqueous and lipid environments enables both water- and lipid-soluble drugs to be carried. The likelihood of tissue toxicity being induced by liposome constituents is low because they are biodegradable.[48] However, much research requires to be done to ensure that the preparation stays at the site of action, delivers a predictable concentration of drug over a prolonged period of time and produces adequate sensory block without motor block or toxicity.

Polymer microspheres

Biodegradable polylactic and lactic–glycolic acid polymers are widely used in drug delivery of implantable contraceptives and sutures. Polylactic-co-glycolic acid (PLGA) is a random copolymer polymerised from lactic and glycolic acids. The ratios 75/25, 65/35 and 50/50 refer to the molar ratios of lactic to glycolic acid repeating units.

Previous clinical uses of microspheres have applied mainly to high-potency drugs which require the release of micrograms per day and which therefore have drug/polymer weight ratios less than 10–12%. Local anaesthetics are comparatively low potency and require several mg per hour to maintain nerve blockade. Thus, to make clinically useful microspheres with local anaesthetics, it has become necessary to develop microsphere formulations with previously unattainably high drug loadings – that is, 50–75% drug to polymer, weight to weight ratio.

In the most-studied formulation, 65/35 PLGA, roughly 20% of the bupivacaine was released in the first 24 hours, and approximately 7% released daily thereafter up to approximately day 10. Even with doses of 600 mg/kg, more than 30–150 times the convulsant dose for aqueous bupivacaine hydrochloride, toxicity was not seen. Incorporation of dexamethasone into bupivacaine microspheres has prolonged blockade by eight to 13 times compared to bupivacaine microspheres alone.[49,50] This would appear to be a local and not a systemic effect of dexamethasone because injections at other remote sites have no effect on the duration of blockade.

Tricyclic antidepressants

The tricyclic antidepressant amitriptyline has analgesic properties in patients with neuropathic pain, probably due to antagonism of *N*-methyl-D-aspartate (NMDA).[51] Amitriptyline is also a potent sodium channel blocker. Recent studies using amitriptyline for peripheral nerve blockade in rats have shown amitriptyline to be less toxic[52] and a more potent blocker[53] of neuronal sodium channels than bupivacaine. A quaternary ammonium derivative, *N*-phenylethyl amitriptyline,[53,54] was also found to be a highly potent sodium channel blocker in vitro and its potency was estimated to be eight times higher than that of the parent drug. Both amitriptyline and *N*-phenylethyl amitriptyline show greater differential blockade in sheep than in rats. This differential blockade in sheep is greater than that produced by lidocaine (lignocaine) or bupivacaine.[55]

Tetrodotoxin

Voltage-gated sodium channels are the molecular targets for a broad range of neurotoxins that act at six or more receptor sites on the channel protein. These toxins fall into three groups according to their site of action – block the pore or alter voltage-dependent gating of sodium channels through binding to intramembranous or extracellular receptor sites.

Tetrodotoxin is a poison found in puffer fish (fugu) and acts by selectively blocking sodium channels at a site and by an action that differs from that of lidocaine (lignocaine). Despite these desirable characteristics, tetrodotoxin has not achieved clinical use as a local anaesthetic because of its perceived systemic toxicity culminating in diaphragmatic paralysis leading to respiratory arrest and death.

In light of the discovery that tetrodotoxin does not cause local neurotoxicity and the lack of enduring CNS or cardiac sequelae (unlike bupivacaine), tetrodotoxin has been investigated as a potential longlasting local anaesthetic.

Tetrodotoxin, when given into a single limb in rats, has a profound systemic effect. The addition of epinephrine (adrenaline) to tetrodotoxin[56] prevented systemic spread and increased the duration of tetrodotoxin-induced nerve blockade compared to bupivacaine alone. Addition of bupivacaine to tetrodotoxin also increased the duration of block. However, no additional benefit was obtained by all three drugs in combination, suggesting that bupivacaine and epinephrine (adrenaline) act via the same mechanism. Bupivacaine possesses vasoconstrictive properties at concentrations of 0.25% and less and, like epinephrine (adrenaline), slows the resorption of tetrodotoxin from the site of injection. All these blocks were achieved with no deaths or signs of respiratory distress or systemic toxicity as indicated by contralateral limb dysfunction.

Capsaicin

Evidence from animal models and studies of human sensory nerves demonstrates that tetrodotoxin-resistant sodium channels are found primarily in small-diameter nociceptor afferent neurons and play an important role in pain conduction and chronic pain. Capsaicin, the pungent ingredient in chilli peppers, is a vanilloid with noxious and analgesic effects that inhibits tetrodotoxin-resistant sodium currents. Sciatic nerve block with capsaicin[57] in male Sprague–Dawley rats produced selective anaesthesia with an increase in thermal latency but no effect on motor strength. The combination of capsaicin and tetrodotoxin was synergistic, prolonging both nociceptive and motor block, with the effect of capsaicin being reversed by the vanilloid antagonist capsazepine. Similar interactions were found between tetrodotoxin and resiniferatoxin (another vanilloid), but much less so between bupivacaine and capsaicin.

References

1. Gokin AP, Philip B, Strichartz GR. Preferential block of small myelinated sensory and motor fibers by lidocaine: in vivo electrophysiology in the rat sciatic nerve. Anesthesiology 2001; 95:1441–1454.

2. Catterall WA. Molecular mechanisms of gating and drug block of sodium channels. Novartis Found Symp 2002; 241:206–218; discussion 218–232.
3. Catterall WA. A 3D view of sodium channels. Nature 2001; 409:988–989, 991.
4. Sato C, Ueno Y, Asai K, et al. The voltage-sensitive sodium channel is a bell-shaped molecule with several cavities. Nature 2001; 409:1047–1051.
5. Nau C, Wang SY, Wang GK. Point mutations at L1280 in Nav1.4 channel D3-S6 modulate binding affinity and stereoselectivity of bupivacaine enantiomers. Mol Pharmacol 2003; 63:1398–1406.
6. Doyle DA, Morais Cabral J, Pfuetzner RA, et al. The structure of the potassium channel: molecular basis of K+ conduction and selectivity. Science 1998; 280:69–77.
7. Valenzuela C, Delpon E, Tamkun MM, Tamargo J, Snyders DJ. Stereoselective block of a human cardiac potassium channel (Kv1.5) by bupivacaine enantiomers. Biophys J 1995; 69:418–427.
8. Hollmann MW, Kurz K, Herroeder S, et al. The effects of S^-, R^+, and racemic bupivacaine on lysophosphatidate-induced priming of human neutrophils. Anesth Analg 2003; 97:1053–1058.
9. Hollmann MW, Wieczorek KS, Berger A, Durieux ME. Local anesthetic inhibition of G protein-coupled receptor signaling by interference with Galpha(q) protein function. Mol Pharmacol 2001; 59:294–301.
10. Volk T, Schenk M, Voigt K, Tohtz S, Putzier M, Kox WJ. Postoperative epidural anesthesia preserves lymphocyte, but not monocyte, immune function after major spine surgery. Anesth Analg 2004; 98:1086–1092.
11. Vanhoutte F, Vereecke J, Verbeke N, Carmeliet E. Stereoselective effects of the enantiomers of bupivacaine on the electrophysiological properties of the guinea-pig papillary muscle. Br J Pharmacol 1991; 103:1275–1281.
12. Nau C, Wang SY, Strichartz GR, Wang GK. Block of human heart hH1 sodium channels by the enantiomers of bupivacaine. Anesthesiology 2000; 93:1022–1033.
13. Moller R, Covino BG. Cardiac electrophysiologic properties of bupivacaine and lidocaine compared with those of ropivacaine, a new amide local anesthetic. Anesthesiology 1990; 72:322–329.
14. Vladimirov M, Nau C, Mok WM, Strichartz G. Potency of bupivacaine stereoisomers tested in vitro and in vivo: biochemical, electrophysiological, and neurobehavioral studies. Anesthesiology 2000; 93:744–755.
15. Valenzuela C, Snyders DJ, Bennett PB, Tamargo J, Hondeghem LM. Stereoselective block of cardiac sodium channels by bupivacaine in guinea pig ventricular myocytes. Circulation 1995; 92:3014–3024.
16. Rutten AJ, Nancarrow C, Mather LE, Ilsley AH, Runciman WB, Upton RN. Hemodynamic and central nervous system effects of intravenous bolus doses of lidocaine, bupivacaine, and ropivacaine in sheep. Anesth Analg 1989; 69:291–299.

17. Huang YF, Pryor ME, Mather LE, Veering BT. Cardiovascular and central nervous system effects of intravenous levobupivacaine and bupivacaine in sheep. Anesth Analg 1998; 86:797–804.

18. Chang DH, Ladd LA, Wilson KA, Gelgor L, Mather LE. Tolerability of large-dose intravenous levobupivacaine in sheep. Anesth Analg 2000; 91:671–679.

19. Ohmura S, Kawada M, Ohta T, Yamamoto K, Kobayashi T. Systemic toxicity and resuscitation in bupivacaine-, levobupivacaine-, or ropivacaine-infused rats. Anesth Analg 2001; 93:743–748.

20. Morrison SG, Dominguez JJ, Frascarolo P, Reiz S. A comparison of the electrocardiographic cardiotoxic effects of racemic bupivacaine, levobupivacaine, and ropivacaine in anesthetized swine. Anesth Analg 2000; 90:1308–1314.

21. Groban L, Deal DD, Vernon JC, James RL, Butterworth J. Cardiac resuscitation after incremental overdosage with lidocaine, bupivacaine, levobupivacaine, and ropivacaine in anesthetized dogs. Anesth Analg 2001; 92:37–43.

22. McLeod GA, Burke D. Levobupivacaine. Anaesthesia 2001; 56:331–341.

23. Scott DB, Lee A, Fagan D, Bowler GM, Bloomfield P, Lundh R. Acute toxicity of ropivacaine compared with that of bupivacaine. Anesth Analg 1989; 69:563–569.

24. Knudsen K, Beckman Suurkula M, Blomberg S, Sjovall J, Edvardsson N. Central nervous and cardiovascular effects of i.v. infusions of ropivacaine, bupivacaine and placebo in volunteers. Br J Anaesth 1997; 78:507–514.

25. Bardsley H, Gristwood R, Baker H, Watson N, Nimmo W. A comparison of the cardiovascular effects of levobupivacaine and rac-bupivacaine following intravenous administration to healthy volunteers. Br J Clin Pharmacol 1998; 46:245–249.

26. Stewart J, Kellett N, Castro D. The central nervous system and cardiovascular effects of levobupivacaine and ropivacaine in healthy volunteers. Anesth Analg 2003; 97:412–416.

27. Cederholm I, Akerman B, Evers H. Local analgesic and vascular effects of intradermal ropivacaine and bupivacaine in various concentrations with and without addition of adrenaline in man. Acta Anaesthesiol Scand 1994; 38:322–327.

28. Newton DJ, Burke D, Khan F, et al. Skin blood flow changes in response to intradermal injection of bupivacaine and levobupivacaine, assessed by laser Doppler imaging. Reg Anesth Pain Med 2000; 25:626–631.

29. Behnke H, Worthmann F, Cornelissen J, Kahl M, Wulf H. Plasma concentration of ropivacaine after intercostal blocks for video-assisted thoracic surgery. Br J Anaesth 2002; 89:251–253.

30. Lee A, Fagan D, Lamont M, Tucker GT, Halldin M, Scott DB. Disposition kinetics of ropivacaine in humans. Anesth Analg 1989; 69:736–738.

31. Sinnott CJ, Cogswell IL, Johnson A, Strichartz GR. On the mechanism by which epinephrine potentiates lidocaine's peripheral nerve block. Anesthesiology 2003; 98:181–188.
32. Albright GA. Cardiac arrest following regional anesthesia with etidocaine or bupivacaine. Anesthesiology 1979; 51:285–287.
33. Brown DL, Ransom DM, Hall JA, Leicht CH, Schroeder DR, Offord KP. Regional anesthesia and local anesthetic-induced systemic toxicity: seizure frequency and accompanying cardiovascular changes. Anesth Analg 1995; 81:321–328.
34. Auroy Y, Narchi P, Messiah A, Litt L, Rouvier B, Samii K. Serious complications related to regional anesthesia: results of a prospective survey in France. Anesthesiology 1997; 87:479–486.
35. Rao RB, Ely SF, Hoffman RS. Deaths related to liposuction. N Engl J Med 1999; 340:1471–1475.
36. Crews JC, Rothman TE. Seizure after levobupivacaine for interscalene brachial plexus block. Anesth Analg 2003; 96:1188–1190.
37. Ala-Kokko TI, Lopponen A, Alahuhta S. Two instances of central nervous system toxicity in the same patient following repeated ropivacaine-induced brachial plexus block. Acta Anaesthesiol Scand 2000; 44:623–626.
38. Dernedde M, Furlan D, Verbesselt R, Gepts E, Boogaerts JG. Grand mal convulsion after an accidental intravenous injection of ropivacaine. Anesth Analg 2004; 98:521–523.
39. Petitjeans F, Mion G, Puidupin M, Tourtier JP, Hutson C, Saissy JM. Tachycardia and convulsions induced by accidental intravascular ropivacaine injection during sciatic block. Acta Anaesthesiol Scand 2002; 46:616–617.
40. Chazalon P, Tourtier JP, Villevielle T, et al. Ropivacaine-induced cardiac arrest after peripheral nerve block: successful resuscitation. Anesthesiology 2003; 99:1449–1451.
41. Reinikainen M, Hedman A, Pelkonen O, Ruokonen E. Cardiac arrest after interscalene brachial plexus block with ropivacaine and lidocaine. Acta Anaesthesiol Scand 2003; 47:904–906.
42. Owen MD, Gautier P, Hood DD. Can ropivacaine and levobupivacaine be used as test doses during regional anesthesia? Anesthesiology 2004; 100:922–925.
43. Tucker GT, Mather LE. Properties, absorption and disposition of local anaesthetic agents. In: Cousins MJ, Bridenbaugh PO, eds. Neural blockade in clinical anaesthesia and management of pain. 3rd edn. Philadelphia: Lippincott-Raven; 1998.
44. Kuhnert BR, Kuhnert PM, Prochaska AL, Gross TL. Plasma levels of 2 chloroprocaine in obstetric patients and their neonates after epidural anesthesia. *Anesthesiology* 1980; 53:21–5.
45. Reynolds F. A comparison of the potential toxicity of bupivacaine, lignocaine and mepivacaine during epidural blockade for surgery. *Br J Anaesth* 1971; 43:567–72.

46. McClure JH. Ropivacaine. Br J Anaesth 1996; 76:300–307.

47. Kissin I, Lee SS, Bradley EL Jr. Effect of prolonged nerve block on inflammatory hyperalgesia in rats: prevention of late hyperalgesia. Anesthesiology 1998; 88:224–232.

48. Boogaerts J, Declercq A, Lafont N, et al. Toxicity of bupivacaine encapsulated into liposomes and injected intravenously: comparison with plain solutions. Anesth Analg 1993; 76:553–555.

49. Castillo J, Curley J, Hotz J, et al. Glucocorticoids prolong rat sciatic nerve blockade in vivo from bupivacaine microspheres. Anesthesiology 1996; 85:1157–1166.

50. Drager C, Benziger D, Gao F, Berde CB. Prolonged intercostal nerve blockade in sheep using controlled-release of bupivacaine and dexamethasone from polymer microspheres. Anesthesiology 1998; 89:969–979.

51. Watanabe Y, Saito H, Abe K. Tricyclic antidepressants block NMDA receptor-mediated synaptic responses and induction of long-term potentiation in rat hippocampal slices. Neuropharmacology 1993; 32:479–486.

52. Srinivasa V, Gerner P, Haderer A, Abdi S, Jarolim P, Wang GK. The relative toxicity of amitriptyline, bupivacaine, and levobupivacaine administered as rapid infusions in rats. Anesth Analg 2003; 97:91–95.

53. Gerner P, Mujtaba M, Khan M, et al. N-phenylethyl amitriptyline in rat sciatic nerve blockade. Anesthesiology 2002; 96:1435–1442.

54. Sudoh Y, Cahoon EE, Gerner P, Wang GK. Tricyclic antidepressants as long-acting local anesthetics. Pain 2003; 103:49–55.

55. Gerner P, Haderer AE, Mujtaba M, et al. Assessment of differential blockade by amitriptyline and its N-methyl derivative in different species by different routes. Anesthesiology 2003; 98:1484–1490.

56. Kohane DS, Lu NT, Crosa GA, Kuang Y, Berde CB. High concentrations of adrenergic antagonists prolong sciatic nerve blockade by tetrodotoxin. Acta Anaesthesiol Scand 2001; 45:899–905.

57. Kohane DS, Kuang Y, Lu NT, Langer R, Strichartz GR, Berde CB. Vanilloid receptor agonists potentiate the in vivo local anesthetic activity of percutaneously injected site 1 sodium channel blockers. Anesthesiology 1999; 90:524–534.

CHAPTER **4.2**

TECHNIQUES OF REGIONAL ANAESTHESIA

GENERAL CONSIDERATIONS

Regional anaesthesia and analgesia, either alone or in combination with general anaesthesia, has the potential to provide excellent operating conditions and prolonged postoperative pain relief, especially when using perineural catheters.

For orthopaedic surgery, the provision of pain relief that enables postoperative mobilisation[1,2] and early feeding may accelerate rehabilitation and return of normal function.

Regional anaesthesia offers better and longer pain relief with fewer side-effects than do opioids. As a result, it is increasingly popular for ambulatory anaesthesia and has contributed to the percentage of day-case patients increasing from less than 10% to around 65% in the US.

Relative indications for regional analgesia

Indications for regional analgesia include:

- to avoid some of the dangers of general anaesthesia, such as known impossible intubation and severe respiratory failure, and where relaxant problems are expected;
- patients who specifically request regional analgesia;
- situations where general anaesthesia is not available (rare);
- to provide high-quality postoperative pain relief;
- as part of a postoperative multimodal rehabilitation programme to enable early return to function.

Relative contraindications for regional analgesia

Contraindications for regional analgesia when used alone include:

- uncooperative or restless patients;
- some psychiatric patients.

Practical considerations when using regional analgesia

Regional analgesia is used less frequently than it might be because of:

- time taken to establish block;
- inexperience of anaesthetists and their fear of failure;
- fear of neurological complications;
- unpopularity of having awake patients at operation;
- concern that a single injection block may wear off in a few hours.

Concern that a single injection block may wear off in a few hours can be overcome, almost anywhere in the body, by inserting a perineural catheter, which can be 'topped up' with local anaesthetic as often as needed.

Preparation before local anaesthetic is injected

Before any local anaesthetic is administered the following should be available:

- an indwelling intravenous cannula;
- a tilting table or trolley;
- facilities for intermittent positive-pressure ventilation (IPPV) with oxygen;
- patient monitoring, including ECG, noninvasive blood pressure, pulse oximetry and end-tidal carbon dioxide (in case of need for general anaesthesia);
- suction equipment and catheters;
- syringes or ampoules of thiopental, propofol, suxamethonium, midazolam and atropine, and pressor agents such as ephedrine, metaraminol and phenylephrine;
- crystalloid and colloid solutions for infusion;
- full resuscitation equipment and drugs, including a defibrillator.

Identification of nerves

Halstead performed the first nerve blocks by open surgical exposure. Now, the quality of peripheral nerve blocks is determined by accurate identification of nerves and precise injection of local anaesthetic into an anatomical space.

Eliciting nerve paraesthesia with a needle has been the traditional means of finding peripheral nerves, but may be associated with block success rates not compatible with modern clinical expectations and, infrequently, with nerve trauma.[3]

New imaging techniques have been introduced to improve the efficacy and safety of regional anaesthesia. They include nerve stimulation, percutaneous electrical guidance (PEG), ultrasound, stimulating catheters and computed tomography (CT) scans. In view of the considerable advances in regional anaesthesia, it is first necessary to discuss these new technological advances in some detail before describing the practice of peripheral regional blockade.

One must remember, however, that new technology only supplements and does not replace detailed knowledge of regional anatomy.

Principles of nerve stimulation

Nerve stimulation was first described by Perthes in 1912. Electrical nerve stimulation of peripheral nerves is now commonly used in clinical practice.

The principle of nerve stimulation is to trigger electrical depolarisation of the nerve and stimulate muscular contractions at the proposed site of surgery.

The nerve membrane obeys Coulomb's law and may be considered to behave like a capacitor, whereby the stimulating charge strength

$$e = k\,(q/r^2)$$

where k is constant, q is the minimum stimulating current and r is the distance of the needle tip from the nerve.

Typical charge strength required to depolarise nerves vary from 120 nanocoulombs (nc) to 1000 nc in elderly diabetics.

The total amount of depolarisation or charge transferred across the membrane is a product of the strength and duration of the stimulus, electrode to nerve distance and electrical impedance of the intervening tissues.

An inverse relationship exists between the strength and duration of electrical stimulation, but differs according to the type of nerve, as illustrated in Figure 4.2.1, from which two important parameters may be defined:

- rheobase – the minimum current that stimulates a nerve, independent of stimulation time;
- chronaxie – the duration necessary to stimulate a nerve when the current is equal to twice the rheobase.

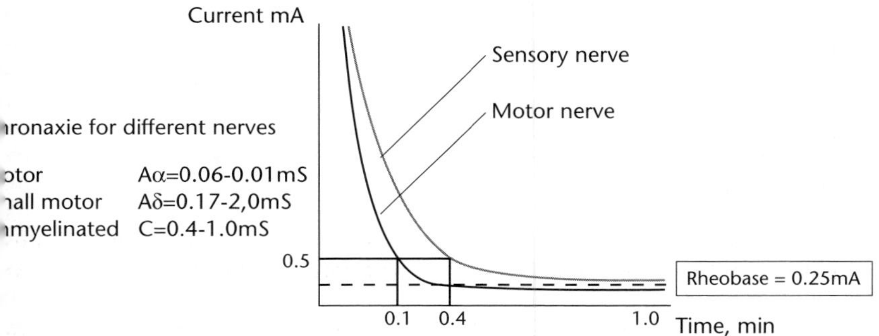

Figure 4.2.1 Strength and duration of electrical nerve stimulation. Illustration shows method of calculating chronaxie.

The chronaxie can be regarded as a measure of the 'excitability of the nerve'.

Stimulation of nerves

The rheobase and chronaxie of nerve fibres are dependent on their function.

The *A*α motor fibres have the shortest chronaxie (0.05–0.1 ms), whereas the fibres of pain sensation (Aδ and C fibres) require a longer pulse (0.15 ms and 0.4 ms, respectively) at minimum current.

Owing to the differences in chronaxie between motor and sensory fibres, mixed peripheral nerves can be localised with short pulses (0.1 ms) without triggering pain sensations. Thus, two different settings of the nerve stimulator are commonly used, depending on clinical circumstance:

- current 1–2 mA, pulse duration 0.1 ms and pulse frequency 2 Hz – stimulates motor fibres without experiencing pain and positions the needle as accurately as possible;
- current 1–2 mA, pulse duration 0.3 ms and pulse frequency 1 Hz – stimulates paraesthesia, but avoids painful muscle contractions in trauma patients.

Needles should be insulated apart from a small area at the tip in order to generate a high current density near the nerve.

When muscle contractions are detected, optimisation of needle position should be sought by incrementally reducing the stimulating current.

When a level between 0.2 mA and 0.5 mA has been reached and muscle contractions are still barely visible, the local anaesthetic may be injected after a negative aspiration test. The anaesthetist should always check the current at which contractions cease. Injection of local anaesthetic at a current less than or equal to 0.2 mA may indicate intraneural injection. If the needle position is correct, the muscle response to injection will disappear instantly. When a significant resistance is noted or paraesthesia is felt, the injection must be stopped immediately. Moreover, aspiration checks should be performed repeatedly during the procedure to exclude inadvertent intravenous injection.

Transcutaneous electrical stimulation

A variety of transcutaneous electrical stimulation devices have been developed in order to reduce the invasive search for the nerves by optimising the needle insertion point over the target nerve.

Urmey and Grossi[4] recently described a technique called percutaneous electrode guidance (PEG). The PEG technique uses a cylindrical transcutaneous electrode with a metallic tip less than 1 mm in width. The electrode indents the skin and underlying subcutaneous tissues toward the nerve, thus reducing the distance to the targeted nerve and tissue electrical impedance. After location of the nerve (current <0.5 mA), a needle is passed through the probe and local anaesthetic is injected. This device is useful for blocking superficial, but not deep, nerves.

Ultrasound

Anatomical knowledge has until recently been based on cadaver dissection but is now being supplanted by ultrasound, owing to progress in transducer technology and image processing.

Ultrasound of peripheral nerves allows imaging of individual anatomy, real-time needle guidance and real-time monitoring of local anaesthetic spread.

Ultrasound involves emission of sound waves (≈20 000 Hz), penetration through tissues, reflection at tissue interfaces and receipt and interpretation of echoes.

Higher frequencies (10–14 MHz) give a higher spatial resolution with low tissue penetration and are better for blocking superficial plexuses.[5] In contrast, localising deeper nerves requires a lower frequency between 4 and 7 MHz .

The sonographic appearance of peripheral nerves varies according to the plane of ultrasound beam.[6] In the transverse plane, nerves are viewed as round/ovoid shapes consisting of hypoechoic bubbles (fascicles) enveloped by hyperechoic elements (epineurium or connective tissue). This is termed a 'honeycomb pattern' and is seen most often in the trunks and proximal cords.

In the longitudinal plane, hypoechoic parallel bands (fascicles) are bordered by hyperechoic striations (epineurium or connective tissue). This is termed a fascicular pattern.

In the transverse view, small vessels, lymph nodes and muscle fascicles can be mistaken for nerves because they have similar size and echogenicity. Colour Doppler mapping of vascular flow is useful to identify blood vessels.

The appearance of needles on ultrasound depends on the direction of needle insertion. When the needle crosses the echo plane (perpendicular to skin) it appears as a hyperechoic dotlike reflex. When the needle is introduced parallel to the echo plane (e.g. at an angle or flat to skin) it appears as a hyperechoic, linear reflex.

Direct visualisation has revealed two new fascinating features of nerve blockade. First, that gentle pressure applied to the skin moves nerves considerably within the subcutaneous tissue and, second, that apparent visual needle contact may not necessarily elicit muscle contractions. In this situation, the needle should not be advanced any further but moved gently sideways.

Claimed benefits[7] of ultrasound-guided regional anaesthesia include reduced complication rates, faster onset times, reduced doses of local anaesthetic, higher and more predictable success rates, documentation and storage (images, video sequences).

Catheter techniques for continuous pain relief

In the days after orthopaedic surgery, the incidence of severe postoperative pain may be between 40 and 70% when using intravenous opioids.

Provision of pain relief nerve by nerve block was first described in 1946 by Asbro, but it was not until recently, with the development of catheter technology and disposable elastomeric infusion devices, that the use of perineural catheters for both ambulatory and inpatients escalated dramatically.

The advantages of continuous perineural nerve block include better pain relief, better mobilisation, improved patient satisfaction, sleep and cognition, and fewer side-effects.[8] Epidural analgesia, although providing comparable pain relief, limits mobilisation and requires urinary catheterisation; patient-controlled analgesia (PCA) offers poorer pain relief, limited mobilisation and increased side-effects such as nausea and vomiting.

Insertion of a perineural catheter is relatively straightforward. The nerve block is performed according to traditional landmarks and with a nerve stimulator and/or ultrasound. Needles are small, insulated and bevelled (Touhy like) to minimise nerve damage. Once the nerve is identified at a current between 0.2 and 0.5 mA, the perineural sheath is dilated with saline or local anaesthetic. No evidence exists regarding the optimal volume of fluid, if any, necessary to dilate the perineural space or whether all the injectate must be given before or after catheter insertion.

The advantage of giving a large volume, albeit in small increments to check for inadvertent intravascular injection, is that if the catheter cannot be threaded, then the patient will have received a single nerve block and postoperative pain relief for 6–24 hours, depending on the type of nerve block.

The author's preference, based on experience, is to dilate the perineural space with 5 mL of 0.5% ropivacaine (also acts as a test dose) or 0.5% levobupivacaine, depending on age and weight, thread a Seldinger wire into the perineural space, then railroad the perineural catheter 5 cm into the nerve sheath. Increments of local anaesthetic are then given through the catheter.

The practical advantages of incremental injection are:

- injection at regular intervals ensures catheter patency, preventing small blood clots from blocking the end hole;
- kinking or blockage is detected by high injection pressures;
- cardiovascular stability is improved, particularly in frail, elderly, cardiovascularly compromised patients presenting for lower limb amputation.

Addition of an electrical stimulating wire to a perineural catheter allows confirmation of the position by stimulating the appropriate muscle bed when the catheter is in position. Use of electrical stimulation to optimise the position of femoral catheters has been shown to improve the quality and depth of femoral block compared to non-stimulating catheters in volunteers.[9]

If a catheter technique is used in for ambulatory surgery, certain criteria must be met:

- patients should understand instructions;
- patients should be accompanied by a responsible person;
- peripheral nerve catheters should be tested for intravascular placement before discharge;
- dilute concentrations of local anaesthetic should be used;
- nerves should be protected from pressure damage;
- a nurse should be available 24 hours a day to answer questions by telephone;
- daily follow-up is mandatory.

Infusion pumps should have a reservoir of 200–400 mL, ensure a constant infusion rate, be tamper proof, and have the option of a patient-controlled bolus function.

Three modes of infusion have been used:

- infusion only – simple, inexpensive and can be disposable, but is incapable of dealing with breakthrough pain or motor block;
- bolus only – ideal for balancing efficacy against side-effects but may be associated with nocturnal pain;
- infusion with patient-controlled bolus – the ideal regimen. In a study of interscalene blocks Singelyn et al. [10] showed that a basal infusion combined with patient-controlled boluses provided pain relief for shoulder surgery equivalent to that of a continuous infusion, but with lower total doses of local anaesthetics.

It is important to note that the optimum concentration and volume of levobupivacaine and ropivacaine for perineural catheters have yet to be determined by dose-finding studies. Furthermore, different nerve plexuses may require varying volumes and concentrations, depending on the anatomical characteristics of the nerves and surrounding perineural space.

Lidocaine (lignocaine), bupivacaine, levobupivacaine and ropivacaine have all been used as the primary local anaesthetic.

The use of bupivacaine (0.1–0.25%) does not result in toxic blood levels when used for postoperative analgesia for 24–72 hours in current regimens.

Typical venous total bupivacaine levels during continuous brachial plexus analgesia are 0.5–1.0 μg/mL and during continuous lumbar plexus analgesia are 0.5–1.8 μg/mL. Plasma levels over 2 μg/mL are considered toxic.

As the optimum concentration and volume mix is not known for perineural infusions of either limb, patients are invariably discharged from hospital with motor block and paraesthesia. This issue remains controversial because patients may be at risk of limb injury.

One large report of 2382 patients having peripheral nerve blocks in an ambulatory setting[11] has shown a low incidence of block failure, rare use of opioids in the recovery unit, high patient satisfaction rate and a low incidence of accidental injury to the blocked arm or leg.

Adjuvants

The role of additives to local anaesthetics blocks has still to be defined.

Additives include opioids, adrenergic agonists (epinephrine [adrenaline] and clonidine), anticholinergics (neostigmine) and *N*-methyl-D-aspartate (NMDA) antagonists (ketamine).

The ideal local anaesthetic adjuvant would reduce onset time, increase the density of the block, prolong analgesia and reduce motor blockade.

Buprenorphine added to an axillary block provided postoperative analgesia three times longer than local anaesthetic block alone, suggesting the existence of peripheral opioid receptors.[12] Addition of epinephrine (adrenaline) both intensifies and prolongs neural blockade blockade by limiting uptake of local anaesthetic into the surrounding vasculature.

A recent human volunteer study has shown concentrations of 1 in 800 000 epinephrine (adrenaline) to be as vasoactive as concentrations of 1 in 400 000 and 1 in 200 000 epinephrine (adrenaline) for cutaneous infiltration when used either alone or with the local anaesthetics, bupivacaine and levobupivacaine.[13]

Clonidine has prolonged motor and sensory block and analgesia for single injection axillary block,[14] but not for interscalene block[15] or infraclavicular infusion.[15,16] Unfortunately, clonidine is associated with significant adverse effects, including hypotension, bradycardia and sedation, all of which limit its use for ambulatory anaesthesia.

In practice, age[17] is actually the major determinant of duration of complete motor and sensory blockade with peripheral nerve block, perhaps reflecting increased sensitivity to conduction blockade produced by local anaesthetic agents in peripheral nerves in the elderly population.

REGIONAL TECHNIQUES

Topical analgesia

The word 'topical' is derived from the Greek word topos, meaning 'a place'. Topical analgesia can be applied:

- on gauze swabs;
- as a liquid in a spray;
- as a cream, gel, or ointment;
- as an aerosol;
- by direct instillation (e.g. conjunctival sac, nose and trachea).

Sites

Sites for topical analgesia are:

- the conjunctival sac – stinging pain on instillation can be eased if the drug is dissolved in methylcellulose;
- the external ear;
- the nasal cavities;
- the upper air passages;
- the perineum and vagina in obstetrics for spontaneous delivery, or for suture of simple lacerations the urethra;
- before open wound closure.

Infiltration analgesia

A weal of local anaesthetic is raised in the skin and through this a larger needle is used to inject the main bulk of solution. Lidocaine (lignocaine) 0.5–1% solution, each with epinephrine (adrenaline), is ideal for this procedure.

For painless skin incisions, infiltration should be intradermal as well as subcutaneous. A slow, gentle technique is important, and the solution should be injected while the needle is moving to reduce the chances of intravenous injection.

As with all forms of local analgesia, the effect is not instantaneous and several minutes must elapse between injection and incision.

HEAD AND NECK

Field block of scalp and cranium

Anatomy

The trigeminal nerve supplies the anterior two-thirds and the posterior divisions of cervical nerves supply the posterior one-third of the scalp and cranium. There are five sensory nerves in front of the ear and four behind it. These nerves all converge towards the vertex of the scalp, so a band of infiltration passing just above the ear through the glabella and the occiput will block them all.

Technique

Injections of 0.5% lidocaine (lignocaine) with epinephrine (adrenaline) solution must be made in three layers:

- skin (intradermal);
- subcutaneous tissues superficial to the epicranial aponeurosis in which the nerves and vessels lie, and also below the aponeurosis;
- periosteum.

In addition, solution should be injected into the substance of the temporalis muscle. The dura is insensitive except at the base of the skull.

Nerve block for eye operations

Retrobulbar and peribulbar blocks are used (see Ch. 5.9).

Nerve block for ear operations

Greater auricular nerve block

The greater auricular nerve is blocked by infiltration of local anaesthetic solution over the mastoid process in the skin fold behind the back of the ear.

Auriculotemporal nerve block

The auriculotemporal nerve is blocked by infiltration of local anaesthetic solution into the skin over the auditory canal in front of the ear.

Blockade of the auriculotemporal and greater auricular nerves together is used for pinnaplasty.

Paracentesis of the eardrum

Two or three metered (10 mg) doses of lidocaine (lignocaine) aerosol spray are applied to the superior wall of the external auditory canal and allowed to trickle down onto the eardrum. This is repeated after 2 minutes and the incision can be made 3 minutes later. It is useful in cooperative children.

Nerve block for nasal operations

Anatomy

The nasal nerve supply is from the first (ophthalmic) division and from the second (maxillary) division of the trigeminal nerve (cranial nerve V). The skin of the nose is supplied by the supratrochlear branch of the frontal nerve (a branch of the ophthalmic nerve), the anterior ethmoidal branch of the nasociliary nerve (another branch of the ophthalmic), and the infraorbital branch of the maxillary nerve. The maxillary nerve via the sphenopalatine ganglion supplies the lining of the maxillary antrum. The frontal nerve supplies the frontal sinus. The anterior and posterior ethmoidal branches of the nasociliary supply the ethmoid region. The anterior ethmoidal branch of the nasociliary nerve supplies sensation to the anterior one-third of the nasal septum and the lateral wall of the nasal cavity. The long sphenopalatine nerves from the sphenopalatine ganglion supply sensation to posterior two-thirds of the nasal septum and the lateral walls of the nasal cavity.

The sphenopalatine ganglion is situated in the pterygopalatine fossa in the upper part of the pterygomaxillary fissure, lateral to the sphenopalatine foramen. Blocking of the sphenopalatine ganglion causes analgesia in the:

- lateral nasal nerve;
- inferior palpebral and superior labial nerves;

- posterior, middle and anterior superior alveolar nerves;
- palatal nerves.

Together these nerves supply the skin of the upper lip, side of the nose, lower eyelid and malar region, the teeth of the upper jaw and the underlying periosteum, the mucosa of the maxillary antrum and of the hard and soft palate, and the posterior part of the nasal cavity.

Techniques

Maxillary nerve and sphenopalatine ganglion block

Maxillary nerve and sphenopalatine ganglion block are useful for operations on the antrum (e.g. Caldwell–Luc) and on the upper lip, palate and upper teeth as far as the bicuspids. A weal is raised 0.5 cm below the midpoint of the zygoma, which is over the anterior border of the coronoid process. Through it a needle is introduced at right-angles to the median plane of the head until it strikes the lateral plate of the pterygoid process at a depth of about 4 cm. The needle is then moved so that its point glances past the anterior margin of the external pterygoid plate. The needle point should be in the pterygomaxillary fissure. The needle has been known to enter the pharynx or the orbit. If the aspiration test is negative, 3–4 mL of 1.5% solution of lidocaine (lignocaine) is injected and a similar amount as the needle is slowly withdrawn.

The anterior ethmoidal nerve is a branch of the nasociliary nerve and is blocked in the medial wall of the orbit as the nerve passes through the anterior ethmoidal foramen. A weal is raised 1 cm above the caruncle at the inner canthus of the eye. A small needle is introduced along the upper medial angle of the orbit for 3.5 cm, keeping near the bone, and 2 mL of 1.5% lidocaine (lignocaine) are injected.

Frontal nerve block

From the same weal as in anterior ethmoid block, the needle is introduced more laterally towards the central part of the roof of the orbit, where the frontal nerve lies between the periosteum and the levator palpebrae superioris.

Lidocaine (lignocaine), 1 mL of 2% solution, is injected in close contact with the bone.

Infraorbital nerve block

The infraorbital nerve, the terminal portion of the maxillary nerve, divides at the infraorbital foramen into inferior palpebral, external nasal and superior labial branches. These supply the side of the nose, the lower eyelid, the upper lip and its mucosa.

The infraorbital foramen is in line with the supraorbital notch and canine fossa, both of which are palpable, or the second upper premolar tooth; it is 1 cm below the margin of the orbit, below the pupil when the eyes look forwards. The mental foramen is in the same straight line, as is also the second bicuspid tooth.

A needle is inserted through a weal 1 cm below the middle of the lower orbital margin, a fingerbreadth lateral to the ala of the nose. Lidocaine (lignocaine), 2 mL of 2% solution, is deposited near the nerve as it issues from the foramen, not while it is in the foramen. The upper lip and tip of the nose are made insensitive by this injection.

For radical operation on the antrum a maxillary block is indicated, together with local infiltration inside the upper lip, over the canine fossa.

For radical operation on the frontal sinus, anterior ethmoidal and frontal blocks are necessary.

For operations for dacryocystitis, anterior ethmoidal and infraorbital blocks are required.

Topical analgesia of the nasal cavities

Topical analgesia of the nasal cavities is useful in cooperative patients with reasonably patent nares.

Spray

The nasal cavities are sprayed with a 2.5 mL mixture of 5% lidocaine (lignocaine) and the vasoconstrictor, phenylephrine hydrochloride 0.5%, aiming dorsally for the mucosa overlying the sphenopalatine ganglion, behind the middle turbinate.

Topical cocaine 4% solution is now rarely used in hospital practice.

Moffett's method

Moffett's method is of historical interest only. The solution is a mixture of 2 mL of 8% cocaine hydrochloride, 2 mL of 1% sodium bicarbonate and 1 mL of 1:1000 epinephrine (adrenaline) solution. It can also be used as 4% cocaine, omitting bicarbonate and epinephrine (adrenaline). A 2 mL syringe with bent cannula is required:

- position 1 – patient lies on the left side with a pillow under the left shoulder and the head in a lateral position at an angle of 45° to the vertical. One-third of the solution is drawn up, half being squirted into each naris along the floor of the nose;
- position 2 – after 10 minutes the second one-third of solution is drawn up and is similarly divided between the two sides of the nose; the patient pinches the nose, turns prone and lies on the face for 10 minutes;
- position 3 – with the remainder instilled the patient rolls on to the right side as in position 1 and remains for 10 minutes. If the septum is to be operated on, 2 mL of 1% lidocaine (lignocaine) and epinephrine (adrenaline) should be injected into the columella and base of the septum in addition, because this area is covered by squamous epithelium which will not absorb the topical agent;

The method gives good analgesia, free from the unpleasantness of gauze packing and its resulting mild trauma.

Nerve block for maxillofacial operations

Local infiltration for dental extraction

Local infiltration for dental extraction can be carried out for all teeth with the possible exception of the lower molars. Lidocaine (lignocaine) 2% with 1: 80 000 epinephrine (adrenaline) solution is commonly used, or alternatively 3% prilocaine with felypressin.

A 26-gauge needle is inserted at the junction of the adherent mucoperiosteum of the gum with the free mucous membrane of the cheek and directed parallel to the long axis of the tooth; 0.5–1 mL of solution is injected superficial to the periosteum on the buccal and either the lingual or the palatal side. Analgesia is tested for after 5 minutes by pushing the needle down the periodontal membrane on each side of the tooth to be extracted. If required, more solution can be injected.

If there is infection involving teeth in the lower jaw, a 5% solution may give better analgesia than the usual 2%. It has a shorter latency but a similar duration of activity.

Mandibular (inferior dental) block

Mandibular (inferior dental) block may be required for extraction of several teeth of the lower jaw or for removal of the second or third molars. Infiltration cannot always be relied on to make these teeth insensitive.

A single well-placed injection renders one-half of the lower jaw and tongue anaesthetic, except for the central incisor, which receives some nerve supply from the other side, and the lateral buccal fold and molar buccal alveolar margin and gum supplied from the buccinator nerve. Both these areas can be infiltrated with a small volume of solution to make them painless.

With the mouth open palpate the anterior border of the ramus of the mandible, the retromolar fossa and the internal oblique ridge.

The needle is inserted just medial to this ridge, lateral to the pterygomandibular ligament for a distance of 1.5 cm, keeping the syringe parallel to the occlusal plane of the lower teeth with its barrel over the premolar teeth of the opposite side; 2 or 3 mL of solution are now injected.

In patients whose orbital blood supply is derived from the middle meningeal artery (a rare anomaly), mandibular nerve block may result in transient amaurosis. This may be due to intra-arterial injection of the local anaesthetic/epinephrine (adrenaline) solution.

Lingual nerve block

The lingual nerve is the only sensory nerve supplying the floor of the mouth between the alveolar margin and the midline.

A finger in the retromolar fossa of the mandible will palpate the internal oblique line. The lingual nerve can be injected, just medial to this line, with 2 mL of 2% lidocaine (lignocaine). This is a useful method of analgesia for removing calculi from the submaxillary duct.

Intraoral nerve blocks

Infraorbital nerve

Infraorbital nerve block is achieved by injection in the mucobuccal fold, just medial to the canine tooth; 1–2 mL of local anaesthetic solution is injected, advancing the needle 1 cm. The entire upper lip is anaesthetised. This can be bilateral.

Mental nerve

Mental nerve block is obtained by injection of 1–2 mL of local anaesthetic solution between the apices of the premolar teeth of the lower jaw. This will anaesthetise the lower lip.

Long buccal nerve

The long buccal nerve can be blocked as it crosses the anterior border of the mandible. Injection is immediately in front of the ramus, in the mucobuccal fold opposite the first molar tooth. The needle is inserted just anterior to the margin of the mandible and 2–3 mL of solution are injected while the needle is withdrawn. This is useful for blocking 'crossover' fibres.

Nerve block for throat operations

Glossopharyngeal nerve block

For glossopharyngeal nerve block the head is fully rotated to the opposite side with the patient lying supine. At the midpoint of a line joining the tip of the mastoid process to the angle of the jaw a needle inserted vertical to the skin makes contact with the styloid process 2–4 cm deep. The needle is partially withdrawn and reinserted 0.5 cm deep to and posterior to the styloid process. Injection of 6 mL of solution at this point will produce analgesia of the posterior one-third of the tongue.

An alternative technique is to deposit solution near the jugular foramen. A 5 cm needle is introduced through a weal just below the external auditory meatus, anterior to the mastoid process. It is advanced perpendicularly to the skin until it meets the styloid process 1.5–2 cm deep and passes it posteriorly for a further 2 cm. Successful block results in analgesia of the posterior one-third of the tongue, uvula, soft palate and pharynx. There is no motor block. The gag reflex is suppressed.

Internal laryngeal nerve block

The superior laryngeal nerve divides into the internal and external laryngeal nerves slightly below and anterior to the greater cornu of the hyoid bone.

The internal laryngeal nerve pierces the thyrohyoid membrane and then separates into terminal twigs, which spread superficially below the mucosa of the piriform fossa.

Block of the internal laryngeal nerve causes analgesia of the lower pharynx, the laryngeal aspect of the epiglottis, the vallecula, the vestibule of the larynx, the aryepiglottic fold and the posterior part of the rima glottidis. There is no motor block.

A 25 g needle is introduced upwards and medially through the thyrohyoid membrane. After aspiration, to exclude entry into the pharynx, 2 mL of 2% lidocaine (lignocaine) solution are injected.

Alternatively, topical application of 2–3 mL of 4% lidocaine (lignocaine) solution to both piriform fossae with a small disposable spray provides good analgesia of the vocal cords for a variety of airway procedures.

Internal laryngeal nerve block by external injection or internal spray techniques is necessary to provide a tubeless field for laser surgery or bronchoscopy (flexible or rigid) when combined with target-controlled infusions (TCI) of propofol.

When combined with topical anaesthesia of the nose using co-phenylcaine spray, and cricothyroid puncture using 3 mL of 4% lidocaine (lignocaine) anaesthesia, excellent conditions are created for awake fibre-optic intubation or tracheal stenting of lung tumours.

Cricothyroid block

The operator stands on the left side of the patient and holds a size 22 G intravenous catheter in the right hand. The index and middle fingers of the left hand hold the cricothyroid membrane steady. A single purposeful stab is made in the relatively avascular midline of the membrane and a marked loss of resistance is felt as the trachea is entered. Gentle probing of the membrane is not recommended because the needle will slide off laterally, increase bleeding, and may traumatise structures in the neck.

After aspiration to confirm the presence of air, the patient is asked to inspire deeply and 3 mL of 4% lidocaine (lignocaine) are rapidly injected into the trachea.

The needle is swiftly removed after injection because the presence of lidocaine (lignocaine) precipitates coughing and spread of local anaesthetic both above and below the vocal cords.

Cricothyroid injection provides the best conditions for fibreoptic intubation.

Food and drink must be prohibited for 3–4 hours after anaesthesia.

Field block for tonsillectomy

Anatomy

The lesser palatine nerve (from the maxillary nerve), the lingual nerve (from the mandibular nerve) and the glossopharyngeal nerve, via the pharyngeal plexus, which gives off filaments that form a plexus called the circulus tonsillaris, supply the tonsil and its immediate surroundings.

Technique

Half an hour before the analgesia is commenced, a tetracaine (amethocaine) lozenge 60 mg is given. Injections of 3–5 mL of 1.5% lidocaine (lignocaine) are now given:

- into the upper part of the posterior pillar;
- into the upper part of the anterior pillar (both pillars must be made oedematous throughout their whole extent);
- into the triangular fold, near the lower pole;
- into the supratonsillar fossa, after drawing the tonsil towards the middle line.

The patient sits, well supported, in a chair. Adequate time must be given for the anaesthetic to act. Fainting sometimes occurs, and depression of the tongue by the spatula may cause discomfort.

Accessory nerve block

Anatomy

The accessory nerve has both cranial and spinal roots. It leaves the skull through the jugular foramen, enters the deep surface of the sternomastoid, pierces it and emerges just above the midpoint of its posterior margin. It crosses the posterior triangle of the neck and enters the anterior border of the trapezius, giving motor fibres to it and to the sternomastoid.

Technique

For accessory nerve block the needle is inserted 2 cm below the tip of the mastoid and 5–10 mL of lidocaine (lignocaine) is injected into the sternomastoid muscle.

Indications

Accessory nerve block is used to relax the sternomastoid and trapezius muscles during physiotherapy for pain in the shoulder and neck (e.g. torticollis).

Cervical plexus block

Anatomy

The cervical plexus is formed by the anterior primary divisions of the upper four cervical nerves, each one of which, after leaving the intervertebral foramen, passes behind the vertebral artery and comes to lie in the sulcus between the anterior and posterior tubercles of the transverse process of the appropriate cervical vertebra.

Each nerve lies between the scalenus medius deeply and the levator anguli scapulae, under cover of the sternomastoid. Each of these four nerves, except the first, divides into upper and lower branches, which form three loops lateral to the transverse processes. The loops are between C1 and C2, C2 and C3, and C3 and C4. The lower branch of C4 joins C5 in the formation of the brachial plexus. The upper loop is directed forwards, the lower two backwards.

Branches of the cervical plexus are superficial (cutaneous), deep (muscular) and communicating. The superficial branches emerging at the posterior border of the sternomastoid, near its midpoint, are:

- ascending branches – the lesser occipital nerve (C2) and great auricular nerve (C2 and C3), which supply the skin of the occipitomastoid region, auricle and parotid;
- transverse branch – the anterior cutaneous nerve of the neck (C2 and C3), which supplies the skin of the anterior part of neck between the lower jaw and the sternum;
- descending branches – the lateral, intermediate and medial supraclavicular nerves (C3 and C4), which supply the skin of the shoulder and upper pectoral region; C1 has no cutaneous branch.

Deep branches of the plexus are:

- the phrenic nerve – C3, C4 and C5;
- anterior (deep) muscular branches;
- posterior muscular branches to sternomastoid, levator scapulae, trapezius and scalenus medius.

Communicating branches are:

- sympathetic – each cervical nerve receives a grey ramus from the cervical sympathetic chain – the upper four nerves from the superior cervical ganglion;
- branch to the vagus;
- branch to the hypoglossal nerve from C1 and C2, the descendens hypoglossi (or superior root of the ansa cervicalis), which joins the descendens cervicalis (or inferior root of the ansa cervicalis) (C2–C3).

The posterior primary divisions of the cervical nerves supply skin and muscles of the back of the neck. Their cutaneous distribution spreads like a cape over the upper thorax and shoulders, and this area is made insensitive in cervical plexus block.

Nerve supplies are as follows:

- thyroid – middle and inferior cervical sympathetic ganglion;
- oesophagus – the vagus (and sympathetic);
- trachea – recurrent laryngeal (and sympathetic);
- sternomastoid – 11th cranial, and second and third cervical nerves.

Technique

For deep cervical block draw a line connecting the mastoid with the transverse process of the sixth cervical vertebra (Chassaignac's tubercle). A second line is drawn parallel and 1.5 cm posterior. A needle is inserted to a depth of 1.5–2 cm perpendicular to all planes of the skin so that the transverse processes are contacted.

Inject into the sulcus between the anterior and posterior tubercles of the transverse processes of the second, third and fourth cervical vertebrae (the sixth, seventh and eighth nerves having no sensory branches in the neck, and the first is purely motor).

For superficial cervical block inject 10 mL of local anaesthetic solution between skin and muscle along the posterior border of the sternomastoid near its midpoint, usually just below the position where it is crossed by the external jugular vein, so as to cut off impulses from the ascending, transverse and descending superficial branches of the plexus.

Cervical plexus block gives analgesia of the front and back of the neck, the occipital region, a cape-like area over the shoulders to below the clavicle, and the skin above the third rib anteriorly and above the upper border of the scapula posteriorly. Its chief indication is in thyroidectomy and awake carotid endarterectomy. Complications include:

- phrenic block;
- intrathecal or intravascular injection;
- vagus and/or recurrent laryngeal nerve block, causing aphonia;
- cervical sympathetic block and Horner's syndrome.

SHOULDER AND UPPER LIMB

Suprascapular nerve block

The suprascapular nerve is the sole pathway of somatic pain from the shoulder and acromioclavicular joints and structures surrounding them. The block does not result in any skin analgesia, but when successful, relieves pain in the shoulder joint.

Technique

The patient should be sitting with arms to the sides and head and shoulders slightly flexed. With a skin pencil the spine of the scapula is lined in – the inferior scapular angle is located and bisected by a line, which crosses the first line. A weal is raised one fingerbreadth from the crossing, in the upper outer angle, and a needle is inserted downwards and medially to make contact with the bone of the supraspinatus fossa, just lateral to the notch. The needle is then withdrawn and reintroduced more medially until its point lies in the notch. Paraesthesia takes the form of pain at the tip of the shoulder, and after aspiration 10 mL of local anaesthetic solution is injected.

The block must be at the suprascapular notch because there the nerve is accessible to a needle and no afferent branches leave it before it passes through the notch.

Types of shoulder pain relieved by this block include subacromial bursitis, painful abduction of the arm and calcified deposits about the capsule of the shoulder joint.

Suprascapular nerve block is used for pain relief, not surgery.

Brachial plexus block

Anatomy

The brachial plexus consists of trunks, divisions and cords (Table 4.2.1) derived from the ventral roots of C5 to C8 and T1 nerves. Variable contributions may also come from C4 and T2 nerves.

The trunks are located between the anterior and middle scalene muscles – the C5 and C6 rami unite to form the upper trunk of the plexus, the C7 ramus becomes the middle trunk, and the C8 and T1 rami unite to form the lower trunk.

At the lateral edge of the first rib, the three trunks separate into anterior and posterior divisions.

The anterior divisions of the superior and middle trunks form the lateral cord of the plexus, the posterior divisions of all three trunks form the posterior cord, and the anterior division of the inferior trunk forms the medial cord.

The lateral cord gives rise to the musculocutaneous nerve and the lateral head of the median nerve; the posterior cord forms the radial and axillary nerves; and the medial cord forms the ulnar nerve, the medial head of the median nerve and the medial cutaneous nerve, which joins with the intercostobrachial nerve to innervate the skin over the ulnar aspect of the arm.

The brachial plexus passes into the axilla, surrounded by a fascial sheath descended from the prevertebral fascia separating the anterior and middle scalene muscles.

Within the axillary sheath, thin septa divide the brachial plexus into separate compartments, thus limiting circumferential spread of injected solutions. Division into compartments accounts for the better results of multiple injection axillary block techniques, and for the relative failure of single-injection techniques.

Anterior scalene

The anterior scalene muscle arises from the anterior tubercles of the transverse processes of the third, fourth, fifth and sixth cervical vertebrae. It is inserted into the scalene tubercle on the inner border of the first rib. The

Nerve origin	Nerve	Motor branches	Sensory branches
Roots	Long thoracic	Serratus anterior	
	Dorsal scapular	Levator scapulae, rhomboids	
	Nerve to subclavius		
Trunks	Suprascapular	Supraspinatus, infraspinatus	
Lateral cord	Lateral pectoral	Pectoralis major and minor	
	Musculocutaneous	Coracobrachialis, biceps, brachialis	Lateral cutaneous nerve of arm
	Lateral head of the median		
Posterior cord	Upper subscapular	Subscapularis	
	Thoracodorsal	Latissimus dorsi	
	Lower subscapular	Subscapularis	
	Axillary	Teres minor, deltoid	Upper lateral cutaneous nerve of of arm
	Radial	Triceps, brachioradialis, extensor carpi radialis longus	Posterior cutaneous nerves of arm and forearm, lower lateral cutaneous nerve of arm
	Posterior interosseous branch of radial	Supinator, extensors of fingers and thumb	
	Superficial branch of radial		Skin dorsum of hand
Medial cord	Medial pectoral		Medial cutaneous nerves of arm and forearm
	Median	Pronator teres, flexor carpi radialis flexor digitorum superficialis, palmaris longus, lateral two lumbricals	Palmar cutaneous branch

Table 4.2.1 Motor and sensory innervation of upper limbs

Continued

Nerve origin	Nerve	Motor branches	Sensory branches
	Anterior interosseous branch	Flexor pollicis longus, flexor digitorum profundus, pronator quadrutus, abductor pollicis brevis, flexor pollicis brevis, opponens pollicis	
	Ulnar	Flexor carpi ulnaris, flexor digitorum profundus, palmaris brevis	Dorsal and palmar cutaneous branches
	Deep terminal branch of ulnar	Flexor and abductor, opponens digiti minimi, four palmar interossei, four dorsal interossei, two lumbricals, adductor pollicis	

Table 4.2.1 Motor and sensory innervation of upper limbs—cont'd

muscle lies anterior to the brachial plexus, being separated from it below by the subclavian artery. Its lateral border, if it is palpable, is a guide to the position of the plexus.

Medial scalene

The medial scalene muscle arises from the posterior tubercles of the six lowest cervical vertebrae and is inserted into the upper surface of the first rib behind the groove made by the brachial plexus and the subclavian artery. The plexus thus lies in front of the muscle.

First rib

The first rib lies in an almost horizontal plane, being inclined slightly downwards and forwards. It passes below the clavicle at about the junction of its inner and middle thirds. The head has a single articular facet, which articulates with the body of the first thoracic vertebra. The tubercle articulates with the transverse process of the same vertebra. The upper surface has two transverse grooves – an anterior one for the subclavian vein and a posterior one for the subclavian artery and the lowest trunk of the brachial plexus. On the inner border, between the grooves, is the scalene tubercle.

The subclavius muscle originates in front of the anterior groove and the scalenus medius is inserted behind the posterior groove.

The lower surface of the first rib has no costal groove – the inner border embraces the dome of the pleura and the outer border gives origin to the first slip of the serratus anterior.

Subclavian artery

The subclavian artery extends from its origin to the outer border of the first rib. The right subclavian artery comes from the innominate artery, the left from the aortic arch.

A major portion of the brachial plexus is located parallel and lateral to the third part of the subclavian and first part of the axillary artery, just above and below the clavicle, respectively.

The third part of the subclavian artery extends from the outer border of the anterior scalene muscle laterally and caudally to the outer border of the first rib, where it becomes the first part of the axillary artery.

The terminal part of the subclavian artery lies behind the clavicle near its midpoint. At this level the inferior trunk of the brachial plexus is posterior to the third part of the subclavian artery. The upper two trunks of the brachial plexus are superior and lateral to the subclavian artery.

Subclavian vein

The subclavian vein is separated from the brachial plexus by the anterior scalene muscle. As it is well protected by the clavicle, it is unlikely to be punctured.

The brachial line

The brachial line runs in a straight line from the transverse process of the sixth cervical vertebra to the axillary artery in the axilla. It runs inferolateral at 45° from the horizontal and slightly forwards at 15°.

Technique

Interscalene block (anterior approach)

To provide satisfactory anaesthesia for shoulder surgery it is necessary to block the upper and middle trunks of the brachial plexus within the interscalene groove. At least five approaches have been developed – the three anterior approaches are the:

- Winnie approach;
- Meier approach;
- modified lateral approach of Borgeat.

The two posterior approaches are the:

- Kappis/Pippa approach;
- Boezaart approach.

For anterior approaches the patient should lie supine, without a pillow, neck extended and turned slightly to the contralateral side and with the arm placed on the abdomen.

Lifting the head readily demonstrates the posterior edge of the sternocleidomastoid muscle.

The initial interscalene block, described by Winnie in 1970,[18] involved gentle palpation of the interscalene groove just behind the sternocleidomastoid at the level of the cricoid cartilage and a single injection of local anaesthetic directed in a medial, dorsal and caudal direction. The needle should be perpendicular to the skin in every plane. The plexus is very superficial (0.7–1.5 cm; in obese patients no more than 2.5 cm).

Only electrical nerve stimulation of muscles below the shoulder is acceptable (biceps or triceps). Alternative twitches arise from muscles innervated by other nerves, which are located in the posterior triangle. These are (from anterior to posterior) – diaphragm (phrenic nerve), rhomboids (dorsal scapular nerve), levator scapulae (nerve to levator scapulae) and trapezius (accessory nerve).

Directing needles medially, however, led in some cases to inadvertent injection into the vertebral artery, epidural space or cerebrospinal fluid (CSF), and Winnie's approach was subsequently modified by Meier et al.[19] In this modification the puncture point is at the posterior edge of the sternocleidomastoid muscle, but located 2–3 cm more cranially, at the level of the superior thyroid notch. The puncture is directed caudal at 30° to the skin and slightly lateral, aiming for the mid to lateral point of the clavicle. This approach is recommended for interscalene catheter insertion.

The modified lateral approach of Borgeat uses the same insertion point as Winnie, but directs the needle along the interscalene space, towards the posterior part of the superior or middle trunk in order to elicit triceps contractions. Using this approach in 700 adults, a catheter was inserted first time in 86% of patients and difficulty threading the catheter was encountered in 6%.[20] For longlasting analgesia, levobupivacaine and ropivacaine are the preferred local anaesthetics.

Injection of 30 mL levobupivacaine 0.5% or ropivacaine 0.5% provides anaesthesia of similar onset, intensity and duration.[21] Lidocaine (lignocaine) provides a faster onset of block, but is associated with poorer pain relief and a longer duration of motor block than ropivacaine.[22]

Interscalene (cervical approach)

The posterior approach to the brachial plexus was initially described by Kappis in 1912 and latterly by Pippa.[23] The advantage of the technique is that the needle only passes through muscle and not nerves or arteries.

The technique involves maximally flexing the head and palpating the spinal processes of the sixth and seventh cervical vertebrae. Differentiating between both is simple. On neck extension, the spinal process of the sixth cervical vertebra moves forward; the more prominent seventh cervical vertebra does not move. Midway between the spinous processes of the sixth and seventh cervical vertebrae, a horizontal line of 3 cm is drawn laterally.

After connecting a nerve stimulator, a 10 cm insulated needle is inserted in a sagittal plane (aiming for the cricoid cartilage) and contact is made with the transverse process of the seventh cervical vertebra after 5–6 cm. The needle is then redirected more cranially and should locate the brachial plexus after 6–8 cm – confirmed by muscle contractions of the shoulder or abduction of the arm, corresponding to upper trunk (C5–C6) stimulation.

The volume of 0.5% bupivacaine, levobupivacaine or ropivacaine sufficient for shoulder surgery is between 0.25 mL/kg and 0.5 mL/kg.

The spread of local anaesthetic after interscalene block may spare the lower nerve roots and is therefore inappropriate for surgery below the elbow.

Injection of local anaesthetic into the higher brachial plexus often leads to incomplete analgesia of skin supplied by the lower brachial plexus. For example, block of the ulnar innervation of the hand may only occur in 70% of patients.

For upper arm surgery, supplementation of an interscalene block is sometimes necessary – subcutaneous infiltration on the inner side of the upper arm blocks the intercostobrachial nerve block, enabling tourniquet use.

With the Boezaart approach,[24] start at the level of the first costovertebral angle and insert the needle into the V-shaped groove between the anterolateral edge of trapezius and the posteromedial edge of levator scapulae, aiming 45° from a parasagittal plane and 30° caudal towards the sternal notch.

Once the bony transverse process of the sixth cervical vertebra is identified, the block needle is repositioned, aiming anteriorly and using a loss of resistance technique.

Both posterior approaches are associated with less motor block than the anterior approaches to the brachial plexus.

For arthroscopic shoulder surgery it is important to block axillary, suprascapular and supraclavicular nerves.

For open surgery, the intercostobrachial nerves may also be blocked.

Prospective, randomised controlled trials have demonstrated that the use of continuous interscalene analgesia provides better pain relief, reduces requirements for postoperative opioids, reduces opioid-related side-effects, and provides better patient satisfaction for at least the first 48 hours after surgery.[25] The benefits of pain relief on physiotherapy and functional outcomes have not been investigated.

The provision of optimal analgesia after shoulder surgery in the ambulatory setting remains difficult.

A single interscalene injection provides pain relief for a mean (range) duration of 22.5 hours (9–48 hours).[26] Administration of local anaesthetic by patient-controlled interscalene analgesia has had mixed results.

A background infusion of 0.2% ropivacaine 4 mL/h with a 6 mL bolus was associated with more breakthrough pain, greater sleep disturbance and a decrease in analgesia satisfaction compared to higher basal rates of infusion 0.2% ropivacaine 8 mL/h with a 2 mL bolus.[27]

Side-effects of all interscalene nerve blocks include phrenic nerve paralysis (85–100%), Horner's syndrome (75%), recurrent laryngeal nerve paralysis (20%), vessel puncture (external jugular vein, internal jugular vein, common carotid artery) and, rarely, pneumothorax (except the Pippa technique). Horner's syndrome consists of miosis, ptosis and anhidrosis. Recurrent laryngeal nerve paralysis consists of hoarseness, difficulty coughing and stridor.

Unilateral diaphragmatic paralysis due to phrenic nerve palsy is an inevitable consequence of interscalene brachial plexus block[28] and is associated with significant reductions in forced vital capacity, forced expiratory volume and peak flow rates. However, the incidence of phrenic nerve paralysis with interscalene catheters is only 20% because the catheter travels 3–5 cm caudally within the sheath. Thus an interscalene catheter should be the technique of choice in patients with impaired respiratory function.

Comparison of the Pippa technique with the Winnie approach to the brachial plexus has shown more complications with the latter technique.

Contraindications to interscalene nerve blocks include contralateral phrenic nerve or recurrent laryngeal nerve paralysis The long-term incidence of neurological complications with the lateral modified approach is 2.4% at 1 month and 0.3% at 3 months.[20]

Supraclavicular block

Three approaches have been developed for supraclavicular block:

- the classic supraclavicular approach of Kulenkampff;
- the subclavian perivascular approach of Winnie and Collins;
- the modified lateral paravascular approach of Moorthy.

The classic supraclavicular approach of Kulenkampff has been largely replaced by upper limb blocks with better success rates and fewer complications.

For supraclavicular block, the patient should be positioned supine and the neck rotated slightly to the contralateral side.

In the midclavicular line, 1 cm posterior to the clavicle and lateral to the axillary artery, the needle is placed and directed posteriorly, medially and caudally until the brachial plexus is located. If it is not found, the needle is 'walked' along the clavicle. However, this approach may be associated with pneumothorax (2–6%), which is suspected by coughing as the dome of the pleura is stimulated.

With the subclavian perivascular approach of Winnie and Collins,[29] the subclavian artery is palpated immediately lateral to the clavicular head of sternocleidomastoid at the level of the cricoid cartilage (sixth cervical vertebra). A 3–4 cm needle is inserted behind the subclavian artery and, after paraesthesia, 40 mL of local anaesthetic is injected.

With the modified lateral paravascular approach of Moorthy,[30] positioning is the same as for the classic approach. The course of the subclavian artery from above to below the clavicle and into the axilla is marked. The needle is advanced along and parallel to the surface marking of the subclavian artery, caudally, laterally, and posteriorly, the tip of the needle being directed towards the axilla and away from the pleura, medial and inferior to the subclavian artery.

Infraclavicular block

The infraclavicular approach to the brachial plexus is the preferred choice for anaesthesia of the elbow and lower arm because spread of local anaesthetic is kept below the clavicle.[31] The brachial plexus is wide at its multi-root origin, but then narrows at the level of the cords as it passes below the clavicle before widening again into its divisions.

Three basic techniques have been described;

- Raj approach;[32]
- coracoid approach;[33]
- vertical infraclavicular approach.[34]

All place local anaesthetic below the clavicle, but on a line passing from the neck, under the clavicle and into the axilla.

The initial Raj technique[32] is associated with technical difficulties and a lower success rate than axillary blocks. The procedure involves insertion of a needle 2.5 cm below the midpoint of the clavicle, aiming at the axillary artery in the 'brachial line' in the axilla.

The coracoid approach involves inserting a needle 2 cm medial and 2 cm caudal to the coracoid process, directly posterior and perpendicular to the skin. The needle, at a mean distance of 4 cm, will contact the cords of the brachial plexus.[35]

Another method has been described based on measurements from cadaver dissection – the vertical infraclavicular approach (VIB).[34] Studies of cadavers have show that the brachial plexus lies at a maximum depth of 4 cm, and lateral to the axillary artery and vein, where the three cords converge at the entrance to the trigonum of the clavipectoral fascia. This corresponds to a skin puncture point corresponding to the halfway point between the ventral apophysis of the acromion and the jugular notch (infraclavicular line).

To identify the ventral apophysis, follow the crest of the scapula laterally to the acromion then ventrally. The correct ventral position is confirmed when the anaesthetist's fingers remain static during movement of the shoulder joint. At the calculated midpoint, the needle is inserted vertically in all planes.

The advantages of the vertical infraclavicular block are that it is simple to learn, it has a high success rate, tourniquets are easily tolerated, patients are positioned comfortably and insertion of a catheter is simple. However, with upper arm blocks, catheters only tend to travel 3–5 cm within neural sheaths.

Despite the close relationship of cords at this level, studies show that identifying the lateral, medial, and posterior cords with either a nerve stimulator[36] or ultrasound guidance[7] improves onset time, duration and overall success rate of infraclavicular block. The advantage of ultrasound guidance is that spread of injectate within the sheath may be seen and a catheter placed exactly under vision.

A modification of the VIB has been suggested. For every 1 cm increase or decrease in the length of the infraclavicular line from a mean of 22 cm, the corresponding site of insertion is shifted 2 mm laterally or medially.[37] An easy guide to evaluating the motor responses to electrical stimulation during infraclavicular block is if the arm is positioned in the anatomical position, the fifth digit moves laterally (pronation of the forearm) when the lateral cord is stimulated, posteriorly (extension) when the posterior cord is stimulated, and medially (flexion) when the medial cord is stimulated.[38]

Maintaining postoperative pain relief with infraclavicular catheters is best served with a combination of background infusion and patient-controlled boluses. Reliance on either constant infusions or boluses alone is associated with more breakthrough pain and less patient satisfaction.[39]

Axillary block

In the axilla, branches of the brachial plexus envelope the axillary artery. The median and musculocutaneous nerves together with their sensory branches are anterior or anterolateral (i.e. above the artery), the ulnar nerve is inferior, and the radial nerve is below and behind the vessel).

The musculocutaneous nerve is given off high in the axilla and resides within the body of the coracobrachialis muscle.

Ultrasound examination of volunteers has increased knowledge of the relationships between the axillary artery and nerves;[40] anatomical variation and asymmetry are common.

As the three main nerves begin to move apart from each other shortly after passing the lateral edge of the pectoralis minor muscle, complete brachial plexus block at the axilla is more likely the more proximal the approach.

The axillary brachial plexus block was first described by Halstead in 1884. Its advantages are the presence of one landmark (the axillary artery), and no possibility of pneumothorax, stellate ganglion block, recurrent laryngeal nerve block or phrenic nerve block.

Techniques described for axillary block include transarterial injection, palpation of fascial clicks, and single and multiple injections.

Common to all techniques is the position of the patient. With the patient lying supine, the arm to be blocked is abducted no more than 90°

and should be positioned on an arm board. Excessive abduction in the shoulder joint should be avoided because it makes palpation of the axillary artery pulse difficult and increases the risk of nerve injury by stretching the brachial plexus.

The anaesthetist's index finger should palpate the pulse of the axillary artery at the midaxillary fossa level. This shortens the distance between the needle insertion site and the brachial plexus block by compressing the subcutaneous tissue and stabilises the position of the artery and needle during performance of the block. This finger should not be moved during multiple injections.

Axillary block techniques using multiple injections[41,42] have reported higher success rates, shorter latency, and/or more complete block than with single-shot techniques. It would appear that ulnar nerve stimulation is not necessary for block success. Although multiple stimulations require more time, readiness for surgery may actually be faster.

Use of high doses (225 mg) of bupivacaine, levobupivacaine and ropivacaine for axillary block has shown slightly better sensory and motor block intensity with ropivacaine.[43] Complete motor block at the elbow was more frequent in the ropivacaine group (67%) than in the bupivacaine (47%) and levobupivacaine groups (30%) ($P < 0.01$).

The incidence of neurological deficits with axillary block is no different between single and multiple injection techniques (<2%).[44] However, the use of multi-injection axillary block is decreasing in modern practice as infraclavicular blocks become more popular.[45]

Bier's block

For Bier's block two cannulae should be inserted, one in the dorsum of the hand and another in a vein in the other limb in case of toxic signs. Veins in the forearm or antecubital fossa are best avoided.

The limb is drained of blood by elevation for 5 minutes, with or without compression of the brachial artery. An Esmarch bandage, the Rhys–Davies exsanguinator (an inflatable pneumatic cylinder, which is easier to apply and less uncomfortable) or an orthopaedic pneumatic splint can all be used for this purpose.

A dedicated double cuff is securely placed on the upper arm, and the upper one is inflated to a pressure a little above the systolic blood pressure, before removal of the compression or pneumatic bandage.

Injection of the local anaesthetic solution follows, and after 5–10 minutes, the lower cuff is inflated and the upper one released, to minimise discomfort. A tourniquet that does not occlude the brachial artery throughout the operation may result in congestion of the limb, absorption of the drug and imperfect analgesia. Close attention to detail and to the efficiency of the apparatus is most important.

The patient is ready for operation after an interval of 10 minutes.

Analgesia and motor weakness continue while the tourniquet remains inflated.

Bier's block has been used successfully in children, and also on the lower limb, in which case the cuff should be placed on the mid-calf.

Local anaesthetic solutions

Preservative-free 0.5% lidocaine (lignocaine) and prilocaine are effective and relatively safe; the usual volume required is 3–4 mg/kg. In contrast, bupivacaine is efficient but potentially toxic, and should not be used.

Cuff deflation

Cuff deflation is best done in stages, although an interosseous leak may occur. Local anaesthetic drug is released into the circulation in a biphasic manner. There is an initial fast release of 30%, but 50% may still be present in the limb 30 minutes later.

Toxic signs include drowsiness, twitches, jactitations or convulsions and bradycardia proceeding to asystole, hypotension and ECG abnormalities. The patient should be carefully observed during the 10 minutes following release of the cuff. Reinflation may be considered if signs of toxicity arise.

Contraindications

Contraindications for Bier's block include:

- Raynaud's disease;
- sickle cell anaemia ;
- scleroderma.

Distal nerve blocks

Distal nerve blocks provide analgesia in the presence of systemic infection or anticoagulation, and are used for day-case surgical procedures such as median nerve decompression, repair of lacerations, tendons or nerves, and excision of small lesions. They also supplement insufficient brachial plexus block.

Elbow blocks

Median nerve

In the cubital fossa the median nerve lies medial and relatively deep to the brachial artery, partially covered by the biceps muscle tendon. It supplies the superficial forearm muscles, passes between the two heads of pronator teres and gives off the anterior interosseous nerve, which supplies the deep forearm muscles.

For median nerve block, the needle is inserted 1 cm medial to the tendon and 2 cm cranial to the intercondylar line. The volume of injectate is the same as radial nerve block at the wrist: 5 mL of local anaesthetic to the nerve and 5 mL within the superficial tissues on withdrawal of the needle in order to block the medial cutaneous nerve of forearm.

Ulnar nerve

The ulnar nerve passes through flexor carpi ulnaris, supplying it, and enters the cubital fossa medially. In the forearm it supplies the ulnar half of flexor digitorum profundus.

For ulnar nerve block, the patient is placed in the supine position and the elbow flexed 30°. The needle is introduced between the median condyle and the olecranon and advanced 1–2 cm proximally in order to avoid nerve damage due to the volume injected.

Radial nerve

The radial nerve lies between the biceps and brachioradialis muscles, 1 cm cranial to a line dissecting the medial and lateral condyles of the humerus (intercondylar line). Below this point, the nerve divides into a deep motor branch (posterior interosseous nerve) to supinator and the wrist and finger extensors, and a superficial cutaneous branch, passing with the radial artery to the dorsum of the wrist and dorsal aspects of the thumb, index and middle fingers.

For radial nerve block, the needle is advanced slightly medial and cephalad between the biceps and brachioradialis muscle, and 5 mL of local anaesthetic solution are injected, with another 5 mL injected on withdrawal into the subcutaneous tissue to block the lateral cutaneous nerve of the forearm.

Wrist blocks

Median nerve

At the wrist, the median nerve lies between the palmaris longus tendon and flexor carpi radialis. The median nerve has a palmar cutaneous branch and a deep nerve, which passes through the flexor retinaculum into the carpal tunnel, supplying thenar muscles and the skin of the thumb and lateral two and a half fingers together with the skin over the dorsal aspects of their terminal phalanges.

A needle is inserted through the deep fascia of the wrist, 1–2 cm proximal to the flexor skin crease of the wrist and immediately lateral to the tendon of the palmaris longus. As the needle is withdrawn, a subcutaneous injection is made to block the palmar cutaneous branch.

Ulnar nerve

The ulnar nerve lies lateral to the flexor carpi ulnaris tendon and superficial to the flexor retinaculum. It supplies the skin of the medial one and a half fingers and has a deep branch, which supplies most of the small muscles in the hand. Ulnar nerve block is performed by inserting a block needle at the level of the ulnar styloid process laterally, under the flexor carpi ulnaris tendon, and injecting 5 mL of local anaesthetic.

Radial nerve

In the lower forearm, the radial nerve passes round to the back of the hand and is sensory to the skin over the first web space, thumb and lateral one and a half fingers.

The radial nerve block is actually a field block of the superficial terminal branches as they pass over the radial side of the carpus.

For radial nerve block, the anatomical 'snuffbox' and the extensor pollicis longus tendon are made prominent by extension of the thumb. A needle are inserted over the tendon opposite the base of the first metacarpal and advanced proximally along the tendon while 2 mL of local anaesthetic solution are injected. The needle is than withdrawn almost to the skin and a subcutaneous injection of 5–8 mL of local anaesthetic solution is made across the dorsal aspect of the wrist (at the level of the ulnar styloid) to block the terminal dorsal branches of the nerve.

Digital nerve block

Two palmar and two dorsal nerves supply each digit. With a fine (25 G) needle an intradermal weal is raised on the dorsum of the finger near its base and 2 mL of 1 or 2% lidocaine (lignocaine) (or one of its congeners) solution are injected into the substance of the finger through this weal between the bone and the skin and repeated on the other side of the digit.

The weals should be connected by 1 mL of solution between skin and bone on the dorsal aspect. Analgesia may take 15 minutes to become established. The palmar skin is not pierced.

Precautions

For digital nerve block:

- epinephrine (adrenaline) should not be used;
- if a tourniquet is used no more than 3 mL of solution should be injected;
- a tourniquet must not remain on the finger for more than 15 minutes and must not used at all in patients with Raynaud's disease.

HIP AND LOWER LIMB

Single-limb anaesthesia is increasing in popularity for ambulatory and major surgery. Block of only one limb enables mobilisation, obviates catheterisation and provides extensive postoperative pain relief. However, the advantages may be overshadowed by increased anaesthetic time, a need sometimes for two injections, and some tourniquet discomfort. Often lower limb blocks are combined with either general or spinal anaesthesia.

Anatomy of the lumbar plexus

The lumbosacral plexus innervates the lower leg. It is formed from the anterior primary rami of T12 to L4 and is enveloped within a sheath between the psoas major muscle and the quadratus lumborum muscle.

The anterior root of L1 divides into the ilioinguinal nerve and the iliohypogastric nerve, and sends a contribution to the genitofemoral nerve.

The L2, L3 and L4 roots divide into anterior and posterior divisions. The anterior division of L2 joins with L1 to form the genitofemoral nerve. The anterior divisions of L2, L3 and L4 descend as the obturator nerve. The posterior divisions of L2, L3 and L4 converge to form the lateral cutaneous nerve of thigh and the femoral nerve.

Iliohypogastric nerve (L1)

The iliohypogastric nerve leaves the psoas major, crosses the quadratus lumborum, perforates the transversus abdominis and then divides into lateral and anterior cutaneous branches. Its lateral cutaneous branch supplies the skin on the anterior part of the gluteal region after piercing the internal and external oblique muscles 5 cm behind the anterior superior iliac spine and just above the iliac crest, while the terminal part of the nerve supplies the skin over the pubic bone after piercing the aponeurosis of the external oblique, 2 cm medial to the anterior superior iliac spine. It does not divide into anterior and posterior branches.

Ilioinguinal nerve (L1)

The ilioinguinal nerve accompanies the iliohypogastric nerve in its early course, lying just inferior to it in close relationship to the iliac crest. About 2 cm anterior and just below the anterior superior spine, it pierces the internal oblique and runs medially behind the aponeurosis of the external oblique. It then passes with the spermatic cord through the inguinal canal and supplies the skin of the upper and medial part of the thigh and the adjacent skin covering the external genitalia. It has no lateral cutaneous branch, unlike the iliohypogastric nerve, and in the inguinal canal is sensory.

Genitofemoral nerve (L1, L2)

The genital branch of the genitofemoral nerve supplies the skin of the scrotum or labium majus, and is motor to the cremaster muscle. The femoral branch supplies an area of skin on the middle of the anterior surface of the upper part of the thigh.

Lateral cutaneous nerve of the thigh (L2, L3 – posterior divisions)

The lateral cutaneous nerve of the thigh supplies the skin of the anterolateral aspect of the thigh as far as the knee anteriorly, but laterally not quite so low after passing behind the inguinal ligament and the sartorius muscle, just medial and slightly inferior to the anterior superior iliac spine.

Femoral nerve (L2, L3, L4 – posterior divisions)

The femoral nerve emerges from the psoas major, passes between it and the iliacus, and enters the thigh behind the inguinal ligament and just lateral to the femoral artery, from which it is separated by a slip of the psoas major. It has anterior and posterior divisions, the former giving rise to the saphenous nerve, which extends to the medial lower leg and the medial and intermediate cutaneous nerves of the thigh.

The femoral nerve supplies the hip joint and knee joint, the skin of the anterior part of the thigh and the anteromedial part of the leg. It is motor to the quadriceps femoris, the sartorius and the pectineus (Table 4.2.2).

Obturator nerve (L2, L3, L4 – anterior divisions)

The obturator nerve emerges from the medial border of the psoas muscle where it is a posterior relation of the external iliac vessels. After running forwards on the lateral wall of the pelvis it pierces the obturator canal and divides into anterior and posterior branches; the former supply the adductor longus and brevis and the gracilis, with a branch going to the hip joint; the posterior branch supplies the adductor magnus and the hip joint.

The obturator nerve supplies an area of skin on the medial aspect of the thigh and sends a small branch to the knee joint.

An accessory obturator nerve is present in about 25% of people and runs a variable course across the superior pubic ramus.

Nerve	Muscle	Function
Femoral	Quadriceps femoris	Flexes hip, extends knee
Obturator nerve	Adductors of thigh	Adduct thigh
Tibial nerve	Biceps femoris muscle	Flexes knee and rotates leg laterally
	Semimembranosus muscle	Flexes knee
	Semitendinosus muscle	Extends thigh, flexes leg and rotates it medially
	Flexor hallucis longus	Flexes foot
	Flexor digitorum longus	Flexes toes
Common peroneal nerve	Tibialis anterior, extensor digitorum muscles, extensor hallucis muscles, peroneal muscles	Dorsiflexion and inversion of foot, extend, evert and pronate the outer foot

Table 4.2.2 Lower leg muscle innervation and function

Femoral block

For lower limb block, combinations of femoral and sciatic nerve blocks are the mainstay of anaesthetic techniques.

Femoral block is ideal for anterior cruciate ligament surgery and knee arthroplasty.

The patient should lie supine. The needle is inserted 1.5 cm lateral to the femoral artery, approximately 2 cm below the inguinal ligament and 30° to the skin and advanced in a cranial direction. Contractions of the quadriceps femoris muscle and movement of the patella are necessary to locate the femoral nerve accurately. Injection of 15 mL is sufficient for femoral block alone.

The technique of simultaneously blocking the femoral, the lateral cutaneous and the obturator nerves by a single injection of local anaesthetic (three in one) was first described in 1973,[46] and it was suggested that the underlying mechanism was one of cephalad spread resulting in a blockade of the lumbar plexus. However, this block is difficult to achieve in practice. Magnetic resonance imaging of 30 mL of bupivacaine 0.5% has shown lateral spread from the femoral nerve to the lateral cutaneous nerve and slight medial spread to the anterior branch of the obturator nerve. No involvement of the proximal and posterior portions of the obturator nerve was observed, nor was there any cephalad spread that could have resulted in a lumbar plexus blockade.[47] Even placing a catheter 15–20 cm within the femoral nerve sheath does not guarantee lumbar plexus block.

In a study of 100 patients,[48] injection of radiographic contrast down the femoral catheter reached the lumbar plexus in only 23%. Of these patients, 91% achieved a three-in-one block by sensory/motor evaluation. Most patients had two nerves blocked depending on the direction of the catheter.

In clinical practice, insertion of a femoral catheter 5 cm provides excellent pain relief and ability to straight leg raise.

Confirmation comes from rehabilitation outcome studies of continuous femoral block for knee arthroplasty. Two studies comparing femoral catheter infusions with epidural infusions and PCA morphine have shown equivalent pain relief to the former and fewer side-effects than the latter.[49,50] Furthermore, the improved pain relief with femoral blocks allowed earlier mobilisation and reduced hospital stay and overall rehabilitation.

Lateral cutaneous nerve of thigh block

For lateral cutaneous nerve of thigh block a weal is raised one fingerbreadth below and medial to the anterior superior spine of the ilium. A needle is inserted perpendicularly to the skin and 1% lidocaine (lignocaine) is deposited between the skin and the iliac bone and along the pelvic brim for two fingerbreadths internally to the anterior superior spine; 10–15 mL of solution are used. The nerve lies deep to the fascia lata of the thigh. When associated with femoral block, adequate analgesia is produced for taking skin grafts from the front of the thigh.

Obturator nerve block

The anterior and posterior divisions of the obturator nerve are blocked as they lie in the obturator canal below the superior ramus of the pubis, between the pectineus and the obturator externus. The following technique can be used – the patient lies supine with the leg slightly abducted. A skin mark is made halfway between the pubic tubercle and femoral artery, 2–3 cm below the inguinal ligament. The pubic ramus is palpated here and a disposable 18 G spinal needle inserted to strike the bone. The needle is then withdrawn slightly and turned through 90° to a point about 2 cm below the superior ramus and parallel to the shaft of the femur. The needle is now advanced into the obturator foramen by a forward movement of 4–5 cm. After aspiration tests, and provided there is no resistance to injection, 10 mL of local anaesthetic solution are deposited.

Psoas compartment block

The lumbar plexus may also be blocked by the psoas compartment approach. This was first described by Chayen et al. in 1976. The technique of Capdevila, based on evidence from CT scanning, is now recommended.[51] With the patient in the lateral decubitus position and operative side up, the needle is inserted 3 cm caudal and 5 cm lateral to the spinous process of the fourth lumbar vertebra, two-thirds of the distance between the midline and the intercristal line, which runs vertically through the posterior superior iliac spines. It is important to contact the transverse process of the fourth lumbar vertebra in order to judge the depth of needle insertion. The needle is then redirected underneath the transverse process.

The lumbar plexus lies 1–2 cm beyond the transverse process of the fourth lumbar vertebra. The median lumbar plexus depth is 85 mm in men and 70 mm in women, but the same distance beyond the transverse process. Contraction of the quadriceps muscle indicates close proximity to the lumbar plexus, and 30 mL of local anaesthetic solution is injected when muscle contraction is stimulated using an electrical current between 0.2 and 0.5 mA A plexus catheter is then advanced 3–5 cm past the needle orifice.

Studies have shown that the plexus lies within the psoas major muscle in three-quarters of patients and between psoas and quadratus lumborum in the other quarter.

The advantages of the posterior approach to the lumbar plexus are that it is easy to perform and provides a more consistent block of the obturator nerve than the femoral approach, greater haemodynamic stability than epidural analgesia, better pain relief and fewer side-effects than PCA, and better overall patient satisfaction.

Despite the large distance between skin and nerves ultrasonic guidance has successfully placed needles onto the lumbar plexus using low-frequency ultrasound.

Comparison of lumbar plexus block and femoral block with PCA morphine has shown reduced pain scores, halving of morphine requirements and a similar pharmacokinetic profile with both regional modalities.[52,53]

Psoas compartment block is associated with two major complications – retroperitoneal haematoma and total spinal anaesthesia. Lumbar plexus catheters, like epidurals, should be removed 12 hours after low molecular weight heparin (LMWH) administration to minimise haematoma formation.

Total spinal anaesthesia is not uncommon with lumbar plexus block, especially when combined with spinal anaesthesia. Large volumes injected around the lumbar plexus may spread back through the intervertebral foramen, compressing the dura and increasing the height of any accompanying spinal block. Typical signs of total spinal injection include difficulty speaking, poor respiratory effort, bilateral arm weakness, bradycardia and hypotension. Patients require intubation, ventilation and general anaesthesia until the spinal block subsides.

Anatomy of the sacral plexus

The sacral plexus is composed of the lumbosacral trunk (L4, L5) and the ventral rami of the upper four sacral nerves (S1–S4). They lie on the posterior wall of the pelvic cavity between the piriformis and the pelvic fascia and have in front the ureter, the internal iliac vessels, and the sigmoid colon on the left. The sacral plexus passes out of the pelvis through the greater sciatic foramen.

Posterior cutaneous nerve of the thigh (S1–S3)

The posterior cutaneous nerve of the thigh supplies the skin of the lower part of the gluteal region, the perineum and the back of the thigh and leg.

Sciatic nerve (L4, L5, S1–S3)

The sciatic nerve leaves the pelvis through the greater sciatic foramen and passes in an arc below the gluteal muscles and down the posterior aspect of the thigh midway between the greater trochanter of the femur and the ischial tuberosity. From the lower margin of piriformis, it passes into the buttock on the posterior surface of the ischium.

From midway between the greater trochanter and the ischial tuberosity, deep to gluteus maximus, the sciatic nerve passes vertically downwards into the hamstring compartment. It lies posterior to obturator internus, the gemelli, quadratus femoris and adductor magnus, but is crossed posteriorly by the long head of biceps femoris. It supplies all the hamstring muscles.

At the upper angle of the popliteal fossa (or occasionally within the pelvis) the sciatic nerve separates into the tibial nerve and the common peroneal nerve; in approximately 3% of people the two may separate at higher levels in the pelvis.

Tibial nerve

The tibial nerve passes down the leg deep to soleus, and at the ankle divides into medial and lateral plantar branches which supply the muscles and deep structures of the sole of the foot. The tibial nerve also gives rise to the medial calcaneal nerve, which supplies the heel.

Common peroneal nerve

The common peroneal nerve turns round the neck of the fibula and divides into the deep peroneal (or anterior tibial) and superficial peroneal nerves.

The superficial peroneal nerve supplies peroneus longus and brevis and emerges between them to supply the skin of the lower leg and much of the dorsum of the foot (except the skin of the first web space and the lateral side of the fifth toe).

The deep peroneal nerve passes into the anterior compartment of the leg to supply the anterior compartment muscles.

Perforating cutaneous nerve (S2 and S3)

The perforating cutaneous nerve supplies the skin over the medial and lower parts of the gluteus maximus.

Pudendal nerve

The pudendal nerve leaves the pelvis through the greater sciatic foramen, crosses the ischial spine medial to the pudendal vessels and goes through the lesser sciatic foramen. With the pudendal vessels it passes upwards and forwards along the lateral wall of the ischiorectal fossa, in Alcock's canal, a sheath of the obturator fascia. It gives off:

- the inferior rectal nerve supplying the external anal sphincter and the skin around the anus;
- the perineal nerve supplying the skin of the scrotum or labium majus;
- the dorsal nerve of the penis or clitoris;
- the medial and lateral posterior scrotal (or labial) nerves;
- visceral branches supplying the rectum and bladder.

Sciatic block

Postoperative pain is generally worse after knee arthroplasty than after hip arthroplasty, and adequate analgesia after knee replacement is difficult to achieve with femoral analgesia alone. Recent studies are now showing that addition of a sciatic block to femoral block in patients after knee replacement improves pain relief and reduces rescue morphine consumption.[54] Sciatic nerve block gives analgesia of the whole foot with the exception of an area of skin over the medial malleolus supplied by the saphenous branch of the femoral nerve

Several posterior, lateral and anterior approaches to the sciatic nerve have been described. Posterior approaches include the transgluteal (Labat), parasacral[55] and subgluteal.[56]

Transgluteal approach

In the transgluteal approach the patient is placed in the lateral position, with the leg to be blocked uppermost. The other leg is extended and a pillow placed between the legs for comfort. The upper leg is bent approximately 30–40° at the hip joint and approximately 90° at the knee joint. A line is drawn 5 cm perpendicularly from the midpoint of the line connecting the greater trochanter and the posterior superior iliac spine and a needle is inserted perpendicularly. Often gluteal muscle contraction will be observed before dorsiflexion of the foot. In thin patients, the sciatic nerve may be palpable.

Parasacral approach

For the parasacral approach[57] a line is drawn between the posterior superior iliac spine and the ischial tuberosity – needle entry is 6 cm inferior to the posterior superior iliac spine.

All patients develop a full sensory block of all three major components of the sciatic plexus (tibial, common peroneal, and posterior cutaneous nerve of the thigh).

Some practitioners prefer this approach for inserting sciatic catheters.

Subgluteal approach

In the subgluteal approach a line is drawn from the greater trochanter to the ischial tuberosity; then, from the midpoint of this line, a second line is extended caudally for 4 cm in the depression between biceps femoris and semitendinosus. The end of this line represents the site of needle entry.

The subgluteal approach provides anaesthesia of similar quality to the transgluteal approach, but with less discomfort.[58] Separate block of the peroneal and tibial components is associated with a faster onset of anaesthesia than with single injection. However, the double injection technique causes more patient discomfort during establishment of the nerve block.[59]

Supine posterior approach

For the supine posterior approach[32] the patient is in a supine position with the leg in slightly more than 90° flexion. The midpoint of a line drawn between the greater trochanter and the ischial tuberosity is located. The 10 cm needle is inserted perpendicularly to the skin and the peripheral nerve stimulator activated. The needle is advanced slowly for about 5–8 cm until plantar or dorsal flexion of the foot is noted and 20 mL of local anaesthetic solution are injected.

If the motor response cannot be obtained after 8 cm depth the needle should be redirected, first slightly medially and than laterally across the drawn line. This block is relatively easy to perform even in the obese patient because the nerve lies more superficially (due to the stretched gluteal muscles) than with other approaches. From the practical point of view the biggest problem is the need for an assistant who is physically able to hold the leg in flexion during the procedure.

Lateral approach

Lateral approaches (Guardini) to the sciatic nerve block have also been described.[60] As the patient remains in the supine position, the lateral approach is a convenient alternative to the posterior approach.

A line is drawn distally from the greater trochanter, on the posterior margin of the femur. Three to 5 cm distal from the greater trochanter, a 12–15 cm needle is inserted through the skin perpendicular to the major axis of the limb, connected to a peripheral nerve stimulator and advanced to contact the bone. The needle is then redirected posteriorly to slide off the bone and advanced under the femur to elicit contraction of the calf or dorsal flexion of the foot, usually at a depth of 8–12 cm. The heads of the biceps femoris may be stimulated while advancing the needle, causing contractions in the thigh and confusing the operator.

Sukhani et al.[61] have described a single injection lateral infragluteal–parabiceps approach, whereby the sciatic nerve is located along the lateral border of the biceps femoris muscle.

Anterior approach

The anterior approach to the sciatic nerve is helpful in patients who cannot be placed in the lateral recumbent position. The line connecting the anterior superior iliac spine and the symphysis is marked and divided into thirds. The greater trochanter is then identified and a line drawn inferomedially and parallel to the first line.

From the first line, a perpendicular line is drawn from the junction of the medial and middle thirds to intersect the second guideline. The puncture is made at this point of intersection and passes between the sartorius laterally and the rectus femoris medially and reaches the sciatic nerve below the lesser trochanter. Internal rotation of the leg may help location of the sciatic nerve and reduce trauma to the femoral nerve and vessels.[62]

Popliteal sciatic blocks

Popliteal sciatic catheters are especially suited for foot operations associated with much pain, such as revision osteotomies of the toes, synovectomies, and amputations of the foot. The posterior popliteal approach is performed with the patient in the prone position.

Three landmarks form a surface triangle – the skin crease behind the knee is the base, with the medial semimembranosus muscle and lateral biceps femoris tendon forming the walls.

Anatomic studies revealed that the sciatic nerve divides into the tibial nerve and the common peroneal nerve at a mean distance (SD) of 61 mm (27 mm) above the popliteal fossa crease. Thus, contrary to traditional teaching that puncture should be 5–7 cm above the crease, a needle should be inserted 10 cm cranial from the base of the triangle and about 1 cm lateral of the median line to block both nerves before division.[63,64] For block, a peripheral nerve stimulating needle is introduced at an angle of 45–60° to the skin to facilitate catheter insertion approximately 3–5 cm past the needle tip. Active mobilisation, however, can kink or break the catheter.

The lateral approach to the popliteal block may offer an advantage for placement of a continuous catheter. A 10 cm insulated Tuohy needle connected to a nerve stimulator is introduced in the groove between the biceps femoris and vastus lateralis 7 cm cephalad to the most prominent point of the lateral femoral condyle.[65] This approach ensures more secure placement of the catheter away from the mobile knee joint. However, the subgluteal and classic posterior approaches have a higher success rate and a significantly faster onset of anaesthesia than the lateral popliteal approach.[66,67]

Anatomy of the foot

Sole of foot

The sole of the foot is supplied by:

- the medial (L4 and L5) and lateral (S1 and S2) branches of the tibial nerve, supplying the medial and lateral anterior part of the sole;
- the sural nerve supplying the posterior and lateral part of the sole and heel;
- the tibial nerve (S1 and S2) supplying the medial part of the heel.

Dorsum of foot

The dorsum of the foot is supplied by:

- the medial terminal branch of the deep peroneal nerve (the adjacent sides of the first and second toes);
- the sural nerve – innervates the lateral side of the fifth toe;
- the superficial peroneal supplies the remainder.

Medial side of foot

The medial side of the foot is supplied by the saphenous nerve from the femoral nerve. It is also supplied by the medial plantar branch of the tibial nerve.

Lateral side of foot

The lateral side of the foot is supplied by the sural nerve from the tibial and common peroneal nerves, which goes to the fifth toe and lateral side of the foot.

Distal nerve blocks

Ankle blocks

Deep peroneal nerve (anterior tibial nerve – S1 and S2)

The deep peroneal nerve is blocked by inserting a needle midway between the most prominent points of the medial and lateral malleoli, on the circular line of infiltration in front of the ankle joint. It is directed medially towards the anterior border of the medial malleolus and local anaesthetic solution (10–15 mL) is injected between the bone and the skin; paraesthesia should be elicited if possible.

Instead of blocking this nerve at the ankle, its parent trunk, the common peroneal nerve, can be blocked at the neck of the fibula, where it can be rolled under the finger.

The deep peroneal nerve supplies the dorsal skin on adjacent sides of the first and second toes.

Superficial peroneal nerve (S1 and S2)

The superficial peroneal nerve, a branch of the common peroneal nerve, can be blocked immediately above the ankle joint by a subcutaneous weal extending from the front of the tibia to the lateral malleolus. It supplies the dorsum of the foot (with the exception of the small area innervated by the tibial nerve).

Sural nerve (L5, S1 and S2)

To block the sural nerve a subcutaneous injection of 5–7 mL is made between the lateral malleolus and the calcaneal tendon; care is necessary to avoid intravenous injection into the short saphenous vein.

Saphenous nerve (L3 and L4)

The saphenous nerve is the terminal branch of the femoral nerve and accompanies the long saphenous vein anterior to the medial malleolus, where it can be blocked by the injection of 10 mL of local anaesthetic solution. It supplies an area of skin just below and above the medial malleolus.

Tibial nerve (S1 and S2)

With the patient in the prone position the tibial nerve is blocked by 10 mL of solution introduced through a point on the circular weal just internal to the calcaneal tendon, deep to the flexor retinaculum near the palpable posterior tibial artery. It is easiest with the patient lying prone. The needle is inserted forwards and slightly outwards towards the posterior aspect of the tibia, near which the solution is deposited.

An alternative technique uses bony landmarks. The sustentaculum tali is a semilunar-shaped prominence and can be palpated about halfway between the medial malleolus and the medial border of the heel. Insert the needle at right-angles to the skin down onto its bony surface, withdraw slightly and then inject 5–7 mL of local anaesthetic. The local anaesthetic spreads under the medial retinaculum of the ankle joint and gives a reliable block of all branches of the tibial nerve.

Ring block of the toe

To achieve a ring block of the toe, plain lidocaine (lignocaine), 1.5 mL of 2% solution, is injected into each side of the proximal phalanx near its base. After an interval of 7–10 minutes the operation can commence.

BLOCK OF THE SYMPATHETIC NERVOUS SYSTEM

Sympathetic blockade is most commonly carried out in the:

- neck (stellate ganglion block);
- upper and lower limbs (intravenous sympathetic block);
- lumbar region (L1–L4);
- abdomen (splanchnic or coeliac plexus block).

Stellate ganglion block

Stellate ganglion block is also referred to as cervicothoracic sympathetic block because when 10–15 mL of anaesthetic solution are injected into the correct plane at the base of the neck, the middle cervical, stellate and the second, third and usually the fourth thoracic ganglia and their rami are blocked. This results in interruption of all sympathetic fibres to most of the thorax, head, neck and arm (except possibly the nerve of Kuntz). Certain visceral afferent fibres are also blocked (e.g. the cervical cardiac nerves).

The stellate ganglion is often blocked by spillover following supraclavicular brachial plexus block.

Anatomy

The stellate ganglion is formed by the fusion of the lowest of the three cervical ganglia with the first thoracic ganglion. It is irregular in size and position, being usually 1–3 cm long, and differs in the same individual on the two sides.

The cervical sympathetic chain and its three ganglia lie in front of the head of the first rib and the seventh cervical and first thoracic transverse processes, just behind the subclavian artery and the origin of the vertebral artery. It lies posterior to the carotid sheath on the longus colli and longus cervicis muscles. It is anterior to the eighth cervical and first thoracic nerves, so paraesthesia involving these nerves shows that the needle is too deeply placed. On the right side, the apex of the lung and the dome of the pleura are anterior relations; on the left side these structures are 2.5 cm lower and so are not in such close relationship to the ganglion.

Vasoconstrictor fibres pass from the stellate and the other cervical sympathetic ganglia to a plexus around the internal carotid artery.

Branches from the second and sometimes also from the third thoracic sympathetic ganglion often go directly to the upper limb via the first thoracic nerve, thus bypassing the stellate ganglion.

The stellate ganglion sends grey rami to the seventh and eighth cervical nerves, gives origin to the inferior cervical cardiac nerve, and supplies branches to the vessels in its vicinity. It may communicate with the vagus.

Postganglionic sympathetic fibres are also distributed to the arm with the somatic nerves of the brachial plexus and are distributed from them to the vessels, supplying vasoconstrictor impulses to the whole limb.

Indications

The most frequent indication for stellate ganglion block is to release vascular tone, and it may need to be repeated several times. Thus stellate ganglion block is used for the management of sympathetically mediated chronic pain in the arm, head or neck. However, there is growing controversy surrounding the role of sympathetic block in chronic regional pain syndromes. Most evidence for efficacy is based on case series. Only one-third of patients attain full pain relief.

Technique

Stellate ganglion block performed on a patient with an increased bleeding time or a decreased clotting time may result in a large haematoma in the deep planes of the neck. Long-acting neurolytic drugs (e.g. 6% phenol or absolute alcohol) are used chiefly to control cardiac pain. Bilateral block should not be carried out at the same time.

Paratracheal approach

For the paratracheal approach the patient lies supine, chin forward, neck extended, without a pillow. A weal is raised two fingerbreadths lateral to the suprasternal notch and a similar distance above the clavicle, which is on the medial border of the sternomastoid overlying the transverse process of the seventh cervical vertebra.

The position can be checked by palpating the tubercle of Chassaignac and the cricoid cartilage, both of which are at the level of the sixth cervical transverse process (i.e. a little higher than the weal).

A fine 5–8 cm needle is inserted directly backwards through the weal, while downward and backward pressure is exerted on the sternomastoid to draw the muscle and the carotid sheath laterally. When contact is made with bone (the seventh cervical vertebra) the needle is withdrawn 0.5–1 cm so that its point lies in front of the longus colli muscle and, after careful aspiration for blood (the vertebral artery is very near) and CSF, 15–20 mL of 0.5% lidocaine (lignocaine) or similar solution is injected. This will, if correctly placed, diffuse up and down in the fascial plane and will block the ganglia and rami from C2 to T_4 inclusive – 30 minutes may elapse before Horner's syndrome and vasodilatation of the arm appear.

Signs of successful block

Signs of successful stellate ganglion block are:

- Horner's syndrome – miosis, enophthalmos and ptosis – this does not guarantee sympathetic paralysis of the vessels of the arm;
- flushing of the cheek, face and neck and arm;
- engorged veins of the arm;
- increase in skin temperature;
- flushing of the conjunctiva and sclera;
- anhidrosis of the face and neck;
- lacrimation;
- stuffiness of the nostril (Guttmann's sign);
- Mueller's syndrome – injection of the tympanic membrane and warmth of the face.

Complications and dangers

Complications and dangers of stellate ganglion block are:

- perforation of the oesophagus, with infection;
- intrathecal injection causing a total spinal block;
- intravascular injection (e.g. sending a volume of solution via the vertebral artery straight up to the medulla);
- pneumothorax;
- cardiac arrest – very rare, although it has resulted from surgical cervicothoracic sympathectomy (a permanent stellate block);
- alteration of the voice from recurrent laryngeal nerve block;
- phrenic nerve block;
- brachial plexus block;
- extradural or intradural block;
- mediastinitis;
- intercostal neuralgia.

Death has been reported after stellate ganglion block, so it should not be undertaken lightly.

Lumbar sympathetic block

Surgical lumbar sympathectomy was first described in 1934. A technique using phenol dissolved in a radio-opaque medium and an image intensifier has been used.

Anatomy

The sympathetic trunk in the lumbar region consists of four ganglia and their interconnecting fibres. It lies on the anterolateral aspect of the bodies of the lumbar vertebrae, immediately medial to the psoas muscle, which fills the triangular space between the vertebral bodies and the transverse processes.

A tendinous arch, which gives part origin to the psoas muscle, connects the upper and lower borders of each lumbar vertebra and forms a tunnel around the side of the bone in which the lumbar vessels and the grey ramus communicans run. The lumbar arteries are posterior, but the veins may be anterior. The fatty tissue occupying this tunnel is an extension of that in the extradural space and it passes through the intervertebral foramina as far forward as the sympathetic chain. The chain lies in a fascial plane bounded by the vertebral column, the psoas sheath and the parietal peritoneum.The first lumbar vertebra is on a level with the intersection of the last rib and the outer border of the erector spinae. The interspace between the fourth and fifth vertebra corresponds to the highest point of the iliac crests in many patients.

In the sacral region, each chain consists of four ganglia with intervening fibres lying medial to the anterior sacral foramina.

Preganglionic fibres (white rami) are derived from the anterior primary rami from T_4 to T12 and each ganglion gives off a grey ramus to the corresponding sacral nerve to supply sympathetic innervation to the lower limbs.

On the coccyx, the two chains unite to form the ganglion impar.

Disturbances of function of the sympathetic nervous system can produce vasospasm, pain and visceral dysfunction.

Sympathetic block can remedy all of these, either temporarily, for diagnosis, or permanently, by interrupting a vicious circle.

Technique

Posterior approach

For lumbar sympathetic block using a posterior approach the patient is placed in the prone position with two pillows flexing the lumbar spine, or in a lateral spinal position with the affected side uppermost and the spine flexed. He or she should be premedicated with a sedative. The procedure can be carried out in the patient's bed if necessary.

Skin weals are raised at points 5 cm lateral to the upper borders of the spinous processes of the second, third and fourth lumbar vertebrae. Successful injection at these points blocks all the vasoconstrictor impulses to the lower limb. These points lie immediately above the transverse processes of the corresponding vertebrae.

A 12–16 cm needle is introduced through each weal at right-angles to the skin for 4–5 cm and should encounter the transverse process; it is slightly withdrawn and directed upwards so that it passes between the transverse processes; it is also directed slightly inwards.

After travelling 3–4 cm from the transverse process, the needle should make contact with the anterolateral aspect of the body of the vertebra.

After careful aspiration to exclude both blood and CSF, 10 mL of 1% lidocaine (lignocaine) are injected at each site and spread out in the retroperitoneal tissue. If force is required, the needle tip is in the anterior vertebral ligament or the psoas muscle and should be withdrawn slightly.

The spinal lumbar nerves run midway between the spinous processes, so if the needle point is kept in relation to the upper border of the transverse process, pain from hitting a nerve should be avoided. The lumbar arteries, branches of the aorta and their veins must also be avoided.

After 5–20 minutes the leg becomes less painful, its temperature increases and it becomes dry, its superficial veins dilate, and there is hyposensitivity to pinprick.

A 12 cm needle is inserted at an angle of 70° through a weal three fingerbreadths lateral to the superior point of the spinous process of the third lumbar vertebra. It should miss the transverse process and come into contact with the body of the vertebra in the psoas tunnel – 15–20 mL of anaesthetic solution are now injected.

Use of X-ray control with an image intensifier greatly adds to the accuracy of needle placement.

For chemical sympathectomy three needles are placed against the bodies of the second, third and fourth lumbar vertebrae and their position verified radiologically – 3 mL of either 6% phenol in water or absolute alcohol, preceded by local analgesia, are injected through each correctly placed needle.

Complications

Complications of lumbar sympathetic block are:

- intradural injection and spinal analgesia;
- intravascular injection;
- hypotension;
- haemorrhage into the sheath of the psoas muscle, with pain referred to the groin and upper and inner part of the thigh;
- neuritis of the genitofemoral nerve.

Caudal block gives the same results as lumbar sympathetic block, but it is not unilateral and produces, in addition to sympathetic paralysis, motor paresis and analgesia, which may be useful objective signs of successful sympathetic block.

Splanchnic analgesia; retrocrural coeliac plexus block

Anatomy

Semilunar or coeliac plexus

There are two semilunar or coeliac plexuses, one on each side of the midline, lying on the aorta and the crura of the diaphragm just above the pancreas, at the level of the first lumbar vertebra between the adrenal glands and behind the stomach and lesser sac.

The renal vessels are inferior to the plexus, whereas the vessels to the adrenals often pass through it. They are connected with each other and with their associated ganglia (superior mesenteric and inferior mesenteric etc.) by a network of nerve fibres around the coeliac artery. These fibres are postganglionic fibres of the greater and lesser splanchnic nerves. From this mass of retroperitoneal nerve tissue fibres pass with the arteries to the abdominal viscera. These plexuses also receive twigs from the right vagus and the phrenic nerves.

The semilunar plexus, with the aorticorenal and superior mesenteric plexus together make up the solar or epigastric plexus.

Afferent fibres from the abdominal viscera, both sympathetic and parasympathetic (vagus), pass through the coeliac ganglia. Afferent fibres from the pelvic viscera, travelling through the nervi erigentes (S2–S4), do not.

The greater splanchnic nerve (the superior thoracic splanchnic nerve), like the lesser and the lowest splanchnic, is composed of preganglionic fibres, which are in effect elongated white rami. Most of its fibres are myelinated. It arises from the union of four or five roots coming from the thoracic sympathetic ganglia, which receive white rami from the fifth to the tenth thoracic nerves, sometimes higher. The greater splanchnic nerve enters the abdomen through the crus of the diaphragm on each side, with the lesser and lowest splanchnic nerves, and enters the corresponding semilunar ganglion. It mainly contains visceral afferent fibres. Within the abdomen the greater splanchnic nerve lies between the diaphragm and the adrenal gland on each side.

The lesser splanchnic nerve (the middle thoracic splanchnic nerve) arises from the lower thoracic ganglia of the sympathetic cord, connected with the tenth and 11th thoracic nerves. It enters the corresponding aortorenal ganglion.

The lowest splanchnic nerve (the inferior thoracic splanchnic nerve) arises from the last thoracic ganglion and enters the renal plexus and the posterior renal ganglion.

The lumbar splanchnic nerves are presumably blocked when the coeliac plexus is blocked, by spreading of solution.

The first lumbar splanchnic nerve arises from the first lumbar ganglion; the second from the second and third ganglia (they join the coeliac plexus); the third from the second, third and fourth ganglia; the fourth from the fourth and fifth ganglia. The last two join the superior hypogastric plexus.

The hypogastric nerve (presacral nerves) extends from the third lumbar vertebra to the first sacral, where it ends by dividing into the right and left hypogastric nerves or plexuses. It lies in front of the lower part of the abdominal aorta, behind the peritoneum.

Superior hypogastric plexus

The superior hypogastric plexus was formerly known as the presacral nerve. It is retroperitoneal, lying on the body of the fifth lumbar vertebra. It receives:

- fibres from the sympathetic trunk via the third and fourth lumbar ganglia;
- fibres known as the intermesenteric plexus coming from the coeliac, mesenteric and pararenal plexuses;
- parasympathetic fibres.

The superior hypogastric plexus innervates the transverse, descending and sigmoid colon with nerve fibres that pass alongside the inferior mesenteric artery.

Inferior hypogastric plexus

The inferior hypogastric plexus is a collection of ganglia and nerve fibres where preganglionic sympathetic fibres synapse. It receives fibres from the inferior hypogastric nerves, together with parasympathetic fibres, and supplies the viscera of the female pelvis (except the ovaries). Its sympathetic element provides sensory and motor fibres to the urinary and anal sphincters; the parasympathetic fibres are motor to the bladder and rectum. Sensory and motor fibres of the inferior hypogastric plexus travel with blood vessels and may be damaged in pelvic operations.

Division of the superior hypogastric plexus (presacral neurectomy) is used in the treatment of dysmenorrhoea.

Afferent pathways from abdominal viscera

Afferent pathways from abdominal viscera travel in within splanchnic nerves from sensory nerve endings in the walls of the viscera and mesentery and enter the spinal cord with the white rami of the lower seven thoracic nerves (and sometimes higher), having their cell stations in the posterior root ganglia of these nerves. Afferent impulses also travel to the CNS within the vagus and phrenic nerves. Visceral afferent fibres, travelling with the sympathetic fibres, enter the cord at the following levels:

- stomach T6–T10;
- small gut T9–T10;
- large gut to middle of transverse colon T11–L1;
- distal colon L1–L2;
- liver and biliary tract T7–T9;
- pancreas T6–T10;
- kidney and ureter T10–L1/L2;
- bladder and prostate T11–T12;
- testis and ovary T10–T11;
- uterus T10–T11.

Preganglionic fibres to the adrenal glands do not synapse in the coeliac or other preaortic plexuses, but pass directly to end around chromaffin cells of the medulla. In addition to the lesser splanchnic nerve, fibres go to the adrenals from nerves T10 to L2.

Technique of splanchnic block

Splanchnic block can be performed from the front (Braun, Wendling), or from behind (Kappis). Braun's method is usually performed by the surgeon.

Braun's method

With the abdomen opened, the liver is gently retracted upwards and the stomach drawn to the left. The anterior aspect of the body of the first lumbar vertebra is located medial to the lesser curvature of the stomach; the aorta is retracted laterally and the long Braun needle is inserted down to the bone and 50 mL of solution injected (e.g. 0.5% lidocaine (lignocaine)).

Kappis's method

For Kappis's method the patient is in the spinal position, sitting or lying prone. The fourth interspace is located, lying on or before the intercristal line; by counting upward, the spine of the first lumbar vertebra is identified. Weals are raised four fingerbreadths (7.5 cm) from this spine, one in each side of the midline. The weals must be below the lateral tip of the 12th rib. A long needle is inserted at an angle of 45° to the median plane through this weal with its bevel facing inwards. It is directed slightly cephalad and thrust in until it makes contact with the body of the 12th thoracic vertebra. It is then partly withdrawn and its point directed more laterally until its bevel is felt to glance past the lateral aspect of the body of the vertebra. The needle is then advanced a further 1 cm and, after a most careful aspiration test, 20–40 mL of solution are injected. The average distance between the skin and the plexus is 7–10 cm. If blood is aspirated into the syringe, the needle point may be in the vena cava or the aorta and must be moved until it is free of these vessels.

Bilateral block is probably unnecessary.

Fluoroscopy aids accurate placement of the needle. CT-aided coeliac plexus block has been described. Insertion of the needle at the level of the second lumbar vertebra has been advocated.

The usual strengths of solution employed are prilocaine 0.5%; lidocaine (lignocaine) 0.5%; tetracaine (amethocaine) 1:2000 to 1:4000. Epinephrine (adrenaline) should be added.

Complications of splanchnic block

Splanchnic block causes a profound fall in blood pressure, which can be partially controlled by an intravenous infusion of fluid or by ephedrine or one of its congeners, should it be considered necessary. It produces analgesia of the abdominal viscera, with the exception of the pelvic viscera (i.e. the sigmoid colon, rectum, bladder and reproductive organs). The bowel becomes contracted and ribbonlike. The patient must be particularly well premedicated, an intravenous narcotic anaesthetic being given until his or her mental state is calm.

The surgeon must be lighthanded, especially when the peritoneal cavity is being explored, because its lateral walls are not rendered insensitive either by the splanchnic block or by the abdominal field block (but by posterior intercostal block).

Therapeutically, splanchnic block is useful in the treatment of carcinoma of the pancreas and acute pancreatitis (perhaps because it relaxes the sphincter of Oddi). It causes a greater blood supply to be diverted to the pancreas. If these conditions are found at laparotomy, splanchnic block with phenol has much to recommend it. The block may be repeated if desirable.

Splanchnic block has also been used in the terminal stages of upper abdominal cancer to relieve pain. Alcohol in saline, 50%, preceded by local anaesthetic solution, has been employed.

ABDOMEN AND PERINEUM

Intraperitoneal anaesthesia

Local anaesthetic can be injected through a laparoscopic surgical port. A local anaesthetic mixture recently described is bupivacaine 0.125% with 1:800 000 epinephrine (adrenaline) and sodium bicarbonate 0.2%. Sodium bicarbonate 0.2% is made up by diluting 0.5 mL of sodium bicarbonate 8.5% with 19.5 mL of local anaesthetic mixture. A total of 100 mL is injected, 80 mL into the peritoneal cavity and 20 mL into the laparoscopic ports. Tilt the table as appropriate.

Abdominal field block

Anatomy

The xiphoid is on a level with the body of the ninth thoracic vertebra. The subcostal plane is at the third lumbar vertebra. The highest part of the iliac crest is on a level with the interspace between the third and fourth lumbar vertebrae.

The superficial fascia in the upper abdomen is a single fatty layer, but from a point midway between the umbilicus and the pubis two layers are described, the deep layer (fascia of Antonius Scarpa) and the superficial layer (fascia of Petrus Camper).

Camper's fascia passes over the inguinal ligament and is continuous with the superficial fascia of the thigh. It is continued over the penis, spermatic cord and scrotum, where it helps to form the dartos muscle. In the female it is continued into the labia majora.

Scarpa's fascia is tougher. It blends with the deep fascia of the thigh and, like Camper's fascia, is continued over the penis and helps to form the dartos. From the scrotum it becomes continuous with Colles' fascia over the perineum.

There is no deep fascia covering the abdomen.

Muscles of the abdominal wall

The external oblique is the largest and most superficial of the muscles of the anterior abdominal wall. The aponeurosis is attached below to the anterior superior spine and to the pubic crest and tubercle – it thus forms the inguinal ligament. In the midline it forms the linea alba, which runs from the symphysis pubis to the xiphisternum. The subcutaneous or external inguinal ring is an opening in the aponeurosis. The fibres of the external oblique pass downwards and inwards, like those of the external intercostal muscles.

The internal oblique is a thinner layer than the external oblique. The fibres of this muscle run upwards and inwards.

The fibres of transversus abdominis run transversely. Between it and the external oblique run the lower intercostal, iliohypogastric and ilioinguinal nerves.

Below the level of the iliac crest the fibres of these three muscles (external oblique, internal oblique and transversus abdominis) are aponeurotic and run downwards and medially.

Each rectus abdominis muscle arises from the crest of the pubis and from the ligaments in front of the symphysis, and is inserted into the anterior aspects of the fifth, sixth and seventh costal cartilages and into the xiphisternum. Three tendinous intersections cross the muscle and are firmly attached to the anterior layer of its sheath, but not to the posterior layer. One is at the level of the xiphisternum, one at the umbilicus and the third one midway between.

Pyramidalis is a small muscle on each side, within the rectus sheath. It serves to strengthen the linea alba.

The rectus sheath contains, in addition to the rectus and pyramidalis muscles, the superior and inferior epigastric vessels and the terminations of the lower six intercostal nerves and vessels. The nerves pierce the lateral margin of the sheath and run in relation to its posterior wall before they enter the substance of the muscle.

The abdominal muscles are supplied by the anterior rami of the lower six thoracic nerves and by the iliohypogastric and ilioinguinal nerves. They are accessory muscles of expiration and help to compress the abdominal viscera, as in defaecation, straining, coughing etc. They are not muscles of normal inspiration.

The transversalis fascia is a thin membrane, continuous with the iliac and pelvic fasciae. In the inguinal region it is stronger and thicker than elsewhere and through it, at the abdominal inguinal (internal inguinal) ring, passes the spermatic cord or the round ligament.

Sensory nerve supply of the abdominal wall

Sensory nerve supply of the abdominal wall is provided by the anterior primary rami of the lower six thoracic nerves, via the intercostal nerves:

- T5 supplies the skin in the region of the nipple;
- T7 nerve supplies skin in the epigastrium;
- T10 supplies skin in the region of the umbilicus;
- T12 supplies skin midway between the umbilicus and the pubis;
- the skin of the groin is supplied by the iliohypogastric nerve (L1).

Intercostal nerves and the last thoracic nerve pass under the costal margin between the slips of the diaphragm and run forwards between the internal oblique and the transversus abdominis before they pierce the lateral margin of the rectus sheath. After lying behind the rectus muscle, they pierce its substance and supply it, and end as anterior cutaneous nerves.

Vessels of the abdominal wall

The only vessels likely to be injured by the anaesthetist are the superior and inferior epigastric arteries and veins:

- the superior artery is the termination of the internal mammary artery and enters the rectus sheath posterior to the seventh costal cartilage;
- the inferior epigastric artery arises from the external iliac artery and enters the rectus sheath behind the arcuate line of Douglas.

Technique of abdominal field block

Local infiltration

In all operations performed under field block analgesia it is necessary to infiltrate the line of incision both subcutaneously and intradermally. The injections should be commenced 15–20 minutes before the incision is to be made. Weals are raised:

- at the tip of the xiphisternum opposite the body of the ninth thoracic vertebra and on each side (weal 1);
- at the ninth costal cartilage, where the rectus muscle crosses it (weal 2);
- at the lateral margin of the rectus, just above the umbilicus (weal 3);
- at the lateral margin of the rectus, below the umbilicus if the incision is to be prolonged (weal 4).

Through weals 2, 3 and 4 a needle is inserted perpendicularly until it meets the resistance of the rectus sheath. If the patient is conscious he or she will experience pain when the anterior layer of the rectus sheath is pierced. The needle is advanced a further 0.5 cm and 5 mL of solution are injected into the sheath. After withdrawal into the subcutaneous tissue, the needle is inclined upwards and downwards so that more solution is deposited into the rectus sheath.

It is important to remember the positions of the tendinous intersection so that solution is deposited between each pair to ensure even distribution of the anaesthetic drug. Posterior to the muscle, these intersections do not impede the spread of solution.

After completion of the deep injections the weals are joined together along the lateral margin of the rectus by lines of subcutaneous injection. Similarly, weal 1 is joined to each weal 2 along the costal margin.

A total of 50–100 mL of solution is used (e.g. 0.5% lidocaine (lignocaine)).

Costoiliac block

Costoiliac block gives a wider zone of analgesia and relaxation than the rectus sheath block outlined below, but is more difficult to carry out successfully.

Weals are raised on each side along the costal margin and vertically downward to the iliac crest. Solution is deposited from needles passed through these weals into the subcutaneous and muscular layers of the abdominal wall, remembering that laterally the intercostal nerves lie between the transversus abdominis and internal oblique. The weals are joined together by subcutaneous infiltration, as described for rectus sheath block. In muscular subjects, in addition, solution can be injected into the rectus sheath. The volume of solution required is 15–200 mL.

Rectus sheath block

Rectus sheath block is an excellent method for producing muscular relaxation when combined with a light general anaesthetic, and if the incision is to be midline or paramedian it is usual to do both sides. Perforation of the peritoneum should be avoided, but in the absence of peritonitis or adhesions no serious harm is likely to result.

The anterior layer of the rectus sheath is detected by the needle throughout its whole extent, but the posterior layer only for about 7.5 cm above and below the umbilicus.

Solution is placed posterior to the muscle so that the intercostal nerves supplying it, together with the zone of skin medial to its outer border, are blocked.

If the abdomen shows the scar of a previous operation, abdominal field block may be difficult and undesirable, and intercostal block or paravertebral block may be indicated if the operation is to be performed under local analgesia.

Abdominal field block renders the abdominal wall and its underlying parietal peritoneum insensitive. To block pain impulses from the viscera and posterolateral parietal peritoneum, either light general anaesthesia or a splanchnic block and posterior intercostal block is required.

Regional analgesia for intra-abdominal surgery, although popular in the past, requires multiple punctures and near toxic doses of local anaesthetic drugs and thus finds little favour today.

Ilioinguinal block for repair of inguinal hernia

Anatomy

The inguinal canal is 4 cm long and extends from the internal inguinal ring laterally to the external inguinal ring medially. It lies above the inner half of the inguinal ligament.

The internal or abdominal ring is just above the midpoint of the inguinal ligament; it is an opening in the transversalis fascia and just medial to it is the inferior epigastric artery.

The subcutaneous or external ring lies above and lateral to the pubic crest. It is an opening in the external oblique, and through it passes the spermatic cord in the male and the round ligament in the female. They lie lateral to the pubic spine.

The walls of the inguinal canal are:

- anteriorly – external oblique and internal oblique in its lateral third;
- posteriorly – transversalis fascia in its whole length; conjoint tendon or falx inguinalis in its inner two-thirds; reflected part of the inguinal ligament in its inner-third; the femoral vessels;
- the floor is formed by the inguinal ligament;
- the roof is formed by arching fibres of the conjoint tendon of the transversus abdominis and the internal oblique.

The contents of the inguinal canal are the ilioinguinal nerve and the spermatic cord (or the round ligament of the uterus).

The spermatic cord comprises the internal and external spermatic arteries and the artery to the vas deferens, the pampiniform plexus of veins, the lymphatic vessels, the autonomic nerve fibres and the vas deferens in the male.

Indirect inguinal hernia

All inguinal hernias are protrusions through the fascia transversalis. An indirect hernia protrudes through the deep inguinal ring, descends into the cord and receives a covering from the external spermatic fascia, cremasteric muscle and internal spermatic fascia (from the fascia transversalis).

Direct inguinal hernia

A direct inguinal hernia protrudes through the fascia transversalis in the more medial part of the posterior wall of the canal through the triangle of Hesselbach, the boundaries of which are laterally, the inferior or deep epigastric artery; medially the outer border of the rectus; inferiorly, the inguinal ligament.

Nerve supply

The nerve supply of the inguinal region is from the last two thoracic and the first two lumbar nerves via the iliohypogastric, the ilioinguinal and the genitofemoral.

The last two thoracic nerves run downwards and inwards, just above the anterior superior iliac spine, between the internal oblique and transversus muscles. They end by piercing the rectus sheath.

The iliohypogastric and ilioinguinal nerves come from the first lumbar root. They are inferior to the last two thoracic nerves and curve round the body just above the iliac crest, gradually piercing the muscles and ending superficially. The ilioinguinal nerve traverses the inguinal canal, lying anterior to the spermatic cord, and becomes superficial through the external ring and supplies the skin of the scrotum. The iliohypogastric nerve, after running between the internal oblique and the transversus abdominis, pierces the internal oblique just above the anterior superior iliac spine and supplies the skin over the pubis.

The genitofemoral nerve comes from the first and second lumbar nerves and divides into a genital and a femoral branch. The genital branch enters the inguinal canal from behind through the internal ring.

Indications

Indications for ilioinguinal block are:

- to avoid the risks of general anaesthesia or the possible risks of hypotension associated with intra- or extradural analgesia in slim, elderly, or poor-risk patients;

- to reduce the risk of aspiration of intestinal contents in cases of strangulation, by having a fully awake patient (bowel resection usually requires other methods of pain relief);
- for day-case surgery;
- for postoperative pain relief;
- used routinely by some surgeons.

Technique

For ilioinguinal block three weals are made as follows:

- one fingerbreadth internal to the anterior superior iliac spine (weal 1);
- over the pubic ramus (weal 2);
- 1.5 cm above the midpoint of the inguinal ligament (weal 3).

Through weal 1, a larger needle is introduced vertically backwards until it is felt to pierce the aponeurosis of the external oblique with a slight click. After aspiration, 20–30 mL of solution (see below) are injected so that both the ilioinguinal and iliohypogastric nerves are surrounded. At this point a needle introduced perpendicularly to the skin will not pierce the peritoneum. Solution is deposited in all layers, including the small area of tissue between the weal and the anterior superior spine.

Through weal 2 a larger needle deposits solution in the intradermal and subcutaneous layers in the direction of the umbilicus. This blocks nerve twigs overlapping from the opposite side.

Through weal 3 a needle is inserted perpendicularly to the skin until it pierces the aponeurosis of the external oblique. At this level 20 mL of solution are injected so that the genital branch of the genitofemoral nerve is blocked.

Intradermal and subcutaneous infiltration along the line of the incision may be necessary to obtain perfect analgesia; in addition, infiltration of the periosteum near the pubic tubercle and Astley Cooper's ligament, the conjoint tendon and the lateral border of the rectus abdominis muscle should be performed in cases of direct inguinal hernia.

The use of 0.5% solution of prilocaine with epinephrine (adrenaline) allows a generous volume of relatively nontoxic local anaesthetic solution to be employed. Otherwise 0.25% bupivacaine or 0.5% lidocaine (lignocaine), both with epinephrine (adrenaline), are suitable. The dose of bupivacaine should not exceed 2 mg/kg. Mixing the anaesthetic with dextran 70 or 150 has been used to prolong the local anaesthetic effect.

If the hernia is strangulated or irreducible, the surgeon should inject deeper layers under vision as he goes along.

The patient may complain of temporary discomfort when the neck of the sac is under tension; this can often be relieved by infiltration of local anaesthetic solution around the neck.

Infiltration analgesia is a perfectly acceptable method of pain relief for elective inguinal and femoral hernias and patients require less postoperative analgesia and vomit less than after general anaesthesia.

Regional analgesia has a number of advantages, as follows:

- it avoids the risks of general anaesthesia;
- it makes the surgeon gentle;
- the patient can cough during the operation if required;
- the surgeon uses less tension in his sutures;
- the patient can walk off the table and be treated as a day case;
- catheterisation is eliminated;
- quicker turnaround of cases.

Field block for repair of femoral hernia

Anatomy

A femoral hernia passes through the femoral canal and the saphenous opening or fossa ovalis, an opening in the deep fascia of the thigh, 3.8 cm (1.5 in) below and 3.8 cm (1.5 in) lateral to the pubic tubercle.

The femoral canal is the most medial of three compartments, the most lateral containing the femoral artery and the intermediate one the femoral vein.

The femoral canal is 1–2 cm long, and at its mouth is the femoral ring. The femoral ring is bounded in front by the inguinal ligament and behind by the pectineus, laterally by the femoral vein, and medially by the lacunar ligament of Gimbernat. Astley Cooper's ligament is a backward extension of the lacunar ligament along the pelvic brim (iliopectineal line) for 1.5 cm. The ring contains the femoral septum or fatty pad.

The coverings of a femoral hernia are, from within outwards, the fat from the femoral septum, the prolongation of the fascia transversalis forming the anterior wall of the femoral sheath, and the cribriform fascia of the fossa ovalis.

Technique

The technique for field block for repair of femoral hernia is similar to that for repair of inguinal hernia. Paravertebral block from T10 to L3 may also be carried out. It is a suitable procedure for operation on strangulated inguinal and femoral hernias.

Iliac crest block

For iliac crest block a weal is raised 4 cm from the anterior superior iliac spine on a line joining this spine to the xiphisternum. A needle is inserted laterally, first just beneath the skin and then deeper until the ilium is touched. Local anaesthetic solution is injected so that it anaesthetises T12 and the iliohypogastric and ilioinguinal nerves as they lie between the internal oblique and the transversus abdominis muscles.

Field block for operations on the anal canal

For field block for operations on the anal canal a weal is made on each side of the anus and 2.5 cm away from it. From these weals a subcutaneous rhomboidal zone of infiltration is made, using 20 mL of 0.5% bupivacaine and epinephrine (adrenaline). Deep injections are now made from the infiltrated zone into each quadrant, 5 mL into each, with a finger in the rectum preventing perforation of the mucous membrane. The nerve to the external anal sphincter is the perineal branch of S4. The operation can be done satisfactorily with the patient in the prone position with the pelvis raised. Heavy premedication should be employed.

Penile block – field block for circumcision

Anatomy

The sensory nerves of the penis are derived from the terminal branches of the internal pudendal nerves. The dorsal nerves of the penis travel beneath the pubic bone, one on each side of the midline, lying against the dorsal surface of the corpus cavernosum. The skin at the base of the organ is supplied by the ilioinguinal and the genitofemoral nerves. In addition, the posterior scrotal branches of the perineal nerves run paraurethrally to the ventral surface and fraenum, so four nerves have to be blocked.

Technique

For penile block an intradermal and subcutaneous ring weal is raised around the base of the penis – the subcutaneous infiltration should precede the intradermal. The dorsal nerve is next blocked on each side by injecting 5 mL of solution (see below) into the dorsum of the organ just below, but not deep to, the symphysis so that the needle point lies against the corpus cavernosum. If the needle pierces the corpus cavernosum, pain is experienced.

For the ventral injection of the paraurethral branches, the penis should be pulled upwards and 2 mL of solution injected near the base into the groove formed by the corpora cavernosa and the corpus spongiosum.

Infiltration of 5 mL of 1% lidocaine (lignocaine) or 0.5% bupivacaine into each dorsal nerve provides good postoperative analgesia. In infants, smaller volumes are used. Postoperative pain can be relieved by repeated penile block in awake patients, even in children, without undue discomfort. Epinephrine (adrenaline) must not be used because it may cause penile necrosis.

Care must be taken not to cause haematoma formation because this may contribute to gangrene of skin – subpubic injection must be avoided.

Pain following circumcision under general anaesthesia can be relieved by sacral extradural analgesia or by infiltrating each dorsal nerve at the root of the penis with 1–3 mL of local anaesthetic solution (e.g. 0.5% bupivacaine, without epinephrine [adrenaline]). This is a satisfactory alternative to extradural sacral block, with fewer complications. Lidocaine (lignocaine) spray or gel applied topically gives useful relief.

THORAX

Thoracic paravertebral block

The reintroduction of paravertebral anaesthetic block in 1979 has improved post-thoracotomy pain and reduced complications compared to epidural anaesthesia performed at the same spinal level.[68] Recently, paravertebral infusions have been used to provide postoperative pain relief for ambulatory surgery.[69] Thoracic paravertebral block involves injecting a local anaesthetic close to the vertebral column where the nerve trunks emerge from the intervertebral foramina.

The paravertebral space is a wedge-shaped compartment, bounded:

- above and below by the heads and necks of adjoining ribs;
- posteriorly by the costotransverse ligament;
- medially it communicates with the extradural space through the intervertebral foramen;
- laterally it is bounded by the parietal pleura and its apex leads into the intercostal space.

The posterolateral aspect of the body of the vertebra and the intervertebral foramen and its contents forms the base The upper aspect of the spinous process coincides with the transverse process of the lower vertebra.

There is no direct communication between one paravertebral space and another, but an indirect communication exists medially through the intervertebral foramen with the extradural space.

Spread from one paravertebral space to another, across the extradural space, is frequent and may involve nerves on the same or opposite sides of the body.

When the first thoracic to second lumbar nerve roots are blocked, their rami communicantes are blocked too.

Technique

For thoracic paravertebral block skin weals are raised 4 cm from the midline. In the thoracic region, the injection point is 2–3 cm lateral to the superior aspect of the spinous process. Through each weal, a needle is inserted perpendicularly 3–5 cm to strike bone near the lateral extremity of the transverse process. It is then redirected to pass below the transverse process and at this point local anaesthetic solution is injected. Insertion of the block needle in a caudal direction reduces the risk of pneumothorax compared to insertion in a cranial direction because the block needle is much more likely to hit the corresponding rib. The block needle is more likely to penetrate pleura when inserted in in a cranial direction.

Never disconnect the syringe to the extension tubing because there is a risk of pneumothorax.

Aspiration tests are essential. If there is resistance to injection, progress 3 mm through the costotransverse ligament.

If several levels are to be blocked, a large 15 mL volume can be injected. The placement of a catheter in turn allows the continuous administration of 3–4 mL/h. The anaesthetic solution spreads in the intercostal, interpleural and epidural directions.

Complications

Complications of thoracic paravertebral block include:

- local anaesthetic toxicity;
- pneumothorax (<1%);
- epidural diffusion (1%);
- hypotension (<5%);
- intravascular injection.

Horner's syndrome indicates achievement of C6–T1 sympathetic block – in such situations the patient should be closely monitored for possible phrenic and/or recurrent laryngeal nerve block.

Intercostal nerve block

Cutaneous nerves of the trunk

Anteriorly

Anteriorly the cutaneous nerves of the trunk are:

- the lateral, intermediate and medial supraclavicular branches of the superficial division of the cervical plexus (C3–C4);
- the anterior rami of the thoracic nerves, excluding T1;
- the iliohypogastric and ilioinguinal nerves (L1).

Posteriorly

Posteriorly the cutaneous nerves of the trunk are:

- the posterior rami of C2–C5, T1–T12 and L1–L3;
- the five sacral and the coccygeal nerves.

Anatomy of spinal nerves

Typical intercostal nerves are the third to sixth thoracic nerves. Each nerve is formed by the union of the anterior (motor) and the posterior (sensory) root – the posterior root has a ganglion on it.

The mixed spinal nerve soon divides into anterior and posterior primary divisions (rami). The thoracic or dorsal nerves are then distributed as follows.

The posterior rami are smaller than the anterior. They turn backwards and divide into medial and lateral branches (except C1, S4 and S5, coccygeal), which supply the muscles and skin of the back.

The anterior rami in the thoracic region of the second to sixth nerves are each connected to the lateral sympathetic chain by a grey and a white ramus communicans. Each crosses the paravertebral space between the necks of contiguous ribs and then enters the subcostal groove where it lies below the vein and artery in a triangular space, bounded above by the rib, the posterior intercostal membrane and the internal intercostal muscle until it reaches the anterior axillary line, at which point the nerves come into direct relationship with the pleura, as the innermost intercostal muscle terminates. There is a communication between each space and those contiguous to it. Each intercostal nerve supplies muscular branches to the intercostal muscles and lateral and anterior cutaneous branches to supply the skin of the chest and abdomen. The seventh to 11th nerves pass below and behind the costal cartilages, between the slips of the diaphragm running between the internal oblique and transversus muscles (again between the second and third layers) to enter the posterior layer of the rectus sheath. They run deep into the rectus, pierce and supply it, and end as anterior cutaneous nerves (Figs 4.2.2 and 4.2.3).

The lateral cutaneous branch emerges in the midaxillary line and divides into anterior and posterior branches, which supply the skin on the lateral wall of the chest as far forward as the nipple line.

The anterior cutaneous branch is the termination of the intercostal nerve; it supplies the skin on the front of the chest, internal to the nipple line.

Exceptions

The first intercostal nerve supplies most of its fibres to the brachial plexus and gives neither lateral nor anterior cutaneous branches, the skin over the first intercostal space being supplied by the descending branches of the cervical plexus (C3–C4).

The lateral cutaneous branch of the second intercostal nerve crosses the axilla and becomes the intercostobrachial nerve, supplying the skin on the medial aspect of the arm.

The lateral cutaneous branch of T12, which does not divide into anterior and posterior branches, crosses the iliac crest to supply the skin of the upper part of the buttock as far as the greater trochanter.

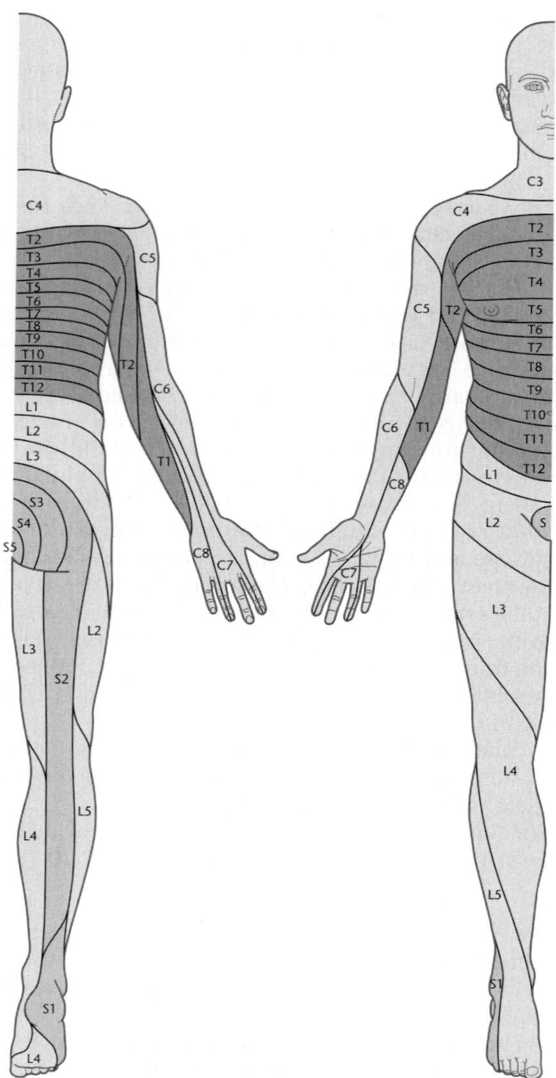

Figure 4.2.2 Sensory dermatomes.

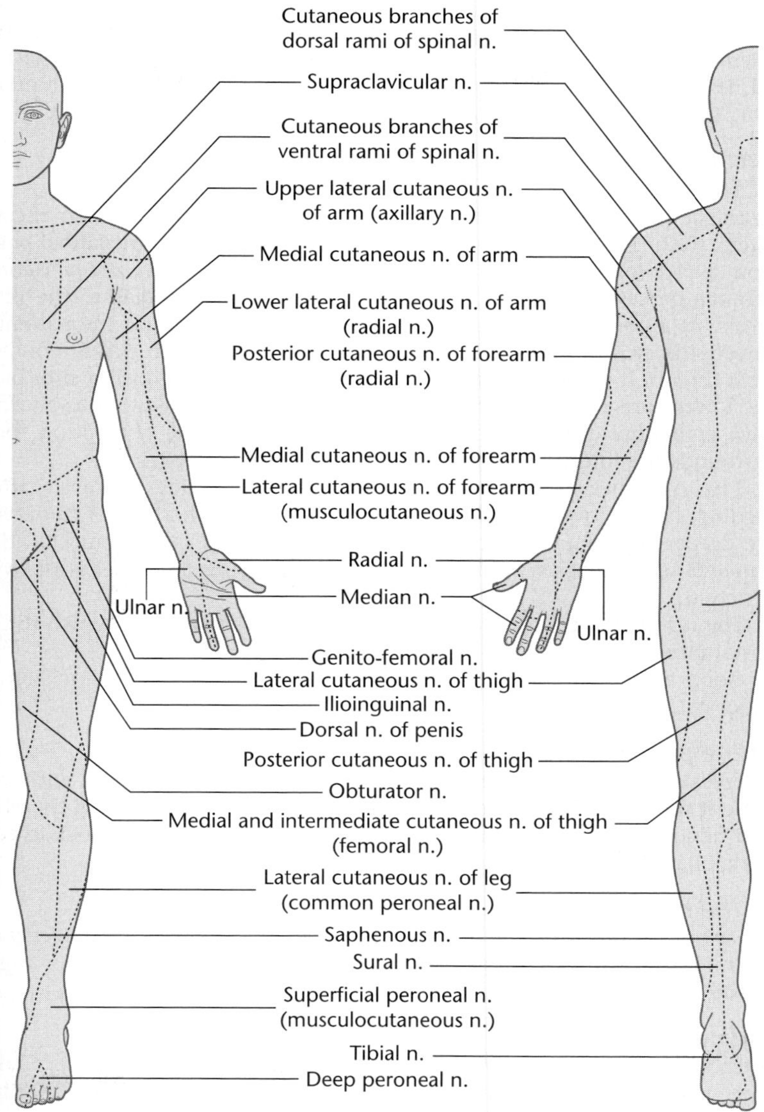

Figure 4.2.3 Sensory innervation.

T12 and L1 nerves supply sensory branches to the anterior chest and anterior abdominal wall, the parietal pleura and the parietal peritoneum. T10, lateral and anterior cutaneous branches, supplies the area of the umbilicus. T9, T8 and T7 supply the skin between the umbilicus and the xiphisternum. T11, T12 and L1 supply the skin between the umbilicus and the pubis.

Technique of intercostal nerve block

At the angle of the ribs

At the angle of the ribs the intercostal nerve becomes relatively superficial, lateral to the erector spinae muscle. The patient is placed in the lateral position and two lines are drawn, four fingerbreadths from the vertebral spinous processes, extending from the spines of the scapulae to the iliac crests. At a point where the lower border of the 11th rib on the patient's upper side crosses the line, a needle is introduced until it makes contact with the rib. It is then partially withdrawn and advanced until it slips past the lower border of the rib for 3 mm; 2–3 mL of local anaesthetic solution with epinephrine (adrenaline) are then injected. A zone of solution thus surrounds the intercostal nerve as it lies in the subcostal groove.

T10 to T6 nerves are now injected on the upper side, followed, after turning, by the lower seven nerves on the patient's other side. T12 nerves are deeper and require special care. Before T6 and T7 can be injected the patient's scapulae must be drawn laterally by crossing his or her arms over his chest.

The needle pierces the trapezius, the latissimus dorsi and the two intercostal muscles.

Good analgesia for up to 12 hours results if the abdominal incision is subcostal.

In the posterior axillary line

Intercostal nerve block in the posterior axillary line is carried out with the patient supine and arms abducted to a right-angle. In this position the ribs, and hence the intercostal nerves, are not so deeply placed. A block in the midaxillary line misses the lateral cutaneous nerve.

In the midaxillary line

It has been shown that the intercostal nerves can be blocked at the level of the midaxillary line in supine patients as effectively as at the posterior angle of the ribs.

Indications

Intercostal block is useful in enabling deep breathing and coughing to take place in patients with postoperative abdominal pain or with fractured ribs, but it does not always produce good results.

Intercostal block has also been used for rib resection and insertion of a drain.

Freezing an intercostal nerve within the thorax using a cryoprobe is now rarely used to reduce post-thoracotomy pain.

Complications

Complications of intercostal block include:

- pneumothorax;
- damage to intercostal vessels;
- toxicity due to excessive absorption of local anaesthetic and associated epinephrine (adrenaline).

Intercostal block is the technique associated with the highest systemic absorption of local anaesthetic and requires patient monitoring for 20 minutes after injection.

It has been proposed that more complications follow intercostal nerve block performed from inside the thorax than percutaneously.

Interpleural block

Technique

For interpleural block the anaesthetic solution is given as a single injection or as an infusion through a cannula inserted between the ribs into the pleural space. Identifying the pleural space without causing a pneumothorax requires care.

The skin may be punctured with a sharp needle just above a rib (at the angle of the rib, or in the axillary line). A semi-blunt needle (e.g. Tuohy) attached to a saline or local anaesthetic-filled syringe is inserted and loss of resistance used to identify the interpleural space. Spontaneous respiration makes puncture of the lung less likely at this point. The needle hub is occluded between detaching the syringe and inserting the catheter, to prevent air entry into the pleural cavity. Twenty mL of 0.5% bupivacaine or ropivacaine will produce a block lasting up to 4 hours. Continuous infusion is less effective than intermittent injection. The technique may be used to control post-cholecystectomy pain and after other abdominal operations. It has been used in chronic pain.[64]

Complications of interpleural block include pneumothorax, damage to intercostal vessels during insertion, and toxic signs of abnormally rapid absorption of drug from the pleural space, although toxic effects are rare after boluses of 20 mL of 0.5% bupivacaine or ropivacaine with epinephrine (adrenaline) 1:200 000.

References

1. Capdevila X, Barthelet Y, Biboulet P, Ryckwaert Y, Rubenovitch J, d'Athis F. Effects of perioperative anaesthetic technique on the surgical outcome and duration of rehabilitation after major knee surgery. Anesthesiology 1999; 91:8–15.

2. Chelly JE, Greger J, Gebhard R, et al. Continuous femoral blocks improve recovery and outcome of patients undergoing total knee arthroplasty. J Arthroplasty 2001; 16:436–445.
3. Selander D, Dhuner KG, Lundborg G. Peripheral nerve injury due to injection needles used for regional anesthesia. An experimental study of the acute effects of needle point trauma. Acta Anaesthesiol Scand 1977; 21:182–188.
4. Urmey WF, Grossi P. Percutaneous electrode guidance: a noninvasive technique for prelocation of peripheral nerves to facilitate peripheral plexus or nerve block. Reg Anesth Pain Med 2002; 27:261–267.
5. Chan VW. Applying ultrasound imaging to interscalene brachial plexus block. Reg Anesth Pain Med 2003; 28:340–343.
6. Perlas A, Chan VW, Simons M. Brachial plexus examination and localization using ultrasound and electrical stimulation: a volunteer study. Anesthesiology 2003; 99:429–435.
7. Sandhu NS, Capan LM. Ultrasound-guided infraclavicular brachial plexus block. Br J Anaesth 2002; 89:254–259.
8. Ilfeld BM, Morey TE, Enneking FK. Continuous infraclavicular brachial plexus block for postoperative pain control at home: a randomized, double-blinded, placebo-controlled study. Anesthesiology 2002; 96:1297–1304.
9. Salinas FV, Neal JM, Sueda LA, Kopacz DJ, Liu SS. Prospective comparison of continuous femoral nerve block with nonstimulating catheter placement versus stimulating catheter-guided perineural placement in volunteers. Reg Anesth Pain Med 2004; 29:212–220.
10. Singelyn FJ, Seguy S, Gouverneur JM. Interscalene brachial plexus analgesia after open shoulder surgery: continuous versus patient-controlled infusion. Anesth Analg 1999; 89:1216–1220.
11. Klein SM, Nielsen KC, Greengrass RA, Warner DS, Martin A, Steele SM. Ambulatory discharge after long-acting peripheral nerve blockade: 2382 blocks with ropivacaine. Anesth Analg 2002; 94:65–70.
12. Candido KD, Winnie AP, Ghaleb AH, Fattouh MW, Franco CD. Buprenorphine added to the local anesthetic for axillary brachial plexus block prolongs postoperative analgesia. Reg Anesth Pain Med 2002; 27:162–167.
13. Newton DJ, McLeod GA, Khan F, Belch JJ. The effect of adjuvant epinephrine concentration on the vasoactivity of the local anesthetics bupivacaine and levobupivacaine in human skin. Reg Anesth Pain Med 2004; 29:307–311.
14. El Saied AH, Steyn MP, Ansermino JM. Clonidine prolongs the effect of ropivacaine for axillary brachial plexus blockade. Can J Anaesth 2000; 47:962–967.
15. Culebras X, Van Gessel E, Hoffmeyer P, Gamulin Z. Clonidine combined with a long acting local anesthetic does not prolong postoperative analgesia after brachial plexus block but does induce hemodynamic changes. Anesth Analg 2001; 92:199–204.

16. Ilfeld BM, Morey TE, Enneking FK. Continuous infraclavicular perineural infusion with clonidine and ropivacaine compared with ropivacaine alone: a randomized, double-blinded, controlled study. Anesth Analg 2003; 97:706–712.

17. Simon MJ, Veering BT, Stienstra R, van Kleef JW, Burm AG. The effects of age on neural blockade and hemodynamic changes after epidural anesthesia with ropivacaine. Anesth Analg 2002; 94:1325–1330.

18. Winnie AP. Interscalene brachial plexus block. Anesth Analg 1970; 49:455–466.

19. Meier G, Bauereis C, Heinrich C. [Interscalene brachial plexus catheter for anesthesia and postoperative pain therapy. Experience with a modified technique]. Anaesthesist 1997; 46:715–719.

20. Borgeat A, Dullenkopf A, Ekatodramis G, Nagy L. Evaluation of the lateral modified approach for continuous interscalene block after shoulder surgery. Anesthesiology 2003; 99:436–442.

21. Casati A, Borghi B, Fanelli G, et al. Interscalene brachial plexus anesthesia and analgesia for open shoulder surgery: a randomized, double-blinded comparison between levobupivacaine and ropivacaine. Anesth Analg 2003; 96:253–259.

22. Casati A, Vinciguerra F, Scarioni M, et al. Lidocaine versus ropivacaine for continuous interscalene brachial plexus block after open shoulder surgery. Acta Anaesthesiol Scand 2003; 47:355–360.

23. Rucci FS, Pippa P, Barbagli R, Doni L. How many interscalenic blocks are there? A comparison between the lateral and posterior approach. Eur J Anaesthesiol 1993; 10:303–307.

24. Boezaart AP. Continuous interscalene block for ambulatory shoulder surgery. Best Pract Res Clin Anaesthesiol 2002; 16:295–310.

25. Ilfeld BM, Morey TE, Wright TW, Chidgey LK, Enneking FK. Continuous interscalene brachial plexus block for postoperative pain control at home: a randomized, double-blinded, placebo-controlled study. Anesth Analg 2003; 96:1089–1095.

26. Wilson AT, Nicholson E, Burton L, Wild C. Analgesia for day-case shoulder surgery. Br J Anaesth 2004; 92:414–415.

27. Ilfeld BM, Morey TE, Wright TW, Chidgey LK, Enneking FK. Interscalene perineural ropivacaine infusion:a comparison of two dosing regimens for postoperative analgesia. Reg Anesth Pain Med 2004; 29:9–16.

28. Urmey WF, Talts KH, Sharrock NE. One hundred percent incidence of hemidiaphragmatic paresis associated with interscalene brachial plexus anesthesia as diagnosed by ultrasonography. Anesth Analg 1991; 72:498–503.

29. Winnie AP, Collins VJ. The subclavian perivascular technique of brachial plexus anesthesia. Anesthesiology 1964; 25:353–363.

30. Moorthy SS, Schmidt SI, Dierdorf SF, Rosenfeld SH, Anagnostou JM. A supraclavicular lateral paravascular approach for brachial plexus regional anesthesia. Anesth Analg 1991; 72:241–244.

31. Rodriguez J, Barcena M, Alvarez J. Restricted infraclavicular distribution of the local anesthetic solution after infraclavicular brachial plexus block. Reg Anesth Pain Med 2003; 28:33–36.

32. Raj PP, Parks RI, Watson TD, Jenkins MT. A new single-position approach to sciatic-femoral nerve block. Anesth Analg 1975; 54:489–493.

33. Whiffler K. Coracoid block – a safe and easy technique. Br J Anaesth 1981; 53:845–848.

34. Mehrkens HH, Geiger PK. Continuous brachial plexus blockade via the vertical infraclavicular approach. Anaesthesia 1998; 53(suppl 2):19–20.

35. Wilson JL, Brown DL, Wong GY, Ehman RL, Cahill DR. Infraclavicular brachial plexus block: parasagittal anatomy important to the coracoid technique. Anesth Analg 1998; 87:870–873.

36. Gaertner E, Estebe JP, Zamfir A, Cuby C, Macaire P. Infraclavicular plexus block: multiple injection versus single injection. Reg Anesth Pain Med 2002; 27:590–594.

37. Greher M, Retzl G, Niel P, Kamolz L, Marhofer P, Kapral S. Ultrasonographic assessment of topographic anatomy in volunteers suggests a modification of the infraclavicular vertical brachial plexus block. Br J Anaesth 2002; 88:632–636.

38. Borene SC, Edwards JN, Boezaart AP. At the cords, the pinkie towards: Interpreting infraclavicular motor responses to neurostimulation. Reg Anesth Pain Med 2004; 29:125–129.

39. Ilfeld BM, Morey TE, Enneking FK. Infraclavicular perineural local anesthetic infusion: a comparison of three dosing regimens for postoperative analgesia. Anesthesiology 2004; 100:395–402.

40. Retzl G, Kapral S, Greher M, Mauritz W. Ultrasonographic findings of the axillary part of the brachial plexus. Anesth Analg 2001; 92:1271–1275.

41. Coventry DM, Barker KF, Thomson M. Comparison of two neurostimulation techniques for axillary brachial plexus blockade. Br J Anaesth 2001; 86:80–83.

42. Sia S, Lepri A, Campolo MC, Fiaschi R. Four-injection brachial plexus block using peripheral nerve stimulator: a comparison between axillary and humeral approaches. Anesth Analg 2002; 95:1075–1079.

43. Liisanantti O, Luukkonen J, Rosenberg PH. High-dose bupivacaine, levobupivacaine and ropivacaine in axillary brachial plexus block. Acta Anaesthesiol Scand 2004; 48:601–606.

44. Fanelli G, Casati A, Garancini P, Torri G. Nerve stimulator and multiple injection technique for upper and lower limb blockade: failure rate, patient acceptance, and neurologic complications. Study Group on Regional Anesthesia. Anesth Analg 1999; 88:847–852.

45. Deleuze A, Gentili ME, Marret E, Lamonerie L, Bonnet F. A comparison of a single-stimulation lateral infraclavicular plexus block with a triple-stimulation axillary block. Reg Anesth Pain Med 2003; 28:89–94.

46. Winnie AP, Ramamurthy S, Durrani Z. The inguinal paravascular technic of lumbar plexus anesthesia: the '3-in-1 block.' Anesth Analg 1973; 52:989–996.

47. Marhofer P, Nasel C, Sitzwohl C, Kapral S. Magnetic resonance imaging of the distribution of local anesthetic during the three-in-one block. Anesth Analg 2000; 90:119–124.

48. Capdevila X, Biboulet P, Morau D, et al. Continuous three-in-one block for postoperative pain after lower limb orthopedic surgery: where do the catheters go? Anesth Analg 2002; 94:1001–1006.

49. Capdevila X, et al. Effects of perioperative analgesic technique on the surgical outcome and duration of rehabilitation after major knee surgery. Anesthesiology 1999; 91(1):8–15.

50. Chelly JE, et al. Continuous femoral blocks improve recovery and outcome of patients undergoing total knee arthroplasty. J Arthroplasty 2001; 16(4): 436–445.

51. Capdevila X, Macaire P, Dadure C, et al. Continuous psoas compartment block for postoperative analgesia after total hip arthroplasty: new landmarks, technical guidelines, and clinical evaluation. Anesth Analg 2002; 94:1606–1613.

52. Kaloul I, Guay J, Cote C, Fallaha M. The posterior lumbar plexus (psoas compartment) block and the three-in-one femoral nerve block provide similar postoperative analgesia after total knee replacement. Can J Anaesth 2004; 51:45–51.

53. Kaloul I, Guay J, Cote C, Halwagi A, Varin F. Ropivacaine plasma concentrations are similar during continuous lumbar plexus blockade using the anterior three-in-one and the posterior psoas compartment techniques. Can J Anaesth 2004; 51:52–56.

54. Cook P, Stevens J, Gaudron C. Comparing the effects of femoral nerve block versus femoral and sciatic nerve block on pain and opiate consumption after total knee arthroplasty. J Arthroplasty 2003; 18:583–586.

55. Mansour NY. Reevaluating the sciatic nerve block: another landmark for consideration. Reg Anesth 1993; 18:322–323.

56. Di Benedetto P, Casati A, Bertini L, Fanelli G. Posterior subgluteal approach to block the sciatic nerve: description of the technique and initial clinical experiences. Eur J Anaesthesiol 2002; 19:682–686.

57. Mansour NY, Bennetts FE. An observational study of combined continuous lumbar plexus and single-shot sciatic nerve blocks for post-knee surgery analgesia. Reg Anesth 1996; 21:287–291.

58. di Benedetto P, Bertini L, Casati A, Borghi B, Albertin A, Fanelli G. A new posterior approach to the sciatic nerve block: a prospective, randomized comparison with the classic posterior approach. Anesth Analg 2001; 93:1040–1044.

59. Taboada M, Alvarez J, Cortes J, Rodriguez J, Atanassoff PG. Is a double-injection technique superior to a single injection in posterior subgluteal sciatic nerve block? Acta Anaesthesiol Scand 2004; 48:883–887.

60. Guardini R, Waldron BA, Wallace WA. Sciatic nerve block: a new lateral approach. Acta Anaesthesiol Scand 1985; 29:515–519.

61. Sukhani R, Candido KD, Doty R, Jr., Yaghmour E, McCarthy RJ. Infragluteal-parabiceps sciatic nerve block: an evaluation of novel approach using a single-injection technique. *Anesth Analg* 2003; 96:868–73.

62. Moore CS, Sheppard D, Wildsmith JA. Thigh rotation and the anterior approach to the sciatic nerve: a magnetic resonance imaging study. Reg Anesth Pain Med 2004; 29:32–35.

63. Vloka JD, Hadzic A, April E, Thys DM. The division of the sciatic nerve in the popliteal fossa: anatomical implications for popliteal nerve blockade. Anesth Analg 2001; 92:215–217.

64. Borgeat A, Blumenthal S, Karovic D, Delbos A, Vienne P. Clinical evaluation of a modified posterior anatomical approach to performing the popliteal block. Reg Anesth Pain Med 2004; 29:290–296.

65. Chelly JE, Greger J, Casati A, Al-Samsam T, McGarvey W, Clanton T. Continuous lateral sciatic blocks for acute postoperative pain management after major ankle and foot surgery. Foot Ankle Int 2002; 23:749–752.

66. Taboada M, Alvarez J, Cortes J, et al. The effects of three different approaches on the onset time of sciatic nerve blocks with 0.75% ropivacaine. Anesth Analg 2004; 98:242–247.

67. Taboada M, Rodriguez J, J AL, Cortes J, Gude F, Atanassoff PG. Sciatic nerve block via posterior Labat approach is more efficient than lateral popliteal approach using a double-injection technique: a prospective, randomized comparison. Anesthesiology 2004; 101:138–142.

68. Richardson J, Sabanathan S, Jones J, Shah RD, Cheema S, Mearns AJ. A prospective, randomized comparison of preoperative and continuous balanced epidural or paravertebral bupivacaine on post-thoracotomy pain, pulmonary function and stress responses. Br J Anaesth 1999; 83:387–392.

69. Greengrass R, Buckenmaier CC, 3rd. Paravertebral anaesthesia/analgesia for ambulatory surgery. Best Pract Res Clin Anaesthesiol 2002; 16:271–283.

Further reading

Brown D, ed. Regional anesthesia and analgesia. Philadelphia: WE Saunders; 1996.

Cousins MJ, Bridenbaugh PO, eds. Neural blockade in clinical anaesthesia and the management of pain. 3rd edn. Philadelphia: JB Lippincott; 1998.

Wildsmith JAW, Armitage EN, McClure J, eds. Principles and practice of regional anaesthesia. 3rd edn. Edinburgh: Churchill Livingstone; 2003.

CHAPTER **4.3**

SPINAL ANAESTHESIA — INTRADURAL AND EXTRADURAL

Intrathecal anaesthesia has been practised for over 100 years. The intrathecal use of cocaine was first described by Bier in 1898 and the use of intrathecal opioids was first described in 1901 by a Romanian surgeon, Racoviceanu-Pitesti. In 1979, Behar et al.[1] published the first report on the extradural use of morphine. Intradural and extradural anaesthesia is widely practised for both surgery and obstetrics.

This chapter outlines the anatomy of the spinal column and the pharmacodynamics of local anaesthetics and opioids, and describes the different modes of spinal and extradural anaesthesia, indications for intervention, clinical efficacy, side-effects, and outcomes associated with neuraxial block.

ANATOMY

Vertebral column

The vertebral column consists of seven cervical, 12 thoracic, five lumbar, five sacral and four or five coccygeal vertebrae. In adults the sacral and coccygeal vertebrae are fused. The vertebral column has four curves – the anterior convexity of the sacrum, the lumbar lordosis, the thoracic kyphosis and the cervical lordosis.

In the supine position the fourth lumbar vertebra marks the highest point of the lumbar curve and the fourth or fifth thoracic vertebra is the lowest point of the dorsal curve. Lordosis, scoliosis and arthritis of the spine change the shape of the curves and increase the difficulty of intrathecal and extradural puncture.

At least one-quarter of the length of the vertebral column is made up of intervertebral discs, each consisting of an outer cover, the annulus fibrosus, enclosing a core of gelatinous material, the nucleus pulposus. The discs give flexibility to the column and act as shock absorbers. The annulus may rupture, usually posteriorly, causing pressure on nerve roots.

The vertebral bodies and intervertebral discs are held together throughout the length of the spine by the anterior and posterior longitudinal ligaments. Posterior to the vertebral bodies and posterior longitudinal ligament are the vertebral canal and the spinous processes.

The spinous processes of the cervical, upper thoracic and lumbar vertebrae are almost horizontal and lie posterior to the bodies of their respective vertebra. The other spinous processes are inclined downwards, their tips being opposite the bodies of the vertebrae immediately below. Maximal inclination is present in the midthoracic region (between the fifth and eighth thoracic vertebrae).

The spinous processes are held vertically together by the interspinous ligament, except in the cervical spine, where it is absent. Anteriorly, it fuses with the ligamenta flava and the laminae. Posteriorly, the interspinous ligament blends with the strong supraspinous ligament that runs along the tips of the spinous processes and blends with the ligamentum nuchae at its superior end. In the elderly the ligament can become ossified, making a midline approach to the extradural space difficult.

The vertebral canal is bordered posteriorly by the spinous processes and interspinous ligaments, laterally by the pedicles and posterolaterally by the laminae and ligamenta flava, a thick, yellow elastic structure that passes from lamina to lamina and connects in the midline. The lateral halves of the ligamenta flava meet variably in the midline at an angle less than 90° and form a steeply arched roof over the lumbar posterior extradural space.

A midsagittal gap between the ligamenta flava in the midline is common (50%) in the thoracic and cervical regions. It may contribute to a variable loss of resistance when the midline approach is used to enter the extradural space.

The vertebral canal ends superiorly in the foramen magnum and inferiorly in the sacral hiatus.

The vertebral canal consists of spinal cord, spinal membranes, adipose tissue, blood vessels, cerebrospinal fluid (CSF) and the roots of spinal nerves.

Degenerative joint disease and ageing can narrow the intervertebral foramina and prevent the spread of local anaesthetic out of the foramina, resulting in greater longitudinal spread in the extradural space.

Spinal cord

The spinal cord is the extension of the central nervous system (CNS) into the upper two-thirds of the vertebral canal. It is 45 cm long in the average adult, extending from the upper border of the atlas to the upper border of the second lumbar vertebra. At its upper end, the spinal cord is continuous with the medulla oblongata and below with the conus medullaris, from which the filum terminale descends as far as the coccyx. There are two enlargements of the cord, one in the cervical, the other in the lumbar region, corresponding to the origins of the nerves of the arms and legs.

In the fetus the spinal cord is the same length as the vertebral canal. During growth and development of children, the canal grows more rapidly than the cord such that nerve roots that pass out transversely in early fetal life become more oblique. In adult life, the cauda equina consists of vertical lumbar and sacral nerves bathed in CSF that descend to meet their respective foramina.

The spinal cord receives its vascular supply from three arteries, one anterior and two posterior. The anterior spinal artery, a single vessel lying in the substance of the pia mater overlying the anterior median fissure, arises at the level of the foramen magnum from the junction of a small branch from each vertebral artery. It receives communications from the intercostal, lumbar and other small arteries and supplies the lateral and the anterior columns, comprising three-quarters of the substance of the cord. Thrombosis of this artery causes anterior spinal artery syndrome.[2]

The posterior spinal arteries, two on each side, branch from the posterior inferior cerebellar arteries at the level of the foramen magnum. They supply the posterior columns that carry fibres responsible for position, touch, and vibration sense. Communicating branches at the level of the first and 11th thoracic vertebrae are larger than the others (arteries of Adamkiewicz) and help to supply the cervical and lumbar enlargements of the cord. The artery at the 11th thoracic vertebra supplies the cord both upwards and downwards; that at the first thoracic vertebra only downwards from this level.

Three membranes (dura, arachnoid and pia mater) ensheath the spinal cord. The dura is the outermost membrane. It is a strong fibrous sheath consisting of collagen and elastin fibres. The fibrous bands forming the structure of the dura mater have hitherto been regarded as longitudinal, and clinical teaching has recommended insertion of needles parallel to the dural fibres to separate rather than cut dural tissue. However, recent electron microscopy has revealed a more complex arrangement. Dural fibres are actually arranged in a complex, overlapping lattice, suggesting that the position of needle bevel has little influence on the size and shape of the dural hole.

Within the cranium, the dura is composed of an outer endosteal component that lies against the bone of the cranium and an inner meningeal layer. Both layers are tightly adherent except where they divide to form the venous sinuses. Within the vertebral column, the dural layers separate. The inner, meningeal layer of the cerebral dura mater forms the spinal dura mater and the cranial endosteal layer continues as periosteum lining the vertebral canal, thus forming the extradural space, closed off from the cranial vault. The extradural space communicates freely with the paravertebral space through the intervertebral foramina and caudally ends at the sacral hiatus.

Extradural space

The extradural space contains loose areolar connective tissue, semiliquid fat, lymphatics, arteries, an extensive plexus of veins, and the spinal nerve roots as they exit the dural sac and pass through the intervertebral foramina.

The anteroposterior dimension of the posterior extradural space varies markedly throughout the length of the extradural space. In the cervical region the posterior extradural space averages 1–2 mm, whereas in the lumbar region it averages 5–6 mm.

Investigation of the anatomy and dynamics of the extradural space with techniques such has epiduroscopy have been supplanted by cryomicrotome sectioning[3] whereby, shortly after death, a cadaver is frozen and dissected in planes 100 μm thick. Artefact is minimised by immediate freezing, allowing relationships between structures to be readily identified. From this work, the lumbar extradural space has been anatomically described as segmented and discontinuous. This is attributable to the predominance of lumbar extradural fat, wedged between dura and the side walls of the vertebral canal, dividing the extradural space into anterior, lateral and posterior segments.

Segmentation may impede the passage of an extradural catheter and promote coiling and misplacement.[3] In addition, direct injection of local anaesthetic into extradural fat may account for a prolonged latency of clinical effect. In more cephalad cervicothoracic regions, the extradural fat disappears and the dura directly contacts lamina. In contrast, the thoracic extradural space is more continuous; it has less fat than the lumbar region and dura is less likely to contact bone. Thus extradural catheters placed in the midthoracic interspaces may pass with greater ease.

When the extradural space is entered off the midline, the Touhy needle is less likely to encounter extradural fat and injection of local anaesthetic may dissect the capsule of the fat pad away from the bony and ligamentous walls of the vertebral canal.

Several studies support the existence of dorsomedian ligamentous strands that draw the dura posteriorly in a dorsomedian dural fold, the plica mediana dorsalis. Latex casts, computed tomography (CT) epidurography and epiduroscopy describe tenting of the dura and a narrowing of the extradural space in the midline. Investigators have proposed that this segmentation of the extradural space may impede extradural catheter placement, or cause maldistribution of local anaesthetics and unilateral or patchy anaesthesia. In contrast to other imaging techniques, cryomicrotome sectioning has not demonstrated any evidence of a dorsomedian fold nor fibrous tissue within the extradural space.[4,5] Thus, it would seem that unilateral block is more likely a result of poor technique – inadequate volume or passage of the extradural catheter through an intervertebral foramen.

Following extradural injection, local anaesthetic spreads as rivulets through many small channels, not unlike fluid spreading between two sheets of polythene.[5] The greater the volume of injectate, the more homogenous the spread as channels open up. Injected solution travels preferentially towards the nerve roots and through the intervertebral foramina, although with some restriction exerted by the fascia of the posterior longitudinal ligament.

A network of valveless veins connecting the head and the pelvis fills the anterior thoracic extradural space. Venous return from the pelvis passes through the extradural venous plexus to the azygos vein, bypassing the inferior vena cava (IVC). Thus any obstruction to IVC flow from an increase in intra-abdominal pressure (coughing or straining) or an intra-abdominal mass (pregnancy or tumour) redirects venous return through the vertebral venous plexus.

Dilated extradural veins pose many problems for the anaesthetist. In particular, the risk of entering veins during extradural catheter insertion and inadvertent intravenous injection is increased. Dilatation of veins decreases extradural space volume, distributing local anaesthetics more widely and increasing the extent of anaesthetic block. Exposure to greater vascular surface area also increases the risk of local anaesthetic toxicity owing to greater absorption from the extradural space.

The arachnoid membrane is a membrane of flat, overlapping cells with tight junctions closely applied to the dura. Although only eight cells thick, the arachnoid membrane presents the greatest barrier to drug transport from the extradural space to the cerebrospinal fluid (CSF).

The space between the dura and arachnoid is termed the subdural space. Although a potential space, malposition of an extradural needle and injection of local anaesthetic between the dura and arachnoid creates a hydrospace, extending widely into thoracic and lumbar regions and providing rapid clinical pain relief. If suspected, the extradural catheter should be immediately removed as migration through the thin arachnoid mater into CSF can easily occur and precipitate total spinal anaesthesia.

The pia is a fenestrated, single layer of flat epithelial cells that is tightly adherent to the spinal cord and sends delicate septa into its substance. From each lateral surface of the pia mater a fibrous band, the denticulate ligament, projects into the subarachnoid space, and is attached by a series of pointed processes to the dura as far down as the first lumbar nerve. The pia mater is separated from the arachnoid by CSF within the subarachnoid space, a continuation of the ventricular system CSF at the base of the brain.

Cerebrospinal fluid lies between arachnoid and the pia within the spinal canal. The total volume of CSF, including CSF within the ventricles and around the cisterns of the brain, is between 100 and 150 mL.

Cerebrospinal fluid is formed from the choroid plexuses of the four cerebral ventricles at a rate of 800 mL/day, five times the total volume of CSF. The choroid plexus is a protrusion of blood vessels covered by a thin epithelial layer. Compared to plasma, sodium and chloride ion concentrations are greater, and glucose and potassium concentrations are lower in

CSF. The pH of CSF is 7.32, but is very responsive to change in carbon dioxide (CO_2). CSF is reabsorbed by arachnoid villi, which project into the venous sinuses of the brain and veins of the spinal cord.

Lumbosacral CSF volume varies considerably (from 43 to 81 mL)[6] and is the principal determinant of intrathecal spread of drugs. No clinical measure of CSF volume is available.

Spinal nerves

There are 31 pairs of spinal nerves – eight cervical, 12 thoracic, five lumbar, five sacral, one coccygeal. Each main spinal nerve is formed in the intervertebral space from the convergence of anterior and posterior roots. The perineurium of the spinal nerves is formed from pia and arachnoid membranes and the epineurium is formed from the dura. The spinal nerve trunks subsequently divide into anterior and posterior primary divisions.

Nerve roots differ in size between the thoracic and lumbar regions.[7] The diameter of thoracic roots is half that of lumbar roots, although much variability in root sizes occurs between individuals.

Arachnoid granulations up to 3 mm in diameter cluster around the nerve roots in the dural cuff region. They emerge through the dura and press into surrounding veins and extradural fat. Arachnoid granulations clear the CSF of foreign particulate material by emptying directly into the extradural venous plexus or by lymphatic drainage. Transport of drugs back into the CSF by this route does not occur.

Sympathetic chain

Efferent fibres arising from cell bodies in the lateral columns of the spinal cord between the first thoracic and the second lumbar segmental levels travel in the anterior primary rami of spinal nerves, then pass in white rami communicantes to the sympathetic chain.

The sympathetic chain consists of two long nerve strands, one on each side of the vertebral column, that extend from the base of the skull to the coccyx. Each trunk consists of a series of ganglia, interconnected by bundles of nerve fibres (interganglionic rami) to form a chain. The sympathetic ganglia contains the cell bodies of postganglionic sympathetic effector neurons. The nonmyelinated axons of the postganglionic neurons are distributed to the periphery by a variety of routes – grey rami communicantes back to the spinal nerves, prevertebral plexuses in front of the vertebral column and periarterial plexuses.

The cervical part of the sympathetic trunk consists of three interconnecting ganglia, the superior, middle and inferior. The latter is fused with the first thoracic ganglion to form the stellate ganglion, positioned between C7 and T1 in front of the seventh cervical transverse process and neck of the first rib. Interruption of preganglionic input or postganglionic outflow from the stellate ganglion produces Horner's syndrome, which includes dropping of the upper eyelid (ptosis), a small pupil, and absence of sweating on the affected side of the head and neck.

The sympathetic trunks enter the thorax from the neck, descend in front of the heads of the ribs and enter the abdomen by piercing the crura of the diaphragm. In the thorax, each trunk has 11 or 12 separate ganglia of varying sizes, including the stellate described above.

The thoracic sympathetic trunks give rise to delicate cardiac and pulmonary mediastinal branches and to larger branches called splanchnic nerves. In the abdomen and pelvis, the two sympathetic trunks descend on the vertebral column, adjacent to the psoas major muscles. The right trunk lies behind the IVC, the left one beside the aorta. The trunks continue into the pelvis, where they lie on the pelvic surface of the sacrum.

Postganglionic fibres within the abdomen form plexuses such as the coeliac plexus, intermesenteric plexus and the superior hypogastric plexus. The coeliac plexus spreads down the abdominal aorta and all its branches, giving rise to subsidiary perivascular plexuses, named according to the blood vessels along which they pass.

Peripheral nerves are comprised of thousands of nerve fibres. They contain either sensory or motor fibres of the somatic and autonomic nervous systems, but sometimes both in combination.

CENTRAL NEURAXIAL BLOCKADE

Central neuraxial blockade is commonly used for abdominal, perineal, gynaecological and lower limb operations. It offers excellent anaesthesia and fewer side-effects than general anaesthesia. Central neuraxial blockade is obtained by:

- intradural anaesthesia;
- extradural anaesthesia;
- combined intradural and extradural anaesthesia;
- continuous intradural anaesthesia.

Intradural anaesthesia

Single-injection intradural (spinal) anaesthesia is simple to administer, with rapid onset and offset of sensory and motor block. It is used as a single technique for ambulatory surgery and for major surgery when combined with long-acting intrathecal opioids, extradural anaesthesia or regional lower limb block. Spinal anaesthesia has a faster onset of action and fewer complications than epidurals, and a more predictable onset, duration and offset than regional limb blocks. The rapid onset of spinal anaesthesia reduces the need for general anaesthesia for urgent caesarean section, thus minimising the risk of failed intubation and acid aspiration. General anaesthesia in pregnancy is associated with a tenfold increase in failure to intubate the trachea and has been shown, since the first audit of maternal morbidity and mortality in 1950, to have contributed to maternal and fetal death.

Extradural anaesthesia

Extradural analgesia is the central neuraxial method of choice for relieving pain in labour, particularly when combined with opioids such as fentanyl or sufentanil.

The advantage of lumbar extradural analgesia is that extension and increased depth of the extradural block for operative delivery is readily obtained by injection of local anaesthetic. Potential side-effects include visceral pain from traction of the peritoneum during caesarean section and local anaesthetic toxicity[8,9] (convulsions, torsades de pointes) after inadvertent intravascular injection.

In contrast, placement of an extradural catheter into a thoracic interspace provides anaesthesia for abdominal and cardiothoracic surgery when combined with general anaesthesia. Postoperative titration of analgesia provides optimal pain relief on awakening from surgery and for several days without recourse to intravenous opioids. Sufficient freedom from pain to allow deep breathing and coughing without restriction goes some way towards attenuating the incidence of hypoxaemic episodes and pulmonary complications experienced after surgery.

Thoracic extradural analgesia is a pivotal intervention, providing early pain-free mobilisation and earlier feeding within accelerated rehabilitation programmes designed to speed up return to 'normal' function.[10]

Combined intradural and extradural anaesthesia

Combined spinal extradural (CSE) anaesthesia is a combination of intradural and extradural techniques. It has a faster onset of action than extradural analgesia for the provision of pain relief in labour. However, common to all techniques that penetrate the dura, the side-effects carry a substantial risk and include post-dural puncture headache (PDPH) and meningitis.

For CSE, the overall balance of benefit versus risk improves when analgesia is requested in late labour or for long arduous labours (dystocia). Combined spinal extradural would not seem to offer significant advantage in terms of mode of delivery compared to extradural analgesia.

Continuous intradural anaesthesia

Continuous spinal anaesthesia (CSA) combines the advantages of a single-dose spinal with that of a continuous technique.[11,12] Advantages include direct application of local anaesthetic and opioid to the CSF, attenuation of the neurohormonal stress response, titration of profound anaesthetic block, relative cardiovascular stability when used in small doses and little risk of toxicity.

Continuous spinal anaesthesia allows the use of regional anaesthesia when extradural anaesthesia is relatively contraindicated (severe cardiac disease) or might be difficult (severe obesity).

PREPARATION FOR CENTRAL NEURAXIAL BLOCKADE

Preparation for central neuraxial blockade consists of:

- assessment, explanation, consent and examination of the patient;
- obtaining venous access;
- commencing intravenous infusion;
- establishing monitoring of the patient (oxygen saturation, ECG, noninvasive blood pressure etc.);
- checking the anaesthetic machine;
- ensuring that the operating table tilts;
- making sure that anaesthetic drugs are available (thiopental or propofol, suxamethonium, atropine);
- ensuring that a defibrillator is available.

A sedative benzodiazepine drug often helps the patient to tolerate the procedure. Ketamine 0.1–0.25 mg/kg has been given when positioning causes pain, such as in fractured hip. The patient can be positioned in the sitting or lateral position. If heavily sedated or ill, the patient should be placed in the lateral position with his or her back parallel to the edge of the table and knees and head flexed. For caesarean section, intrathecal injection is frequently performed in the right lateral position to avoid unilateral left-sided spinal anaesthesia when women are turned supine with a left lateral tilt after the injection. Many anaesthetists find the sitting position easier than the lateral position. The patient is placed across the table or bed with their feet resting comfortably on a stool – the spine should be flexed with the chin pressed on to the sternum. A pillow on the knees gives helpful support to the arms.

Examination of the patient's back, identification of bony landmarks and use of aseptic technique are essential for good practice.

Site of insertion

Spinal anaesthesia, CSE and continuous spinal catheters should be inserted between the third and fourth lumbar vertebrae. However, identifying the correct lumbar interspace is fraught with error. Tuffier's line joining the posterior superior iliac spines is unreliable as it does not always pass through the body of the fourth lumbar vertebra. Seven cases of conus medullaris syndrome were recently reported after spinal anaesthesia between the second and third lumbar vertebrae,[13] characterised by unilateral lumbosacral paresthesia, motor block and, in three patients, bladder symptoms. The tip of the conus usually lies between the first and second lumbar vertebrae, but it may extend further. Ultrasound guidance has recently shown that only 13 out of 17 anaesthetists correctly identified the L3/4 interspace and four selected an interspace higher than they thought.[14]

Thoracic extradural catheters should be inserted at the interspace corresponding to the middle of the surgical wound. Although the decision to perform regional anaesthesia on a patient under general anaesthesia remains contentious, it is preferable to perform thoracic extradural anaesthesia while the patient is lightly sedated. Insertion of a spinal or extradural needle in an awake patient has two principal benefits – lancinating pain warns the anaesthetist of any potential neurological damage, and the extent of sensory analgesia can be measured before inducing general anaesthesia. Classic landmarks are the root of the spine of scapula at the level of the third thoracic vertebra and the inferior angle of scapula at the level of the seventh thoracic vertebra. Always counts up interspaces from that between the third and fourth lumbar vertebrae as a check.

An aseptic technique should be used for all neuraxial blocks. The technique should be the same as for any invasive surgical procedure – hat, mask, handwashing, donning of sterile gown and gloves. The insertion site should be carefully prepared and draped and sterility maintained throughout the procedure. Pain can be minimised by the infiltration of local anaesthetic into the subcutaneous and deeper tissues, especially during the paramedian approach, onto the lamina through the Touhy needle.

Preparation of all drugs should be with a filter needle. Care should be taken not to contaminate intrathecal local anaesthetics with skin preparation fluid. Injection of intrathecal drug is easier with a Luer lock 3 mL syringe. This prevents dripping and loss of contents on injection.

Approach for spinal anaesthesia

Two approaches exist to the intrathecal or extradural space – midline or paramedian. In the elderly, supraspinal and interspinal ligaments are often calcified, and intervertebral spaces are narrowed. The author's preference is to use the paramedian approach for spinal anaesthesia in the elderly. The spinal introducer is inserted 1–1.5 cm lateral to the midline at the inferior aspect of the intervertebral space and directed slightly caudally about 20° to the midline.

Approach for extradural anaesthesia

For extradural anaesthesia, the midline approach is no more difficult in the lower thoracic region compared to lumbar epidurals because of the similar angulation of the spinous processes. In the mid and high thoracic regions, however, extreme upward angulation of the Tuohy needle directed through a small space makes insertion more difficult in the midline. The inferior tip of the spinous process corresponding to the vertebra above should be palpated and, 1 cm lateral to this point, local anaesthetic injected into both skin and the lamina of the vertebral body below. The approach of the needle is about 15° to the midline and 60–65° from the coronal plane. It may be preferable to use the paramedian approach because the bony lamina of the vertebra below acts as a depth finder and there is a definite 'rubbery' feel as the Tuohy needle passes from bony lamina to ligamentum flavum. The thoracic extradural space is identified by two methods – loss of resistance to saline/air, or hanging drop. Use of saline is associated with a reduced dural puncture rate.

Contraindications to central neuraxial blockade

Absolute

Absolute contraindications to central neuraxial blockade are:

- raised intracranial pressure (papilloedema, cerebral oedema, tumours in the posterior fossa, suspected subarachnoid haemorrhage);
- coagulopathy, blood dyscrasias or full anticoagulant therapy;
- skin sepsis or marked spinal deformity;
- patient refusal;
- hypovolaemia.

Relative

A relative contraindication to central neuraxial blockade is mildly impaired coagulation.

The risk of spinal haematoma should be weighed against the benefits of avoiding general anaesthesia in patients with platelets less than 80 000/mL. If coagulation is impaired, spinal anaesthesia should be preferred over extradural anaesthesia because of the reduced risk of haematoma formation.

Site of action of local anaesthetics

Local anaesthetics probably act on nerve roots, although some molecules reach the substance of the spinal cord.

Site of action of opioids

Unlike an equivalent intravenous injection, an opioid, when administered into the extradural space, must pass down a concentration gradient and negotiate several different tissue spaces, each with different properties, to reach the spinal cord.

Bioavailability

Extradural

The extent to which drugs reach their site of action is termed bioavailability.[15] Bioavailability is determined by the pharmacological properties of drugs and the relative hydrophobic and hydrophilic properties of tissues.

Pharmacological properties of a drug include not only its lipid solubility, but also the amount of free, non-protein-bound unionised drug available to diffuse down a concentration gradient. The higher the p*K*a of a local anaesthetic or opioid, the greater its ionisation at physiological pH and the less non-ionised drug available to diffuse through tissues.

Within the extradural space, the relationship between permeability and lipid solubility is biphasic,[15] with optimal permeability around an octanol: water coefficient of 125. As the water coefficient of morphine is 6 and that of fentanyl is 813, neither can be considered a permeable drug when administered via the extradural space. Diamorphine (diacetyl morphine) with an octanol: water coefficient of 280 represents a drug with good permeability because it is able to pass through both lipid- and water-soluble environments. The protein binding of diamorphine is only 40%. Of the remaining unbound fraction, 27% is available for transfer across membranes, equivalent to 16% of the total mass of diamorphine available for diffusion.

Little difference is evident between diamorphine and morphine concerning protein binding and free diffusible drug. In contrast, only 16% of fentanyl is not protein bound, of which only 9% is unionised, representing only 1.4% of administered fentanyl free for tissue transfer. Thus, 11 times more diamorphine molecules are available for diffusion compared to fentanyl.

Intradural

Although the dura is a relatively tough, avascular fibrous membrane, the arachnoid,[17] with its tight overlapping cells, represents 90% of resistance to drug permeability and keeps CSF confined to the subarachnoid space. Drugs are removed primarily from the rich capillary network of subdural vessels apposed to and supplying the underlying arachnoid. Animal studies have shown that epinephrine (adrenaline) reduces capillary blood flow in line with reduced clearance of drugs from extradural space.[18] Epinephrine (adrenaline) has a more pronounced effect on more vasodilatatory drugs such as lidocaine (lignocaine) compared to bupivacaine.

Within the CSF, drugs move by diffusion and bulk flow. Diffusion is proportional to the temperature of solution and inversely to the square of mass. As the mass of drugs administered into CSF is similar, diffusion alone does not explain movement in CSF. Why drugs move cephalad in CSF is attributable to the movement of CSF itself. As arterial blood flows into the brain, compression of the cranial CSF pushes spinal CSF caudally down the posterior surface of the spinal cord then cephalad up the anterior surface of the spinal cord.

The differences in rates of respiratory depression between intrathecal opioids are attributable to clearance into the dorsal horn. Clearance into the dorsal horn or systemic vasculature is dependent on lipid solubility. Lipid-soluble drugs, such as fentanyl, penetrate poorly into the dorsal horn and keep to lipid-soluble white matter. Their volume of distribution is high owing to partitioning within white matter, or into plasma. Water-soluble drugs, such as morphine, penetrate deep into grey matter (lacks myelin) where opioid receptors exist. Thus, water-soluble drugs such as morphine have a greater potency when injected into CSF than do lipid-soluble drugs such as fentanyl.

Recent evidence from two studies in women in labour suggest that fentanyl has a spinal cord action and reduces local anaesthetic EC_{50} (median effective concentration) compared to a concomitant intravenous injection.[19,20] Similar evidence exists for extradural administration of fentanyl after surgery, and an increased sensitivity in labour to opioids may explain these findings.

Clinical efficacy

Selective central neuraxial blockade

Spinal and extradural anaesthesia with local anaesthetic[21] blocks the following:

- autonomic (sympathetic) preganglionic b fibres;
- sensory fibres (Aβ, Aδ, C, conveying temperature, pinprick, touch, pressure, vibration and proprioception);
- motor fibres (Aα, Aγ).

During central neuraxial blockade, the height of the sympathetic, sensory and motor block follows the same order.[22] Thus, sympathetic block is higher than sensory block, the extent of which varies according to testing modality. A block of T5 to light touch is recommended for confirmation of adequate anaesthesia before caesarean section. However, the corresponding block heights to testing modalities such as ice or pinprick in the same patient may be two to three sensory segments higher. The duration of sensory block is greater than that of motor block.

The rank order of sensitivity to neural block is in the order $A\gamma > A\delta = A\alpha > A\beta > C$,[21] with faster-conducting C fibers (conduction velocity >1 m/s) more sensitive than slower ones (conduction velocity <1 m/s).

Predictors of successful central neuraxial blockade

De Filho et al.[23] have investigated the chances of successful spinal or epidural block in 1481 patients. Success was defined as locating the epidural space or CSF at the first attempt. For each block the following factors were recorded: gender, age, height, weight, body habitus, ability to palpate the spinous processes, spinal anatomy, patient positioning, premedication, needle type and gauge, approach, spinal level of the block, and the provider's level of experience. The results showed that the success rate of entering CSF or the epidural space first time was 61.51%. Multivariate logistic regression analysis identified independent predictors of initial success as the quality of anatomical landmarks odds ratio (OR [95% CI]) 1.92 (1.6–2.4), experience of the anaesthetist 1.2 (1.2–1.3) and the adequacy of patient positioning 3.8 (2.84–5.2).

SPINAL ANAESTHESIA

Efficacy of spinal anaesthesia

Prediction of spread

The best predictor of spread of intrathecal solutions is CSF volume.[6] This parameter cannot be measured in practice. Clinically, spread of intrathecal local anaesthetic is determined principally by the baricity of the solution and the position of the patient.[24] Baricity is the density of solution relative to CSF. The density of a solution is the mass of drug (g) per mL of solution.

Other determinants of spread of local anaesthetic include age, height, body mass index, pregnancy, spinal anatomy, site of injection, direction of needle aperture and tissue fixation.

Age

There is a tendency to increased spread of spinal anaesthesia with increased age, probably owing to decreased CSF volume and increased susceptibility to local anaesthetic block in the elderly.

Height

There is no significant correlation between height and spread of spinal anaesthesia within the normal range of adult heights. At the extremes of height there is a tendency to increased spread because the solution has greater distances to cover.

Body mass

Body mass expressed as the relative weight to surface area (kg/m^2) has an effect on the spread of spinal anaesthesia. Increased spread occurs in obese patients owing to engorgement of extradural veins and compression of the subarachnoid space, and reduction in CSF volume.

Pregnancy

Pregnant patients have a more extensive cephalad spread of spinal block than nonpregnant patients. Several factors may account for this. Progesterone is found in greater amounts in CSF and sensitises nerves to local anaesthetics.

Inferior vena cava (IVC) obstruction by the pregnant uterus redirects cardiac return via the extradural venous plexus to the azygous vein and, as in obese patients, compresses CSF. Venous return via the IVC is favoured if the patient lies in a lateral position. The density of local anaesthetics only influences spread of block height in the lateral decubitus position because the effect of IVC obstruction is minimised. However, if the patient is placed in the left tilted 15° position, IVC obstruction becomes the predominant influence on spread and overwhelms the effect of density.[25] Solutions of hypobaric, isobaric and hyperbaric bupivacaine spinal agents all spread to similar high sensory dermatomes in the pregnant patient.

Phenylephrine can decrease rostral spread of spinal anaesthesia in pregnancy, compared to intravenous ephedrine.[26]

Technique

Anatomy of the spine and site of injection

During pregnancy there may be kyphosis, with flattening of the lumbar curvature, or alternatively accentuation of the curvature in addition to the wider female pelvis. Injection in the lateral decubitus position at the interspace between the second and third lumbar vertebrae has a tendency to higher block. However, as with all hypobaric plain solutions, the interindividual spread is irrespective of the chosen interspace. For caesarean section no differences exist between right lateral and left lateral positions and spread of spinal block.[27]

Direction of the needle aperture

The direction of the orifice of a pencil-point needle influences the spread of anaesthesia. Spread is less when local anaesthetic is injected caudally compared to cranial orientation of the needle opening. Injection of hyperbaric solution through a lateral orifice can provide unilateral anaesthesia if the patient is maintained in the lateral position. Combined spinal extradural is associated with greater spread, and a greater incidence of hypotension and vasoconstrictor administration than are single-injection spinals.[28]

Fixation

Intrathecal local anaesthetic takes 1–2 hours to fix to tissues, not 15 minutes as was previously thought.

Factors influencing onset, spread and duration of spinal anaesthesia

Baricity

Hypobaric solutions

A hypobaric local anaesthetic is defined as a solution with a density more than three standard deviations (SD) below mean human CSF density. Hypobaric solutions manifest as an unpredictable median sensory block height with a large interindividual spread and are occasionally associated with block failure when the spinal block has not spread high enough for surgery.

Hyperbaric solutions

Hyperbaric solutions are technically solutions with a density more than 3 SD above mean human CSF density. However, this is difficult to define because there are many different influences on the density of local anaesthetics.

Density

Human CSF density is not uniform and varies according to age, sex, pregnancy and illness (Table 4.3.1).[29,30]

Densities of local anaesthetics

The densities of bupivacaine, levobupivacaine and ropivacaine are shown in Table 4.3.2. All plain solutions of bupivacaine and ropivacaine are hypo-

Group	CSF density (g/mL) (SD)
Men	1.00067 (0.00018)
Postmenopausal women	1.00060 (0.00015)
Premenopausal women	1.00047 (0.00008)
Pregnant women	1.00033 (0.00010)

Table 4.3.1 Density of CSF

Solution	Density at 23°C g/mL (SD)	Density at 37°C g/mL (SD)
Bupivacaine 0.25%	1.00345 (0.00003)	0.99921 (0.00009)
Bupivacaine 0.5%	1.00376 (0.00002)	0.99944 (0.00012)
Bupivacaine 0.75%	1.00369 (0.00002)	0.99938 (0.00017)
Levobupivacaine 0.25%	1.00418 (0.00001)	0.99985 (0.00002)
Levobupivacaine 0.5%	1.00419 (0.00002)	1.00024 (0.00009)
Levobupivacaine 0.75%	1.00482 (0.00002)	1.00056 (0.00010)
Ropivacaine 0.2%	1.00372 (0.00002)	0.99960 (0.00006)
Ropivacaine 0.5%	1.00380 (0.00002)	0.99953 (0.00013)
Ropivacaine 0.75%	1.00380 (0.00003)	0.99953 (0.00014)
Ropivacaine 1%	1.00381 (0.00002)	0.99950 (0.00010)

Table 4.3.2 Density of plain solutions of local anaesthetic.[30] Data represent mean (SD)

baric at 37°C (>3SD from the density of CSF).[31] The density of levobupivacaine 0.5% with and without dextrose is significantly greater than the corresponding densities of bupivacaine 0.5% and ropivacaine 0.5% at both 23°C and 37°C. The mean (±SD) density of levobupivacaine 0.75% is 1.00056 (0.00003) g/mL, and it can be regarded as an isobaric solution.

Factors influencing density of local anaesthetics

The density of local anaesthetics is influenced by temperature, electrolyte composition and the addition of dextrose and opioids. Although changes in density may seem minimal and clinically unnecessary, a change in density as low as 0.0006 g/mL may influence spread of local anaesthetic.

Temperature

As the temperature of bupivacaine, levobupivacaine or ropivacaine is reduced, density increases. All concentrations of bupivacaine and ropivacaine are hypobaric when measured at 37°C, but hyperbaric when measured at 23°C.

Electrolyte composition

The increased density of levobupivacaine may be attributable to its higher sodium ion content and higher osmolality compared to bupivacaine and ropivacaine.[31] As the concentration of levobupivacaine is increased, sodium concentration is held constant, whereas as the concentration of bupivacaine or ropivacaine is increased, sodium concentration is reduced. In addition, there is a 13% additional contribution to osmolarity by levobupivacaine compared to bupivacaine. Ampoules of 0.75% levobupivacaine contain 7.5 mg/mL free base (26.0 mmol/L), whereas corresponding ampoules of 0.75% bupivacaine contain 6.66 mg/mL free base, and 7.5 mg hydrochloride (23.1 mmol/L), and ampoules of 0.75% ropivacaine 6.63 mg/mL 7.5 mg hydrochloride (24.1 mmol/L).

Dextrose

Several studies of spinal anaesthesia for lower limb, urological surgery and caesarean section with bupivacaine,[32] ropivacaine[33] and tetracaine (amethocaine)[34] show that addition of a small amount of dextrose to local anaesthetics increases the density of injectate provides a reliable and sufficient sensory block within a small range of median maximal block height.

Opioids

Opioids are often added to spinal preparations of local anaesthetics to improve anaesthesia and prolong postoperative analgesia. Opioids such as fentanyl are hypobaric (0.9933 g/mL), and when added to a local anaesthetic will render the subsequent mixture even more hypobaric. The degree to which this occurs is proportional to the respective densities and volumes of individual drugs.

Sensory spread of spinal block

The clinical efficacy of a local anaesthetic may be measured as:

- time of onset (usually time to attain predefined dermatomal level or maximal block height);
- duration of action (usually time to predefined block height or time to complete resolution of block);
- upper and lower sensory levels to sensory testing over time (usually pinprick).

Hypobaric solutions exhibit a variable, unpredictable and unreliable block.[35] Block height varies between L2 and T_4 and occasionally is inadequate for surgery. Hyperbaric solutions of bupivacaine (8% dextrose) provide a reliable, but high block height (T_4) associated with hypotension and bradycardia. In contrast, addition of small quantities of dextrose to bupivacaine provides a reliable but not excessive block[33] (T7/8) (Fig. 4.3.1).

Duration of spinal block

The duration of spinal anaesthesia is dependent on the mass of drug – the greater the mass of local anaesthetic injected, the longer the duration. For

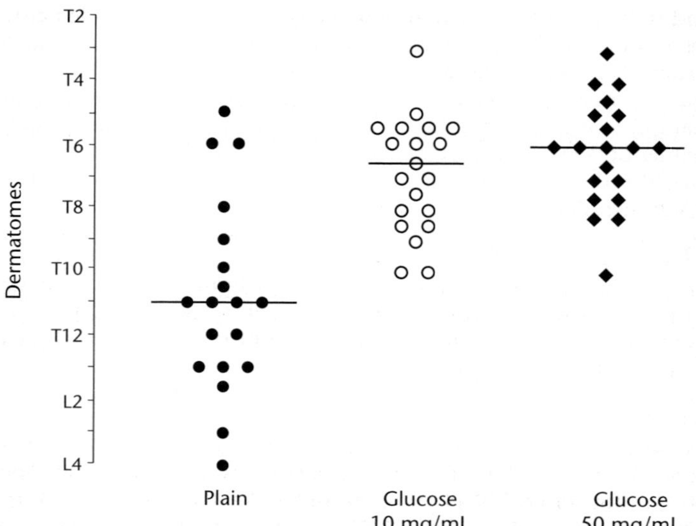

Figure 4.3.1 Sensory spread of spinal ropivacaine with dextrose compared to that of plain bupivacaine. Each point represents maximal spread for each patient.

ambulatory surgery, very small doses of bupivacaine (5 mg) have been successfully used, with duration of block of 60 minutes. On the other hand, the mean duration of spinal anaesthesia after 20 mg of bupivacaine is 3–4 hours. For caesarean section, doses of 10–12.5 mg provide adequate anaesthesia, whereas doses below 10 mg are associated with peritoneal pain.

Potency of intrathecal local anaesthetics

In order to objectively compare the onset, duration and offset of local anaesthetics, knowledge of their relative potencies is required for both intradural and extradural administration. The method commonly used to determine relative potency is that of sequential allocation,[36] whereby the concentration of drug administered in a fixed volume to a patient is determined according to the response of the previous patient. Three outcomes exist:

- visual analogue scale (VAS) score ≤10 mm at any time within 30 minutes of initial injection: extradural is regarded as successful and the next patient is given a smaller concentration of drug;
- VAS score >10 mm at all times within 30 minutes of initial injection and subsequent rescue extradural analgesia provides pain relief: the extradural is regarded as unsuccessful and the next patient is given a higher concentration of drug;
- VAS score >10 mm at all times within 30 minutes of initial injection and subsequent rescue extradural analgesia does not provide pain relief: the extradural is regarded as a technical failure and the next patient is given the same concentration of drug.

Plotting the sequential response of patients shows an oscillating pattern from which a median effective concentration (EC_{50}) is calculated and a dose–response curve derived.

Sensory block

Using this methodology, no differences were seen when levobupivacaine and ropivacaine were injected intrathecally with fentanyl 10 μg and morphine 0.2 mg for elective caesarean section as part of a CSE technique. The ED_{50}s for attaining a bilateral block height of T6 and successful anaesthesia were 6.7 and 7.6 mg, and ED_{95}s were 11.0 and 11.2 mg for levobupivacaine and ropivacaine, respectively.[37]

Motor block

The motor blocking capacity of both drugs was also compared in a similar cohort of patients undergoing CSE for elective caesarean section.[37] The ED_{50} (95% CI) for motor block at 5 minutes was 4.8 (4.49–5.28) mg for levobupivacaine and 5.9 (4.82–6.98) mg for ropivacaine. The estimated ED_{95} motor block was 5.9 (5.19–6.71) mg for levobupivacaine and 8.3 (6.30–10.44) mg for ropivacaine, potency ratio 0.83.

Intrathecal drugs

Local anaesthetics

Lidocaine (lignocaine)

Lidocaine (lignocaine) has a rapid onset of action, intermediate duration and low toxicity with minimal side-effects, allowing rapid discharge and high levels of patient satisfaction. There is a dose-dependent increase in duration. Reduction of the intrathecal dose of lidocaine (lignocaine) 2% to 40 mg decreased duration of anaesthesia for outpatient surgery without compromising quality of spinal block. Disadvantages include its neurotoxicity, with transient neurological symptoms (TNS) as frequent as 33%. TNS are less frequent in the pregnant population.

Bupivacaine

Bupivacaine is the amide local anaesthetic most commonly used for spinal anaesthesia for caesarean section. It exhibits a sensory/motor split, but is toxic in overdose. Its relative toxicity compared to that of lidocaine (lignocaine) is greater than its relative potency. A dose of 10–12.5 mg is required for caesarean section. It can be used for ambulatory surgery if doses of 7.5 mg are given. The frequency of TNS after plain or hyperbaric bupivacaine is small. It is also safe in CSA. In low concentrations (0.1–0.125%) it can also be used alone or in combination with opioids to provide postoperative analgesia.

Ropivacaine

No cases of TNS have been described with ropivacaine. Hyperbaric spinal solutions are more reliable. The duration of motor blockade observed is similar to that with intrathecal lidocaine (lignocaine).

Significant differences have emerged between bupivacaine and ropivacaine for intrathecal anaesthesia. Initial studies of intrathecal hypobaric ropivacaine showed a variable and inadequate sensory block, particularly using lower doses of 15 mg. However, recent studies of hyperbaric ropivacaine have shown that the drug can provide predictable and reliable anaesthesia for surgery. Compared to bupivacaine[39] (with 8% dextrose), ropivacaine (with 5% dextrose) had a longer onset of block to T10 (5 min vs 2 min), lower median maximum block height (T7 vs T5), shorter regression of sensory block to T10 (56.5 min vs 118 min), quicker mobilisation 253.5 min vs 331 min and earlier micturition (276 min vs 340.5 min).

Ropivacaine has the potential to replace lidocaine (lignocaine) for ambulatory anaesthesia. For caesarean section, when combined with with sufentanil 2.5 μg sensory block has been shown to be more effective with 8 mg bupivacaine (97%) than with 8 mg levobupivacaine (80%) or 12 mg ropivacaine (87%) and to be associated with longer motor block.[40]

Levobupivacaine

Very little difference exists in the spread, duration and offset of intrathecal block between bupivacaine and levobupivacaine as the plain[41] or hyperbaric solutions[42] over a range of doses from 4 mg to 12 mg.

Procaine

Procaine has been used for spinal anaesthesia for almost 100 years. As a short-acting agent it was substituted by lidocaine (lignocaine), which provided a faster onset and longer duration of anaesthesia. Recent concern about TNS after the use of spinal lidocaine (lignocaine) has renewed the interest in procaine spinal anaesthesia. It is associated with nausea and a longer duration of action than lidocaine (lignocaine).

Prilocaine

Prilocaine is available in only a few countries. The incidence of TNS after prilocaine is only 3%.

Tetracaine (amethocaine)

Tetracaine (amethocaine) is a long-acting amino ester with a duration of action greater than that of bupivacaine. It is associated with poor tolerance of a limb tourniquet compared to bupivacaine.

Mepivacaine

Mepivacaine as 20–40 mg hyperbaric solutions has been safely used for spinal anaesthesia since 1961. It is associated with a high frequency of TNS. Its duration of action is 50% greater than that of lidocaine (lignocaine).

Opioids

Addition of opioids such as fentanyl (12.5 μg), sufentanil (2.5–5 μg), diamorphine (0.3 mg) and morphine (0.1–0.2 mg) improves analgesic quality, prolongs sensory block, reduces local anaesthetic requirements, reduces the duration of motor blockade and improves haemodynamic stability. Intraoperative analgesic supplementation in caesarean section is reduced from 24% to 4%. Fentanyl, sufentanil, diamorphine and morphine all increase the duration of postoperative analgesia.

Morphine

Morphine improves the quality of spinal anaesthesia and postoperative pain relief lasts over 18 hours. The small dose of morphine used in local anaesthetics for spinal has an additive effect.

Diamorphine

Diamorphine is only available in the UK. Diacetylmorphine breaks down quickly to morphine within the spinal cord. The CSF clearance is twice that of morphine.

Fentanyl

Fentanyl has high lipid solubility, a very large volume of distribution in the spinal cord and rapid clearance from the CSF. The dose is 10–25 μg. Pruritus is common with a higher dose. The addition of 10 μg fentanyl to 5 mg bupivacaine for day-case surgical knee arthroscopy increased success from 75–100% without prolonging discharge time or time to micturition. It may decrease the incidence of TNS with lidocaine (lignocaine). There is little difference in the extradural and intrathecal doses of fentanyl and sufentanil. It does not reduce patient-controlled analgesia (PCA) morphine consumption. Some studies have shown an increase in PCA requirements after intrathecal fentanyl compared to controls.

Sufentanil

Sufentanil has high lipid solubility, a very large volume of distribution in the spinal cord and rapid clearance from CSF. Intrathecal sufentanil in 2.5–7.5 μg doses has been found to relieve labour pain and improves the quality of caesarean section spinal anaesthesia.

Pethidine (Meperidine)

Pethidine is a unique opioid analgesic that possesses local anaesthetic properties. It is rapidly taken up and cleared from the spinal cord in the rat, so there is less risk of respiratory depression. It produces little motor block. It is inadequate for peripheral nerve block – in a study of volunteers pethidine did not produce a median nerve block.

Adjuvants

Epinephrine (adrenaline)

Epinephrine (adrenaline) prolongs the duration of spinal anaesthesia. It causes antinociceptive effects on the level of the spinal cord via direct activation of descending inhibitory pathways. Addition of 0.2 mg epinesphrine (adrenaline) to 60 mg isobaric intrathecal lidocaine (lignocaine) significantly prolongs sensory and motor blockade and time to micturition.

Clonidine

Clonidine is commonly added to local anaesthetics in spinal, extradural and peripheral blocks. Doses of 15–45 μg intrathecal clonidine prolong the duration of sensory analgesia. Side-effects such as hypotension and sedation have restricted its more extensive use.

Neostigmine

Neostigmine inhibits the breakdown of acetylcholine, the endogenous neurotransmitter in descending inhibitory fibres. Doses are 5–100 μg. A dose-dependent increase in the incidence of nausea and vomiting occurred in patients who received neostigmine.

EXTRADURAL ANAESTHESIA AND ANALGESIA

Spread of extradural anaesthesia

Prediction of spread

Multivariate regression analysis of 803 ASA class 1–2 patients[43] undergoing lumbar extradural anaesthesia has shown that spread of extradural analgesia, as defined by dose per spinal, significantly increases with increasing age, weight, body mass index, dose of local anaesthetic, addition of fentanyl, higher extradural site of injection, and decreasing body height. The relationship between volume and spread is not linear because a stepwise increase in volume results in a relatively small increase in spread (Fig. 4.3.2).

Multivariate analysis of patients with thoracic extradural analgesia after abdominal surgery has shown independent predictors of longer time to first experience of pain with increasing age, use of diamorphine-containing solutions (compared to fentanyl) and, when excluding technical failures, type of surgery.[43a] Patients after oesophageal surgery experienced pain significantly earlier than vascular surgery patients.

Age

Spread of extradural solutions increases with age (see Fig. 4.3.2). Dose requirements fall by 40%.[44] Greater falls occur in heart rate and blood pressure in the elderly.[45] A fall in epidural fat content with age improves compliance and reduces the resistance to spread of local anaesthetics. In addition, a reduction in the number of axons and a fall in conduction velocity increases the sensitivity of nerves to local anaesthetic.

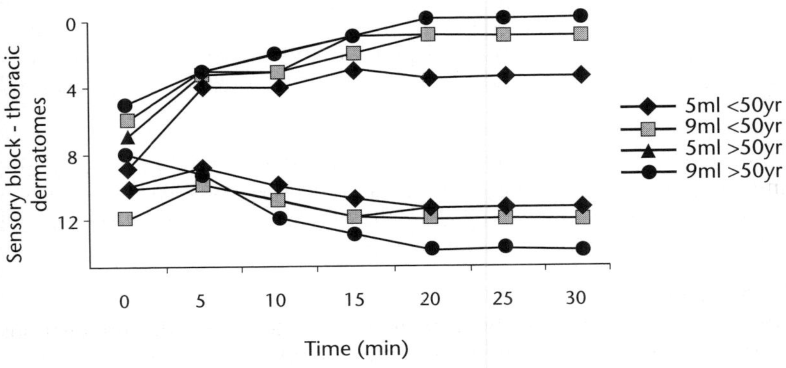

Figure 4.3.2 Spread according to age and volume of injectate when injected at the interspace between the seventh and eighth thoracic vertebrae.

Site of injection

Spread depends on the site of injection and type of operation:

- lumbar extradural for labour;
- lumbar extradural for caesarean section;
- thoracic extradural for abdominal surgery;
- lumbar extradural for abdominal surgery.

Dermatomal spread of analgesia to pinprick of lumbar extradural after injection of 10 mL 0.25% bupivacaine and levobupivacaine[45] for pain in early labour is similar. Median block extends from T9 to L2. When the first bolus wears off, a further injection of 10 mL 0.25% bupivacaine and levobupivacaine extents the block from T8 to S2. Mean VAS is shown to decrease with each contraction. It can be seen that good pain relief in labour is compatible with a VAS less than or equal to 10 mm.

Dermatomal spread of analgesia to pinprick of lumbar extradural after injection of 25–30 mL 0.5% bupivacaine and levobupivacaine[46] for elective caesarean section is also similar. Median block extends from T_3 to S3. Regression of extradural block to T10 takes over 300 minutes.

For abdominal surgery dermatomal sensory spread of extradural local anaesthetics varies according to the site of injection.[48,49] As illustrated in Figure 4.3.3, high thoracic epidurals have minimal cranial spread but marked caudal spread. Conversely, more cranial spread occurs following low thoracic epidurals compared with the high and midthoracic epidurals. This phenomenon is attributable to a progressive increase in the width of the extradural space from 1–1.5 mm at C5 (due to cervical cord expansion) to 2.5–3 mm at T6 and to 5–6 mm at L2. Thus, insertion of a low thoracic extradural should be at a level corresponding to the midline of the surgical incision, whereas a high thoracic extradural should be inserted at a relatively cranial point with respect to the incision.

Insertion of a lumbar extradural for abdominal surgery may compromise outcome compared to a well-managed thoracic epidural. Lumbar sensory block for abdominal surgery is difficult to maintain, rescue analgesia is required more often and motor block is inevitable. As sympathetic blockade is extended to the lower limbs, baroreceptor-mediated reflex vasoconstriction is limited to areas cephalad to the block, increasing the likelihood of coronary vasoconstriction and myocardial ischaemia. Furthermore, following large blood loss, decreases in mean arterial pressure, systemic vascular resistance and base excess are significantly larger in the presence of extensive thoracolumbar blockade compared to selective thoracic blockade or general anaesthesia alone. The Bezold–Jarisch reflex, characterised by bradycardia, vasodilation and hypotension is also more common with extensive lumbar epidural blocks. Only by restricting spread to the lumbar and low thoracic regions can lumbar epidural block restrict splanchnic sympathetic blockade, maintain venous return and lessen

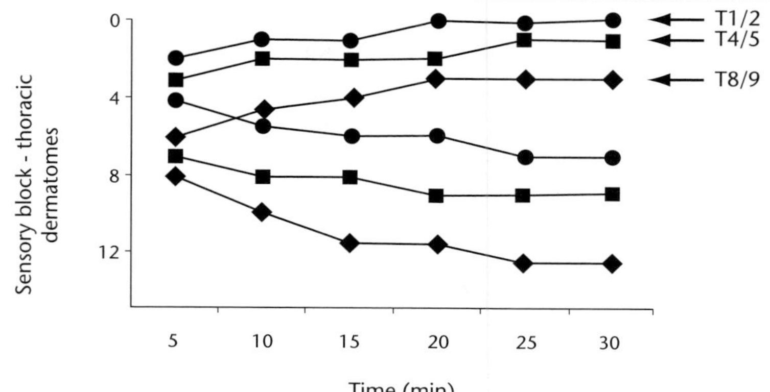

Figure 4.3.3 Spread of injectate from three different sites of injection: T1/2 (circles), T4/5 (squares), and T8/9 (diamonds).

hypotension. Therefore, the evidence suggests that lumbar epidural anaesthesia should be avoided in patients undergoing abdominal or thoracic procedures.

Dose of extradural local anaesthetic

Traditionally, mass (the product of volume and concentration) has been regarded as the primary determinant of extradural spread and efficacy.

Scott et al.[50] found that increasing the mass of bupivacaine and etidocaine for epidural block, by increasing concentration and keeping the volume constant, resulted in a more rapid onset and duration of sensory and motor blockade with better pain relief.

Two recent studies have challenged the claim that the mass of local anaesthetic determines efficacy. Sakura et al.,[51] using quantitative sensory analysis and the same mass of lidocaine (lignocaine) (200 mg), showed that 10 mL of 2% lidocaine (lignocaine) increased the intensity of sensory block compared to 20 mL of 1% lidocaine (lignocaine) anaesthesia.

Furthermore, the first MLAC (minimum local anaesthetic concentration) study of chlorprocaine for labour analgesia showed, with increasing volumes, that sequential oscillation between patients occurred at low concentrations of chlorprocaine, suggesting that the efficacy of local anaesthetics is concentration dependent. The impact of the volume dependency of local anaesthetics using MLAC has never been studied. Thus, it is not known if the relationship between concentration and volume is linear or curvilinear when assessed over large volumes.

Large versus small concentrations

A large concentration and small volume of levobupivacaine given as a continuous thoracic extradural infusion provides an equal quality of postoperative analgesia as a small-concentration and large-volume infusion and induces less motor blockade and fewer haemodynamic repercussions.[52]

Mode of delivery

Three modes of delivery of local anaesthetic can be used:

- continuous infusion;
- patient-controlled extradural analgesia (PCEA);
- intermittent bolus.

Continuous infusion, despite being the most popular means of administration, is associated with sensory block regression, particularly with local anaesthetic alone. Addition of opioid increases the time to first analgesic rescue. The continued popularity of infusion stems from the perception that it is has fewer cardiovascular and respiratory side-effects than bolus alone.

Patient-controlled extradural analgesia, usually with a background infusion, allows patient self-titration and sparing of local anaesthetic consumption by up to one-third.[53] The main advantage of PCEA compared to infusion is comparable efficacy, but with a marked reduction in side-effects. However, this technique is dependent on an awake, cooperative patient and is not suitable for patients sedated following general anaesthesia. Patient-controlled extradural analgesia using large boluses (15 mL) of bupivacaine 0.1% and fentanyl 2 μg/mL, without a background infusion, is recommended for labour pain.

Intermittent bolus administration at fixed time intervals has been shown to minimise block regression compared to the same concentration of local anaesthetic given as an infusion after pelvic surgery and during labour.

Choice of local anaesthetic

The choice of local anaesthetic may vary when used for:

- labour;
- caesarean section;
- surgery.

Extradural bupivacaine 0.1%, levobupivacaine 0.1%[54] and ropivacaine 0.1%[55] appear equipotent when combined with fentanyl 2 μg/mL and using PCEA for labour analgesia. However, differences in motor block between levobupivacaine, ropivacaine and bupivacaine are clinically apparent during caesarean section. With levobupivacaine 0.5% for extradural anaesthesia, 39% of patients achieved a modified Bromage score of 0 compared to only 10% with the use of 0.5% bupivacaine, but without detriment to the quality of surgical operating conditions.[56]

For surgery levobupivacaine 0.5% produces an extradural block of similar onset, quality and duration as that produced by the same volume of

0.5% bupivacaine, with a motor block deeper than that produced by 0.5% ropivacaine. Two of five patients with ropivacaine had an intraoperative Bromage score less than 2, compared to one out of five patients with levobupivacaine and none with bupivacaine. When prolonging the block for the first 12 hours after surgery with a patient-controlled extradural infusion, 0.125% levobupivacaine provides adequate pain relief after major orthopaedic surgery, with similar recovery of motor function as with 0.125% bupivacaine and 0.2% ropivacaine.[57] When used as PCEA and combined with small-dose extradural morphine, 0.1% levobupivacaine and 0.1% ropivacaine produce comparable postoperative analgesia with a similar incidence of side-effects.[58]

Combinations of extradural drugs

Many comparisons have been made of local anaesthetic alone, opioid alone or combinations of the two. The overall findings suggest that the combination of local anaesthetic and opioid provides best analgesia on movement, has less hypotension compared to local anaesthetic alone and halves the duration of ileus compared to extradural opioid alone or PCA. Knowledge of the optimal mix of local anaesthetic and opioid would improve pain relief and minimise side-effects associated with both drugs. One study so far has attempted this in 190 patients receiving thoracic extradural analgesia for 48 hours after major abdominal surgery.[59] Combinations of bupivacaine, fentanyl and infusion rate were investigated by a stepwise optimisation model until there was the best balance of analgesia and side-effects. Optimisation techniques use groups of three or six patients and take into account side-effects as well as efficacy to determine the new concentrations and volume of local anaesthetic and opioid. The optimal combinations were bupivacaine 8 mg/h plus fentanyl 30 μg/h at an infusion rate of 9 mL/h, and bupivacaine 13 mg/h plus fentanyl 25 μg/h at an infusion rate of 9 mL/h.

Alternative adjuvants include clonidine, epinephrine (adrenaline) and ketamine. Clonidine is an α_2-agonist associated with hypotension and sedation. Using the same optimisation model, the best dose of clonidine is 5 μg/h when combined with bupivacaine 9 mg/h and fentanyl 21 μg/h at an infusion rate of 9 mL/h.

Addition of epinephrine (adrenaline) to mixtures of local anaesthetic and fentanyl improves pain relief, probably by a spinal cord α_2-agonist effect, attenuates sensory block regression, and reduces serum fentanyl concentrations.[60]

Ketamine is an *N*-methyl-D-aspartate (NMDA) receptor antagonist and has been used as an adjuvant to opioids and local anaesthetics within the extradural space. However, evidence now exists that intravenous intraoperative administration of ketamine reduces secondary hyperalgesia at 6 months following surgery. This does not occur with extradural ketamine.

Type of operation

Type of operation was an independent predictor of time to first experience of pain when excluding all patients with technical failure. Longer pain relief was obtained in patients undergoing, in rank order, pelvic, vascular, splenic, hepatopancreatic, bowel, abdominal wall, gastro-oesophageal and renal surgery.

Potency of extradural local anaesthetics

Sequential allocation studies (Fig. 4.3.4) of the minimum effective local analgesic concentration (MLAC) for extradural analgesia in the first stage of labour have shown the EC_{50} (95% CI) of levobupivacaine to be 0.083 (0.065–0.101)% compared to 0.081 (0.055–0.108)% for bupivacaine.[36]

Using the same methodology, the EC_{50} for ropivacaine was 0.111 (0.100–0.122)%[61] and 0.156 (0.136–0.176)%[62] when compared to bupivacaine[59] 0.067 (0.052–0.082)% and 0.093 (0.076–0.110)%,[62] respectively. Recent direct comparisons of levobupivacaine and ropivacaine have shown respectively a 2% and a 19% difference in potency.

The calculated EC_{50}s for levobupivacaine were consistent with previous studies – 0.077 (0.058–0.096)%[63] and 0.087 (0.081–0.094)%,[64] but for ropivacaine were much lower than had previously been shown 0.089 (0.075–0.103)%[64] and 0.092 (0.082–0.102)%.[63] However, interpretation of these results should take into account the expression of levobupivacaine concentration as mg/mL base in contrast to preparations of bupivacaine and ropivacaine where the dose is expressed as mg/mL of hydrochloride. Levobupivacaine contains 13% more active local anaesthetic than bupivacaine.

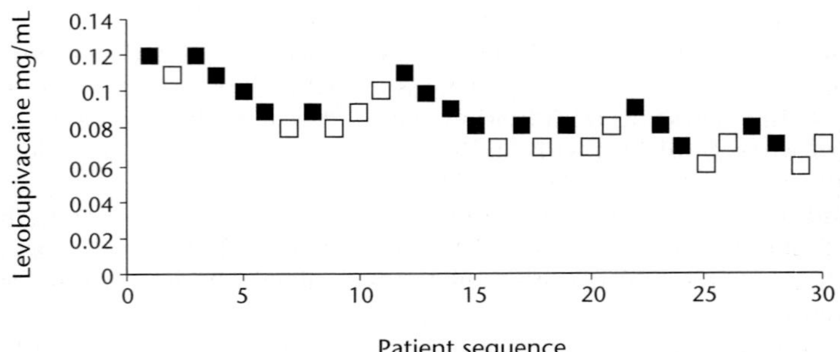

Figure 4.3.4 Example of sequential allocation technique. The *y* axis represents the concentration of local bupivacaine. The *x* axis shows each successive patient. The blocked squares represent successful block, the empty squares represent unsuccessful block. Data from Ninewells Hospital.

Potency of extradural adjuvants

The effect of adding epinephrine (adrenaline), fentanyl and sufentanil has also been shown using sequential allocation. The addition of epinephrine (adrenaline) 1:300 000 reduced the EC_{50} of bupivacaine by a third from 0.091 (0.081–0.102)% to 0.060.5 (0.047–0.083)%.[65] Fentanyl at concentrations of 2 μg/mL and 3 μg/mL significantly reduced the MLAC of levobupivacaine from 0.091 (0.052–0.130)% to 0.047 (0.023–0.072)% and 0.050 (0.035–0.060.5)%, respectively.[66] The addition of sufentanil at doses of 0.5 μg/mL, 1 μg/mL and 1.5 μg/mL resulted in significant reductions in the MLAC of bupivacaine to 0.048 (0.030–0.060.5)%, 0.021 (0–0.050.5)%, and 0.009 (0–0.023)%, respectively.[67]

Motor block

Motor block is measured by two subjective scales:

- modified Bromage scale (0, full power; 1, unable to straighten leg; 2, just able to flex knees; 3, foot movement only);
- Medical Research Council (MRC) straight leg raising score (0, no active contraction; 1, visible palpable contraction without active movement; 2, movement possible with gravity eliminated, 3, movement possible against gravity; 4, movement possible against gravity plus resistance, but weaker than normal; 5, normal power).

Sensory–motor split of extradural local anaesthetics

Ropivacaine

An early in-vitro study[68] in isolated rabbit vagus nerve was the first to show a preferential blockade of sensory to motor fibres with ropivacaine. The results showed that the depressant effect of bupivacaine was 16% greater than that of ropivacaine on motor fibres, but only 3% greater on sensory fibres. The enhanced differential between sensory and motor blockade was given further standing from an extradural infusion study on volunteers using 0.1%, 0.2%, 0.3% ropivacaine, 0.25% bupivacaine or saline.[69] Over the 21-hour study period, sensory block and isometric quadriceps function were measured. The results showed that ropivacaine 0.2% and 0.3% were associated with less motor block than 0.25% bupivacaine (Fig. 4.3.5). However, the extent of sensory spread was concentration dependent for ropivacaine and receded much more quickly than for bupivacaine (Fig. 4.3.6).

Levobupivacaine

Widening of the sensory motor split with ropivacaine and levobupivacaine compared to bupivacaine corroborates clinical studies of analgesia in labour using extradural and intrathecal levobupivacaine. Using the same MLAC methodology, and definition of motor block according to the Bromage

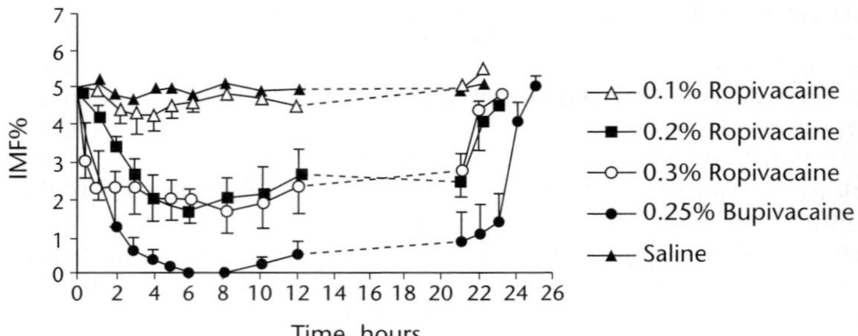

Figure 4.3.5 Quantitative isometric motor function (IMF) as a percentage of pre-epidural measurement for saline, ropivacaine 0.1%, 0.2%, 0.3%, and bupivacaine 0.25%.

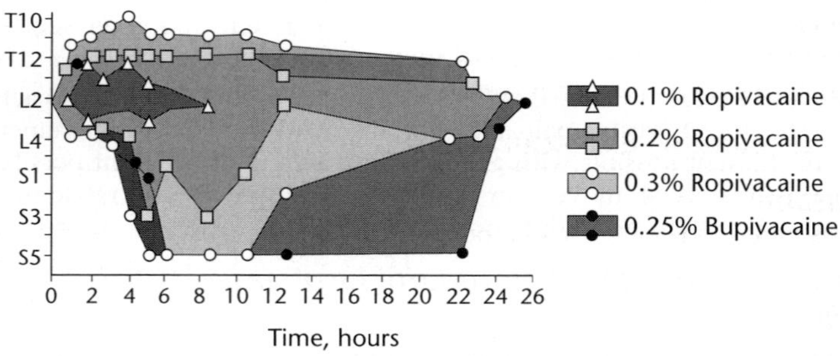

Figure 4.3.6 Sensory spread of ropivacaine 0.1%, 0.2%, 0.3%, and bupivacaine 0.25%.

scale, both ropivacaine and levobupivacaine have been shown to have less propensity for motor block than bupivacaine.

Comparative potency of local anaesthetics for motor block

During extradural analgesia for labour, the motor block minimal local analgesic concentration (MLAC) for bupivacaine[70] was 0.33% (0.28–0.37) and for ropivacaine was 0.49% (0.43–0.56%), potency ratio 0.66 (0.52–0.82). The EC_{50} for levobupivacaine was 0.31% (0.29–0.34%) compared to 0.27% (0.25–0.30%) for bupivacaine, potency ratio 0.87 (0.77–0.98).[71]

The relative importance of motor block depends on the type of surgical procedure, and the depth and duration required of postoperative analgesia. This should be balanced against the clinical properties of each local anaesthetic, such as time of onset, duration of analgesia and motor block and propensity for rescue analgesia. Limb operations, for example, need not only an immobile surgical field, but also postoperative pain relief of such depth that rapid mobilisation is possible without motor block to accelerate postoperative function and rehabilitation.

Combination of general anaesthesia and extradural anaesthesia

Induction of general anaesthesia following the establishment of thoracic extradural anaesthesia can precipitate hypotension, particularly with propofol. Hypovolaemia following fasting and or bowel preparation for surgery will accentuate any drop in blood pressure. Therefore it is good practice to restore blood volume with intravenous fluids and establish general anaesthesia with intravenous etomidate under direct arterial pressure monitoring. When the patient is anaesthetised, fluids can be titrated according to central venous pressure or oesophageal Doppler monitor. Extradural top-ups of 3–5 mL bupivacaine 0.75% or equivalent are administered judiciously throughout the operation and on wound closure. Alternatively, a constant infusion of extradural solution can be run intraoperatively to minimise fluctuations in blood pressure. Little evidence exists regarding intraoperative management of extradural anaesthesia.

Sacral (caudal) extradural block

Anatomy

The sacrum is a large triangular bone formed by the fusion of the five sacral vertebrae, articulating above with the fifth lumbar vertebra and below with the coccyx. The posterior surface is convex and down its middle line runs the median sacral crest with its three or four rudimentary spinous processes. The laminae of the fifth and sometimes of the fourth sacral vertebrae fail to fuse in the midline; the deficiency thus formed is known as the sacral hiatus. The tubercles representing the inferior articular processes of the fifth sacral vertebra are prolonged downwards as the sacral cornua. These cornua, with the rudimentary one of the fourth vertebra above, bound the sacral hiatus.

The four posterior sacral foramina correspond with the anterior foramina. Each transmits a sacral nerve posterior ramus and communicates with the sacral canal.

The sacral canal is a prismatic cavity running through the length of the bone and following its curves. Superiorly it is triangular in section and is continuous with the lumbar vertebral canal. Its lower extremity is the sacral hiatus, closed by the posterior sacrococcygeal membrane. Fibrous strands sometimes occur in the canal and divide the extradural space into compartments. These may account for some cases of failure to produce uniform analgesia. Its anterior wall is formed by fusion of the bodies of the sacral vertebrae, its posterior wall by fusion of the laminae. On each lateral wall of the canal, four foramina are present that divide in the form of a Y into anterior and posterior sacral foramina.

The contents of the sacral canal are:

- the dural sac that ends at the lower border of the second sacral vertebra, on a line joining the posterior superior iliac spines; the pia mater is continued as the filum terminale;
- the sacral nerves and the coccygeal nerve, with their dorsal root ganglia;
- a venous plexus formed by the lower end of the internal vertebral plexus – these vessels are more numerous anteriorly than posteriorly and so the needle point should be kept as far posteriorly as possible;
- areolar and fatty tissue – more dense in males than in females.

Anatomical abnormalities of the sacrum are not uncommon. They include:

- upward and downward displacement of the hiatus;
- pronounced narrowing or partial obliteration of the sacral canal, making needle insertion difficult;
- ossification of the sacrococcygeal membrane;
- absence of the bony posterior wall of the sacral canal, owing to failure of laminae to fuse;
- dural extension to the level of the third sacral vertebra;
- the hiatus may be of many different shapes, ranging from long and narrow to broad. The extradural space below it may range from being deep to excessively shallow – its average length is 10–15 cm.

When a local anaesthetic solution is injected into the sacral canal it ascends upwards in the extradural space for a distance proportional to the volume of solution, the force of injection, the amount of leakage through the eight sacral foramina and the consistency of the connective tissue in the space. The first two are controllable but the last are not, so precise placement of the solution is impossible and sometimes leads to unexpected results.

Technique

Before commencing it is important to examine the patient, explain the procedure and obtain consent. Premedication may be necessary. An intravenous infusion should be set up, monitoring commenced and the presence of safety resuscitation equipment checked. The patient should be asked to lie in the prone position with hips slightly flexed over two pillows, or in the lateral position with hips flexed. It is important to use a full aseptic technique with cleansing of the skin before insertion of the needle.

The triangular sacral hiatus is palpated at the top of the natal cleft. A weal is raised over the hiatus, with a fine intradermal needle using no more than two drops of solution because oedema obscures the landmarks. A 5-cm needle is inserted through the sacrococcygeal membrane at 45°. After aspiration tests for blood and CSF have proved negative, injection is performed. When the needle is correctly placed, injection is easy with no great force being required to depress the plunger of the syringe.

Advantages

Excellent postoperative analgesia is obtained with caudal extradural block. The dose of 0.25% bupivacaine is 0.5–0.75 mL/kg. Caudal extradural block is popular for postoperative analgesia in children (e.g. after circumcision and orchidopexy). It is also useful in adults undergoing haemorrhoidectomy, urological or vaginal procedures, usually combined with light general anaesthesia.

Disadvantages

Disadvantages of caudal extradural block are:

- length of time taken for development of analgesia;
- lack of accurate control of height of analgesia;
- muscular relaxation not maximal in mid and high blocks, although it is excellent in low blocks;
- technical difficulty if anatomy is abnormal;
- risk of inadvertent subarachnoid injection if the dura extends downwards;
- hypotension and possible signs of drug toxicity;
- complete flaccidity of the anal sphincters (a condition unpopular with some surgeons) has been reported;
- urinary retention may occur, but is difficult to assess;
- may cause temporary inability to ejaculate in males.

Technical failure of extradural anaesthesia

The benefits of extradural analgesia are limited by technical failure in up to one in seven patients. There are three reasons for failure:

- epidural never worked;
- technical problem occurred with the catheter during epidural infusion;
- epidural analgesia failed despite a functioning catheter.

Two centres have reported technical problems with thoracic extradurals. Epidurals that never worked, catheter technical problems and failure of epidural analgesia despite a functioning catheter comprised 2.4%, 6.8% and 1.4% respectively of Dundee patients[72] versus 1.3%, 10% and 3.6% respectively of Boston patients.[72a] The most common problem in Dundee was leaking at the epidural site (3.5% of all epidurals). Common to both centres was the timing of technical failure: the majority occurred after 24 hours of infusion. In Dundee, 79 (56%) occurred following the first 24 hours, median (interquartile range) time to technical failure 27 hours (14–46 hours). Clinical application of a technical intervention with such a high failure rate is a cause for concern.

COMBINED SPINAL EXTRADURAL

The CSE technique was introduced in an attempt to combine the reliability of spinal anaesthesia with the flexibility of epidural anaesthesia. The introduction of pencil-point Whitacre and Sprotte needles in the early 1990s and reduction of PDPH to less than 0.5% allowed routine CSE for labour analgesia.[73]

Historically, four methods of CSE have been used:

- single-needle single-interspace. First described in 1937 by Soresi, a New York surgeon.He first establised epidural anaesthesia. If insufficient, the needle was inserted into the CSF and local anaesthetic injected to obtain spinal anaesthesia;
- double-needle, separate interspaces. Curelaru 1979 and Brownridge 1981;
- needle-through-needle. Described in 1982 by Coates and Mumtaz for orthopaedics and Carrie for obstetrics – long-shafted spinal needle inserted through standard epidural needle;
- needle-beside-needle single-interspace.

Combined spinal extradural anaesthesia is used regularly in obstetrics for pain relief in labour and anaesthesia for caesarean section. For labour, the standard needle-through-needle approach is taken. Intrathecal injection of 1 mL 0.25% bupivacaine with 15–25 μg of fentanyl provides rapid pain relief, which lasts 45–75 minutes. Use of sufentanil 5 μg instead of fentanyl extends analgesia up to 120 minutes. Extradural top-ups with 15 mL bupivacaine 0.1% and fentanyl 2 μg/mL provide extended pain relief.

A meta-analysis of 14 CSE studies in labour (2047 women)[74] showed a 5-minute reduction in establishment of analgesia and improved maternal satisfaction, but a greater incidence of pruritus compared to extradural block. No difference was found between CSE and epidural techniques with regard to maternal mobility, rescue analgesia requirements, the incidence of PDPH, or admission of the baby to the neonatal intensive care unit. CSE analgesia was not associated with a higher incidence of emergency caesarean delivery. Emergency caesarean section for fetal distress within 90 minutes of the administration of intrathecal sufentanil occurred only in association with obstetric factors.[75]

Combined spinal extradural is associated with more hypotension than extradural anaesthesia. Compression of the dural sac by extradural drug extends intrathecal spread of local anaesthetic. One study[76] has suggested that the incidence and severity of hypotension during induction of CSE anaesthesia could be reduced if the injection of local anaesthetic was performed in the lateral as opposed to the sitting position.

CONTINUOUS SPINAL ANAESTHESIA

Continuous spinal anaesthesia was first described by a British surgeon, Dean, in 1907, who left the needle in place during surgery. In 1939, Lemmon split the operating table mattress to reduce the incidence of needle trauma. Touhy in 1944 used a no. 4 ureteral catheter through a 15G needle. Hurley and Lambert in 1989 described the continuous spinal microcatheter.

The use of micro spinal catheters in the late 1980s and early 1990s led to 12 cases of cauda equina syndrome, culminating in the banning of microcatheters by the US Food and Drug Administration. Characteristic of each case of neurological injury was poor efficacy of block despite an unremitting requirement for local anaesthetic. The reason was that microcatheters had unknowingly turned caudal and 5% lidocaine (lignocaine) was repeatedly given. A pool of high-concentration lidocaine (lignocaine) surrounded the cauda equina, leading to irreversible damage to sacral nerves and permanent bowel and bladder dysfunction.

Continuous spinal catheters have been used in Europe and have provided good analgesia for major abdominal, orthopaedic and vascular surgery.[77,78]

Continuous spinal anaesthesia provides continuous access to the subarachnoid space where factors such as baricity and position of the patient can be used to influence the spread, duration and extent of anaesthesia and analgesia. However, the subarachnoid space is markedly less forgiving of errors than the extradural space.

Continuous spinal anaesthesia requires small doses of local anaesthetics to achieve anaesthesia and analgesia. Doses are approximately one-tenth the amount of local anaesthetic used in the extradural space.

Doses for CSA can be further reduced from those needed for single-dose spinal anaesthesia by 25–33%. This translates into small doses of lidocaine (lignocaine) (12.5–25 mg) or bupivacaine (2.5–5.0 mg). Additional incremental doses, using 2.5 mg, will expand the block.

Paraesthesias have been reported in as many 50% of spinal catheter placements. It also appears that neurological injury will occur more frequently after spinal anaesthesia when a paraesthesia is elicited. The number of paraesthesias observed varies little with different-sized needles and catheters and different microspinal catheter systems. The relationship between paraesthesia and neurological outcome is not known.

Rates of post dural puncture headache (PDPH) after CSA have been lower than predicted, probably owing to an inflammatory reaction to the catheter.

It seems prudent to choose the smallest catheter that is practical for the patient or population.

ADVERSE EFFECTS OF CENTRAL NEURAXIAL BLOCKADE

The recognition of the benefits and risks of sympathectomy with regard to cardiac, respiratory gastrointestinal and metabolic function is necessary to manage patients optimally.

Cardiovascular

Sympathetic activation associated with surgery and postoperative pain manifests as tachycardia, hypertension and increased contractility, all of which serve to increase myocardial oxygen consumption. Injured tissues require more oxygen after surgery for repair. However, the response of patients with coronary atherosclerosis to surgical stress differs from that of healthy patients. Sympathetic stimulation may constrict post-stenotic coronary arteries and reduce blood supply to the subendocardium. The uncoupling of oxygen delivery and demand presents as postoperative silent myocardial ischaemia, the intensity of which predicts long-term severe myocardial events. Meta-analysis has demonstrated a statistically significant reduction in postoperative myocardial infarction, thromboembolism and death with the use of thoracic extradural analgesia.

Intrathecal and extradural block each provide a selective sympathectomy that is associated with cardiovascular complications such as bradycardia (even asystole) and other arrhythmias and hypotension.

Bradycardia

The Bezold–Jarisch reflex, characterised by bradycardia, vasodilation and hypotension, is associated with extensive lumbar extradural blocks. In contrast, placement of an extradural catheter in an interspace equivalent to the midline of the surgical incision provides a selective sympathectomy and, in patients at risk of perioperative ischaemia, dilates constricted coronary vessels, decreases heart rate and improves cardiac function by reducing preload and afterload and optimising myocardial oxygen delivery. Only by restricting spread to the lumbar and low thoracic regions can lumbar extradural block restrict splanchnic sympathetic blockade, maintain venous return and lessen hypotension. Therefore, the evidence suggests that lumbar extradural anaesthesia should be avoided in patients undergoing abdominal or thoracic procedures.

When extended to high thoracic levels, spinal anaesthesia may be associated with bradycardia and asystole. The overall incidence of moderate bradycardia (defined as a heart rate <50 beats/min) from prospective studies is 8.9–13%. High sympathetic block to the level of cardiac sympathetic innervation ($T1–T_4$) reduces venous return and exposes unopposed vagal parasympathetic tone, leading to marked bradycardia and asystole.

The cardiac response to poor venous return is mediated via three cardiac reflexes:

- the atrial or Bainbridge reflex, whereby decreases in venous return result in decreased efferent outflow to the cardioaccelerator fibres, and a reduction in heart rate;
- sinoatrial node stretch reflex, whereby stretch receptors in the sinoatrial node respond proportionally to venous return;
- the Bezold–Jarisch reflex, whereby baroreceptors located in the inferoposterior wall of the left ventricle respond to increases in ventricular contractility induced by reductions in preload and ventricular volume. Stretching of these baroreceptors paradoxically increases vagal output from the vasomotor centre, resulting in severe bradycardia.

Predictors of bradycardia during spinal anaesthesia

Independent predictors of bradycardia (<50 beats/min) during spinal anaesthesia include baseline heart rate of less than 60 beats/min (OR 4.9), ASA I (OR 3.5), prolonged PR interval (OR 3.2), use of β-blockers (OR 2.9) and block height T5 or higher (OR 1.7).

Hypotension

The overall incidence of hypotension during spinal anaesthesia is reported to be 8–33% and the overall incidence of bradycardia is reported to be 9–16%. Four out of five of episodes (81%) of episodes of hypotension and almost three out of four (74%) of episodes of bradycardia occur when the peak sensory block height is higher than T5.

Hypotension after spinal or extradural anaesthesia can be attributed to reduction in systemic vascular resistance and/or a fall in cardiac output.[79] Bilateral sympathectomy dilates venous capacitance vessels below the level of the spinal block. As two-thirds of the blood volume is contained within the venous capacitance vessels, venous return decreases and consequently reduces cardiac output.

The physiological response to hypotension is compensatory vasoconstriction of veins above the level of the sympathectomy. Thus, the degree to which hypotension occurs is dependent on the height of the block, the extent of venous pooling, particularly within the splanchnic capacitance vessels, and the degree of upper extremity vasoconstriction.

Unlike the venous vasculature, the arterioles retain a significant degree of vasomotor tone during sympathetic blockade. In young healthy subjects with good myocardial function, systemic vascular resistance decreases only moderately (15–18%), even with significant sympathetic blockade.

Preservation of cardiac output during spinal anaesthesia allows maintenance of oxygen delivery to vital organs such as the brain, as demonstrated by lack of change in jugular venous oxygen saturation, and decreases total body oxygen consumption by up to 20.5%.

The cardiovascular response to spinal anaesthesia changes with the height of the block and age. In young healthy subjects, reductions in blood pressure are mild because of compensatory upper extremity vasoconstriction. However, when spinal anaesthesia is extended to high thoracic and cervical levels, upper extremity and splanchnic vasoconstriction is abolished and hypotension ensues. The elderly have a more profound drop in blood pressure owing to an exaggerated decrease in systemic vascular resistance to sympathetic blockade compared to younger patients. Typically, with T4–T6 sensory levels of spinal anaesthesia, systemic vascular resistance decreases by 23–26%, central venous pressure decreases by 2–3 mmHg, and left ventricular end-diastolic volume decreases by 20%.

For abdominal surgery, insertion of a lumbar extradural catheter and upwards extension of the block is not recommended because the consequences on patient outcome may be worse than with a well-managed thoracic extradural. Lumbar sensory block for abdominal surgery is difficult to maintain, rescue analgesia is required more often and motor block is inevitable. As sympathetic blockade is extended to the lower limbs, baroreceptor-mediated reflex vasoconstriction is limited to areas cephalad to the block, increasing the likelihood of coronary vasoconstriction and myocardial ischaemia. Furthermore, following large blood loss, decreases in mean arterial pressure, systemic vascular resistance and base excess are significantly larger in the presence of extensive thoracolumbar blockade than with selective thoracic blockade or general anaesthesia alone.

Caesarean section

Sudden hypotension under spinal anaesthesia has been associated with a decline in uteroplacental blood flow and significant fetal acidosis compared to extradural anaesthesia, which may compromise neonatal wellbeing. Nevertheless, a decrease in fetal pH has not been shown to reduce neonatal Apgar or neurobehavioural assessment scores.

The treatment of hypotension is left uterine displacement, volume preload, preferentially with colloids, and vasopressors in low doses. A recent meta-analysis indicates that fetal gas exchange may be preserved even more effectively with the use of phenylephrine. α-Adrenergic drugs increase maternal cardiac output by increasing preload when given to treat hypotension caused by neuraxial blockade.

The incidence of hypotension is no greater in severe pre-eclampsia and spinal anaesthesia may also be safely performed in this patient group.

Compression of the great vessels within the abdomen by the pregnant uterus, abdominal tumours or abdominal packs may cause severe hypotension in the presence of central neural blockade. Hypovolaemia or sepsis amplify drops in blood pressure after spinal anaesthesia. Systemic absorption of the local anaesthetic drug can depress vascular smooth muscle and myocardial function, with a fall in cardiac output.

Predictors of hypotension during spinal anaesthesia

Independent predictors of hypotension (systolic <90 mmHg or 30% decrease from baseline) during spinal anaesthesia include maximal sensory block at T5 or higher (OR 3.8) age over 40 years (OR 2.5), systolic blood pressure less than 120 mmHg (OR 2.4), combined spinal/general anaesthesia (OR 1.9) and dural puncture at the interspace between the second and third lumbar vertebrae or higher (OR 1.8).

Another survey showed additional risk factors to be chronic alcohol consumption (OR 3.1), emergency surgery (OR 2.8) and hypertension (OR 2.2). Patients with a history of alcohol abuse are more likely to have underlying autonomic dysfunction and patients with hypertension have mild intravascular volume depletion and are more vulnerable to the redistribution of the central blood volume to the capacitance vessels.

Treatment of hypotension

Treatment of hypotension should be directed towards the underlying mechanisms of decreased cardiac output and systemic vascular resistance. Clinical interventions include 100% oxygen, elevation of the legs, rapid infusion of fluids and intravenous sympathomimetic drugs.

Positioning of patient

One study has shown that hypotension during CSE could be reduced if intrathecal injection was performed in the lateral as opposed to the sitting position. Placing the patient in the left lateral position significantly reduced the amount of ephedrine required and the duration of hypotension.

Fluid management

Crystalloid

Numerous studies of prophylactic volume loading to prevent hypotension have largely failed in all patient populations – surgical, elderly, obstetric.

Studies of large volumes (12–30 mL/kg) of crystalloid infusion before spinal anaesthesia have shown no difference in the incidence of hypotension probably because large volumes of crystalloid quickly redistribute from the intravascular to the extravascular compartment.

Colloids

In contrast to crystalloid solutions, prophylactic volume loading with colloid solutions (500–1000 mL) prior to spinal injection has consistently maintained blood pressure and volume expansion in both surgical and obstetric patients owing to a sustained increase in intravascular volume, maternal cardiac output and uteroplacental blood flow. The improved efficacy of colloid therapy must be weighed against its increased cost and the small but significant risk of anaphylaxis. Additionally, there is little evidence that prophylactic volume loading improves either maternal or fetal outcome, as long as significant hypotension is recognised and treated early. Combining a low-dose spinal anaesthetic technique with colloid preloading minimises the haemodynamic consequences and vasopressor requirements of neuraxial anaesthesia for caesarean section.

Sympathomimetics

The relative selectivity of sympathomimetics for adrenergic receptors depends on the chemical structure of the drug. Maximal α- and β-adrenergic receptor activity is dependent on the presence of hydroxyl groups on the 3 and 4 positions of the benzene ring of β-phenylethylamine.

The four most commonly used sympathomimetics are:

- epinephrine (adrenaline);
- phenylephrine;
- metaraminol;
- ephedrine.

Epinephrine (adrenaline) has the optimal physical structure for producing α- and β-adrenergic effects and represents the prototype drug among the sympathomimetics. Release from the adrenal medulla stimulates:

- myocardial contractility;
- heart rate;
- vascular and bronchial smooth muscle tone;
- glandular secretions;
- glycogenolysis and lipolysis.

Epinephrine (adrenaline) is the most potent activator of α-adrenergic receptors, being two to ten times more active than norepinephrine (noradrenaline). In increasing doses, it stimulates β_2, β_1 and α_1 receptors.

Epinephrine (adrenaline)-induced stimulation of β_2 receptors produces peripheral vasodilation and increased flow to skeletal muscle. Stimulation of β_1 receptors increases systolic blood pressure, heart rate and cardiac output. There is a modest reduction in diastolic blood pressure, reflecting vasodilation from activation of β_2 receptors. The net effect is an increase in pulse pressure and minimal change in mean arterial pressure. Higher doses stimulate α_1 receptors in the skin, mucosa and hepatorenal vasculature, producing intense vasoconstriction. Increases in heart rate accelerate the rate of spontaneous phase 4 depolarisation, increasing the likelihood of cardiac arrhythmias.

Phenylephrine is a synthetic non-catecholamine. Structurally, it is a 3-hydroxy phenylethylamine differing from epinephrine (adrenaline) only in lacking a 4-hydroxyl group on the benzene ring. Phenylephrine directly and indirectly (by release of norepinephrine [noradrenaline]) stimulates α- adrenergic receptors ($\alpha_1 > \alpha_2$). It also has a small effect on β-adrenergic receptors. Clinically, it mimics the effects of norepinephrine (noradrenaline), but is less potent and longer lasting. Central nervous system stimulation is minimal. Intravenous phenylephrine produces intense peripheral vasoconstriction, increased systolic and diastolic blood pressure, and reflex bradycardia. Reflex heart rate slowing can result in a decrease in cardiac output. Renal, splanchnic and cutaneous blood flows are reduced, but coronary blood flow is increased. Pulmonary arterial pressure is elevated.

Metaraminol is a synthetic non-catecholamine that, like ephedrine, acts on α- and β-adrenergic receptors by indirect and direct effects. However, it produces more intense peripheral vasoconstriction and a smaller increase in myocardial contractility than ephedrine. Intravenous administration of metaraminol, 0.5–2 mg produces a sustained increase in systolic and diastolic blood pressure that is due almost entirely to peripheral vasoconstriction. Vasoconstriction decreases renal and cerebral blood flow and is accompanied by a reflex reduction in heart rate and cardiac output.

Ephedrine is a nonselective direct- and indirect-acting synthetic non-catecholamine acting on α- and β-adrenergic receptors. Its principal mode of action is increased myocardial contractility and rate due to activation of β_1 receptors. Higher doses produce α-receptor-mediated peripheral vasoconstriction. Ephedrine has until recently been the choice of vasopressor in obstetric anaesthesia, given in aliquots of 3–6 mg or as a variable infusion of 60 mg ephedrine in 500 mL crystalloid. Subsequent doses of ephedrine are associated with tachyphylaxis. Ephedrine has been administered intramuscularly to prevent maternal hypotension during spinal anaesthesia. However, ephedrine may contribute to fetal acidosis, and phenylephrine has now been recommended as the vasoconstrictor of choice for caesarean section. A decrease in uteroplacental blood flow has been observed with larger doses as indicated by increases in pulsatility indices.[27] If high doses of vasopressors are used, the uterine artery will constrict and uteroplacental blood flow will decline.

Treatment plan

Hypotensive patients with accompanying tachycardia should be given increments of phenylephrine 100 μg or metaraminol 0.5–1 mg. Hypotension with bradycardia may be treated with intravenous ephedrine (3–6 mg). For severe bradycardia, unresponsive to either ephedrine or atropine or in the setting of a precipitous decrease in heart rate, epinephrine (adrenaline) (10–25 μg) should be administered. Higher doses in increments of 100 μg may be required up to 1 mg for cardiac arrest to perfuse coronary arteries.

Respiratory

The muscles responsible for breathing are the diaphragm, the intercostal muscles and the abdominal muscles. After central neuraxial block, changes in inspiratory function are minimal except for slight decreases in vital capacity. In the absence of sedation, minute ventilation, tidal volume, respiratory rate, mean inspiratory flow rates, arterial oxygen tension or carbon dioxide tensions change little, even with high to mid thoracic blocks.

In contrast, expiratory muscle function is decreased in proportion to the level of spinal anaesthesia, demonstrated by reductions in maximal expiratory pressure and flow rates. An 11% decrease in peak expiratory flow occurs with a block to T8 compared to a 17% fall with a block to T4. These changes are attributable to paralysis of abdominal muscles used in forced exhalation. Thus, coughing and clearing of secretions may be impaired after spinal anaesthesia, particularly in patients with pre-existing lung disease. During spinal analgesia breathing becomes quiet and tranquil, due not only to motor blockade but also to deafferentation, with reduction of sensory input to the respiratory centre.

Hypoxaemia during or after spinal anaesthesia is associated with sedative drugs given intravenously or neuraxially. Monitoring of respiratory rate, oxygen saturation, blood pressure and sedation levels during and after spinal anaesthesia is warranted.

Extradural block attenuates reduction in FRC after abdominal surgery[80] better than intravenous opioids, lessens the work of the heart and tends to relieve any pre-existing pulmonary vascular congestion. The effect of block is largely on the cardiovascular system.

Postoperative decrements in respiratory function are common following abdominal surgery and several studies have investigated the effect of thoracic epidural anaesthesia on postoperative respiratory function. An observational study by Flisberg et al.[81] investigated 15 ASA 1 and 2 patients receiving thoracic epidural infusions of bupivacaine and morphine for abdominal surgery. Of the 15 patients, 11 registered abnormal breathing patterns or short episodes of apnoea, four of which were associated with a raised Pa_{CO_2} over 6.5 kPa (48.8 mmHg).

Madej et al.[82] compared three groups of patients randomised to epidural bupivacaine and diamorphine infusion, epidural diamorphine bolus and PCA morphine for analgesia following abdominal hysterectomy. Compared to the other two groups, patients receiving the epidural solution were more prone to oxygen desaturation. The pathophysiological reason for the deterioration in respiratory function, even in the presence of thoracic extradural analgesia, is complex. High thoracic extradural anaesthesia increases functional residual capacity by a caudal motion of the diaphragm and a concomitant decrease in intrathoracic blood volume. Diaphragmatic function is impaired by stimulation of inhibitory phenic nerves within the abdomen.

In the elderly, significant reductions in minute ventilation and tidal volume occur, but the ventilatory responses to hypercapnia and hypoxia are maintained when using thoracic extradural anaesthesia.[83, 84]

Apnoea during spinal and extradural anaesthesia

Causes of apnoea during spinal and extradural analgesia include:

- inadequate medullary blood flow due to inadequate cardiac output – a serious situation demanding immediate cardiorespiratory support;
- total spinal analgesia with denervation of all the respiratory muscles – true phrenic paralysis is uncommon because the motor roots are large;
- accidental subdural injection: a small volume of solution may travel to an unexpectedly high level in this potential space;
- toxic effects of the local analgesic drug;
- injection of a opioid analgesic drug.

Treatment

Treatment of apnoea during spinal and extradural anaesthesia is to:

- control the airway and ventilate the lungs with 100% oxygen;
- diagnose the cause and monitor other vital signs (e.g. arterial pressure, oxygen saturation, level of consciousness, level of block, pupil size, skin rashes).

Gastrointestinal

Preganglionic sympathetic fibres from T5 to L1 are inhibitory to the gut. Innervation of the oesophagus is vagal. Removal of sympathetic activity to the gut reveals unopposed gut vagal activity – sphincters are relaxed, peristalsis is active and the pressure within the bowel lumen is increased. Stimuli arising in the upper abdomen may ascend along the unblocked vagus and phrenics, and cause discomfort if the patient is conscious.

The sympathectomy of thoracic extradural anaesthesia has been shown to benefit bowel function by reducing the duration of postoperative ileus,[85] enhancing bowel blood flow and preventing falls in gastric intramucosal pH (pHi) in patients undergoing major abdominal surgery. The increase in bowel motility from unopposed parasympathetic activity is not associated with any significant increase in anastomotic dehiscence.[86]

Splanchnic blockade may also have deleterious haemodynamic consequences because the splanchnic veins contribute substantially to the control of overall venous capacitance. Hence, sympathetic block during intrathecal and extradural anaesthesia vasodilates mesenteric vessels and is associated with hypotension because of reduced venous return. The degree to which blood pressure falls is dependent on the relative extent of splanchnic sympathetic blockade and the degree of baroreceptor-induced vasoconstriction in unblocked regions of the body.

Hypotension can compromise gut mucosal integrity as well as myocardial blood flow. Translocation of endotoxin from the gut lumen and release of inflammatory mediators are the basis of the systemic inflammatory response, leading to increases in capillary permeability and multiorgan failure. Therefore it is important to prevent gut hypoperfusion.

The extent to which splanchnic blood flow is flow or pressure dependent has been examined recently by measuring inferior mesenteric artery flow and serosal flux using laser Doppler imaging.[87] From this work it would appear that correction of mean perfusion pressure is inotropes is more likely to correct bowel blood flow than is excessive fluid resuscitation.

Ephedrine (mixed α and β) or metaraminol (α) in small aliquots is often used to correct hypotension. A low-dose infusion of dopamine or dopexamine (β and δ) at 3–5 μg/kg/min may also be infused to increase mesenteric and hepatic blood flow.

During hemorrhagic hypotension and after resuscitation, thoracic extradural anaesthesia has beneficial effects on intestinal microvascular perfusion. Because of blockade of sympathetic nerves, thoracic extradural anaesthesia prevents perfusion impairment of the muscularis during hypotension and attenuates leucocyte rolling after resuscitation.[88]

Thoracic extradural anaesthesia (TEA) is associated with a decreased mean arterial blood pressure, but no change in total hepatic blood flow[89] or intestinal oxygenation.[90] Extradural anaesthesia and postoperative analgesia for major abdominal surgery increases oxygen tension in the wound[91] and unblocked tissue[92] compared to general anaesthesia and intravenous morphine analgesia.[87,91]

Nausea and vomiting

Gastric emptying time is quicker when extradural block is employed for postoperative pain relief than when narcotic analgesics are used. Causes of nausea are:

- hypotension – correction using a pressor drug may relieve nausea;
- increased peristalsis;
- traction on nerve endings and plexuses, especially via the vagus;
- presence of bile in the stomach due to relaxation of the pyloric and bile duct sphincters;

- opioid analgesics (premedication);
- psychological factors;
- hypoxaemia.

Genitourinary

Sympathetic supply to the kidneys is from T11 to L1 via the lowest splanchnic nerves. Any effects on renal function are due to hypotension. Autoregulation of renal blood flow is impaired if mean arterial pressure falls below about 50 mmHg. Bladder sphincters are not relaxed during sympathetic block and so soiling of the table by urine is not seen, and the tone of ureters is not greatly altered. The penis is often engorged and flaccid owing to paralysis of the nervi erigentes (S2 and S3); this is a useful positive sign of successful block. The second, third and fourth sacral spinal nerves (S2–S4) contain the afferent and efferent pathways responsible for control of the bladder and urethral sphincters. Distention of the bladder sends afferent signals (via the pelvic nerve to the sacral segments of the spinal cord), which are transmitted to the frontal lobe. Voluntary micturition is initiated by efferent impulses from the higher cortical centres to the pontine micturition centre, which then activates preganglionic motor fibres in the sacral (S2–S4) spinal cord that initiate contraction of the detrusor muscle.

After the induction of spinal anaesthesia, the urge to void (normal detrusor function) is abolished within 60 seconds. The ability to void normally does not return until sensory anaesthesia has regressed to S3. Prolonged inhibition of normal detrusor function with the use of long-acting local anaesthetics, such as bupivacaine, may allow bladder over-distension and urinary retention. In a study of healthy male patients undergoing non-urological surgery after spinal anaesthesia comparing 100 mg lidocaine (lignocaine) with 10 mg bupivacaine, the time to return of normal detrusor function after spinal injection was significantly longer in the bupivacaine group (233 minutes versus 462 minutes). The patients in the bupivacaine group generated an average of 875 mL urine. In contrast, the patients in the lidocaine (lignocaine) group had generated an average of 498 mL urine by the time they regained normal detrusor function.

Postoperative urinary retention may result in hypertension, hypotension, bradycardia and damage to the detrusor, leading to incomplete emptying of the bladder and an increased long-term risk of urinary tract infections.

A recent study of ambulatory surgery patients (considered at low risk of urinary retention) discharged before voiding after short-acting spinal anaesthesia demonstrated significantly shorter discharge times and no reports of urinary retention.

Metabolic

Muscle wasting occurs after surgery because the rate of muscle protein breakdown exceeds the rate of synthesis.[93] Amino acids provide the substrate for gluconeogenesis in the liver, resulting in an elevation in plasma glucose levels and increased insulin resistance. Sympathetic blockade of adrenal catecholamine release restores the balance between muscle synthesis and breakdown,[94] attenuating the rise in plasma glucose.[95] Provision of oral energy substrates before and after surgery, combined with early mobilisation, serves to limit muscle and fat breakdown and accelerate rehabilitation.[94]

Hypothermia

Mild perioperative hypothermia can occur with spinal anaesthesia, particularly in the elderly and with extensive blocks. Perioperative hypothermia has been shown to adversely affect the incidence of myocardial ischaemia, cardiac morbidity wound infection, surgical bleeding and patient discomfort. Core hypothermia with spinal anaesthesia develops primarily from a redistribution of heat from core tissues, which are well-perfused tissues such as the head and trunk, to the peripheral tissues, or arms and legs. Therefore, to minimise the risk of intraoperative hypothermia during spinal anaesthesia, the following strategies are recommended:

- first, core temperature should be monitored;
- second, active warming with forced air warmers should be used if core hypothermia occurs – or its prophylactic use considered in extended operations or high-risk patients;
- third, intravenous fluids should be warmed to approximately 37°C if large volumes are to be administered.

Endocrine

The release of antidiuretic hormone during surgery is suppressed by central neural blockade. The rise in blood cortisol levels associated with surgery performed under general anaesthesia may be less marked if afferent impulses are blocked by spinal or extradural anaesthesia compared to operations under general anaesthesia, particularly for lower limb or pelvic surgery,[96] Lumbar extradural block prevents lymphocytopenia and granulocytosis after operation, thereby preventing immunosuppression.

Central nervous system

Increased sensitivity to the sedating effects of midazolam has been reported with spinal anaesthesia in unpremedicated patients, the degree of sedation corresponding to the level of sensory block. Decreased afferent input may make the reticular activating system more susceptible to the sedative actions of drugs. Recently Pollock et al. reported that spinal anaesthesia is accompanied by significant sedation compared with controls, most pronounced at 60 minutes, possibly favouring direct rostral spread of local anaesthetics to the CNS with direct action on the brain, or redistribution of blood flow and increasing cerebral concentrations of local anaesthetics. Sedative drugs should be administered cautiously in patients with central neuraxial anaesthesia.

Neurological

Two large surveys of the neurological complications of regional anaesthesia practice have been undertaken. In a large prospective survey[97] of the complications of regional anaesthesia conducted in France, the incidence of neurological injury (5.9/10 000) and cardiac arrest (6.4/10 000) was three and six times greater respectively with intradural anaesthesia compared with extradural anaesthesia (see Table 4.1.3). Two-thirds of the patients with neurological deficits had either a paresthesia during needle placement or pain on injection. Seventy-five percent of the neurological deficits after nontraumatic spinal anaesthesia occurred in patients who had received hyperbaric lidocaine (lignocaine), 5%. Seizures due to local anaesthetic toxicity occurred in 23 patients, but were four times more common after regional blockade.

The second survey[98] identified 56 major complications in 158 083 regional anaesthesia procedures performed (3.5/10 000). Again, spinal anaesthesia was associated with a greater incidence of cardiac arrest, and lidocaine (lignocaine) spinal anaesthesia was associated with more neurological complications than was bupivacaine spinal anaesthesia (14.4/10 000 vs 2.2/10 000).

One of the most thorough studies of neurological damage following thoracic extradural analgesia complications has been conducted by Giebler et al.[99] No permanent neurological sequelae were reported in 4185 patients, although unsuccessful catheter placement occurred in 1 in 93, and self-limiting peripheral nerve lesions in 1 in 174 patients. The incidence of dural tap was 1 in 140 patients, but was less common at higher insertion sites.

The largest study of neurological complications using 603 macro- and microcatheter (smaller than 24 G) catheters[100] reported two paraesthesias, one aseptic meningitis and one cauda equina syndrome and a 9.6% incidence of PDPH, one-third of whom were pregnant patients with size 28 G microcatheters.

Post-dural puncture headache (PDPH)

Post-dural puncture headache was recognised after first spinal anaesthetic in 1898 by Bier and his surgical resident Hildebrandt, who performed spinal anaesthesia on each other. Typical location of the headache is bifrontal and/or occipital. Occasionally, the symptoms involve the neck and upper shoulders. The intensity ranges from mild to excruciating. PDPH rate is worse in the upright position or during coughing or straining. There is associated nausea, photophobia, tinnitus, diplopia and cranial nerve palsy, and rarely cortical vein thrombosis, subarachnoid haemorrhage or subdural haematoma. It is more common in young pregnant patients, and with accidental dural puncture rate during epidural anaesthesia using Touhy needles (60%–80%). Reduced by the introduction of size 25 G and 27 G Whitacre pencil-point needles, which replaced cutting needles. Treatments include caffeine, sumatriptan and adrenocorticotropic hormone, but there is little evidence to support their use. The autologous epidural blood patch was first described by Gormley in 1960.

Epidural blood patch

The epidural blood patch requires two clinicians and an aseptic technique. The epidural is performed at the same space as the previous spinal or epidural if possible. Once the epidural is in place, withdraw 20 mL of blood from the forearm. The blood is carefully and aseptically transferred to the anaesthetist, who injects it slowly through the epidural needle or until pain is felt in the back. Patients should be placed supine for 1–2 hours following the procedure to reduce the leakage of CSF from the dural hole. It is successful in 70% of patients and may have to be repeated.

Cranial nerve palsies

Paralysis of every cranial nerve except the first, ninth and tenth has been reported after spinal anaesthesia, and transient deafness or tinnitus is not uncommon. Paralysis of the sixth cranial nerve, which innervates the lateral rectus, causes diplopia. The onset is commonly between the fifth and 11th postoperative days and is associated with headache. It may be delayed for 3 weeks. Paralysis is never complete. About 50% of patients recover within a month.

Cauda equina syndrome

Concerns about the use of spinal lidocaine (lignocaine) began in the early 1990s with published reports of cauda equina syndrome (Table 4.3.3) after CSA and a case report of four patients who experienced aching and pain in the buttocks and lower limbs after spinal anaesthesia. Of the 11 cases of cauda equina syndrome, 10 patients had received doses of lidocaine (lignocaine) up to 300 mg, and one patient had received tetracaine (amethocaine). The cause of toxicity was inadvertent caudal placement of microcatheters and pooling of local anaesthetic around the sacral roots. In response to a lower than expected extent of anaesthesia, large doses of drug were given via the intrathecal catheters and exacerbated sacral pooling. In 1992, because of safety concerns, spinal microcatheters were removed from the US market.

Syndrome	Onset	Duration	Pain	Neurological symptoms	Treatment
TNS – Transient Neurological Syndrome	6–36 h	1–7 days	Unilateral or bilateral pain in the anterior or posterior thighs extension into legs	Nil	NSAIDs, opioids, warm heat
Chlorprocaine back pain	Immediate onset after extradural regression	1–4 h	Low back pain	Nil	NSAIDs, oral opioids
Extradural haematoma	0–2 days	Requires surgery	Radicular back pain	Muscle weakness, sensory deficit	CT scan, laminectomy
Extradural abscess	2–7 days	Requires surgery	Backache, fever	Progressive neurologic symptoms	Antibiotics, possible surgical drainage
Spinal nerve injury	0–2 days	1–12 weeks	Pain during insertion of needle or catheter	Paraesthesia over distribution of nerve root	EMG
Anterior spinal artery syndrome	Immediate		Painless	Paraplegia	?Vasodilators
Adhesive arachnoiditis		Chronic	Pain on injection	Variable degree of neurologic	CT or MRI
Cauda equina syndrome		Chronic		Loss of bowel and bladder function, paraplegia, motor weakness, sensory	

Table 4.3.3 Neurological complications of central neuraxial block

Transient neurological syndrome

In 1993 Schneider et al. published a case report of patients undergoing spinal anaesthesia in the lithotomy position and who, postoperatively, experienced aching and pain in the buttocks and lower limbs. This is now termed transient neurological syndrome (TNS).

Several different laboratory models have proved that all local anaesthetics can be neurotoxic when applied to neural tissues in clinically relevant concentrations, but that lidocaine (lignocaine) and tetracaine (amethocaine) are potentially more neurotoxic than bupivacaine. Neurotoxicity of lidocaine (lignocaine) is both concentration- and time-dependent, but is not related to sodium channel blockade or the addition of glucose.

Surgical position has an important influence on the incidence of TNS. For example, patients undergoing surgery in the lithotomy position have an incidence of TNS of approximately 30–36%, patients undergoing arthroscopic knee surgery have an incidence of 18–22% and patients undergoing surgery in the supine position have an incidence of 4–8%. It is important to emphasise that if a patient presents with an abnormal neurological examination or motor weakness, causes other than TNS must be eliminated.

Extradural haematoma

Anticoagulants such as heparin, low molecular weight heparin (LMWH) or warfarin are given prophylactically to patients in the perioperative period to prevent deep vein thrombosis. However, if neuraxial anaesthesia is administered when a patient is anticoagulated, catastrophic bleeding may occur within the spinal canal during needle or catheter placement or removal. Bleeding inside the spinal canal may lead to spinal cord compression and untoward motor deficit, necessitating immediate CT scan and surgical laminectomy to prevent paraplegia. In 1998, the US Food and Drug Administration reported 43 cases of spinal haematomas in patients who had received spinal or extradural anaesthesia and who had received enoxaparin 30 mg twice daily. Sixteen patients did not recover from paraplegia despite emergency surgery. This was probably due to higher doses administered (enoxaparin 30 mg twice daily) compared to European protocols (enoxaparin 40 mg once daily). In 1998, consensus conference guidelines were published and recommended lower doses of LMWH. Overall, the incidence of bleeding complications due to neuraxial blocks is estimated to be less than 1/150 000 for extradural and less than 1/220 000 for spinal anaesthesia. Associated risks include use of anticoagulants, thrombocytopenia, chronic alcohol use, chronic renal failure and difficult blocks.

Heparin

Heparin has a half-life of 1–2 hours. Unfractionated heparin inhibits factor II (thrombin) as well as factor X. Its bioavailability is weak and unpredictable because endothelial cells and fibrinogen show a high affinity for the unfractionated heparin molecule. Activity is measured by the activated partial thromboplastin time (PTT). Current Ameriacn Society of Regional Anesthesia (ASRA) guidelines[101] recommend that intravenous heparin should be delayed 1 hour after needle placement, and catheters should be removed at least 1 hour before the next heparin administration or 4 hours after the last heparin dose. An activated PTT should be checked for normal coagulation before performing spinal anaesthesia in patients who have been anticoagulated for a long time, especially in debilitated patients.

Low molecular weight heparins

Low molecular weight heparins have a slow onset (90 minutes) and a half-life of 4 hours. Their effects last 12 hours.

Low molecular weight heparins are the gold standard in the prevention of postoperative venous thromboembolism. They have shorter chains than unfractionated heparin and show no interaction with endothelial cells or fibrinogen. Thus, their bioavailability is higher and more reliable than that of standard heparin. Peak anti-X activity occurs 3–4 hours after a subcutaneous injection of LMWH. The plasma half-life of LMWH is two to four times that of standard heparin and increases in patients with renal failure. As their activity is more focused on factor X, monitoring of activated PTT is not recommended. Monitoring of anti-Xa activity is advised only in the elderly and in patients with renal failure.

As the plasma half-life of LMWH is 4 hours, 12 hours is the recommended safe interval following LMWH prophylaxis for placement of a central neuraxial block or removal of an extradural catheter. Nevertheless, a delay of 24 hours is recommended in cases of administration of LMWH in higher doses (e.g. enoxaparin 1 mg/kg twice daily) for treatment of deep venous thrombosis and pulmonary embolism.

It appears that there is no clear advantage of administering LMWH before surgery. The results of a recent meta-analysis show that the effectiveness and safety of starting LMWH prophylaxis after surgery are comparable to those observed with preoperative prophylaxis. The administration of LMWH before surgery may lead to an increase in the amount of bleeding during surgery compared to the same dose started early postoperatively. LMWH may be administered 1–2 hours after neuraxial blockade.

Warfarin

Oral anticoagulant prophylaxis remains a common practice in the United States for patients undergoing hip or knee arthroplasty. Warfarin blocks factors II, VII, IX and X as well as proteins C and S. As the plasma half-lives of these proteins are different (7 hours for factor VII, 36 hours for factor X, and 50 hours for factor II), we can observe an early increase in prothrombin time (PT) and international normalised ratio (INR) due to a decrease in factor VII, whereas the fully anticoagulant effect is not achieved before 72–96 hours (factor II, IX and X decrease). The ASRA Consensus Conference agreed that an INR value should be less than 1.4 before performing a neuraxial block and before removal of a spinal or extradural catheter. In patients receiving chronic warfarin medication, the PT and INR require 3–5 days to normalise after discontinuation of the drug. It is mandatory to document normal coagulation status before performing any neuraxial block in such a setting.

Antiplatelet drugs

The effects of new antiplatelet drugs such as ticlopidine and clopidogrel seem more pronounced than those of aspirin or nonsteroidal anti-inflammatory drugs (NSAIDs). In addition, the mechanisms of inhibiting platelet functions differ – aspirin and NSAIDs inhibit cyclo-oxygenase, leading to a decrease in thromboxane A_2 synthesis by platelets and a decrease in prostacyclin synthesis by endothelial cells. Ticlopidine inhibits the ADP pathway necessary for platelet aggregation. Moreover, the duration of inhibition of platelet function differs between these classes of drugs. Inhibition of cyclo-oxygenase is reversible after NSAID treatment because this effect is related to plasma concentration of the drug, whereas it is permanent with aspirin until platelet regeneration (7 days).

As there is no accurate test that will reliably guide the anti-aggregant effect of antiplatelet drugs, clinicians must rely on the weak notion of 'time interval' between the last ingestion of the drug and the timing of central neuraxis anaesthesia. For example, whereas 7 days are necessary to eliminate any antiplatelet effect of aspirin or clopidogrel, 10–14 days are required for ticlopidine. The COX-2 inhibitor drugs, which are known to preserve platelet function (because COX-2 enzyme is not expressed on platelets), should not delay the performance of spinal or extradural anaesthesia.

Neither aspirin alone nor NSAIDs without additional factors are considered significant factors for the development of spinal haematoma after central neuraxial anaesthesia. Horlocker et al.[100] showed in their prospective study that there was no correlation between antiplatelet medications and bloody needle or catheter placement during neuraxial blocks. However, when these drugs are associated with other drugs affecting coagulation (heparin, antiplatelet drugs etc.) or with multiple and difficult punctures, they may increase the bleeding risk inside the spinal canal, thus making possible the occurrence of a compressive spinal haematoma. In elective cases, aspirin and ticlopidine should be stopped 7 and 10 days before surgery, respectively. If the underlying medical disease is serious (e.g. carotid stenosis, recent coronary event), they should be replaced with subcutaneous heparin or LMWH until 12 hours before surgery.

Recent consensus statements[101] have recommended that the decision to perform neuraxial block should be made on an individual basis, balancing benefit versus risk. The patient's coagulation status should be optimised at the time of spinal or extradural needle or catheter placement, and the level of anticoagulation must be carefully monitored during the period of extradural catheterisation. Indwelling catheters should not be removed in the presence of therapeutic anticoagulation because this appears to significantly increase the risk of spinal hematoma. Vigilance in monitoring is critical to allow early evaluation of neurological dysfunction and prompt intervention.

CENTRAL NEURAXIAL BLOCKADE AND OUTCOME

Recognition of the link between severe pain, impaired rehabilitation and poor long-term outcomes was made by an American surgeon, George Crile, over 90 years ago.[102] He proposed, on the basis of clinical observations, that preventing pain impulses from reaching the CNS could improve surgical outcome and that this could be facilitated by the use of regional anaesthetic blocks in addition to general anaesthesia. He suggested that separation of tissue injury from the neural and behavioural response to surgical trauma is necessary to aid healing, and that this 'anoci-association' could accelerate and improve recovery.

Awareness of the ability of epidural analgesia to modify the neuroendocrine response to surgery and attenuate postoperative elevations in plasma glucose levels[103] stimulated researchers to investigate the impact of epidural anaesthesia and analgesia on postoperative morbidity and mortality.[104] Subsequently, many studies compared the application of thoracic epidural analgesia to traditional intravenous and intramuscular morphine analgesia.

The first two studies by Yaeger et al.[105] and Tuman et al.[106] provided encouraging evidence that good postoperative analgesia reduced cardiac, pulmonary and infectious complications following surgery. This was attributed to a reduction in the neuroendocrine stress response as measured by urinary cortisol. However, subsequent studies increasingly failed to show differences in outcome.[107,108]

Meta-analyses

Pooling the results of many underpowered studies to derive a single estimate of effect is called meta-analysis. Meta-analyses of the impact of thoracic epidural analgesia on single organ function have shown significantly improved respiratory, cardiac and gastrointestinal outcomes.

In the meta-analysis by Ballantyne et al.,[109] epidural local anaesthetics increased Pao_2 and decreased theincidence of pulmonary infections and overall pulmonary complications compared to systemic opioids. Compared to systemic opioids, epidural opioids halved the incidence of atelectasis.

A meta-analysis of 11 randomised controlled studies by Beattie et al.[110] showed a significant reduction in postoperative myocardial infarction with thoracic epidural analgesia when administered for more than 24 hours.

Furthermore, Jorgenson et al.[111] consistently showed reduced time to return of gastrointestinal function, measured as time to first flatus or defaecation, in the epidural local anaesthetic group compared to groups receiving systemic or epidural opioid.

In order to determine the influence of central neuraxial block on morbidity and mortality after surgery, a meta-analysis of 141 studies of regional anaesthesia versus general anaesthesia was undertaken.[112] Overall, 247 deaths occurred in 9559 patients, a mortality rate of 2.6%. Patients receiving regional anaesthesia had a lower mortality rate, a lower incidence of pulmonary embolism, less need for transfusion and a lower incidence of myocardial infarction and renal failure. Criticisms of the study were its heterogeneity (it included both spinals and epidurals), that over two-thirds of deaths came from nine studies with at least 10 deaths per study, and that the greatest reductions in mortality rate were associated with orthopaedic surgery (the group most likely to have received spinal anaesthesia).

Routine clinical use of thoracic epidural anaesthesia followed by prolonged postoperative analgesia in the 1990s prompted two large multicentre studies of high-risk surgical patients randomised to either epidural block or intravenous PCA morphine. Neither found differences in mortality rate between groups, although analysis of subgroups in the study by Park et al.[113] showed reductions in myocardial infarction, stroke and respiratory failure after abdominal aortic surgery. In the study by Rigg et al.[114] there were reductions in the incidence of respiratory failure.

Why are less convincing results being found? Profound changes have taken place in anaesthetic, medical and surgical practice in the past decade. Preoperative fluid optimisation,[115] use of shorter-acting drugs such as remifentanil and esmolol, and improved monitoring such as the oesophageal Doppler have all changed practice. Fewer postoperative patients are referred to the intensive care unit (ICU) as more patients are managed on postoperative surgical wards. New medical treatments such as β-blockade[116,117] and angiotensin-converting enzyme (ACE) inhibitors, and better thomboprophylaxis have all served to reduce mortality rates over the past decade. New surgical procedures are less invasive and associated with less blood loss.

In 1993, Kehlet and Dahl[118] proposed a similar hypothesis to Crile, but within a modern multimodal framework of preoperative optimisation, minimisation of intraoperative stress using regional anaesthesia, aggressive early pain-free mobilisation and early oral feeding. Few randomised controlled studies have been published to support Kehlet's hypothesis, although initial studies have shown benefits to patients. An audit of abdominothoracic oesophagectomy[119] investigated a multimodal approach using intense analgesia, early feeding and early mobilisation. This showed shorter times to extubation, mobilisation and ICU discharge compared to a historical control group.

A prospective randomised study by the same group subsequently investigated the impact of a multimodal approach on patients undergoing radical cystectomy.[120] In the first part of the study, 30 patients were randomised to receive general anaesthesia followed by systemic opioids or general anaesthesia followed by thoracic epidural analgesia. Parenteral nutrition was provided to both groups for 5 days after surgery. An additional 15 patients were treated with a multimodal approach consisting of intraoperative general anaesthesia and thoracic epidural analgesia, early oral nutrition, and enforced mobilisation. The results showed that patients in the latter group had lower levels of urinary catecholamines, better nitrogen balance, less fatigue and better overnight recovery.

The feasibility of an accelerated 48-hour postoperative stay programme after colonic resection[121] was conducted by Kehlet's group to try and reduce the length of hospital stay after colonic resection. Sixty consecutive patients undergoing elective colonic resection were studied using a well-defined postoperative care programme. Normal gastrointestinal function returned within 48 hours in 57 patients, and the median hospital stay was 2 days. There were no cardiopulmonary complications. The readmission rate was 15%, including two patients with anastomotic dehiscence; other readmissions required only short-term observation.

To accelerate recovery, the initial 'pain-free state' has to be taken advantage of in such a way that obstacles to recovery, such as drains and central venous lines, are removed, and patients encouraged to 'return to normal function' with early feeding and mobilisation.[10,122] Providing good pain relief without accelerated rehabilitation offers no extra advantage to patient outcomes.

Fulfilling Kehlet's goal of pain-free movement and 'normal function' on successive postoperative days, however, requires unremitting, complete high-quality pain relief, which is only available with well-managed continuous regional blockade.[123] Therefore, also implicit within Crile's and Kehlet's hypotheses, is the notion of not only providing pain relief of such intensity that patients are able to feed and mobilise, but that this state should be sustained without impediment until wounds have started to heal. Breakthrough pain requiring rescue analgesia impairs feeding, increases nausea and vomiting, and limits mobilisation (Fig 4.3.7).

Quality of life

Few studies, unfortunately, have investigated the benefits of epidural analgesia on long-term function and evaluated health status from the patient's perspective – that is, an assessment of health-related quality of life (HQL). In the most prominent study,[124] 64 patients undergoing elective colonic resection were randomised to either thoracic epidural analgesia using a mixture of bupivacaine and fentanyl or intravenous PCA with morphine.

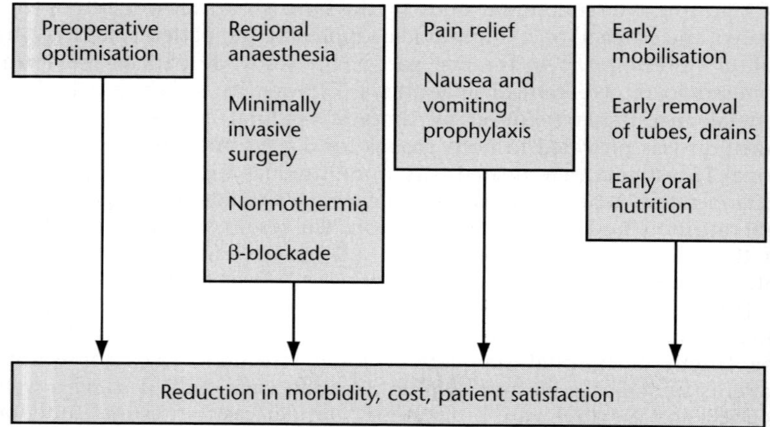

Figure 4.3.7 Fast-track surgery and accelerated rehabilitation.

All patients received the same early feeding and mobilisation opportunities. Primary outcome was functional exercise capacity, as measured by the 6-minute walking test, and the secondary outcome was health-related quality of life, as measured by the SF-36 health survey. Both measures were assessed before surgery and at 3 and 6 weeks after hospital discharge. After 6 weeks, patients in the PCA group had a significantly greater decrement in walking distance than patients in the epidural group. The latter group had lower postoperative pain and fatigue scores, allowing improved mobilisation. The results of this study corroborate data from another study by Capdevila et al.[125] demonstrating that the perioperative use of epidural analgesia and perineural catheters shortens rehabilitation time after major knee surgery (Fig. 4.3.8).

Chronic pain

The relationship between surgery and chronic pain is now recognised.[126] Chronic pain can follow amputation, thoracotomy, cardiac surgery, mastectomy, cholecystectomy and inguinal hernia repair. The development of chronic pain can be attributed to two perioperative events, nerve injury or ligation at the time of operation, and the severity of postoperative pain. This latter factor suggests that aggressive pain therapy to suppress early postoperative pain could reduce the intensity and the occurrence of chronic pain. However, only one study has compared the effect of pre-emptive versus post-incisional epidural analgesia on the incidence of chronic pain. Twenty-eight patients undergoing thoracotomy were ran-

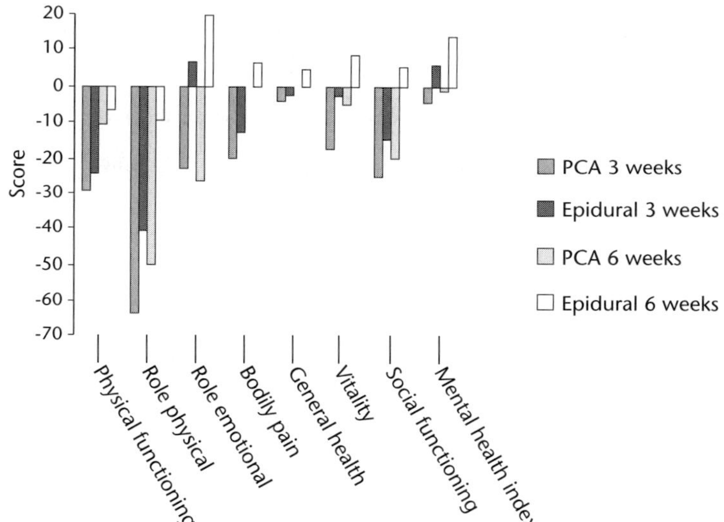

Figure 4.3.8 Quality of life parameters 3 and 6 weeks after thoracic epidural anaesthesia.

domly allocated to pre- or post-incisional mepivacaine followed by epidural infusion for 72 hours. In the pre-emptive group, pain scores were significantly reduced on the second and third post operative days and the number of pain-free individuals was significantly reduced after 3 and 6 months.

References

1. Behar M, Magora F, Olshwang D, Davidson JT. Epidural morphine in treatment of pain. Lancet 1979; 1:527–529.
2. Djurberg H, Haddad M. Anterior spinal artery syndrome. Paraplegia following segmental ischaemic injury to the spinal cord after oesophagectomy. Anaesthesia 1995; 50:345–348.
3. Hogan QH. Epidural anatomy examined by cryomicrotome section. Influence of age, vertebral level, and disease. Reg Anesth 1996; 21:395–406.
4. Hogan Q, Toth J. Anatomy of soft tissues of the spinal canal. Reg Anesth Pain Med 1999; 24:303–310.
5. Hogan Q. Distribution of solution in the epidural space: examination by cryomicrotome section. Reg Anesth Pain Med 2002; 27:150–156.

6. Carpenter RL, Hogan QH, Liu SS, Crane B, Moore J. Lumbosacral cerebrospinal fluid volume is the primary determinant of sensory block extent and duration during spinal anesthesia. Anesthesiology 1998; 89:24—29.
7. Hogan Q. Size of human lower thoracic and lumbosacral nerve roots. Anesthesiology 1996; 85:37–42.
8. McClure JH. Ropivacaine. Br J Anaesth 1996; 76:300–307.
9. McLeod GA, Burke D. Levobupivacaine. Anaesthesia 2001; 56:331–341.
10. Wilmore DW, Kehlet H. Management of patients in fast track surgery. Br Med J 2001; 322:473–476.
11. Bevacqua BK. Continuous spinal anaesthesia: what's new and what's not. Best Pract Res Clin Anaesthesiol 2003; 17:393–406.
12. Denny NM, Selander DE. Continuous spinal anaesthesia. Br J Anaesth 1998; 81:590–597.
13. Reynolds F. Damage to the conus medullaris following spinal anaesthesia. Anaesthesia 2001; 56:238–247.
14. Watson MJ, Evans S, Thorp JM. Could ultrasonography be used by an anaesthetist to identify a specified lumbar interspace before spinal anaesthesia? Br J Anaesth 2003; 90: 509-11.
15. Camu F, Vanlersberghe C. Pharmacology of systemic analgesics. Best Pract Res Clin Anaesthesiol 2002; 16:475–488.
16. Bernards CM. Understanding the physiology and pharmacology of epidural and intrathecal opioids. Best Pract Res Clin Anaesthesiol 2002; 16:489–505.
17. Bernards CM, Hill HF. Morphine and alfentanil permeability through the spinal dura, arachnoid, and pia mater of dogs and monkeys. Anesthesiology 1990; 73:1214–1219.
18. Bernards CM, Shen DD, Sterling ES, et al. Epidural, cerebrospinal fluid, and plasma pharmacokinetics of epidural opioids (part 2): effect of epinephrine. Anesthesiology 2003; 99:466–475.
19. Polley LS, Columb MO, Naughton NN, Wagner DS, Dorantes DM, van de Ven CJ. Effect of intravenous versus epidural fentanyl on the minimum local analgesic concentration of epidural bupivacaine in labor. Anesthesiology 2000; 93:122–128.
20. D'Angelo R, Gerancher JC, Eisenach JC, Raphael BL. Epidural fentanyl produces labor analgesia by a spinal mechanism. Anesthesiology 1998; 88:1519–1523.
21. Gokin AP, Philip B, Strichartz GR. Preferential block of small myelinated sensory and motor fibers by lidocaine: in vivo electrophysiology in the rat sciatic nerve. Anesthesiology 2001; 95:1441–1454.
22. Brull SJ, Greene NM. Zones of differential sensory block during extradural anaesthesia. Br J Anaesth 1991; 66:651–655.

23. de Filho GR, Gomes HP, da Fonseca MH, Hoffman JC, Pederneiras SG, Garcia JH. Predictors of successful neuraxial block: a prospective study. Eur J Anaesthesiol 2002; 19:447–451.

24. Connolly C, Wildsmith JA. Intrathecal drug spread. Can J Anaesth 1998; 45:289–292.

25. Connolly C, McLeod GA, Wildsmith JA. Spinal anaesthesia for Caesarean section with bupivacaine 5 mg ml^{-1} in glucose 8 or 80 mg ml^{-1}. Br J Anaesth 2001; 86:805–807.

26. Cooper DW, Jeyaraj L, Hynd R, et al. Evidence that intravenous vasopressors can affect rostral spread of spinal anesthesia in pregnancy. Anesthesiology 2004; 101:28–33.

27. Law AC, Lam KK, Irwin MG. The effect of right versus left lateral decubitus positions on induction of spinal anesthesia for cesarean delivery. Anesth Analg 2003; 97:1795–1799.

28. Goy RW, Sia AT. Sensorimotor anesthesia and hypotension after subarachnoid block: combined spinal-epidural versus single-shot spinal technique. Anesth Analg 2004; 98:491–496.

29. Richardson MG, Wissler RN. Density of lumbar cerebrospinal fluid in pregnant and nonpregnant humans. Anesthesiology 1996; 85:326–330.

30. Lui AC, Polis TZ, Cicutti NJ. Densities of cerebrospinal fluid and spinal anaesthetic solutions in surgical patients at body temperature. Can J Anaesth 1998; 45:297–303.

31. McLeod GA. Density of spinal anaesthetic solutions of bupivacaine, levobupivacaine, and ropivacaine with and without dextrose. Br J Anaesth 2004; 92:547–551.

32. Sanderson P, Read J, Littlewood DG, McKeown D, Wildsmith JA. Interaction between baricity (glucose concentration) and other factors influencing intrathecal drug spread. Br J Anaesth 1994; 73:744–746.

33. Whiteside JB, Burke D, Wildsmith JA. Comparison of ropivacaine 0.5% (in glucose 5%) with bupivacaine 0.5% (in glucose 8%) for spinal anaesthesia for elective surgery. Br J Anaesth 2003; 90:304–308.

34. Lee A, Ray D, Littlewood DG, Wildsmith JA. Effect of dextrose concentration on the intrathecal spread of amethocaine. Br J Anaesth 1988; 61:135–138.

35. Wildsmith JA. Predicting the spread of spinal anaesthesia. Br J Anaesth 1989; 62:353–354.

36. Lyons G, Columb M, Wilson RC, Johnson RV. Epidural pain relief in labour: potencies of levobupivacaine and racemic bupivacaine. Br J Anaesth 1998; 81:899–901.

37. Ginosar Y, Mirikatani E, Drover DR, Cohen SE, Riley ET. ED50 and ED95 of intrathecal hyperbaric bupivacaine coadministered with opioids for cesarean delivery. Anesthesiology 2004; 100:676–682.

38. Camorcia M, Capogna G, Lyons G, Columb M. Epidural test dose with levobupivacaine and ropivacaine: determination of ED50 motor block after spinal administration. Br J Anaesth 2004; 92:850–853.

39. Whiteside JB, Burke D, Wildsmith JA. Spinal anaesthesia with ropivacaine 5 mg ml^{-1} in glucose 10 mg ml^{-1} or 50 mg ml^{-1}. Br J Anaesth 2001; 86:241–244.

40. Gautier P, De Kock M, Huberty L, Demir T, Izydorczic M, Vanderick B. Comparison of the effects of intrathecal ropivacaine, levobupivacaine, and bupivacaine for Caesarean section. Br J Anaesth 2003; 91:684–689.

41. Glaser C, Marhofer P, Zimpfer G, et al. Levobupivacaine versus racemic bupivacaine for spinal anesthesia. Anesth Analg 2002; 94:194–198.

42. Alley EA, Kopacz DJ, McDonald SB, Liu SS. Hyperbaric spinal levobupivacaine: a comparison to racemic bupivacaine in volunteers. Anesth Analg 2002; 94:188–193.

43. Curatolo M, Orlando A, Zbinden AM, Scaramozzino P, Venuti FS. A multifactorial analysis of the spread of epidural analgesia. Acta Anaesthesiol Scand 1994; 38:646–652.

43a. McLeod G. Thoracic epidural analgesia: Influences on time to first experience of pain Reg Anesth Pain Med 2003; 6:590, A24

44. Hirabayashi Y, Shimizu R. Effect of age on extradural dose requirement in thoracic extradural anaesthesia. Br J Anaesth 1993; 71:445–446.

45. Simon MJ, Veering BT, Stienstra R, van Kleef JW, Burm AG. The effects of age on neural blockade and hemodynamic changes after epidural anesthesia with ropivacaine. Anesth Analg 2002; 94:1325–1330.

46. Burke D, Henderson DJ, Simpson AM, et al. Comparison of 0.25% S–bupivacaine with 0.25% RS– bupivacaine for epidural analgesia in labour. Br J Anaesth 1999; 83:750–755.

47. Faccenda KA, Simpson AM, Henderson DJ, Smith D, McGrady EM, Morrison LM. A comparison of levobupivacaine 0.5% and racemic bupivacaine 0.5% for extradural anesthesia for caesarean section. Reg Anesth Pain Med 2003; 28:394–400.

48. Visser WA, Liem TH, van Egmond J, Gielen MJ. Extension of sensory blockade after thoracic epidural administration of a test dose of lidocaine at three different levels. Anesth Analg 1998; 86:332–325.

49. Okutomi T, Hashiba MM, Hashiba S, Masubuchi A, Morishima HO. The effects of single and fractionated doses of mepivacaine on the extent of thoracic epidural block. Reg Anesth Pain Med 2001; 26:450–455.

50. Scott DB, McClure JH, Giasi RM, Seo J, Covino BG. Effects of concentration of local anaesthetic drugs in extradural block. Br J Anaesth 1980; 52:1033–1037.

51. Sakura S, Sumi M, Kushizaki H, Saito Y, Kosaka Y. Concentration of lidocaine affects intensity of sensory block during lumbar epidural anesthesia. Anesth Analg 1999; 88:123–127.

52. Dernedde M, Stadler M, Bardiau F, Boogaerts J. Comparison of different concentrations of levobupivacaine for post-operative epidural analgesia. Acta Anaesthesiol Scand 2003; 47:884–890.

53. Limberi S, Markou N, Sakayianni K, et al. Coronary artery disease and upper abdominal surgery: impact of anesthesia on perioperative myocardial ischemia. Hepatogastroenterology 2003; 50:1814–1820.

54. Purdie NL, McGrady EM. Comparison of patient-controlled epidural bolus administration of 0.1% ropivacaine and 0.1% levobupivacaine, both with 0.0002% fentanyl, for analgesia during labour. Anaesthesia 2004; 59:133–137.

55. Lee BB, Ngan Kee WD, Ng FF, Lau TK, Wong EL. Epidural infusions of ropivacaine and bupivacaine for labor analgesia: a randomized, double-blind study of obstetric outcome. Anesth Analg 2004; 98:1145–1152.

56. Faccenda KA, Simpson AM, Henderson DJ, Smith D, McGrady EM, Morrison LM. A comparison of levobupivacaine 0.5% and racemic bupivacaine 0.5% for extradural anaesthesia for caesarian section. RAPM.2003; 91(5): 684-9

57. Casati A, Santorsola R, Aldegheri G, et al. Intraoperative epidural anesthesia and postoperative analgesia with levobupivacaine for major orthopedic surgery: a double-blind, randomized comparison of racemic bupivacaine and ropivacaine. J Clin Anesth 2003; 15:126–131.

58. Senard M, Kaba A, Jacquemin MJ, et al. Epidural levobupivacaine 0.1% or ropivacaine 0.1% combined with morphine provides comparable analgesia after abdominal surgery. Anesth Analg 2004; 98:389–394.

59. Curatolo M, Schnider TW, Petersen-Felix S, et al. A direct search procedure to optimize combinations of epidural bupivacaine, fentanyl, and clonidine for postoperative analgesia. Anesthesiology 2000; 92:325–337.

60. Niemi G, Breivik H. Epinephrine markedly improves thoracic epidural analgesia produced by a small-dose infusion of ropivacaine, fentanyl, and epinephrine after major thoracic or abdominal surgery: a randomized, double-blinded crossover study with and without epinephrine. Anesth Analg 2002; 94:1598–605.

61. Polley LS, Columb MO, Naughton NN, Wagner DS, van de Ven CJ. Relative analgesic potencies of ropivacaine and bupivacaine for epidural analgesia in labor: implications for therapeutic indexes. Anesthesiology 1999; 90:944–950.

62. Capogna G, Celleno D, Fusco P, Lyons G, Columb M. Relative potencies of bupivacaine and ropivacaine for analgesia in labour. Br J Anaesth 1999; 82:371–373.

63. Benhamou D, Ghosh C, Mercier FJ. A randomized sequential allocation study to determine the minimum effective analgesic concentration of levobupivacaine and ropivacaine in patients receiving epidural analgesia for labor. Anesthesiology 2003; 99:1383–1386.

64. Polley LS, Columb MO, Naughton NN, Wagner DS, van de Ven CJ, Goralski KH. Relative analgesic potencies of levobupivacaine and ropivacaine for epidural analgesia in labor. Anesthesiology 2003; 99:1354–1358.

65. Polley LS, Columb MO, Naughton NN, Wagner DS, van de Ven CJ. Effect of epidural epinephrine on the minimum local analgesic concentration of epidural bupivacaine in labor. Anesthesiology 2002; 96:1123–1128.

66. Lyons G, Columb M, Hawthorne L, Dresner M. Extradural pain relief in labour: bupivacaine sparing by extradural fentanyl is dose dependent. Br J Anaesth 1997; 78:493–497.

67. Polley LS, Columb MO. Comparison of epidural ropivacaine and bupivacaine in combination with sufentanil for labor. Anesthesiology 2000; 92:280–281.

68. Bader AM, Datta S, Flanagan H, Covino BG. Comparison of bupivacaine- and ropivacaine-induced conduction blockade in the isolated rabbit vagus nerve. Anesth Analg 1989; 68:724–727.

69. Zaric D, Nydahl PA, Philipson L, Samuelsson L, Heierson A, Axelsson K. The effect of continuous lumbar epidural infusion of ropivacaine (0.1%, 0.2%, and 0.3%) and 0.25% bupivacaine on sensory and motor block in volunteers: a double-blind study. Reg Anesth 1996; 21:14–25.

70. Lacassie HJ, Columb MO, Lacassie HP, Lantadilla RA. The relative motor blocking potencies of epidural bupivacaine and ropivacaine in labor. Anesth Analg 2002; 95:204–208.

71. Lacassie HJ, Columb MO. The relative motor blocking potencies of bupivacaine and levobupivacaine in labor. Anesth Analg 2003; 97:1509–1513.

72. McLeod G, Davies H, Munnoch N, Bannister J, MacRae W. Postoperative pain relief using thoracic epidural analgesia: outstanding success and disappointing failures. Anaesthesia 2001; 56:75–81.

72a. Ballantyne JC, McKenna JM, Ryder E Epidural analgesia – experience of 5628 patients in a large teaching hospital derived through audit *Acute Pain* 2003; 4:89–97.

73. Rawal N, Holmstrom B. The combined spinal–epidural technique. Best Pract Res Clin Anaesthesiol 2003; 17:347–364.

74. Hughes D, Simmons SW, Brown J, Cyna AM. Combined spinal-epidural versus epidural analgesia in labour. Cochrane Database Syst Rev 2003:CD003401.

75. Albright GA, Forster RM. Does combined spinal-epidural analgesia with subarachnoid sufentanil increase the incidence of emergency cesarean delivery? Reg Anesth 1997; 22:400–405.

76. Yun EM, Marx GF, Santos AC. The effects of maternal position during induction of combined spinal-epidural anesthesia for cesarean delivery. Anesth Analg 1998; 87:614–618.

77. Michaloudis D, Petrou A, Bakos P, et al. Continuous spinal anaesthesia/analgesia for the perioperative management of high-risk patients. Eur J Anaesthesiol 2000; 17:239–247.

78. Vercauteren MP, Geernaert K, Hoffmann VL, Dohmen D, Adriaensen HA. Postoperative intrathecal patient-controlled analgesia with bupivacaine, sufentanil or a mixture of both. Anaesthesia 1998; 53:1022–1027.

79. McCrae AF, Wildsmith JA. Prevention and treatment of hypotension during central neural block. Br J Anaesth 1993; 70:672–680.

80. Warner DO, Warner MA, Ritman EL. Human chest wall function during epidural anesthesia. Anesthesiology 1996; 85:761–773.

81. Flisberg P, Jakobsson J, Lundberg J. Apnea and bradypnea in patients receiving epidural bupivacaine-morphine for postoperative pain relief as assessed by a new monitoring method. J Clin Anesth 2002; 14:129–134.

82. Madej TH, Wheatley RG, Jackson IJ, Hunter D. Hypoxaemia and pain relief after lower abdominal surgery: comparison of extradural and patient-controlled analgesia. Br J Anaesth 1992; 69:554–557.

83. Sakura S, Saito Y, Kosaka Y. The effects of epidural anesthesia on ventilatory response to hypercapnia and hypoxia in elderly patients. Anesth Analg 1996; 82:306–311.

84. Sakura S, Saito Y, Kosaka Y. Effect of extradural anaesthesia on the ventilatory response to hypoxaemia. Anaesthesia 1993; 48:205–209.

85. Carli F, Trudel JL, Belliveau P. The effect of intraoperative thoracic epidural anesthesia and postoperative analgesia on bowel function after colorectal surgery: a prospective, randomized trial. Dis Colon Rectum 2001; 44:1083–1089.

86. Holte K, Kehlet H. Epidural analgesia and risk of anastomotic leakage. Reg Anesth Pain Med 2001; 26:111–117.

87. Gould TH, Grace K, Thorne G, Thomas M. Effect of thoracic epidural anaesthesia on colonic blood flow. Br J Anaesth 2002; 89:446–451.

88. Adolphs J, Schmidt DK, Mousa SA, et al. Thoracic epidural anesthesia attenuates hemorrhage-induced impairment of intestinal perfusion in rats. Anesthesiology 2003; 99:685–692.

89. Vagts DA, Iber T, Puccini M, et al. The effects of thoracic epidural anesthesia on hepatic perfusion and oxygenation in healthy pigs during general anesthesia and surgical stress. Anesth Analg 2003; 97:1824–1832.

90. Vagts DA, Iber T, Szabo B, et al. Effects of epidural anaesthesia on intestinal oxygenation in pigs. Br J Anaesth 2003; 90:212–220.

91. Buggy DJ, Doherty WL, Hart EM, Pallett EJ. Postoperative wound oxygen tension with epidural or intravenous analgesia: a prospective, randomized, single-blind clinical trial. Anesthesiology 2002; 97:952–958.

92. Kabon B, Fleischmann E, Treschan T, Taguchi A, Kapral S, Kurz A. Thoracic epidural anesthesia increases tissue oxygenation during major abdominal surgery. Anesth Analg 2003; 97:1812–1817.

93. Carli F, Halliday D. Modulation of protein metabolism in the surgical patient. Effect of 48-hour continuous epidural block with local anesthetics on leucine kinetics. Reg Anesth 1996; 21:430–435.

94. Lattermann R, Carli F, Schricker T. Epidural blockade suppresses lipolysis during major abdominal surgery. Reg Anesth Pain Med 2002; 27:469–475.

95. Lattermann R, Carli F, Wykes L, Schricker T. Epidural blockade modifies perioperative glucose production without affecting protein catabolism. Anesthesiology 2002; 97:374–381.

96. Brandt M, Kehlet H, Binder C, Hagen C, McNeilly AS. Effect of epidural analgesia on the glycoregulatory endocrine response to surgery. Clin Endocrinol (Oxf) 1976; 5:107–114.

96a. Pollock JE, Neal JM, Liu SS, Burkhead D, Polissar N. Sedation during spinal anesthesia. *Anesthesiology* 2000. 93:728–34.

97. Auroy Y, Narchi P, Messiah A, Litt L, Rouvier B, Samii K. Serious complications related to regional anesthesia: results of a prospective survey in France. Anesthesiology 1997; 87:479–486.

98. Auroy Y, Benhamou D, Bargues L, et al. Major complications of regional anesthesia in France: The SOS Regional Anesthesia Hotline Service. Anesthesiology 2002; 97:1274–1280.

99. Giebler RM, Scherer RU, Peters J. Incidence of neurologic complications related to thoracic epidural catheterization. Anesthesiology 1997; 86:55–63.

100. Horlocker TT, McGregor DG, Matsushige DK, Chantigian RC, Schroeder DR, Besse JA. Neurologic complications of 603 consecutive continuous spinal anesthetics using macrocatheter and microcatheter techniques. Perioperative Outcomes Group. Anesth Analg 1997; 84:1063–1070.

101. Horlocker TT, Wedel DJ, Benzon H, et al. Regional anesthesia in the anticoagulated patient: defining the risks. Reg Anesth Pain Med 2004; 29(suppl 2):1–12.

102. Katz J. George Washington Crile, anoci-association, and pre-emptive analgesia. Pain 1993; 53:243–245.

103. Naito Y, Tamai S, Shingu K, et al. Responses of plasma adrenocorticotropic hormone, cortisol, and cytokines during and after upper abdominal surgery. Anesthesiology 1992; 77:426–431.

104. Liu S, Carpenter RL, Neal JM. Epidural anesthesia and analgesia. Their role in postoperative outcome. Anesthesiology 1995; 82:1474–1506.

105. Yeager MP, Glass DD, Neff RK, Brinck-Johnsen T. Epidural anesthesia and analgesia in high-risk surgical patients. Anesthesiology 1987; 66:729–736.

106. Tuman KJ, McCarthy RJ, March RJ, DeLaria GA, Patel RV, Ivankovich AD. Effects of epidural anesthesia and analgesia on coagulation and outcome after major vascular surgery. Anesth Analg 1991; 73:696–704.

107. Baron JF, Bertrand M, Barre E, et al. Combined epidural and general anesthesia versus general anesthesia for abdominal aortic surgery. Anesthesiology 1991; 75:611–618.

108. Norris EJ, Beattie C, Perler BA, et al. Double-masked randomized trial comparing alternate combinations of intraoperative anesthesia and postoperative analgesia in abdominal aortic surgery. Anesthesiology 2001; 95:1054–1067.

109. Ballantyne JC, Carr DB, deFerranti S, et al. The comparative effects of postoperative analgesic therapies on pulmonary outcome: cumulative meta-analyses of randomized, controlled trials. Anesth Analg 1998; 86:598–612.

110. Beattie WS, Badner NH, Choi P. Epidural analgesia reduces postoperative myocardial infarction: a meta-analysis. Anesth Analg 2001; 93:853–858.

111. Jorgensen H, Wetterslev J, Moiniche S, Dahl JB. Epidural local anaesthetics versus opioid-based analgesic regimens on postoperative gastrointestinal paralysis, PONV and pain after abdominal surgery. Cochrane Database Syst Rev 2000:CD001893.

112. Rodgers A, Walker N, Schug S, et al. Reduction of postoperative mortality and morbidity with epidural or spinal anaesthesia: results from overview of randomised trials. Br Med J 2000; 321:1493.

113. Park WY, Thompson JS, Lee KK. Effect of epidural anesthesia and analgesia on perioperative outcome: a randomized, controlled Veterans Affairs cooperative study. Ann Surg 2001; 234:560–569; discussion 569–571.

114. Rigg JR, Jamrozik K, Myles PS, et al. Epidural anaesthesia and analgesia and outcome of major surgery: a randomised trial. Lancet 2002; 359:1276–1282.

115. Wilson J, Woods I, Fawcett J, et al. Reducing the risk of major elective surgery: randomised controlled trial of preoperative optimisation of oxygen delivery. Br Med J 1999; 318:1099–1103.

116. Mangano DT, Layug EL, Wallace A, Tateo I. Effect of atenolol on mortality and cardiovascular morbidity after noncardiac surgery. Multicenter Study of Perioperative Ischemia Research Group. N Engl J Med 1996; 335:1713–1720.

117. Poldermans D, Boersma E, Bax JJ, et al. The effect of bisoprolol on perioperative mortality and myocardial infarction in high-risk patients undergoing vascular surgery. Dutch Echocardiographic Cardiac Risk Evaluation Applying Stress Echocardiography Study Group. N Engl J Med 1999; 341:1789–1794.

118. Kehlet H, Dahl JB. The value of "multimodal" or "balanced analgesia" in postoperative pain treatment. Anesth Analg 1993; 77:1048–1056.

119. Brodner G, Pogatzki E, Van Aken H, et al. A multimodal approach to control postoperative pathophysiology and rehabilitation in patients undergoing abdominothoracic esophagectomy. Anesth Analg 1998; 86:228–234.

120. Brodner G, Van Aken H, Hertle L, et al. Multimodal perioperative management – combining thoracic epidural analgesia, forced mobilization, and oral nutrition – reduces hormonal and metabolic stress and improves convalescence after major urologic surgery. Anesth Analg 2001; 92:1594–600.

121. Basse L, Hjort Jakobsen D, Billesbolle P, Werner M, Kehlet H. A clinical pathway to accelerate recovery after colonic resection. Ann Surg 2000; 232:51–57.

122. Kehlet H, Wilmore DW. Multimodal strategies to improve surgical outcome. Am J Surg 2002; 183:630–641.

123. Bromage PR. 50 years on the wrong side of the reflex arc. Reg Anesth 1996; 21(suppl 6):1–4.

124. Carli F, Mayo N, Klubien K, Schricker T, Trudel J, Belliveau P. Epidural analgesia enhances functional exercise capacity and health-related quality of life after colonic surgery: results of a randomized trial. Anesthesiology 2002; 97:540–549.

125. Capdevila X, Barthelet Y, Biboulet P, Ryckwaert Y, Rubenovitch J, d'Athis F. Effects of perioperative analgesic technique on the surgical outcome and duration of rehabilitation after major knee surgery. Anesthesiology 1999; 91:8–15.

126. Macrae WA. Chronic pain after surgery. Br J Anaesth 2001; 87:88–98.

Section 5

Anaesthesia for various procedures

CHAPTER 5.1

ABDOMINAL SURGERY

The provision of anaesthesia for abdominal surgery covers the full range of presentations, from the elective day-case patient to the very urgent emergency patient. The anaesthetic techniques used have to mirror this diversity. The vast majority of patients will require general anaesthesia, often combined with thoracic epidural blockade because epidural blockade can provide other benefits as well as postoperative analgesia for the patient. Other operations, particularly in the pelvis and on the abdominal wall, can be carried out under central neuraxial blockade or even regional nerve block.

The requirements for general anaesthesia are unconsciousness (unless regional analgesia is used), suppression of the surgical response, good relaxation to provide surgical access and the prevention of gastric contents entering the glottis.

The preoperative assessment of abdominal surgical patients must be comprehensive. The perioperative period must incorporate close observation and monitoring. Analgesia is vital to the quality of postoperative recovery.

GENERAL CONSIDERATIONS

Primary problems

Many primary problems can lead to abdominal surgical intervention.

Bleeding

Although bleeding may arise from anywhere in the gastrointestinal (GI) tract, 75% occurs in the upper tract.

Common causes of bleeding are gastritis, gastric and duodenal ulcers and oesophagitis. Oesophageal varices are less common, but can result in an emergency presentation with dramatic bleeding, characterised by haematemesis, malaena and varying degrees of shock.

Lower GI tract bleeding is more common in the elderly, is more insidious in onset and the site of bleeding more difficult to find.

Perforation

Perforation is often associated with sudden onset of abdominal pain and signs of peritonism. A common cause is perforation of a peptic ulcer, appendix or diverticulum. Malignant or inflammatory bowel disease presenting with perforation has a worse outcome.

Obstruction

Obstruction can occur anywhere in the GI tract, most commonly secondary to adhesions, often in the small bowel. Vomiting, constipation and abdominal distension are the classic features. Other causes include hernias, inflammatory bowel disease and malignancies.

Infarction

Infarction may be secondary to torsion, strangulation, thromboembolic occlusion or vasculitis. Patients present with pain and signs of peritonism.

Inflammation

Inflammation can occur throughout the GI tract, with some disease involving large parts of the bowel, such as Crohn's disease or ulcerative colitis.

Secondary problems

The secondary problems associated with abdominal procedures are common to many disease states. Emergencies may be complicated by hypovolaemic shock with endotoxaemia, leading to a generalised inflammatory response and sepsis. The bowel, is considered by many as the source of multi-organ dysfunction syndrome.

Thermoregulation

Thermoregulation under anaesthesia is affected by several mechanisms and is characterised by a three-phase response:

- the first is a rapid reduction in temperature attributable to vasodilation, the compensatory vasoconstrictor response having been reset to a lower temperature;
- the second phase is slower, contributed to by the heat loss from radiation, convection and evaporation. These losses are a significant factor in abdominal surgery;
- during the third phase, a plateau occurs when metabolic heat production becomes activated at the new lower set threshold.

Hypothermia is exacerbated in general anaesthesia by epidural and spinal anaesthetic techniques and also in the elderly patient who has impaired thermoregulation.

The consequences of moderate hypothermia include myocardial ischaemia or arrhythmias, increased intraoperative blood loss, poor wound healing and increased nitrogen breakdown. Drug metabolism is also affected, causing prolonged action of muscle relaxants. There is an overall tendency for patients with postoperative hypothermia to have a longer hospital stay. Therefore it is imperative that techniques are used to maintain core temperature above 36.5°C, and forced-air convective warmers are the most efficient.

Respiration

Respiratory function can be affected in several ways by abdominal disease and intra-abdominal procedures.

The occurrence of postoperative respiratory complications has long been recognised and many ways have been sought to minimise this potentially serious adverse event. There are multifactorial causes – even the presenting emergency patient can already be compromised by aspiration, splinting of the diaphragm and basal lung collapse from increased abdominal pressure. This can be further compromised by the supine position and postoperative pain, which will contribute to further atelectasis. The overall presentation is of reduced functional residual capacity and ventilation–perfusion mismatch.

Minimally invasive techniques using pneumoperitoneum can also influence respiratory function by reducting chest compliance and functional residual capacity.

There are several opportunities for the anaesthetic technique to adversely influence respiratory function, such as the use of nitrous oxide, opiates and aspiration of abdominal contents at the onset of anaesthesia. One of the outcome benefits of epidural analgesia is in the reduction of postoperative chest complications.

Circulation

The splanchnic circulation is under the control of the sympathetic nervous system, humoral factors and local factors. In the fasting state only one-fifth of capillary beds are open, leaving a large reserve to meet any increased metabolic demands. Around 30% of the cardiac output is delivered to the splanchnic circulation. Liver blood flow is 25–30% of cardiac output at rest and increased during increased hepatic activity. The splanchnic flow is a fine balance and is often reduced early in hypotension to enable blood flow to be diverted to other organs. Splanchnic perfusion is increasingly compromised in the elderly patient and in operations involving bowel obstruction and perforation.

Several techniques, both preoperative and intraoperative, have been proposed to maximise splanchnic blood flow and perfusion. This 'optimisation' has been shown to improve outcome in high-risk elective surgical patients. Post-epidural hypotension and therefore reduction of splanchnic blood flow must be rigorously corrected.

Biochemistry

Fluid and electrolyte derangements can be seen not only in the emergency patient, but also in patients presenting for elective abdominal surgery. Patients presenting for colonoscopy who have had bowel preparation can show significant morbidity, especially in the elderly. Correction of the imbalance is imperative before the start of surgery, even in emergency cases. Monitoring of fluid replacement will often require invasive techniques.

The emergency patient can have significant imbalance created by vomiting, diarrhoea or fluid sequestration. Fluid sequestration can be masked – losses into the obstructed bowel, or caused by third-space shifts of fluid created by changes in vascular permeability and colloid osmotic changes in hypoalbuminaemic patients. Loss of gastric secretions can result in hypochloraemic alkalosis with hypovolaemia and hypokalaemia. Loss of lower GI secretions from massive diarrhoea or losses from fistulae are commonly associated with hypovolaemia and metabolic hyperchloraemic acidosis.

TECHNICAL CONSIDERATIONS

Preparation for abdominal surgery

Preparation for abdominal surgery is as important for elective cases as it is for the high-risk emergency case.

Every patient should be assessed by an anaesthetist before surgery. The diverse nature of abdominal surgery will require special input on top of the routine assessment of the patient's fitness for surgery. The standard routine of history, examination and investigation will apply from the outset. Colorectal patients often have 'bowel prep' before surgery, and patients, in particular the elderly, can be significantly dehydrated to warrant intravenous fluids before induction.

Hiatus hernia and reflux disease will necessitate precautions to prevent aspiration of gastric contents. In these cases preoperative use of antacids, proton pump inhibitors or H_2-receptor antagonists should be considered. There may be a requirement for rapid sequence induction in symptomatic patients to prevent aspiration.

Day-case patients will require close screening and careful selection. Emergency patients may require significant resuscitation (as discussed in the intestinal obstruction section, p. 550). High-risk elective abdominal surgical patients have been shown to have an improved outcome if they undergo pre-optimisation before surgery. Targets for pre-optimisation are:

- cardiac index – 4.5 L/min/m^2;
- oxygen delivery index – 600 mL/min/m^2;
- oxygen consumption index – 170 mL/min/m^2.

To achieve these targets a pulmonary artery catheter is required to monitor the parameters. However, central venous oxygen saturations have been used as a surrogate marker to guide resuscitation.

Patients with myocardial disease undergoing high-risk surgery can benefit from preoperative β-blockade. The improved outcome has been shown in patients with high cardiac risk indices. It is not known whether patients with lower risk would benefit from preoperative β-blockade.

The two approaches to pre-optimisation demonstrate that the whole of the perioperative period is important in determining better outcomes. Identifying which patients would benefit is important, but as yet this has not been absolutely quantified. The two methods are not mutually exclusive – patients with severe coronary artery disease will benefit from circulation optimisation as well as a reduction in cardiac work.

Avoidance of aspiration of gastric contents into the airway is important. The consequence of aspiration may be obstruction by solid material, bronchospasm, laryngospasm, pneumonitis, bronchopneumonia or adult respiratory distress syndrome. Vomiting presents a problem at induction and regurgitation presents a problem immediately after induction.

The patient should be prepared preoperatively with nasogastric tube drainage, gastric acid neutralisation and reduction of volume by inhibition of gastric secretions and enhanced emptying of the stomach.

The induction of anaesthesia will involve preoxygenation followed by rapid sequence induction with cricoid pressure to prevent potential aspiration. Although cricoid pressure is a simple technique, incorrect application can cause serious problems. This can be avoided by the correct training of assistants.

Open abdominal surgery

Anaesthetic technique

Monitoring

Before the start of anaesthesia the minimal standard of monitoring is commenced – electrocardiogram, noninvasive blood pressure, oximetry, capnography, oxygen and volatile agent analysis, temperature and airway pressure.

Induction of anaesthesia

The inspired/end-tidal oxygen difference is the best monitor of the adequacy of preoxygenation and consequent denitrogenation. An agent most suitable to the condition of the patient should be used for intravenous induction of anaesthesia.

Muscle relaxation

The choice of muscle relaxant will depend on patient factors and the specifics of the abdominal operation. If there is a risk of regurgitation and consequent aspiration, a depolarising agent such as suxamethonium is preferred to allow more rapid control of the airway. A modified approach might use rocuronium. Otherwise a non-depolarising drug can be used from the outset, so long as assessment of the airway indicates that intubation is unlikely to be difficult.

Tracheal intubation

Tracheal intubation should be followed by identification of correct placement of the endotracheal tube using both clinical signs and capnographic traces. The laryngoscopic reflex can be obtunded by prior injection of opioid, such as alfentanil. Increasingly laryngeal mask airways (LMAs) are being used, but there must be no regurgitation risk when these airways are used.

Maintenance of anaesthesia

Maintenance of anaesthesia is with a volatile agent in either air/oxygen mix or nitrous oxide/oxygen mix. Nitrous oxide is now used less often because of the increased risk of postoperative nausea and vomiting, and also because the increase in bowel distension makes the gas undesirable.

Opioids and nonsteroidal anti-inflammatory drugs (NSAIDs) are used to provide multimodal analgesia. A total intravenous technique can be used, commonly propofol and a short-acting opioid such as remifentanil.

Aliquots of muscle relaxants can be given according to the response from the nerve stimulator.

Conclusion of surgery

At the end of the procedure, with the guidance of a nerve stimulator, the neuromuscular blockade is reversed using an anticholinesterase preceded by atropine or glycopyrronium to counteract muscarinic-like effects.

Tracheal extubation

When spontaneous respiration is established the tracheal tube is removed after pharyngeal suction and toilet. The tube is removed in the lateral recovery position and high-flow oxygen administered. The patient is then transferred to a recovery area on oxygen and close observation, and monitoring is continued for as long as necessary. Prolonged close observation may take place in a critical care area.

Postoperative analgesia

Postoperative analgesia is increasingly provided by thoracic epidural; however, this technique is only a part of what should be a multimodal regimen. No single regimen will reduce postoperative morbidity and mortality. Multimodal interventions may lead to a reduction of postoperative sequelae and improved quality of recovery and outcome.

Deep venous thrombosis prophylaxis

Prophylaxis against deep venous thrombosis should relate to risk; intra-abdominal surgery, especially pelvic procedures, conveys an increased risk. This is reduced by the use of anticoagulants and support stockings or pneumatic compression devices. Most centres use low molecular weight heparin. There must be strict guidelines regarding the use of regional techniques when anticoagulants are used.

Alternative local anaesthetic techniques

Alternative local anaesthetic techniques for abdominal surgical operations fall under two main headings:

- central neuraxial blockade;
- regional or field blockade.

Central neuraxial blockade may be achieved with epidural analgesia or with spinal analgesia. Field blockade may be achieved with inguinal, interpleural or intervertebral techniques. Central neuraxial and field blocks may be used on their own or to supplement general anaesthesia.

Epidural analgesia

Epidural analgesia for abdominal surgery provides good operating conditions and good postoperative analgesia. There is a reduced neuroendocrine stress response, a shortened period of postoperative ileus and enhancement of bowel blood flow. The increased bowel motility is not associated with an increase in breakdown of anastomoses. Thoracic epidurals vasodilate splanchnic veins and the associated hypotension can, if not corrected, compromise gut mucosal integrity. Gut hypoperfusion must be prevented, and vasoconstrictors are more likely to correct bowel blood flow than is excessive fluid resuscitation.

The optimal mix of local anaesthetic and opioid remains to be determined. The use of opioid will help reduce the concentration of local anaesthetic, which will enable earlier mobilisation of the postoperative patient. The addition of an opioid improves the quality of the block but can lead to respiratory depression. The addition of other adjuvants such as the selective α_2-adrenergic agonist clonidine has been recommended. Lumbar blockade for abdominal surgery is difficult to maintain and should be used for pelvic and abdominal wall procedures only. The Bezold–Jarisch reflex of bradycardia, vasodilatation and hypotension is more common with extensive lumbar blockade. Selective thoracic epidural blockade should be used for patients undergoing intra-abdominal procedures. The establishment of epidural blockade ideally should occur before commencing general anaesthesia, but there may be some circumstances where insertion of the epidural catheter is carried out in the anaesthetised patient.

The use of epidurals should be part of strict guidelines involving close monitoring by trained nurses to identify potential dangerous side-effects. Local guidance should be enforced for the use of epidurals in patients taking anticoagulants, removal of the catheter being as important an issue as insertion. The most common side-effect is a failed epidural, where 20% of patients will experience severe pain. This must be eliminated by having sufficiently trained staff and monitoring by a dedicated pain team.

There are several side-effects, such as hypotension, urinary retention, respiratory depression and pruritus. The most feared – neurological damage, especially paraplegia – is fortunately rare.

There is proven benefit in the quality of postoperative recovery. The elusive outcome benefit remains controversial. Thus a risk–benefit analysis must be applied to each case.

Spinal anaesthesia

Spinal anaesthesia is restricted to operations performed below the umbilicus. Unlike with epidural blockade the duration of surgery is an important consideration. Risk–benefit analysis should be made in each case. Many of the contraindications apply to other forms of regional block, including coagulopathy, concurrent anticoagulants, patient refusal, sepsis, hypovolaemia and raised intracranial pressure.

The fine-gauge pencil-point needle is now the most widely used. This should produce minimal trauma and the smallest hole in the dura. This will reduce the incidence of post-dural puncture headache. The insertion site is between the third and fourth lumbar vertebrae, and the extent of the block is determined by the baricity of the solution, the position of the patient and the dose rather than the volume of the local anaesthetic. Adjuvants include opioids, which can prolong the duration of analgesia; the selective α_2-adrenergic agonist clonidine will also prolong the block.

Lumbar block using hyperbaric solution (2.5–3 mL 0.5% 'heavy' bupivacaine) is suitable for all lower abdominal surgery, including hernia repair. Saddle (perineal) block is indicated for perineal surgery and can be achieved by establishing the block in the sitting position.

Inguinal field block

Inguinal field blockade aims to block the ilioinguinal, iliohypogastric, subcostal and genitofemoral nerves. The first three lie close to each other between the abdominal muscle layers at the level of the anterior superior iliac spine, and they may be conveniently blocked here. This block alone will provide good postoperative analgesia. If the patient is to be awake there should be additional skin infiltration along the incision site with local anaesthetic agent. Once the cord is exposed, the cord and hernial sac should be infiltrated with local anaesthetic.

Interpleural block

Interpleural block is indicated for open cholecystectomy. Equipment is available to allow passage of the catheter through a seal to prevent air entry. The pleural space is identified by a collapsing balloon or free flowing of fluid from a bag attached to the side arm. The catheter is then inserted into the intercostal space. There is spread of local anaesthetic over several dermatomes from this space. Pneumothorax may occur.

Paravertebral block

Paravertebral block can be used for open cholecystectomy and for thoracotomy (oesophagectomy).The paravertebral space is triangular and situated at the head and necks of the ribs, and solution can pass over several dermatomes. The space can be found by the 'loss-of-resistance' technique, 2–3 cm lateral to the appropriate spinous process. Once identified, a catheter can be inserted. This block is a useful adjuvant in a multimodal approach when epidural blockade is contraindicated.

Minimally invasive abdominal surgery

Laparoscopic surgery is a major advance in modern surgical techniques and increasing numbers of surgical procedures will be replaced by the minimally invasive approach. The increase in laparoscopic minimally invasive surgery has resulted in reduced postoperative pain, reduced inflammatory response to surgery and faster discharge from hospital. The advantages of minimally invasive surgery are reduced ileus, reduced pain and reduced aftermath of the stress response to surgery.

Laparoscopic techniques are well established in gynaecological procedures and now increasingly in surgery. Laparoscopic cholecystectomy was the first to be widely accepted, and several others are now well established (e.g. Nissen fundoplication, splenectomy and adrenalectomy).

Laparoscopy

Pneumoperitoneum

Pneumoperitoneum is achieved by insufflating carbon dioxide via a Veress needle at a rate of 1–6 L/min into the peritoneal cavity to a pressure of 10–18 mmHg. This is necessary to create the space to visualise the surgical area through the laparoscope. Carbon dioxide use adds to the safety of the techniques because it is highly soluble in blood and does not support combustion. Carbon dioxide is carried in blood and rapidly eliminated.

Changes in respiratory pressures and haemodynamic parameters are caused by the increased intra-abdominal pressures. The respiratory changes are caused by the cephalad displacement of the diaphragm, leading to a reduction in tidal volume and functional residual capacity. There is decreased compliance and increased airway resistance, leading to a potential increased risk of barotrauma. Uneven distribution leads to ventilation–perfusion mismatch and atelectasis can predispose to postoperative chest infections.

Cardiovascular changes are manifested by a drop in venous return and hence a fall in cardiac output. There is an increase in systemic vascular resistance and a reflex tachycardia. Arrhythmias may occur on gas insufflation, and bradycardia can be induced by stretching of the peritoneum. Hypercarbia can also exacerbate arrhythmias.

Other effects of the pneumoperitoneum are caused by the increased intra-abdominal pressure, which if it exceeds 20 mmHg is associated with a reduction in renal blood flow and urine output. One of the benefits of laparoscopic surgery is a reduction in the hormonal stress response to surgery.

Anaesthetic technique

Careful preoperative assessment is required, focusing on cardiac and respiratory reserve. There are still indications for open procedures. Liver and renal function must be assessed because these organs may be affected by the increased intra-abdominal pressure.

Intravenous induction followed by muscle relaxation, intubation and ventilation is preferable for laparoscopic surgery. This protects the airway and allows ventilation at higher tidal volumes, which are used to prevent hypercarbia and help reduce atelectasis. In upper abdominal procedures a nasogastric tube improves the surgical view.

Intraoperative maintenance of anaesthesia can be by total intravenous or inhalational anaesthesia. A multimodal approach to pain relief is used. Monitoring of the patient should be the minimum standard plus the addition of pressure–volume loops to provide closer observation of lung mechanics. Patients with reduced cardiac reserve will require invasive techniques such as arterial line, central venous pressure (CVP) and estimates of perfusion via central venous oxygenation. Cardiac output can be monitored with pulmonary artery catheters or the less invasive techniques, such as oesophageal Doppler.

Ventilation is adjusted to maintain normocarbia by adjusting tidal volumes; positive end-expiratory pressure (PEEP) may be applied to reduce basal atelectasis. Airway pressures should be carefully monitored and vigilance for pneumothorax maintained.

Postoperative pain relief is aided by local anaesthetic infiltration of the port sites and local anaesthetics applied directly to the operative site. Pain can be quickly controlled by a systemic multimodal approach. Shoulder tip pain is reduced by sitting the patient up early in recovery.

Complications of laparoscopic surgery include surgical emphysema, basal atelectasis with chest infection and an increased tendency for postoperative nausea and vomiting.

SPECIFIC OPERATIONS

Upper GI tract

Oesophagogastrectomy and gastrectomy

Oesophagogastrectomy and gastrectomy both deliver a major physiological challenge to the patient. There are three commonly used approaches for oesophageal surgery:

- an upper midline laparotomy followed by right thoracotomy with anastomosis in the chest (Ivor Lewis procedure);
- a three-stage procedure of right thoracotomy followed by upper midline laparotomy and right-sided cervical incision to allow the anastomosis in the neck;s
- a transhiatal approach allowing anastomosis in the neck without thoracotomy, but this approach does not permit lymph node dissection.

The laparotomy can be performed laparoscopically and there has been an increase in a thoracoscopic approach. Preoperative selection and staging are key to the improved outcome of these patients. The investigations required will be the usual preoperative work-up plus lung function tests and arterial blood gas analysis if one-lung ventilation is required. Echocardiography may be required to ensure correct patient selection.

General anaesthesia supplemented by thoracic epidural analgesia is commonly used. A multimodal regimen of analgesia based on the continuous epidural is used postoperatively. Perioperative monitoring is the routine monitoring with invasive arterial and CVP measurement. Pressure–volume loops provide a breath-by-breath picture of respiratory mechanics. A thoracic approach is a relative indication for one-lung anaesthesia to allow optimal surgical access.

There can be several position changes and double-lumen tube placement must be rechecked after movement. Temperature loss can be a problem and great efforts should be made to maintain normothermia. The procedure is prolonged and care of pressure points must be taken.

Postoperatively the majority of patients are extubated and all should be managed in a critical care area. Good analgesia is vital, and this can be provided by thoracic epidural with judicious use of systemic opioids and NSAIDs. Alternative methods of pain relief can be provided by paravertebral, intercostal nerve blocks with patient-controlled analgesia (PCA).

Biliary tract surgery

Biliary tract surgery can be open or laparoscopic. The indications for the open procedure are a patient unfit for pneumoperitoneum and previous upper GI tract surgery (relative). The effect of opioids on the sphincter of

Oddi is unclear. Pethidine is still used by some in preference to other opioids in the belief that there is less contraction of the sphincter.

Preoperative jaundice is an additional risk; good hydration should be maintained throughout the perioperative period to help avoid renal failure. Vitamin K is advisable preoperatively. Postoperative analgesia is important to aid recovery. This can be via thoracic epidural or PCA using intravenous opioids.

Pancreatic surgery

Pancreatic surgery is sometimes carried out for necrotising pancreatitis, chronic pancreatitis, trauma and neoplastic lesions. There has been a reduction in surgical intervention in acute pancreatitis, but necrosectomy may be indicated if necrotising pancreatitis is detected.

Whipple's procedure involves pancreaticoduodenectomy for lesions in the head of the pancreas. Diabetes mellitus will complicate the perioperative procedure. The operation is long and suitable precautions are taken for temperature loss and protection of pressure points. A thoracic epidural provides good analgesia, and postoperatively patients should be managed in a critical care area.

Lower GI tract

Colorectal surgery

Colorectal surgery involves a wide range of surgical procedures with varying complexity; most involve laparotomy, bowel resection, anastomosis of the remaining segments or stoma formation.

The anaesthetic technique will usually be intravenous induction, muscle relaxation with ventilation, thoracic epidural and perioperative monitoring. Nitrous oxide is avoided to prevent bowel distension. There is often a requirement for large infusions of intravenous fluid. Major blood loss will require blood transfusion. However, transfusion in cancer surgery has provoked debate. Transfusion has been linked with increased tumour recurrence and increased infection rates. White cell-depleted blood is used in an attempt to minimise this effect.

Analgesia may be provided with continuous thoracic epidural and supplemental simple analgesics. Opioids can be used via a PCA system, and NSAIDs added for their opioid-sparing effect. Use of anticholinesterase drugs has been a concern because of the possibility of increased peristaltic activity. This may cause a theoretical risk of bowel anastomosis dehiscence, but conclusive evidence is lacking.

Acute obstruction and perforation

Acute obstruction and perforation of the small or large bowel is a common surgical emergency. It can affect all ages and causes significant morbidity and mortality. The causes of obstruction are many; however, 45–60% of cases are due to adhesions, the small bowel being involved in 90% of cases. Large bowel obstruction is commonly caused by carcinoma.

The sequence of events is identical regardless of the area involved, but the clinical signs may vary. In the early stages, bowel activity above the obstruction increases in an attempt to overcome the blockage. If this is not relieved the bowel will dilate, eventually causing flaccidity of bowel motion. There is proximal bowel distension by gas and fluid, the bowel wall becomes oedematous, and eventually there is fluid leak into the peritoneum causing contamination and peritonitis.

Fluids and electrolytes are sequestered in the lumen and absorption is impeded causing hypovolaemia and electrolyte imbalance, and eventually the patient becomes shocked. As further distension occurs the blood supply becomes compromised, leading to ischaemia, necrosis, and eventally perforation.

The increased intra-abdominal pressure occuring in obstruction can cause diaphragmatic splinting, which can lead to basal lung atelectasis. With prolonged vomiting there will be sodium and water loss, and chloride loss, by creating a metabolic alkalosis, will increase potassium loss. The resultant metabolic abnormality will be a hypovolaemic, hypokalaemic, hypochloraemic metabolic alkalosis. The predominant metabolic derangement associated with obstruction further down the GI tract and in the large bowel is a metabolic acidosis.

Although these patients require urgent surgery, time must be made for full resuscitation, and even in cases of perforation aggressive resuscitation must be commenced.

Resuscitation is aided by invasive monitoring and may necessitate admission to a critical care unit. All patients require a nasogastric tube to empty the stomach. Analgesia should be provided, and thromboprophylaxis if there is no coagulopathy. The decision to provide regional analgesia with continuous epidural must be made on an individual patient basis; the presence of the following may influence the decision:

- coagulopathy;
- sepsis;
- profound hypotension intraoperatively.

Anaesthetic technique

Operations to relieve intestinal obstruction will invariably require general anaesthesia, with perioperative monitoring, which may need invasive arterial and CVP monitoring. After careful assessment and resuscitation, rapid sequence induction is used. A large-bore cannula will be in situ and the nasogastric tube on free drainage. The choice of agents is not important, apart from not using nitrous oxide, which may increase intra-abdominal pressure in the early postoperative period. The risk–benefit of an epidural is assessed on an individual basis.

Large fluid volumes may be required and intraoperative management of fluids can be aided by CVP measurement, oesophageal Doppler and pulmonary artery catheter.

In high-risk elective patients pre-optimisation to a fixed target has been shown to improve outcome – the targets are reached using fluids, blood and inotropes. The benefits in this group of patients are as yet not evidenced based, unlike those of high-risk elective abdominal surgery.

Postoperative management for the majority of patients should be in a critical care area. There are continued fluid shifts and heat loss can be significant. There is also the high risk of patients deteriorating, most commonly with sepsis.

Perineum and abdominal wall

Perianal surgery

Perianal surgery can result in severe pain, which may precipitate reflex responses such as laryngospasm (Brewer–Luckhardt reflex) and arrhythmias.

General anaesthesia with spontaneous breathing can be used, employing potent analgesic agents such as fentanyl or alfentanil to suppress the painful stimuli. The lithotomy or Trendelenburg positions are used, which can predispose to regurgitation and will influence the choice of airway control.

Spinal and caudal extradural anaesthesia have both been used, thus avoiding general anaesthesia and providing good postoperative analgesia. A 'saddle' block aiming to anaesthetise S2–S5 using small volumes (0.5–1.5 mL) of 0.5% heavy bupivacaine is used. Local blocks, such as posterior perineal nerve blockade and local infiltration, can supplement general anaesthesia and provide good perioperative analgesia.

Hernia repair

Hernia repair can occur at several sites in the abdominal wall. A hernia is a bowel protrusion from its normal position through an opening in the abdominal wall. After excision of the sac, the defect is repaired with either sutures or polypropylene mesh. There can be an emergency presentation with strangulation, which may require bowel resection.

Inguinal hernia is the most common hernia, accounting for 75–85% of hernias in both sexes, and can occur at almost any age. Early repair is advised to reduce the risk of strangulation. There is a 3% recurrence rate and the procedure for redo repair is more complex and prolonged. Other hernias include femoral hernias, which can strangulate more easily. Paraumbilical hernias are acquired and are associated with middle age, obesity and multiparity. There is a high risk of strangulation. Incisional hernias are a late complication of abdominal surgery.

A high proportion of repairs are now performed as day-case procedures. There is the occasional presentation as an emergency with symptoms of bowel obstruction. Elective repair can be performed laparoscopically, but at present the benefits over the conventional approach have not materialised.

The anaesthetic technique will depend on presentation, type and size of the hernia. All strangulated hernias should have general anaesthesia with rapid sequence induction and application of cricoid pressure. For other types of repair there is a wide choice of ways to proceed: general anaesthesia with multimodal analgesia based on local field block, field block alone, and regional anaesthesia.

Further reading

Ball J, Rhodes A, Bennett E. Reducing the morbidity and mortality of high risk surgical patients. Yearbook Intens Care Med Emerg Med 2000;331–342.

Darzi A, Mackay S. Recent advances in minimal access surgery. Br Med J 2002; 324:31–34.

Gemmell L, Rincon C. Anaesthetic management of intestinal obstruction. Br J Anaesth CEPD Rev 2001; 5:138–141.

Horlocker T, Wedel D, Benzon H, et al. Regional anaesthesia in the anticoagulated patient: defining the risks. Reg Anaesth Pain Med 2003; 28:172–197.

McCrossan L, Masterson G, Blood transfusion in critical illness. Br J Anaesth 2002; 88:6–9.

Rigg J, Jamrozik K, Myles P, et al. Epidural anaesthesia and analgesia and outcome of major surgery: a randomised trial. Lancet 2002; 359:1276–1282.

Rodgers A, Walker S, Schug S, et al. Reduction of postoperative mortality and morbidity with epidural or spinal anaesthesia: results from overview of randomised trials. Br Med J 2000; 321:1493–1505.

Vanner R, Asai T. Safe use of cricoid pressure. Anaesthesia 1999; 54:1–4.

Wildsmith J, Armitage E, McClure J. Principles and practice of regional anaesthesia. Edinburgh: Churchill Livingstone; 2003.

Williams B, Wheatley R. Epidural analgesia for postoperative pain relief. Royal College of Anaesthetists Bulletin July 2000.

CHAPTER **5.2**

CARDIAC SURGERY

Adult patients present for cardiac surgery and anaesthesia from a variety of sources and can be broadly subdivided into the following groups:

- coronary revascularisation procedures – accounting for around 80% of all cases;
- procedures involving the cardiac valves and their supporting structures that can be either recanalised, repaired or replaced;
- procedures to close defects between the right and left sides of the heart (e.g. atrial and ventricular septal defects);
- surgery for intractable arrhythmias, in particular atrial fibrillation;
- heart and lung transplantation;
- circulatory support procedures as a bridge to myocardial recovery or transplantation – for example ventricular-assist device (VAD) placement, extracorporeal membrane oxygenation (ECMO) and intra-aortic balloon pump (IABP);
- heart failure surgery with excision of excess or non-functioning myocardium to improve ventricular performance;
- operative procedures involving the pericardium and great vessels, both arterial and venous, within the thoracic cavity (e.g. replacement of the ascending aorta, pulmonary embolectomy etc.);
- grown-up congenital cardiac (GUCC) – requiring further surgical correction or revision of a partially corrected congenital anomaly.

GENERAL CONSIDERATIONS

Anaesthetic problems and cardiac surgery

Anaesthetic-related problems in cardiac surgery result either from a direct consequence of the precipitating condition or from associated co-morbidities, for example renal dysfunction, diabetes mellitus, pulmonary disease and the interaction of perioperative drugs with cardiac medications, or as a consequence of the process of cardiopulmonary bypass (CPB).

Effects of the disease process

- Impaired ventricular function may be further depressed by anaesthetic agents and exacerbated by hypotension, hypoxia and acidosis;
- valvular stenosis or regurgitation restricts cardiac output with limited ability to compensate for changes in pre- or afterload. Anaesthetic agents must therefore be given with caution;
- surgical manipulations of the heart may cause arrhythmias and hypotension;
- the function of other organs, especially lungs, liver and kidney, may be impaired and this may result in a reduced ability to maintain normal physiological homoeostasis, including the metabolism and excretion of anaesthetic drugs.

Effects of cardiopulmonary bypass

Isolation of the heart from the circulation is a necessary requisite for most cardiac surgical procedures. The physiological maelstrom resulting from this affects many normal homoeostatic processes and may:

- promote a cytokine-mediated systemic inflammatory response similar to that seen in sepsis;
- affect coagulation and clotting mechanisms adversely, resulting in increased requirements for blood product replacement;
- result in neurological dysfunction, either as a result of the effects of CPB or secondary to an embolic event – air, clot or plaque disruption – produced as a result of surgical manipulation of the heart and aorta;
- result in myocardial damage due to inadequate intra-bypass myocardial protection.

Preparation for cardiac surgery

Patients present for adult cardiac surgery following a cardiological assessment and work-up.

The cardiac assessment process is based on history, examination and special investigations, most commonly cardiac catheterisation and echocardiography assessment of myocardial and valvular function. Preoperative anaesthetic consultation is most commonly performed either at the bedside or in the cardiac pre-admission clinic. A full pre-anaesthetic history and examination should be performed, with particular reference to those areas affecting anaesthetic management.

History

Presenting condition

Key points to note in the history include the presenting condition, for example coronary disease, valvular problem. Where referral for surgery is for angina then the following should be ascertained.

- Is the condition stable or unstable with a continuing requirement for anti-anginal medication (e.g. nitrate or heparin infusions)?
- Is there associated dyspnoea secondary to systolic or diastolic dysfunction?
- Is there a history of recent myocardial infarction or episodes of cardiac failure?
- Time in hospital or transfer from another centre?

Co-existing disease

Co-existing disease increases the morbidity of cardiac surgery, and particular note should be taken of chronic respiratory disease, peripheral and neurovascular disease, renal impairment and diabetes mellitus.

Drugs and allergies

Ascertain the patient's current cardiovascular medications for control of angina, cardiac failure, blood pressure and cardiac arrhythmias. Patients with a recent history of acute coronary syndrome may have been treated with antifibrinolytic agents – streptokinase or powerful antiplatelet drugs with no reversibility (e.g. abciximab). Most patients with a history of angina will be taking antiplatelet drugs (e.g. aspirin, clopidogrel etc.) – these should be stopped 5–7 days preoperatively. Patients in chronic atrial fibrillation will be on warfarin – this should be stopped 3 days before surgery and substituted with low molecular weight heparin

Is there a history of an allergic reaction to heparin, protamine, iodine or antibiotics? If the patient has been on a heparin infusion up to the time of surgery, is there any evidence of heparin-induced thrombocytopenia (HITS)? In cases of redo cardiac surgery was aprotinin used at the first operation?

Dentition

Has a dental check been performed in patients presenting for valve replacement?

Oesophageal disease

If intraoperative transoesophageal echocardiography (TOE) is contemplated any past history of oesophageal disease should be sought to prevent inadvertent oesophageal damage during placement of the probe.

Examination

A problem-focused full examination of the patient is essential, and of particular relevance are the following.

Cardiorespiratory reserve

Look for evidence of the severity of any cardiorespiratory disease and the degree of cardiorespiratory reserve.

Bruits

Listen for bruits in the carotid arteries, especially if cannulation of the internal jugular vein is contemplated.

Peripheral arteries

Where radial arteries are to be used as conduits it is essential to perform an Allen's test to determine vascular sufficiency.

Airway assessment for anticipated difficult intubation

Up to 25% of patients presenting for cardiac surgery are diabetic, and this group has a higher than normal incidence of difficult intubation.

Investigations

Patients presenting for cardiac surgery will have undergone an extensive work-up before operation. Routine preoperative investigations should include the following.

Haematology

A full blood count, coagulation and crossmatch profile.

Biochemistry

Blood chemistry, including urea and electrolytes, liver function tests and random blood sugar. All of these may be abnormal, as a consequence of either the primary disease or drugs used to treat it, such as diuretic therapy. Cardiac-specific enzymes, including troponin T, may be elevated where there is a recent history of myocardial infarction.

Electrocardiography

An electrocardiograph (ECG) may demonstrate abnormalities of rate, rhythm or conduction and show evidence of ischaemic injury or ventricular hypertrophy.

Radiology

The chest radiograph may indicate cardiac abnormalities (e.g. atrial enlargement or cardiomegaly), pulmonary pathology (e.g. chronic obstructive airways disease), or a combination of the two, such as cardiac failure.

Cardiac-specific investigations

Cardiac-specific investigations include cardiac catheter and echocardiography data – in some circumstances, patients may have further investigations to determine myocardial viability or reserve (e.g. positron emission tomography and thallium scans).

Cardiac catheterisation produces a 'road map' of the coronary vasculature, delineating the sites, severity and number of stenotic lesions. Left ventricular function can be assessed by a ventriculogram, allowing an estimate of left ventricular ejection fraction to be made. The gradient across a stenotic valve can also be measured via a catheter pull-through technique.

Echocardiography is most easily performed via the transthoracic (TTE) route. Further information can be obtained by the more invasive transoesophageal echo (TOE), a modality increasingly deployed for intraoperative evaluation by anaesthetists. Echocardiographic investigations give an indication of the severity of valvular pathology as well as allowing an assessment of ventricular systolic and diastolic function. Typical values are listed in Table 5.2.1.

Risk stratification

Risk stratification has been pioneered and used extensively in cardiac surgery, and retrospective analysis of outcome data has led to the development of a number of prospectively validated outcome risk stratification scores (e.g. Parsonett et al.[1] and Euroscore[2]). The following factors have been shown to increase the risk of mortality and morbidity associated with cardiac surgery:

- demographic factors – female gender and age;
- cardiac status – cardiac failure or cardiogenic shock, ejection fraction less than 40%, valve surgery, left ventricular aneurysm;
- co-morbid disease – renal dysfunction, diabetes mellitus, hypertension (systemic or pulmonary) and obesity;
- redo or emergency surgery.

In addition, most cardiac units collect and analyse individual and institutional outcome data, using cumulative risk-adjusted mortality (CRAM) or

Valve	Normal area (cm^2)	Mild stenosis area (cm^2)	Severe stenosis area (cm^2)	Gradient (mmHg)
Mitral	4–6	<2	<1	>15
Aortic	3–5	<1	<0.75	>50

Table 5.2.1 Valve area measurements and gradients in normal and disease states

variable life-adjusted display (VLAD) plots to monitor surgical performance and to allow realistic predications of outcome to be given to patients.

Premedication

Patients presenting for cardiac surgery have high levels of anxiety regarding the procedure. This may result in increased levels of stress-related hormones, which may contribute to the development of ischaemia preoperatively. There are two aspects of premedication to consider.

Provision of anxiolysis

Provision of anxiolysis is best achieved by the administration of a benzodiazepine hypnotic the night before surgery, such as temazepam 10–20 mg or lorazepam 2–4 mg. A further dose may be given up to an hour and a half before operation, or alternatively a opioid-based intramuscular premedication can be administered (e.g. morphine 5–15 mg), depending on the patient's weight and premorbid status.

It is advisable in patients with critical coronary artery disease to prescribe supplemental oxygen via a facemask following premedication.

In the anaesthetic room a short-acting hypnotic, diazepam 0.1 mg/kg or midazolam, can be given to facilitate arterial and central vein cannulation.

Management of current medications

All antianginal, antiarrhythmic and antihypertensive drugs should be taken up to and including the morning of operation.

It is necessary to stop warfarin at least 3 days before surgery and to closely monitor the fall in the international normalised ratio (INR). In patients at increased risk of embolism (e.g. patients with mitral valve disease and atrial fibrillation) anticoagulant cover can be provided by low molecular weight heparins.

Where patients present to surgery still on warfarin, reversal of the effect is best managed by the administration of fresh frozen plasma rather than vitamin K.

Patients on platelet-inhibiting drugs such as aspirin should be advised to stop taking them 3–7 days before surgery. In addition, patients should be told to stop nonsteroidal anti-inflammatory drugs in the week before surgery.

Patients with acute coronary syndromes requiring heparin or nitrate infusions should have these continued up until the time of surgery.

Tight homoeostatic control of blood glucose levels has been shown to improve outcome in critically ill patients[3] and those undergoing cardiac surgery.[4] It is important to establish and maintain normoglycaemia – blood sugar levels between 4.5 and 6.0 mmol/L – within the perioperative period. This should start for all diabetic patients – both type 1 and type 2 – the night before surgery. Intravenous 10% glucose at 100 mL/h should be coadministered with an appropriate sliding scale insulin regimen to maintain these parameters. Following admission to theatre the 10% glucose is changed to 50% to reduce the fluid load, at a rate of 10–20 mL/h, with continuous insulin infusions adjusted to maintain normoglycaemia. It is necessary to maintain tight control until the patient is able to resume normal basic activity and be re-established on their preoperative medication.

TECHNICAL CONSIDERATIONS

Prior to anaesthesia

On admission to the anaesthetic room, ECG and pulse oximetry monitoring should be attached to the patient. Oxygen is administered via a Hudson facemask. A large-bore peripheral cannula is inserted under local anaesthetic. Supplemental sedation may be administered, if required for further line insertions.

Before performing arterial cannulation it is important to ascertain whether the left, right or both radial arteries are to be used as conduit and to select the site of cannulation appropriately – in the latter case a femoral arterial line will need to be sited and additional venous access via a central vein, because both arms will be inaccessible during surgery.

A multi-lumen central venous catheter (CVC) should be placed in an appropriate central vein – most commonly the right internal jugular, under sterile conditions. It has been stated that two-dimensional imaging ultrasound guidance is recommended as the preferred method for insertion of CVCs into the internal jugular vein in adults and children in elective situations.[5]

In high-risk patients, for example those having redo surgery, those with poor ventricular function and patients with endocarditis, further haemodynamic data can be obtained by placement of a pulmonary artery catheter or the use of other direct cardiac output monitoring devices. Caution should be exercised during this procedure because malignant arrhythmias may occur with catheter manipulations.

In patients with established chronic renal failure or acute renal dysfunction, it is advisable to place a vascular access catheter before surgery to allow early postoperative institution of renal support, such as haemofiltration.

External defibrillation pads need to be placed on the back and left lateral chest wall for patients having redo surgery and high-risk cases.

Additional monitoring includes body temperature, urine output, and in cases where circulatory arrest is required, cerebral function monitoring.

Techniques of anaesthesia

Patients are almost always induced on the operating table, fully monitored and pre-oxygenated. Never induce a patient without a surgeon who can put them onto bypass being present in the theatre suite, nor without a perfusionist and a bypass pump available in case the patient's condition deteriorates on induction. Standard anaesthetic machine check and set-up as for all procedures is essential.[6,7]

No one anaesthetic technique has been demonstrated to be better for patients undergoing cardiac surgical procedures. The choice lies between a opioid- or an inhalational-based technique, with most anaesthetists favouring the former. In addition to induction drugs it is essential to prepare a range of agents to control haemodynamics – that is, hypo- or hypertensive episodes. These may be for administration by intermittent bolus or by continuous infusion.

Induction drugs

Thiopental

Thiopental is used in hypnotic doses (1–2 mg/kg) and is still the most commonly employed induction agent, although others are used.

Ketamine

Ketamine is given to the patient in extremis – particularly in those cases where there is cardiovascular decompensation secondary to cardiac tamponade – but should be used cautiously in those with pulmonary hypertension.

Opioid

The opioid of choice is most commonly fentanyl (5–50 μg/kg), although techniques using other opioids (e.g. alfentanil, morphine, remifentanil, sufentanil) have been described.

Muscle relaxant

Traditionally cardiac anaesthetists have used pancuronium (0.1 mg/kg) for intubation and maintenance of muscle relaxation, believing that the slight tachycardia from the pancuronium antagonised the bradycardia from the fentanyl. With the onset of 'fast-track' surgery and early extubation there is a move to the use of shorter-acting muscle relaxants.

Prophylactic antibiotics

Generally three to five doses of prophylactic antibiotics are prescribed in the perioperative period according to local protocols, usually of the cephalosporin type. In patients suspected of having a methicillin-resistant *Staphylococcus aureus* (MRSA) infection or colonisation, vancomycin or teicoplanin should be given before skin incision and continued until negative screening results are obtained. In patients with infective endocarditis a longer period of postoperative chemoprophylaxis with appropriate antibiotics is required.

Anti- and procoagulant drugs

Heparin

Heparin (300 units/kg or 90 mg/m^2 body surface area) by intravenous injection is given for anticoagulation at the request of the surgeon before insertion of the aortic cannula, and in coronary cases following internal mammary artery dissection. If the patient is not heparinised before bypass, the pump and oxygenator will clot. Always use a central line for heparin – aspirate blood from the line before and after administration; verbally confirm to the surgeon that you have given the heparin. Heparin should be given as a bolus over 10–15 seconds.

Heparin is an indirect anticoagulant that interacts with antithrombin III, enhancing its inhibitory action on thrombin generation, thereby inducing a state of anticoagulation.

Heparin may adversely affect platelet function, and in some patients following a period of continuous administration can produce thrombocytopenia (HITS); in addition it can modulate a number of other processes (e.g. inflammatory response, aldosterone production and lipid metabolism[8]).

Where heparin cannot be used as the primary anticoagulant (e.g. in cases of HITS), alternative direct thrombin inhibitors such as lepirudin can be used.[9]

The degree of anticoagulation is measured using the activated clotting time (ACT) – the control level before heparin administration is 90–130 seconds, and it should exceed 400 seconds before starting bypass. Additional heparin during bypass is given according to the ACT.

Serine protease inhibitors

Coagulation-modifying agents and antifibrinolytics such as aprotinin and tranexamic acid are increasingly used to modulate bypass-mediated effects on coagulation and thereby reduce the amount of transfused blood given. These agents are generically known as serine protease inhibitors (Serpins) and produce their action by inhibiting the serine protease-dependent reactions within the clotting cascade.

Aprotinin is administered as an initial test dose of 2500 units (5 mL), followed by a bolus of 195 000 units (195 mL) and an intravenous infusion of 50 000 units/h until 3 hours after surgery. The incidence of anaphylactic reactions with aprotinin is high (1 in 200) and it should be used with caution in patients having had previous exposure to the drug. An ACT over 750 seconds is required before bypass if aprotinin is being used.

Tranexamic acid is given as an intravenous bolus before heparinisation at a dose of 10–50 mg/kg.

Protamine

Protamine (3 mg/kg) should not be drawn up until the patient is off bypass to minimise the risk of potentially fatal administration. Protamine produces its effect by directly antagonising the actions of heparin via an electrochemical antagonism.

Protamine should be administered over a period of 4–5 minutes following separation from bypass and at the request of the surgeon. It is important to inform the perfusionist verbally when you start to give the drug, so that suction devices linked to the bypass machine can be turned off. If it is given too fast hypotension may occur as a result of systemic vasodilatation, or intense pulmonary arterial constriction following the release of thromboxane A_2 in the lung. Patients who are allergic to salmon, have been on isophane insulin, or have had a vasectomy may be allergic to protamine.

Vasoactive and antiarrhythmic drugs

Anaesthesia, surgical stimulation (and manoeuvres) and the process of bypass can promote haemodynamic instability in the patient with cardiac disease. The anaesthetist must be prepared for every eventuality and requires ready access to drugs to modulate all circulatory parameters to control blood pressure, enhance contractility and treat arrhythmias. This may be achieved by bolus administration to achieve a short-term gain, or may require continuous infusions.

Vasopressor drugs suitable for bolus administration include metaraminol, phenylephrine, norepinephrine (noradrenaline) and vasopressin; vasodilators include glyceryl trinitrate and phentolamine; atropine can be administered to increase heart rate. All drugs should be diluted to a concentration such that the incremental administration of 1–2 mL produces the desired effect.

Acute arrhythmias in the peri-bypass period are treated by correcting any precipitating factors and DC cardioversion – if the chest is open – in cases of haemodynamic instability. Persistent arrhythmias may need to be treated with magnesium or amiodarone (300 mg by slow intravenous injection over 10 minutes).

General anaesthesia

In the pre-bypass period anaesthesia can be maintained by either a conventional inhalational or a total intravenous anaesthetic (TIVA) technique using controlled ventilation.

Nitrous oxide is generally avoided because of potential problems with expansion of gaseous emboli and intraluminal air in open heart procedures.

Inhalational agents, in particular isoflurane, are known to be cardioprotective and can prevent intraoperative myocardial damage,[10] although some can affect the conduction pathways and precipitate arrhythmias.

Haemodynamic stability, to prevent unwanted myocardial ischaemic events, is maintained by modulating cardiovascular parameters by the pharmacological manipulation of heart rate, contractility, preload and afterload.

During the bypass period – when ventilation is stopped – anaesthesia is maintained by TIVA, most commonly propofol infusion (3–5 mg/kg/h).

Volatile agents can be introduced into the bypass circuit to maintain anaesthesia during extracorporeal circulation; this should only be undertaken where scavenging and exhaust gas monitoring systems are available.

Regional anaesthesia

Regional anaesthesia, and in particular thoracic epidural anaesthesia, has some benefits in reducing the risk of untoward perioperative myocardial events in patients with cardiac disease presenting for noncardiac surgery.[11] Controversy exists surrounding the risk–benefit in patients undergoing surgery with full heparinisation and the risk of epidural haematoma formation precipitating spinal cord compression leading to paraplegia.[12]

Where thoracic epidurals are to be used as part of the anaesthetic technique in cardiac surgery they should always be placed in the awake patient with a normal clotting profile, and preferably the night before surgery.

Monitoring

ECG and pacing

The ECG warns of myocardial ischaemia and arrhythmias. It is normal practice in cardiac anaesthesia to use a five-lead ECG with ST segment analysis. When blood flow to the myocardium is insufficient a wall motion abnormality develops within 5–10 seconds. At 60–90 seconds the ECG ST–T wave starts to change.

In cases of severe bradycardia an endocardial pacemaker wire may be inserted preoperatively. More commonly, epicardial atrial and ventricular pacing wires are used intra- and postoperatively to achieve atrioventricular concordance and a stable rhythm in the immediate postoperative period.

Transoesophageal echocardiography

Transoesophageal echocardiography (TOE) has a number of specific indications[13] and should be performed in an ordered fashion.[14] It is useful in delineating valvular and septal pathologies and allowing real-time assessment of surgical repairs, in particular of the mitral valve. It provides an early detector of abnormalities of ventricular wall motion, usually due to ischaemia. Information regarding volume and contractile status of the ventricles can help in the choice of inotropes or need for mechanical support to wean from bypass, and TOE is able to delineate residual intracardiac air or atrial thrombus.

The TOE probe is inserted at the time of intubation (unless there is a contraindication). It can be easily damaged and it is advisable to use a biteblock and latex sheath on the probe. TOE can be detrimental to patient care if one ignores the patient while using it.

Pulse oximetry

Peripheral measurement is routine, and mixed venous measurements are available if an oximetric pulmonary artery or CVC is being used.

Arterial pressure

Arterial pressure measurements are available following cannulation of an artery – most commonly the dominant radial artery, although femoral, brachial and ulnar arteries can be used. Flow is nonpulsatile during bypass. Rapid changes may occur.

Central venous pressure

Central venous pressure (CVP) is an indicator of right ventricular filling pressure. During bypass, a rise in CVP suggests obstruction or malposition of the venous lines. At the end of operation high pressure may be caused by overtransfusion or myocardial insufficiency and low pressure by inadequate transfusion.

Left atrial pressure

Left atrial pressure can be measured directly via a catheter inserted by the surgeon at the time of operation, but is more commonly assessed using a pulmonary arterial catheter measurement of wedge pressure.

Cardiac output

Cardiac output can be measured continuously or intermittently using a variety of means, including pulmonary artery catheters and transoesophageal Doppler.

Capnography

It is important to maintain normocapnia during all phases of the operation. Rapid alterations of $Pa\text{CO}_2$ can be harmful and compromise cerebral perfusion.

Temperature

Temperature can be measured in the nasopharynx for core (or brain) temperature. Toe or bladder temperature may be used for peripheral temperature and gives an index of peripheral vasodilatation.

It is vital during the rewarming phase of bypass that cerebral blood temperature does not exceed normal body temperature because this can exacerbate cerebral injury.

In off-pump cardiac surgery it is important to maintain normothermia by minimising heat losses and providing external heat sources (e.g. forced-air warming and heated fluids).

Urine flow

Urine flow is a simple indicator of adequate renal function. Urine output should be recorded every half hour, and should exceed 0.5 mL/kg/h. Initially during bypass the output may be reduced, but increases as rewarming occurs and the priming solution is excreted.

Biochemistry

Regular measurements of serum potassium are necessary and serum potassium should be maintained at over 4.0 mmol/L to minimise arrhythmias.

Glucose levels should be within normal physiological limits (see above, p. 560).

Lactate concentration is a marker of peripheral perfusion and an indirect reflector of cardiac output. Serial estimations can indicate whether a patient's condition is improving or deteriorating in response to a given intervention.

Arterial blood gases

See below.

Cardiopulmonary bypass

The extracorporeal circulation incorporates a pump(s), a heat exchanger and a membrane oxygenator for gaseous exchange.

On initiating bypass, the perfusionist removes the clamp from the venous line and blood drains by gravity or a siphon effect from the right atrium and vena cavae into the venous reservoir. Right ventricular blood flow is reduced and as a result cardiac output drops. The bypass pump returns the blood via the arterial cannula into the patient's aorta or femoral artery. The blood can be heated/cooled and oxygenated in its passage through the bypass machine.

The perfusionist will inform the surgeon and anaesthetist when 'full flow' has been reached – this is the optimal flow (2.2 L/min/m^2) for the patient and is related to the patient's surface area. Flow is usually non-pulsatile, with peri-bypass mean arterial pressures being maintained at 40–80 mmHg. This pressure can be adjusted with small doses of vasoconstrictor or vasodilator drugs.

These procedures are reversed when weaning the patient from CPB on completion of the case.

The CPB machines are operated by a trained perfusionist.

During bypass a number of parameters should be monitored continuously and intermittently (Box 5.2.1).[15]

The following measurements should be available nearby. Local protocols dictate the frequency of measurements:

- activated clotting time to confirm anticoagulation status should be measured at intervals during CPB;
- blood gases – most operations are performed under moderate hypothermia at 28–32°C. Carbon dioxide is more soluble at low

Box 5.2.1

Cardiopulmonary bypass parameters requiring continuous monitoring

Venous oxygen saturation of the blood in the venous return line of the cardiopulmonary bypass circuit

Arterial oxygen tension or saturation of the blood in the arterial line of the CPB circuit

Continuity of the fresh gas flow to the oxygenator using an in-line flowmeter or rotameter

Oxygen concentration of the fresh gas flow to the oxygenator using an oxygen analyser with alarms and sited after the oxygen blender and vaporiser if used

Blood flow rate generated by the arterial pump of the CPB circuit

Arterial line pressure of the CPB circuit

Cardioplegia delivery line pressure when cardioplegia is delivered using the heart–lung machine

Temperature of the blood in the CPB circuit and the water in the heater/cooler system

temperatures and so the $Pa\text{CO}_2$ drops and the pH rises, if the values measured in the blood gas machine at 37°C are corrected to body temperature. Carbon dioxide may be added to the oxygenator gas mixture to avoid this apparent respiratory alkalosis. This is the 'pH-stat' approach. Allowing $P\text{CO}_2$ to fall (and pH to rise) as body temperature falls maintains electrochemical neutrality or the ratio of H^+ to OH^- constant. This means that the fraction of the histidine imidazoles in proteins that are unprotonated is constant. This is the 'alpha-stat' approach, because this fraction is called alpha. It keeps the major buffer systems, and perhaps enzyme function, at their most effective. In practice it means that $P\text{CO}_2$ and pH should not be corrected for temperature when considering acid–base status, and that the apparent respiratory alkalosis should be accepted despite the possibility of cerebral vasoconstriction;

- red cell concentration (haemoglobin or haematocrit) – the pump is primed with crystalloid, colloid or blood if the pre-bypass haemoglobin is less than 10 g/dL, or a mixture of both and an additional 10 000 units of heparin. On initiation of bypass the haematocrit falls to 20–25%. Red blood cell transfusion is only necessary if the on-bypass haemoglobin falls to less than 6 g/dL;

- serum potassium;
- blood sugar;
- filtrate volume – should be measured when a haemofilter/concentrator is being used.

The following measurements should be available at an on-site facility:

- clotting studies, including thromboelastography (TEG) – a means of assessing the clotting capability of the blood to facilitate targeted blood product replacement;
- Serum calcium, lactate and magnesium.

Myocardial protection

The heart is arrested and the myocardium protected against ischaemic damage by the use of cardioplegia. There are many different regimens described for injection into the coronary circulation, but the only essential ingredient is potassium – to induce diastolic arrest.

Cardioplegia can be delivered as warm or cold, blood or crystalloid solutions, via an antegrade route into the aortic root or retrogradely via the coronary sinus. For short periods of reduced cardiac movement ventricular fibrillation may be induced.

In operations on the aortic root involving the coronary ostia and in complex repairs, hypothermic circulatory arrest at temperatures of 15–20°C may be necessary. Under deep hypothermia (15°C) cell metabolism is so low that total circulatory and ventilatory arrest is safe, and the operating field is still and dry. The period of circulatory arrest should be kept as short as possible to minimise cerebral damage. On rewarming, the heart can be defibrillated above 30–32°C.

Blood loss

Although there is no venous return to the heart during bypass, blood reaches the heart from a number of sources, including the coronary circulation, bronchial arteries via pulmonary veins, and in cases of aortic incompetence, across the valve. This heparinised blood is returned via suckers to the bypass reservoir. Suction causes blood cell damage. It is important to use a cell-saver at all times during cardiac surgery and to salvage any remaining blood from the bypass circuit – this will reduce the requirements for autologous blood transfusion.[16]

Complications of cardiac bypass

Complications of cardiac bypass[17] can be divided into those associated with perfusion and the bypass circuit and those resulting from the process of CPB and its effect on the patient. The former include venous airlock, arterial gas embolism, clotting of the bypass circuit and failure of oxygen delivery. The latter include the following.

Awareness

The risk of awareness is inherent in the technique of bypass. Peri-bypass anaesthesia can be maintained by a TIVA technique or by having a vaporiser in the bypass circuit. Depth of anaesthesia can be monitored using techniques such as bispectral index.

Cerebral damage

Cerebral damage[18] may be global or focal, and caused by ischaemia, embolism of gas bubbles, blood clot and calcific fragments from a stenosed aortic valve. Most emboli occur on aortic cannulation, cross-clamp or side-clamp placement or removal, weaning from bypass, and aortic cannula removal.

More subtle neuropsychiatric sequelae and personality changes can occur in up to 30% of patients.

Dysfunction may be worsened by hypocapnia before bypass, low perfusion pressure and hyperglycaemia.

Cerebral autoregulation may be better preserved with the alpha-stat approach to acid–base balance.

The contribution that drugs can make to the lessening of brain damage is slight. Nitrous oxide should be avoided in the immediate post-bypass period because it has the potential to increase the size of any gaseous emboli. Excessive rewarming may worsen neurological damage.

Lung changes

Activation of the complement and kallikrein cascades causes neutrophils to aggregate in the pulmonary circulation. These activated neutrophils affect vascular tone and capillary permeability.

Gas and particulate emboli also contribute to the development of an inflammatory response, which can progress to full-blown adult respiratory distress syndrome (ARDS) in about 2% of patients – perivascular oedema and haemorrhage, congestion and thickening of interalveolar walls, patchy collapse, intra-alveolar haemorrhage, and disturbance of ventilation–perfusion relationships.[19]

Postoperative bleeding

Postoperative bleeding (Box 5.2.2) occurs especially with repeat or prolonged surgery. Bleeding usually responds to meticulous surgical technique, clotting analysis and targeted replacement of clotting factors and platelets. Further protamine is indicated in the presence of a prolonged ACT. Following chest closure, continued bleeding with clot formation may lead to cardiac tamponade, evidenced by hypotension and a rising CVP.

Renal dysfunction

Although haemolysis and haemoglobinuria can occur during bypass, it usually clears spontaneously. Development of renal failure is more related to the cardiovascular state of the patient before and after the operation

Box 5.2.2

Possible causes of postoperative bleeding in a patient following cardiac surgery

Preoperative bleeding diathesis, including treatment with anticoagulant, antiplatelet or thrombolytic drugs

Inadequate neutralisation of heparin

Fibrinolysis and fibrinogen depletion (less than 100 mg/dL)

Platelet sequestration and dysfunction

Failure of surgical haemostasis

Hypothermia

and may occur in response to the inflammatory response of bypass. In the presence of established renal failure peri-bypass haemofiltration can be employed to control fluid balance and facilitate solute and acid clearance

Separation from cardiopulmonary bypass

To achieve an uneventful and successful separation from CPB it is important to have a plan that has been agreed to by the surgeon, anaesthetist and perfusionist. There are a number of conditions which need to be met (Table 5.2.2) before weaning from CPB can be attempted. Most patients (80–90%) undergoing first time coronary surgery will wean from bypass without the need for inotropic support. Acceptable parameters following separation from CPB are given in Table 5.2.3.

Condition	Acceptable	Action required if not met
Patient temperature	>36.5°C	Further rewarming
Rhythm	Sinus rhythm >60 bpm	Pacing to establish atrioventricular synchrony
Serum potassium	>4.0 mmol/L	Give potassium
Acid–base status	Normal	Consider possible causes and correct if necessary
Ventilator	Turned on	
Monitors and alarms	Turned on	
Weaning plan	Agreed	

Table 5.2.2 Conditions that need to be met before attempting to separate from CPB

Parameter	Acceptable level
CVP	<15 mmHg
Systolic blood pressure	90–110 mm/Hg
Cardiac index	2.5–3.0 L/min/m^2
Systemic vascular resistance.	≈1000 dynes/s/cm^5

Table 5.2.3 Acceptable haemodynamic variables following separation from CPB

In cases where preoperative ventricular function is poor, where there has been a prolonged cross-clamp time or inadequate myocardial protection then inotropic or mechanical support may be required. The choice of inotrope or the need for an intra-aortic balloon pump (IABP) will be guided by experience and possible TOE assessment of the ventricle. Increasingly the phosphodiesterase drugs are being used as the first line of treatment for the failing ventricle, and evidence suggests that in many cases a single dose given before weaning from CPB can be effective.

SPECIFIC CARDIAC OPERATIONS

Coronary artery revascularisation

Coronary artery revascularisation can be performed either on or off bypass. Suitable conduits include the internal mammary and radial arteries and the saphenous vein.

In on-pump cases the distal ends of the coronary grafts are sutured to the heart during asystolic arrest at moderate hypothermia, whereas the proximal aortic anastomoses are performed following removal of the aortic cross-clamp during the rewarming phase.

Off-pump coronary artery bypass (OPCAB) surgery has become increasingly popular and has been facilitated by the introduction of suction tissue stabilising devices, which minimise cardiac movement during suturing. Proponents of this technique stress its advantages in high-risk patients with significant co-morbidities.

In the anaesthetic management of these cases the anaesthetist faces two major problems:

- first the maintenance of haemodynamic stability with the heart in a non-physiological and abnormal anatomical position necessary to access each coronary artery to be grafted;
- second, the management of intraoperative myocardial ischaemia, which might develop during the process of grafting.

Choice of anaesthetic technique is less important than a good understanding of the procedure and a close working relationship between surgeon and anaesthetist.[20] In some patients where a single graft to the left anterior descending artery (LAD) is needed this can be performed by a left thoracotomy without bypass – minimally invasive direct coronary artery bypass (MIDCAB). The procedure requires a double-lumen tube and one-lung ventilation. The heart is stabilised by placing sutures under the LAD proximal and distal to the site of the anastomoses while a small footplate rests on the myocardium. External defibrillator pads must be attached to the patient because the heart cannot easily be defibrillated internally via this incision. On-table extubation is usually possible. Anaesthetic management is as for a thoracotomy.

Valvular surgery

Valvular heart disease may be congenital or acquired and more commonly affects the left side of the heart, resulting in haemodynamic disturbances of ventricular function producing pressure-related disorders secondary to stenotic lesions, or volume-related disorders secondary to regurgitant lesions. Corrective surgical procedures can involve recanalisation, repair or replacement of the valve. There is an increasing trend towards conservative surgery, facilitated by the diagnostic use of intraoperative TOE.

Closed mitral valvotomy

Closed mitral valvotomy is performed in some cases of pure mitral stenosis in the presence of an uncalcified valve. Other closed valvotomies are very unusual.

Mitral valve repair

Many surgeons favour mitral valve repair over replacement for mitral regurgitation. Basic techniques involve partial resection of redundant valve leaflets and stabilisation of the valve annulus with a D-shaped ring.

Mitral valve replacement

Mitral valve replacement is indicated when repair of a regurgitant valve is impossible and for cases of endocarditis – involving the mitral valve – and mitral stenosis. A variety of tissue (porcine) and mechanical valves is available for implantation according to surgical preference. Patients with mechanical valves will require life-long anticoagulation to prevent clot formation occurring on the prosthesis.

Aortic valve surgery

Indications for aortic valve replacement are similar to those for the mitral valve. Where the ascending aorta is widened with associated valvular dysfunction, it can be replaced with a tissue valve and graft conduit, homograft or a composite graft. In such cases there is a requirement for the coronary arteries to be dissected off from the native aorta and re-implanted into the graft. In some cases left ventricular outflow obstruction secondary to subvalvular muscle hypertrophy can mimic aortic stenosis; the treatment for patients with this condition is a myomectomy.

Trans-septal defects

Trans-septal defects arise between the right and left sides of the heart and can be atrial or ventricular in origin. Increasingly atrial communications – atrial septal defects (ASDs) and patent foramen ovale (PFO) – can be closed using atrial closure devices introduced and deployed transvenously in the cardiac catheter laboratory. Ventricular septal defects (VSDs) may be congenital (e.g. in association with Down's syndrome) or acquired (following myocardial infarction). Ischaemic VSDs – which can be anterior or inferior – require surgical closure if associated with haemodynamic instability. This operation is associated with high morbidity and mortality rates.

Arrhythmia surgery

Accessory conducting pathways causing intractable arrhythmias may be ablated by radiofrequency delivered down a special cardiac catheter via a transcutaneous route in the cardiac catheter laboratory. Alternatively, subendocardial resection or cryosurgery is carried out requiring CPB. Either method requires extensive electrophysiological mapping of the conducting pathways. In patients with persistent atrial fibrillation secondary to atrial enlargement associated with mitral valve disease, surgical scarring of the atria is performed in the Maze procedure in an attempt to interrupt atrial pathways.

Cardiac transplantation

The main indication for cardiac transplantation is cardiomyopathy, which may be ischaemic, hypertrophic or dilated in nature. Recipients are normally under 50 years of age. Phosphodiesterase inhibitors and mechanical assist devices have been useful in 'bridging' patients to transplantation as donor availability continues to fall. Anaesthetic problems are similar to those for other cardiac operations in a seriously ill patient. Active infection or malignant disease are contraindications. Elevated pulmonary vascular resistance is a relative contraindication, and if acute in nature can be treated with prostaglandin infusions or nitric oxide. The immunosuppressive action of ciclosporin has greatly improved results, but may result in postoperative impairment of renal function.

Heart failure surgery

With the decline in numbers of suitable donors for cardiac transplantation and in the presence of an increasing number of patients with end-stage cardiac failure there has been renewed interest in surgery for heart failure. Operative procedures are aimed at remodelling the ventricle in an attempt to improve performance, and include the Batista and Dor procedures. These are often coupled with the use of mechanical assist devices and biventricular pacing, with the aim of producing a sustained improvement in cardiac output.

Aortic surgery

Thoracic aorta

Thoracic aorta surgery is most commonly performed for aneurysmal dilatation or dissection. The former may be a consequence of aortic stenosis or occur as a result of a connective tissue disorder, such as Marfan's syndrome, whereas the latter arises as a result of intimal disease and is associated with hypertension and smoking.

In aortic dilatation where the coronary ostia and aortic valve are not involved the aneurysmal section of the aorta can be replaced by an interposition woven graft.

Aortic dissection in the ascending aorta (type A) is a surgical emergency and requires an operation to replace the diseased segment and isolate the dissection flap. Dissections in the arch or descending aorta (type B) can be treated conservatively, or in some cases by endovascular stenting.

Ligation of patent ductus arteriosus

If closure of patent ductus arteriosus does not occur after birth, blood flows from the aorta to the pulmonary artery – the reverse of flow in intrauterine life. The left side of the heart dilates to cope with the increased flow through it. Less blood flows down the aorta and the diastolic blood pressure is low. Cyanosis only occurs if pulmonary vascular disease has developed or if other congenital abnormalities exist. There is a continuous murmur, and there may also be pulmonary regurgitation. Endocarditis is a hazard. The ductus is easily torn when it is ligated, especially in an adult, with major bleeding.

Coarctation of the aorta

Surgery for coarctation of the aorta is more risky in an adult than a child because of associated hypertension, coronary artery disease and cerebral aneurysms. Enlarged collaterals in the chest wall prevent a severe rise in pressure when the aorta is clamped. Induced hypotension has a place to reduce blood loss from these collaterals and make the actual suturing of the aorta easier. The blood pressure should be rising again when the clamps are removed. If the collaterals are poorly developed (as in children) and the pressure distal to the coarctation is therefore low, the blood supply to the spinal cord may be at risk.

Pericardium

Constrictive pericarditis

Constrictive pericarditis limits diastolic expansion of the heart. The rise in atrial pressure leads to venous congestion, ascites, peripheral oedema and sometimes atrial fibrillation. The blood pressure may also fall on inspiration (pulsus paradoxus). These patients present considerable anaesthetic risks. Cardiac output may not be able to increase if there is a sudden fall in peripheral resistance, and intravenous induction agents should be administered with caution. The surgical procedure is lengthy and involves considerable manipulation of the heart. Blood loss can be considerable and should be replaced precisely because the circulation is easily overloaded.

Cardiac tamponade

Cardiac tamponade can be defined as the accumulation of fluid, including blood and blood clot, around the heart, resulting in a state of haemodynamic compromise as venous return is reduced. The patient depends on a tachycardia and vasoconstriction to maintain the blood pressure.

Treatment of medical cases is normally by aspiration and insertion of a pericardial drain, but in postoperative and trauma cases open drainage is needed, with mediastinal exploration. Intermittent positive-pressure ventilation may cause severe hypotension before the pericardium is opened, and vasopressors may be required. Chronic pericardial infusions can be drained into the pleural space by creating a pericardial window – this can usually be done via a thoracoscopic approach.

Grown-up congenital cardiac disease

The number of children surviving into adulthood with congenital cardiac lesions – in many of whom there has only been a partial correction – is increasing. Further revision procedures in adult life are often indicated and require specialised multidisciplinary management.

Cardiac catheter laboratory procedures

Most procedures in adult patients are carried out under local anaesthesia with sedation as required. General anaesthesia is required for complex and potentially prolonged electrophysiological procedures and all procedures in children.

Cardioversion is carried out under general anaesthesia and can in most cases be successfully completed following a single dose of an appropriate induction agent.

EARLY POSTOPERATIVE CARE

There is an increasing trend towards a ‘fast-track’ approach to the postoperative care of cardiac surgical patients. In non-complex cases, patients can be nursed in a postoperative anaesthetic care unit (PACU) and transferred to the ward on the day of surgery.[21] More formal intensive care is still required for the more difficult cases.

Artificial ventilation is maintained until cardiovascular stability and rewarming are complete, although some patients who have had uneventful coronary artery surgery can be extubated immediately following the end of surgery.

Arrhythmias

Arrhythmias are common in the immediate postoperative period and can be atrial or ventricular in origin.

Atrial fibrillation is the most frequently occurring post-bypass arrhythmia and affects up to 30% of patients, generally presenting 24–72 hours postoperatively. The incidence is reduced in those patients who continue their cardiac medications – particularly β-blockers – up until the time of operation.[22] Treatment strategies are aimed at correcting any aggravating causes (e.g. hypokalaemia), followed by pharmacological therapies – usually with amiodarone – or DC cardioversion if there is haemodynamic compromise.

Bradycardia can be treated by the administration of atropine, or if recurrent and associated with hypotension, atrial or sequential pacing.

Blood product replacement

After bypass blood is given according to the clinical state and the haemodynamic status of the patient. In general there is no need to transfuse a patient unless the haemoglobin is less than 8 g/dL. In addition blood conservation strategies can be used (e.g. the administration of aprotinin).[23]

Cardiovascular support

Inotropic drugs and vasodilators are sometimes needed after discontinuing bypass and are usually continued into the postoperative period.

Where there is an increased requirement for circulatory support there is a necessity to acquire further information on cardiac status from haemodynamic and echocardiographic data.

Hypotensive episodes are managed by volume loading, followed by vasopressor infusions, most commonly norepinephrine (noradrenaline) titrated to a targeted endpoint.

Where impaired ventricular contractility is the cause of a low cardiac output and hypotension, there is a need to enhance ventricular performance with an inotropic agent. There is an increasing trend away from the use of catecholamines such as epinephrine (adrenaline) and dobutamine towards the use of phosphodiesterase inhibitors such as milrinone, enoximone and levosimendan to achieve this. Phosphodiesterase inhibitors enhance ventricular diastolic relaxation as their primary action in improving contractility. There may be associated vascular relaxation, which may require the use of a vasopressor infusion to maintain blood pressure, by bolus administration followed by a continuous infusion.

Hypertension is generally managed by ensuring adequate levels of sedation and analgesia, followed by infusions of glyceryl trinitrate, supplemented in intractable cases by infusion of a short-acting β-blocker (e.g. esmolol). Post-extubation hypertension can be treated with calcium channel blockers such as nifedipine administered via the sublingual route.

If drug therapy fails to maintain cardiac output, mechanical circulatory support should be considered in the form of an IABP. This is inserted percutaneously into the femoral artery and advanced to the descending aorta. The balloon is inflated in diastole (to help coronary perfusion) and deflated in systole (to reduce afterload). It can increase the output of a failing heart by 10–20%, is relatively simple and provides useful, but limited assistance. In some centres ventricular support can be provided by the use of an implantable ventricular assist device, allowing manipulation of the ventricular preload to optimise cardiac performance.[24]

Postoperative hypothermia

Patient temperature tends to fall following separation from bypass as a result of redistribution of blood flow to cooler peripheral vascular beds and continued heat loss while the chest is open before closure. As a result patients are often admitted to the PACU with a core temperature less than 35°C. To prevent further losses, added heat to the patient is provided by warming infusion fluids and the use of forced-air heating blankets.

Postoperative pain

Pain from a median sternotomy is not severe and is treated by continuous infusion of conventional analgesics supplemented by rectal paracetamol.

Renal dysfunction

Low urine output is common in the immediate post-bypass period and generally responds to a volume challenge. Where urine volumes are less than 0.5 mL/kg/h in the presence of a normal blood pressure and adequate filling pressure 5–10 mg of frusemide can be given intravenously to promote diuresis. A sustained diuresis may be achieved by continuous infusion of low-dose furosemide 0.1 mg/kg/h. The role of 'low-dose' dopamine infusions in preventing renal dysfunction is controversial. Early haemofiltration is necessary when hypervolaemia, acidosis and hyperkalaemia occur.

References

1. Parsonnet V, Dean D, Bernstein AD. A method of uniform stratification of risk for evaluating the results of surgery in acquired adult heart disease. Circulation 1989; 79:I3–I12.
2. Roques F, Nashef SAM, Michel P, et al Risk factors and outcome in European cardiac surgery: analysis of the EuroSCORE multinat onal database of 19030 patients. Eur J Cardiothorac Surg 1999; 15:816–823. Available at www.euroscore.org.
3. van den Berghe G, Wouters P, Weekers F, et al. Intensive insulin therapy in the critically ill patients. N Engl J Med 2001; 345:1359–1367.
4. Furnary AP, Gao G, Grunkemeier GL, et al. Continuous insulin infusion reduces mortality in patients with diabetes undergoing coronary artery bypass grafting. J Thorac Cardiovasc Surg 2003; 125:1007–1021.
5. Technology Appraisal No. 49. Guidance on the use of ultrasound locating devices for placing central venous catheters. Issue date: September 2002. Review date: August 2005. ISBN: 1-84257-213-X .The National Institute for Clinical Excellence, 2002. Available at www.nice.org.uk.
6. Recommendations for standards of monitoring during anaesthesia and recovery. 3rd edn. London: The Association of Anaesthetists of Great Britain and Ireland; 2000. Available at www.aagbi.org.
7. Checking anaesthetic equipment 3. London: The Association of Anaesthetists of Great Britain and Ireland; 2004. Available at www.aagbi.org.
8. Day JRS, Landis RC, Taylor KM. Heparin is much more than just an anticoagulant. J Cardiothorac Vasc Anesth 2004; 18:93–100.
9. Koster A, Kukucka M. Anticoagulation of patients with heparin-induced thrombocytopenia in cardiac surgery. Curr Opin Anaesth 2004; 17:71–74.
10. De Hert SG. Cardioprotection with volatile anesthetics: clinical relevance. Curr Opin Anaesth 2004; 17:57–62.
11. Moè llhoff T, Theilmeier G, Van Aken H. Regional anaesthesia in patients at coronary risk for noncardiac and cardiac surgery. Curr Opin Anaesth 2001; 14:17–25.
12. Gravlee GP. Epidural analgesia and coronary artery bypass grafting: the controversy continues. J Cardiothorac Vasc Anesth 2003; 17:151–153.
13. Cheitlin MD, Armstrong, WF Aurigemma GP, et al. ACC/AHA/ASE 2003 Guideline update for the clinical application of echocardiography: summary article: a report of the American College of Cardio ogy/American Heart Association Task Force on Practice Guidelines (ACC/AHA/ASE Committee to Update the 1997 Guidelines for the Clinical Application of Echocardiography). Circulation 2003; 108:1146–1162.
14. Shanewise JS, Cheung AT, Aronson S, et al. ASE/SCA Guidelines for performing a comprehensive intraoperative multiplane transesophageal echocardiography

examination: recommendations of the American Society of Echocardiography Council for Intraoperative Echocardiography and The Society Of Cardiovascular Anesthesiologists Task Force For Certification In Perioperative Transesophageal Echocardiography. Anesth Analg 1999; 89:870–884.

15. Glenville B, Graham T, Kneeshaw J, et al. Recommendations for standards of monitoring and alarms during cardiopulmonary bypass (2002). Available at www.acta.org.uk/publications_cpb.asp.
16. McGill N, O'Shaughnessy D, Pickering R, et al. Mechanical methods of reducing blood transfusion in cardiac surgery: randomised controlled trial. Br Med J 2002; 324:1299–303.
17. Gravelee GP. Update on cardiopulmonary bypass. Curr Opin Anaesth 2001; 14:11–16.
18. Arrowsmith JE, Grocott HP, Reves JG, Newman MF. Central nervous system complications of cardiac surgery. Br J Anaesth 2000; 84:378–393.
19. Ng CSH, Wan S, Yim APC, Arif AA. Pulmonary dysfunction after cardiac surgery. Chest 2002; 121:1269–1277.
20. Chassot PG, van der Linden P, Zaugg M, et al. Off-pump coronary artery bypass surgery: physiology and anaesthetic management. Br J Anaesth 2004; 92:400–413.
21. Cheng DC. Fast track cardiac surgery pathways. Early extubation, process of care and cost containment. Anesthesiology 1998; 88:1429–1433.
22. Mathew JP, Fontes ML, Tudor IC, et al A multicenter risk index for atrial fibrillation after cardiac surgery. JAMA 2004; 291:1720–1729.
23. Perioperative blood transfusion for elective surgery. Publication No. 54. Glasgow: Scottish Intercollegiate Guidelines Network; 2001. Available at www.sign.ac.uk/guideline.
24. Collard E,van Dyck MJ, Jacquet LM. Ventricular assist devices. Curr Opin Anaesth 2003; 16:33–43.

Further reading

Gothard JWW, Kelleher A, Haxby E. Cardiovascular and thoracic anaesthesia. London: Butterworth Heinemann; 2003.

Hensley FA Jr, Martin DE, Gravlee GP. A practical approach to cardiac anesthesia. 3rd edn. Philadelphia: Lippincott Williams & Wilkins: 2003.

Kaplan JA, Reich DL, Konstadt SN. Cardiac anesthesia. 4th edn. Philadelphia: WB Saunders; 1999.

McKay J, Arrowsmith J. Core topics in cardiac anaesthesia. London: Greenwich Medical Media Ltd; 2004.

CHAPTER **5.3**

DAY SURGERY

GENERAL CONSIDERATIONS

Indications

Previously seen as a form of minor surgery suitable for highly selected patients, day surgery should now be regarded as the treatment of choice for a wide range of elective surgical procedures. It is only contraindicated where there is a clear benefit from pre- or postoperative hospital admission.

Day surgery affords high-quality care on an agreed date, thorough pre-assessment and preparation for surgery, rapid recovery with attention paid to effective analgesia and minimising side-effects, preparation for discharge with appropriate information and subsequent support and follow-up.

Economics

Day surgery has the clear financial advantage of avoiding an overnight stay. Appropriate pre-assessment and freedom from emergency pressures also reduce cancellations and minimise waste. Day surgery may require more expensive drugs and equipment, but this is always outweighed by savings elsewhere. A significant financial burden is not transferred into primary care.

Selection of patients

Patients should be selected based on surgical, social and medical criteria (Box 5.3.1). A wide range of surgical procedures are possible (Boxes 5.3.2 and 5.3.3).

Changes in surgical technique, allowing patients home with drains or catheters for subsequent removal by district nurses, and more sophisticated forms of analgesia, can extend the range even further. Surgeons are often overcautious in their selection of day-surgery patients, and all those having suitable operations should be pre-assessed as soon as the decision to operate is made.

Pre-assessment is usually nurse-run, with advice from consultant anaesthetists, and frequently involves questionnaires and protocols. Investigations are only performed where clinically indicated. Early pre-assessment

Box 5.3.1

Selection criteria for day surgery (see also current guidelines from the NHS Modernisation Agency[1])

Surgical (a list of suitable operations is given in Box 5.3.2)

Thoracic or abdominal cavities not involved (unless minimally invasive)

Pain manageable with oral analgesia

Continuing blood loss or need for fluid replacement unlikely

No expected interruption of blood supply to major organs

Social

Responsible adult to accompany patient home and for 24 hours after general anaesthesia or sedation

Reasonable access to a telephone

GP back-up available

Medical

No upper age limit

American Society of Anesthesiologists grade 1–3 acceptable unless other contraindications

Body mass index <35 acceptable unless other contraindications; 35–40 unacceptable for most procedures

Diabetes mellitus is not a contraindication if well controlled; if on insulin, surgery should not prevent early resumption of normal diet

Contraindications

Marked dyspnoea on mild exertion or at rest

Angina markedly limiting activity or at rest

Myocardial infarction within 6 months

Uncontrolled hypertension (systolic >170 mmHg, diastolic >100 mmHg)

Renal failure on dialysis (fistula formation and minor procedures may be possible)

Severe hepatic disease

allows time for further investigation, specialist referral and corrective action to be undertaken without delaying surgery.

All patients having general anaesthesia require a responsible escort during the journey home and for about 24 hours afterwards. Short travelling times may be more comfortable, but guidelines should be flexible. Emergency care should be available, but this need not be in the same centre as that performing the surgery.

Box 5.3.2

UK Audit Commission (2001)[2] basket of 25 procedures where day surgery should be the preferred option

1. Orchidopexy
2. Circumcision
3. Inguinal hernia repair
4. Excision of breast lump
5. Anal fissure dilatation or excision
6. Haemorrhoidectomy
7. Laparoscopic cholecystectomy
8. Varicose vein stripping or ligation
9. Transurethral resection of bladder tumour
10. Excision of Dupuytren's contracture
11. Carpal tunnel decompression
12. Excision of ganglion
13. Arthroscopy
14. Bunion operations
15. Removal of metalware
16. Extraction of cataract with or without implant
17. Correction of squint
18. Myringotomy
19. Tonsillectomy
20. Submucous resection
21. Reduction of nasal fracture
22. Operation for bat ears
23. Dilatation and curettage/hysteroscopy
24. Laparoscopy
25. Termination of pregnancy

Many of the previous medical selection criteria were somewhat arbitrary and have been modified in the light of experience (see Box 5.3.1).[1] Elderly patients and those with obesity, diabetes mellitus and a variety of other conditions may not only undergo day surgery safely, but may actually benefit from this form of care.

Box 5.3.3

British Association of Day Surgery (1999)[3] trolley of procedures (excluding those now included in the 2000 basket) — about 50% of each procedure should be possible as day surgery

1. Laparoscopic herniorrhaphy
2. Thoracoscopic sympathectomy
3. Submandibular gland excision
4. Partial thyroidectomy
5. Superficial parotidectomy
6. Breast cancer wide excision and axillary clearance
7. Urethrotomy
8. Bladder neck incision
9. Laser prostatectomy
10. Transcervical resection of endometrium
11. Eyelid surgery (tarsoplasty, blepharoplasty)
12. Arthroscopic meniscectomy
13. Arthroscopic shoulder surgery
14. Subcutaneous mastectomy
15. Rhinoplasty
16. Dentoalveolar surgery
17. Tympanoplasty

Selection should focus on the patient's functional limitation and whether he or she would benefit from hospitalisation, rather than looking at just the presence of a disease process.

Preparation for day surgery

Following pre-assessment, patients should agree a date for their surgery. If this is not for several months, they may require brief telephone re-evaluation nearer the time to check that their condition has not worsened. Patients should be given information specific to their procedure. They also need to be told where to come, what to bring and what to expect. Information should be given, verbally and in writing, about regular medication, fasting, need for an escort, postoperative limitations and likely time off work. Dehydration is a major cause of postoperative morbidity and patients should be encouraged not to abstain from clear fluids for more than 2 hours preoperatively.

Premedication may be given to particularly anxious patients, but there can be limited time for it to work. Careful explanation and moving them to the start of the list may be more effective. Administering oral analgesia about 30 minutes before surgery ensures adequate blood levels by the end of the procedure and avoids the disadvantages of rectal, intramuscular and intravenous administration of nonsteroidal anti-inflammatory drugs (NSAIDs).

Facilities

The ideal model is a self-contained day surgery unit within a larger hospital with a separate entrance and identity, dedicated 'ward' areas, operating theatres and recovery. Independent, freestanding day-surgery units are becoming more common. An alternative is a dedicated ward area, using existing theatres. Patients should be on dedicated day-surgery lists. Mixing day cases with inpatients may result in cancellations if the day cases are late on the list and less available medical supervision if they are early. Day cases managed through regular inpatient wards are far less likely to be successfully and comfortably discharged on the day of surgery.

Extended day surgery, or the 23-hour stay facility, is an evolving model of care. Benefits and disadvantages are summarised in Box 5.3.4. If fully integrated with an established day-surgery unit, with the same principles of care, these units can provide a useful additional service, especially where successful discharge is difficult to predict. However, if day surgery is not well established, or if the unit is separate, they can lead to a reduction in true day surgery.

TECHNICAL CONSIDERATIONS

Techniques of general anaesthesia appropriate for day surgery

General anaesthesia for day surgery should use agents that are rapidly eliminated and titratable. Most of those in common use are appropriate. Intravenous propofol or inhaled sevoflurane are both highly suitable for induction of anaesthesia in adults and children. Patients should probably be allowed to choose.

Anaesthesia may be maintained with isoflurane, sevoflurane, desflurane or propofol infusions. Although all have their enthusiastic advocates, good results can be achieved with each in experienced hands. Careful titration of the level of anaesthesia to match the degree of surgical stimulation is probably more important than the specific drug used. Nitrous oxide is often used as an analgesic supplement, especially with volatile anaesthetics. Although it may increase the incidence of postoperative nausea and vomiting (PONV), alternatives, such as opioid analgesics or a deeper level of inhaled anaesthesia, may have the same effect.

Box 5.3.4
Advantages and disadvantages of extended (23-hour) day surgery
Advantages
Accommodates patients who meet day-surgery criteria but who: have surgery too late in the day to permit same-day discharge have no home support require a short period of intensive support
Allows development of new day-case procedures with 'safety net' of overnight stay
Simplifies management of day cases with a high unanticipated admission rate or where the need for overnight stay is unpredictable
Still achieves separation of elective and emergency work and provides most other benefits of day-surgery care
Disadvantages
Where day surgery is not well established, it may promote an overcautious attitude
May encourage poor management of operating list order
Surplus overnight capacity can attract emergency outliers and block beds
Antisocial hours may deter day-case nursing staff

The laryngeal mask provides a simple and effective form of airway for the majority of day surgery and has the additional advantage of being well tolerated at light levels of anaesthesia. Spontaneous ventilation is usually appropriate and the respiratory pattern may aid in anaesthetic titration, and the ability to move protects against awareness. Tracheal intubation and controlled ventilation are acceptable, however, provided that neuromuscular blocking drugs of appropriate duration are used and adequate reversal is ensured. Suxamethonium is best avoided because of muscle pains. Alternatives include a non-depolarising agent or intubation under deep propofol–opioid or sevoflurane anaesthesia.

Intravenous fluids should be administered far more commonly than is currently practised. Although fluid loss may be minimal, hydration with about 1 L of crystalloid has been shown to substantially reduce drowsiness, dizziness and PONV during the recovery period and into the next day.[4]

Intraoperative opioids are a major cause of PONV[5] and their routine use should be avoided as much as possible. Morphine is especially undesirable because it may cause somnolence in addition to PONV, but even modest doses of fentanyl or alfentanil substantially increase PONV. As postoperative pain is usually manageable with other means (see below, p. 590), prophylactic opioids should not be necessary, and the response to intra-operative noxious stimuli should be blunted by adjusting the main anaesthetic agent. Propofol may give some protection against opioid-induced PONV compared to inhaled anaesthetics.

Techniques of local analgesia appropriate for day surgery

A great many minor day-case operations can be performed after infiltration of local anaesthetic. This technique can be extended to some more significant procedures, such as adult circumcision and inguinal hernia repair, making virtually every case suitable for day surgery.

A variety of regional nerve blocks may be used in orthopaedic surgery. Spinal analgesia may be appropriate for inguinal hernia repair, as well as some orthopaedic, urological and gynaecological procedures. It can permit patients with significant obesity or respiratory disease to undergo day surgery. To ensure that prolonged motor and sympathetic block do not delay recovery, a low-dose technique must be used, typically 5 mg bupivacaine and 10 μg fentanyl diluted to a volume of 3 mL. Fine-gauge, pencil-point needles can reduce the incidence of headache after dural puncture to about 1%.

Whatever is used during the procedure, local analgesia makes a major contribution to postoperative pain relief. For many operations, simple wound infiltration (or topical application following circumcision) is as effective as a nerve block and may reduce complications. For example, femoral nerve block, which delays or even prevents discharge, complicates ilioinguinal nerve block in about 5% of hernia repairs. Pain relief should be provided using 0.5% bupivacaine or levobupivacaine in a volume appropriate to the size of the wound. Vasoconstrictors may slightly prolong the duration of analgesia, but their effect is not that significant. Vasoconstrictors should not be used when infiltrating areas with an end-artery blood supply (e.g. digits and other extremities).

Regional nerve blocks are useful after extensive shoulder or knee surgery.

Continuous or intermittent delivery of local anaesthetic agents through a catheter when the patient has returned home[6] may permit more extensive day-surgery operations.

Alternative techniques (sedation, sedoanalgesia)

Local or regional analgesia may be made more acceptable by the addition of anxiolytic, sedative and analgesic adjuvants. Before drug administration, simple measures such as verbal reassurance and the playing of music (of the patient's choice) should be tried. A gentle surgeon is also important. A small dose (typically 1–2 mg) of midazolam can provide appropriate anxiolysis and an initial degree of sedation, supplemented if necessary by small bolus doses (10 mg) or a low-dose infusion (1–2 mg/kg/h) of propofol, which prolongs sedation while allowing titration and does not compromise recovery as much as a higher dose of midazolam.

Pain should primarily be treated with additional local analgesia, but systemic analgesics may be useful to overcome the initial pain of injection or from pressure or traction on deeper structures. Small doses of short-acting opioids are usually appropriate, but care must be taken to avoid respiratory depression, which is especially likely with combinations of opioids and benzodiazepines.

Specific operations

A wide range of procedures can safely and successfully be performed as day surgery (see Box 5.3.2). The proportion of these actually carried out as day cases currently varies widely between hospitals, and even between different surgeons at the same hospital. This variation cannot be explained just by the clinical status of the patient. Where a particular procedure can be performed as a day case, attempts should be made to continually increase the proportion of patients managed in this way. The development of day surgery is a continually evolving process (Box 5.3.5), with procedures moving from inpatient care to day surgery and others moving out into outpatients and primary care.

Laparoscopic cholecystectomy

Laparoscopic cholecystectomy is increasingly being performed as a day case, but concerns persist over pain management and the risks of bleeding and bile leaks. In practice, complications are either apparent within a few hours or occur after a few days, when inpatient cases would also be at home. Pain is usually very well managed by day-surgery units. Patients undergoing day-case cholecystectomy may be better supported than those discharged after an overnight stay in an inpatient ward. Complications leading to increased postoperative pain and conversion to an open procedure are

Box 5.3.5
Continuous evolution of day surgery — developments may require a combination of new surgical techniques, alteration in anaesthetic management, revised working practices and questioning of established practice
Reduce length of stay of inpatient procedures
Convert inpatient procedure into overnight stay
Convert overnight stay into day surgery
Move minor day surgery into outpatient department or primary care

difficult to predict, and there may be advantages in managing all cholecystectomies in a day unit that also has the capacity to keep patients overnight (or even longer) if required.

Tonsillectomy

Tonsillectomy is commonly performed as a day case in North America and parts of Europe, but much less commonly in the UK. The arguments about whether it is unsafe or unwise to perform day-case tonsillectomy (in the UK) are similar to those for laparoscopic cholecystectomy, and again bleeding typically occurs early or very late. Pain is usually manageable. Use of the laryngeal mask improves recovery and virtually eliminates the risk of postoperative laryngospasm.

Future developments

Alternatives to standard diathermy can reduce bleeding after transurethral prostatectomy and may increase the proportion of patients who can be discharged on the day of surgery without a catheter. Sending patients home with a catheter, or for a trial without catheter at home, may further extend day-case prostatectomy, albeit with greater involvement of district nurses.

Allowing patients to go home with drains in situ can also considerably expand the scope of day surgery.

Technological developments, such as the two-incision hip replacement and single-compartment knee replacement, can allow short-stay major joint surgery.

POSTOPERATIVE CONSIDERATIONS

Recovery from anaesthesia

Initial recovery of consciousness, haemodynamic stability and protective reflexes should occur in a properly equipped recovery room. Some patients may reach a satisfactory level while still in the operating theatre and so may safely bypass the recovery room, going straight back to the day-surgery unit (fast-track recovery).

Before discharge, patients should have recovered to the level shown in Box 5.3.6. Scoring systems may sometimes be used, but assessment of recovery is a clinical process and is not aided by psychomotor tests. Following regional analgesia, patients should have minimal sympathetic or motor block. Temporary numbness of a limb or extremity may be acceptable, provided it can be protected against injury.

Patients will not be sufficiently recovered to be able to drive or undertake complex or hazardous tasks in safety and so must be accompanied home and for about 24 hours. Patients should not drive until the pain and immobility from their operation are reduced sufficiently to allow them to control

Box 5.3.6
Clinical criteria for recovery from day-case anaesthesia sufficient to permit safe discharge with an accompanying adult
Oriented to time, place and person
Haemodynamic stability demonstrated
Minimal bleeding or wound drainage
Acceptable control of pain, nausea and dizziness
Ability to dress and walk where appropriate (able to manage, with help, if a single limb is temporarily incapacitated)
Has passed urine (if appropriate)
Provided with appropriate written information and analgesia
Responsible adult to take patient home and provide care for next 24 hours
Community support arranged (if appropriate)
Knows arrangements for follow-up (if appropriate)
Knows emergency arrangements and contact telephone number

their car safely and perform an emergency stop. This may take several weeks, as after inguinal hernia repair. Return to work will depend substantially on the procedure performed, the level of pain and the nature of the work.

Pain management

Prophylactic analgesia should be administered whenever pain is anticipated. NSAIDs are the drug of choice unless there are contraindications (known worsening of asthma, recent gastrointestinal pathology). COX-2 selective NSAIDs probably offer little advantage. Paracetamol and/or codeine are useful alternatives or supplements. Long-acting local analgesia should be used wherever possible.

Severe postoperative pain should be treated with opioid analgesics if required, but not routinely, and the lowest effective dose should be used. Analgesia should be supplied for 3–5 days after most operations. Infusions of local anaesthetic agents through a catheter may allow more extensive operations to be managed as day cases.

Postoperative nausea and vomiting

Effective analgesia, avoiding opioids, adequate hydration and careful drug titration all reduce PONV. Patients at increased risk of PONV may benefit from prophylaxis, but this should not be used routinely. Dexamethasone, cyclizine or a $5HT_3$ antagonist are all suitable for prophylaxis. Multimodal prophylaxis, using combinations of antiemetics from different classes, can be effective in preventing PONV in patients at high risk.

If PONV occurs, it should be treated aggressively unless it is transient. $5HT_3$ antagonists and intravenous fluids are useful. Intractable PONV is usually self-limiting. Admission will not offer a cure if maximal therapy has already been given and patients may be offered the choice of going home, provided they have been adequately hydrated.

Unanticipated admission

Approximately 1–2% of patients will not be able to be discharged as planned, usually for surgical reasons. Unanticipated admission rates are higher after more complex procedures. A similar proportion of patients are likely to be readmitted within 1 month, but many are for unrelated reasons.

Admission rates, pain, PONV and satisfaction rates should be constantly monitored as performance indicators. Anaesthetists should follow up patients before discharge, and monitor their own results.

References

1. NHS Modernisation Agency. National good practice guidelines on pre-operative assessment for day surgery. Modernisation Agency; London 2002.
2. Audit Commission. Day Surgery: Review of national findings. London: Audit Commission Publications, 2001.
3. Cahill CJ. Basket cases and trolleys. Day surgery proposals for the Millenuim. Journal of One-day Surgery 1999; 9:11–12.
4. Yogendran S, Asokumar B, Cheng DCH, et al. A prospective randomized double-blind study of the effect of intravenous fluid therapy on adverse outcomes on outpatient surgery. Anesth Analg 1995; 80:682–686.
5. Apfel CC, Laara E, Koivuranta M, et al. A simplified risk score for predicting postoperative nausea and vomiting: conclusions from cross-validations between two centers. Anesthesiology 1999; 91:693–700.
6. Rawal N. Analgesia for day-case surgery. Br J Anaesth 2001; 87:73–87.

Further reading

Smith I. Day care anaesthesia. London: BMJ Books; 2000.

CHAPTER **5.4**

ENDOCRINE SURGERY

THYROID GLAND

The thyroid gland is the largest endocrine gland. Surgery can vary in complexity, from the simple removal of a nodule to excision of a long-standing retrosternal goitre to relieve tracheal compression and requiring the sternum to be split. The close proximity of the superior and recurrent laryngeal nerves requires special surgical attention.

The thyroid secretes three hormones – thyroxine (T_4), tri-iodothyronine (T_3) and calcitonin. The latter is involved in calcium metabolism. T_4 is produced in the thyroid gland, whereas the more potent T_3 is produced both in the thyroid gland and from extrathyroidal enzymatic deiodination of T_4. Both hormones are regulated by thyroid-stimulating hormone (TSH) secreted by the pituitary, which in turn is regulated by thyrotropin-releasing hormone (TRH) secreted by the hypothalamus. The secretion of both is regulated by negative feedback of plasma levels of free T_3 and T_4. The vast majority of both hormones are bound to plasma proteins such as thyroxine-binding globulin (TBG) and albumin. Free (unbound) levels should be measured to distinguish thyroid disease from abnormalities of the carrier proteins (raised in pregnancy, for example).

The effects of thyroid hormones include regulation of metabolic rate, brain development and function, and growth. They also increase the concentration of adrenergic receptors, which may account for their cardiovascular effects.

HYPERTHYROIDISM

The most important relevant clinical features of excess thyroid hormones are weight loss, palpitations, breathlessness, proximal myopathy (although respiratory muscle involvement has not been reported), mild anaemia and thrombocytopenia. Cardiovascular symptoms and signs include sinus tachycardia or atrial fibrillation, increased cardiac output, precipitation of ischaemic heart disease and cardiac failure, and mitral valve prolapse due to occasional papillary muscle dysfunction.

The key to the management of patients with hyperthyroidism is that they should be euthyroid before surgery, except in an emergency situation. This is achieved by the use of β-blockade, carbimazole and radioactive iodine. These treatments take between 2 and 10 weeks for a clinical effect.

It is also important to note that anaesthetic drugs may be affected by the hypermetabolic state. The clearance and distribution of propofol, for example, are increased.

Preoperative assessment

In addition to the usual preoperative history, examination and investigations it is important to:

- assess thyroid status;
- check for associated conditions;
- assess the (upper) airway;
- perform indirect laryngoscopy.

Thyroid status

Thyroid status can be assessed by measurement of total plasma levels of T_3 and T_4 (thyroxine), free (unbound) levels of T_3 and T_4, and plasma level of TSH before and after giving TRH. Radioactive iodine uptake may be measured and a thyroid scans may also be performed.

Associated conditions

Myasthenia gravis and rheumatoid arthritis are associated with Graves' disease, and phaeochromocytoma is associated with medullary carcinoma of the thyroid.

Airway assessment

A significant mass effect is suggested by positional dyspnoea, dysphagia, and stridor. On chest radiography check for tracheal deviation and narrowing. Lateral thoracic inlet views may be necessary to exclude retrosternal extension and to detect tracheal compression. Tracheal deviation or more than 50% narrowing on chest radiography suggests difficulties with intubation. A computed tomography (CT) scan is indicated in such cases and can give accurate assessment of the degree and site of airway distortion and may also indicate tracheal invasion by malignancy. Plain radiographs overestimate diameters owing to magnification effects, and are unreliable in predicting endotracheal tube diameter and length. Magnetic resonance imaging (MRI) has the advantage of providing images in the sagittal and coronal planes as well as transverse views.

On examination, an enlarged tongue may add to airway difficulty and a lingual thyroid may interfere with laryngoscopy. A goitre may make emergency tracheostomy difficult and retrosternal spread can cause superior vena caval obstruction.

In malignancy, vocal cord palsies are possible. Subsequent distortion and rigidity of the surrounding structures means that the lumen of the trachea may not allow a standard endotracheal tube to pass.

Indirect laryngoscopy

Indirect laryngoscopy should be undertaken by an ear, nose and throat surgeon to assess vocal cord movement and the function of the laryngeal nerves. If indirect laryngoscopy is unsuccessful and a fibreoptic instrument is necessary, the anaesthetist should be alerted to the possibility of a difficult intubation.

Anaesthetic management

The goal is to achieve a depth of anaesthesia to prevent an exaggerated response to surgical stimulation. Ketamine and pancuronium are best avoided. A regional technique may help reduce sympathetic stimulation and for similar reasons benzodiazepine premedication is useful. Extra care and attention should be paid to protecting the eyes from towels and drapes.

The options for airway management include straightforward intravenous induction with tracheal intubation if there is no anticipated difficulty, inhalational induction (especially since the introduction of sevoflurane) or fibreoptic intubation. Sevoflurane with heliox may have a role in cases where the airway is markedly narrowed. However, if there is concern that the airway may be lost after induction of anaesthesia, an awake fibreoptic intubation is the technique of choice. Care needs to be employed, however, because the narrowed airway may become obstructed by the instrument. Tracheostomy under local anaesthesia is only possible if the tracheostomy can easily be performed below the level of the obstruction. Ventilation can be performed through a rigid bronchoscope when attempts to pass an endotracheal tube down the trachea fail.

Hyperextension of the neck is unnecessary. A 25° upward tilt reduces venous oozing. Respiration may be controlled or spontaneous. Some centres monitor the recurrent laryngeal nerve intraoperatively.

At the end of the operation the surgeon may ask for the cords to be inspected if there is any concern regarding recurrent laryngeal nerve damage. However, inspecting the cords at this point is difficult and unreliable. A laryngeal mask airway to maintain the airway and a fibreoptic scope to inspect the cords can be used.[1] It is advisable to aim to reduce coughing on extubation.

It is also possible to perform thyroidectomy under bilateral deep or superficial cervical plexus blocks[2] if patients are unfit for general anaesthesia.

Postoperative complications

There are several potential postoperative complications. Those of most concern acutely threaten the airway. A patient complaint of 'being unable to breathe properly' should be taken seriously. Any respiratory difficulty on extubation may require reintubation.

Recurrent laryngeal nerve damage

Recurrent laryngeal nerve damage may be transient or permanent. Unilateral nerve damage may not be clinically apparent due to compensatory overadduction of the opposing cord. However, a vocal change and slight stridor can be present and it is possible for glottic incompetence, ineffective cough and aspiration to occur.

Of much greater concern is bilateral nerve damage. It is far less common (approximately 1 in 30 000) and may not be immediately apparent on extubation. Bilateral damage causes stridor and laryngeal obstruction due to unopposed adduction of the vocal cords, resulting in complete airway obstruction and requiring immediate reintubation and possibly tracheostomy.

Haematoma

Postoperative haematoma can compromise the airway by a direct mass effect. If this occurs the patient should be reintubated and the haematoma evacuated. It is frequently deep in the tissues of the neck and thus not relieved by mere removal of skin sutures. Reintubation can be very difficult because of swollen and distorted tissues.

Laryngeal oedema

Laryngeal oedema is usually seen on the second or third day postoperatively. It may be secondary to a traumatic intubation or extensive surgery. Diagnosis is by indirect laryngoscopy.

Tracheomalacia

A longstanding goitre may result in the tracheal rings becoming weakened, but it is rare for the trachea to collapse. The absence of a leak before extubation should alert the anaesthetist to the possibility of this complication. Immediate reintubation is required.

Hypocalcaemia

Hypocalcaemia typically develops 24–48 hours postoperatively and is related to damage or resection of the parathyroid glands, most frequently after total thyroidectomy. If the serum calcium is below 2 mmol/L then parenteral calcium replacement is necessary. It is worth remembering that laryngeal stridor progressing to laryngospasm may be one of the first indications of hypocalcaemic tetany.

Other complications

Other complications of surgery for hyperthyroidism include hypothyroidism (and occasionally hyperthyroidism) and hypoparathyroidism.

HYPOTHYROIDISM

Hypothyroidism is commonly due to autoimmune thyroid disease, but may be secondary to pituitary or hypothalamic disease, previous thyroid surgery, or treatment with radioactive iodine. The most relevant features from an anaesthetic viewpoint are hypothermia, anaemia, reduced plasma volume and impaired hepatic drug metabolism (both affecting drug pharmacokinetics), hypoglycaemia, impaired clearance of free water (with or without hyponatraemia), an enlarged tongue, nerve compression due to myxoedema and delayed gastric emptying.

Cardiac and respiratory symptoms and signs include bradycardia, heart failure, pericardial and pleural effusions, abnormal baroreceptor function and coronary artery disease. The electrocardiogram (ECG) can show low voltage and ischaemia.

Patients are susceptible to profound hypotension on induction of anaesthesia, which may be relatively resistant to the effects of catecholamine therapy. The metabolic effects can also make patients more sensitive to depressant drugs (and their effects may last significantly longer). Surgery should be delayed if possible until a euthyroid state is achieved. If surgery is urgent then synthetic T_3 (liothyronine sodium) 50–100 μg can be given slowly intravenously under ECG control, followed by 25 μg 8-hourly.

THYROID CRISIS

Thyroid crisis is due to uncontrolled release of thyroid hormones. The onset is usually rapid and triggered by surgery, trauma and infection. Its occurrence is now rare owing to the use of antithyroid drugs, but clinical features include fever, hypercapnia, acidosis, hyperventilation, tachycardia, arrhythmias, shock, congestive cardiac failure, agitation, tremor, delirium, coma, diarrhoea, abdominal pain, vomiting and jaundice. An acute abdomen may be suspected.

Management of thyroid crisis involves oxygen supplementation, active cooling, β-blockade, hydrocortisone (recommended for possible adrenocortical exhaustion), intravenous fluids (care is needed because cardiac failure may be precipitated in the elderly) and potassium iodide. Some authorities recommend the use of broad-spectrum antibiotics. There is also a possible role for dantrolene[3] because a key differential diagnosis is malignant hyperpyrexia. Metabolic acidosis and hypercarbia are more pronounced in malignant hyperpyrexia than in thyroid storm. Another differential diagnosis is a phaeochromocytoma, where β-blockade alone is contraindicated (see below, p. 600).

PARATHYROID GLANDS

There are usually four parathyroid glands. Each is heavily vascularised. The chief cells synthesise and secrete parathyroid hormone (PTH), which is the major hormone in the control of calcium homoeostasis.

Hyperparathyroidism can be subdivided into primary, secondary and tertiary. In these conditions the clinical features are heavily dependent on the serum calcium level.

PRIMARY HYPERPARATHYROIDISM

Primary hyperparathyroidism results from excessive secretion of PTH, usually from an adenoma (80%). It is associated with renal stones, bone pain and cysts. The raised PTH causes a raised plasma calcium and lowered plasma phosphate. The raised calcium can impair the function of the proximal tubule and also lead to nephrogenic diabetes insipidus. Dehydration can be profound. Peptic ulceration and pancreatitis can occur. Very high calcium levels cause a short QT interval and severe and intractable cardiac arrhythmias.

Preoperative management involves correction of the intravascular volume and electrolyte irregularities. Intraoperatively there may be an unpredictable response to muscle relaxants. Careful positioning of the osteopenic patient is required.

Postoperatively the calcium may drop. Clinical effects usually manifest themselves when the total plasma calcium is under 2.0 mmol/L. Features include paraesthesia, muscle cramps, tetany, spasm (which can result in stridor), convulsions, a prolonged QT interval on ECG (which can predispose to heart block), and decreased cardiac output. The two classic clinical tests are Trousseau's and Chvostek's signs. The clinical features are exacerbated by hypomagnesaemia.

SECONDARY HYPERPARATHYROIDISM

Secondary hyperparathyroidism is most commonly associated with chronic renal failure when PTH secretion increases in response to a chronically low serum calcium. Parathyroid hyperplasia causes a normal or low calcium level and a high phosphate level. In 80% of cases bone and joint pain, pruritus and malaise are likely to improve with parathyroidectomy.

TERTIARY HYPERPARATHYROIDISM

Occasionally parathyroid hyperplasia progresses to autonomous secretion.

HYPOPARATHYROIDISM

The most common cause of hypoparathyroidism is secondary to parathyroid and thyroid surgery. Others include post-radiotherapy and idiopathic causes. Treatment is medical, with calcium replacement (intravenous if severe) and possibly magnesium replacement because a coexisting low serum magnesium is not uncommon.

Postoperatively recurrent laryngeal nerve damage and haematoma can occur in the same manner that was previously discussed for thyroid surgery. Hypocalcaemia can occur and calcium levels should be checked at 6 and 24 hours postoperatively.

ADRENAL GLANDS

The adrenal cortex secretes glucocorticoids, mineralocorticoids and androgens. The major biological effects of adrenal cortex hyper- or hypofunction occur as a result of cortisol or aldosterone excess or deficiency. Tumours of the adrenal medulla produce and secrete catecholamines.

CUSHING'S SYNDROME

Most cases of hypersecretion of cortisol are due to a pituitary adenoma secreting excess adrenocorticotropic hormone (ACTH). Other causes are an adrenal adenoma or carcinoma, or tumours such as an oat cell carcinoma of bronchus that secrete ACTH-like hormones. The most common cause of the syndrome, however, is prolonged administration of high doses of exogenous corticosteroids.

The clinical features of Cushing's syndrome are obesity, hypertension, proximal myopathy, gastro-oesophageal reflux, hypokalaemia and diabetes mellitus. The skin and veins may be extremely fragile. There is an increased susceptibility to infection.

Treatment of Cushing's syndrome may involve adrenalectomy or hypophysectomy. The incidence of postoperative complications and perioperative mortality is highest in patients undergoing bilateral adrenalectomy.

Preoperative preparation involves treatment of hypertension and correction of electrolyte and fluid imbalance and high glucose levels. Antireflux medication and a rapid sequence induction may be indicated. Extra care should be taken positioning the patient on the operating table because of the fragile skin and obesity, particularly if the patient is placed in the lateral position for a unilateral adrenalectomy. If significant skeletal muscle weakness is present, a conservative approach to the use of muscle relaxants is warranted. Intra- and postoperative hydrocortisone cover is required.

Fludrocortisone is required after bilateral adrenalectomy, usually on day 5, because the high doses of hydrocortisone used intraoperatively and in the immediate postoperative period exert significant mineralocorticoid activity.

CONN'S SYNDROME

Conn's syndrome is caused by the secretion of excessive amounts of aldosterone, either by an adenoma of the adrenal cortex (75%) or from bilateral adrenal hyperplasia. An adenoma is treated surgically, whereas hyperplasia is usually treated medically. Clinical features include hypertension, hypokalaemia, metabolic alkalosis and renal tubular damage (leading to nephrogenic diabetes insipidus).

Preoperative management of Conn's syndrome involves the use of spironolactone, which corrects the electrolyte and metabolic effects. Intraoperative management may be complicated by cardiovascular instability when the gland is handled. Postoperatively the patient may need fludrocortisone.

PHAEOCHROMOCYTOMA

Phaeochromocytomas are functionally active catecholamine-secreting tumours of chromaffin cells. They are conveniently referred to as the 10% tumour because roughly 10% are familial, 10% are bilateral, 10% are extra-adrenal and 10% are malignant. They present most frequently in the fourth decade.

Phaeochromocytomas are biochemically very active. The normal medulla secretes mainly epinephrine (adrenaline). *N*-methylation of norepinephrine (noradrenaline) to epinephrine (adrenaline) occurs only in the adrenal medulla, and depends on cortisol received via an intact portocapillary circulation, which can be disrupted by tumour. In contrast, extra-adrenal phaeochromocytomas mainly produce norepinephrine (noradrenaline).

Phaeochromocytomas can present as part of uncommon clinical syndromes. These autosomal dominant inherited conditions include:

- multiple endocrine neoplasia (MEN) type 2 syndrome or Sipple's syndrome – the triad of phaeochromocytoma or adrenal medullary hyperplasia, medullary thyroid carcinoma and hyperparathyroidism;
- MEN type 3 syndrome – characterized by phaeochromocytoma, medullary thyroid carcinoma, mucosal neuromas, ganglioneuromas of the gastrointestinal tract, thickened corneal nerves and marfanoid body habitus;
- neurofibromatosis – an autosomal dominant condition with a 1% incidence of phaeochromocytoma;
- von Hippel–Lindau disease – the coexistence of cerebellar hemangioblastoma and retinal angioma with a 14% incidence of phaeochromocytoma.

Clinical features

The predominant feature of phaeochromocytoma is severe hypertension, which may be sustained, paroxysmal or both. True paroxysmal hypertension is only seen in 35% of cases. Early diagnosis is essential. The rare event of a phaeochromocytoma presenting unexpectedly during an unrelated procedure has a mortality rate exceeding 60%, compared to less than 2% for elective excision.

The hallmark of phaeochromocytoma is the paroxysmal crisis presenting with marked hypertension, severe headache, drenching perspiration, palpitations, facial pallor, anxiety, tremor, weakness and chest pain. Precipitants include changing position, abdominal pressure, coitus, sneezing, voiding, defaecation, exercise, anxiety and certain alcohol beverages. Iatrogenic factors include anaesthetic agents, histamine-releasing drugs, suxamethonium, metoclopramide, nicotine, naloxone, β-blockade, phenothiazines, tricyclic antidepressants and glucagon. Induction of anaesthesia, endotracheal intubation, arteriography, lumbar puncture and labour may also lead to a crisis. Complications of such crises range from myocardial ischaemia, arrhythmias, neurogenic pulmonary oedema and cerebrovascular events to acute abdominal pain with shock following haemorrhage into a tumour.

Diagnosis of phaeochromocytoma is by estimation of urinary and plasma catecholamines. Radiological investigations (CT or MRI) are also vital. An abdominal–pelvic CT or MRI should identify 97% of phaeochromocytomas. This may be followed by meta-iodobenzylguanidine (MIBG) radioisotope studies if no tumour is visualised. MIBG is an iodinated analogue of norepinephrine (noradrenaline) that is actively taken up by tissues involved in catecholamine synthesis.

Preoperative assessment

Clinical assessment of phaeochromocytoma must include a detailed history to elucidate symptoms of cardiac origin because catecholamine induced cardiomyopathy has been diagnosed in up to 50% of such patients.

On examination evidence of hypertensive end-organ damage and the presence of familial conditions must be identified. The ECG may reveal ventricular hypertrophy, arrhythmias and myocardial ischaemia, and echocardiography will determine myocardial function. An elevated haematocrit level indicates significant intravascular volume depletion.

Medical treatment

α-Adrenergic antagonists form the basis of management of phaeochromocytoma, leading to control of high blood pressure, progressive restoration of normovolaemia and reversal of catecholamine cardiomyopathy.

Phenoxybenzamine irreversibly alkylates α-receptors and prevents the clinical response to catecholamine release. However, it also blocks the

α_2-receptors causing tachyarrhythmias via disinhibition of cardiac sympathetic neurons, thereby requiring therapeutic β-blockade. It is commonly started at least 14 days before surgery and continued until 48 hours preoperatively. Stopping the drug a couple of days before surgery reduces the risk of postoperative hypotension. Dosage is started at 10 mg twice daily and increased, depending on blood pressure control, postural hypotension and nasal stuffiness, to between 60 mg and 200 mg daily. The duration of action is longer than its half-life of 24 hours as it reflects receptor resynthesis and may explain the refractory hypotension seen postoperatively in some patients treated with this drug until the immediate preoperative period.

Selective α_1-receptor antagonists, such as prazosin and doxazosin, may be preferred because they are not associated with tachyarrhythmias and sedation. However, although preoperative control of blood pressure is comparable to that with phenoxybenzamine, they may not be as effective during surgery, when massive catecholamine levels can competitively displace the α_1-receptor antagonist from its receptor.

β-Blockade should never be started before α-blockade is established because the hypertensive action of catecholamines on α-receptors is then unopposed by the vasodilator effect of peripheral β_2-receptor stimulation, and the negatively inotropic effect of β-blockade further compromises a dysfunctional myocardium.

Criteria for optimal preoperative control are:

- consistent blood pressure readings below 160/90 mmHg;
- postural hypotension not lower than 80/45 mmHg;
- absence of ST–T changes on the ECG for 7 days;
- no more than one premature ventricular contraction every 5 minutes;
- nasal stuffiness.

Anaesthetic management

Full invasive vascular monitoring is usual and is established under local anaesthesia. Agents that cause sympathetic stimulation are to be avoided. Drugs that release histamine should also be avoided because this stimulates the release of catecholamines. An isoflurane–fentanyl general anaesthetic is an accepted standard technique.

Secretion of huge excesses of catecholamines is most likely during:

- induction of anaesthesia;
- endotracheal intubation;
- tumour manipulation.

Vasodilators such as 1–5 mg phentolamine boluses and sodium nitroprusside or nicardipine infusions should be immediately available.

Magnesium sulphate infusions have also been used successfully because magnesium inhibits catecholamine release, exerts a direct vasodilator effect and reduces α-receptor sensitivity.

Tachyarrhythmias are ideally controlled with esmolol or labetalol boluses or infusions, whereas lidocaine (lignocaine) and amiodarone are very infrequently required for ventricular arrhythmias.

Laparoscopic surgery allows more precise dissection, diminishes the stress response, minimises blood loss and leads to a significantly faster recovery and shorter hospital stay. However, a specific complication is the dramatic catecholamine response to the creation of the pneumoperitoneum. This is considered to result from mechanical stimulation of the tumour, decreased preload, increased afterload and chemical stimulation by carbon dioxide absorbed transperitoneally.

Final ligation of the tumour's venous drainage is associated with a sudden drop in catecholamine levels, often precipitating rapid refractory hypotension, which should initially be treated with fluid loading as directed by central venous or pulmonary artery wedge pressure measurements. This is caused by the combination of downregulation of α-receptors, suppression of the contralateral adrenal medulla, persistence of preoperative adrenergic-receptor blockade, relative hypovolaemia and catecholamine cardiomyopathy. When fluids are not fully effective, vasopressors such asangiotensin are more useful than the commonly used α-agonists

The blood sugar should be checked because hypoglycaemia may occur, especially with β-blockade.

In the emergency situation, if surgery cannot be stopped, the depth of anaesthesia should be increased, help summoned, invasive monitoring started and appropriate antihypertensive therapy administered. Therapeutic heparinisation may be considered.

The most important aspect in the management of a patient with a phaeochromocytoma is the close preoperative co-operation between endocrinologist, anaesthetist and surgeon.

References

1. Maroof M, Siddique M, Khan RM. Post-thyroidectomy vocal cord examination by fibreoscopy aided by the laryngeal mask airway. Anaesthesia 1992; 47:445.
2. Kulkarni RS, Braverman LE, Patwardhan NA. Bilateral cervical plexus block for thyroidectomy and parathyroidectomy in healthy and high risk patients. J Endocrinol Invest 1996; 19:714–718.
3. Bennett MH, Wainwright AP. Acute thyroid crisis on induction of anaesthesia. Anaesthesia 1989; 44:8–30.

Further reading

Breivik H. Perianaesthetic management of patients with endocrine disease. Acta Anaesthesiol Scand. Suppl; 1996; 40:1004–1015.

Farling P.A. Thyroid disease. Br J Anaesth 2000; 85:15–28.

Pace N, Buttigieg M. Phaeochromocytoma. BJA CEPD Rev 2003; 3:20–23.

CHAPTER **5.5**

GYNAECOLOGICAL SURGERY

ANATOMICAL AND PHYSIOLOGICAL CONSIDERATIONS

The pelvis is a congested part of the body's anatomy that contains the urinary tract, the gastrointestinal tract and the genital tract, each with its own blood supply. In addition there are lumbosacral nerves crossing against the sidewall of the pelvis, as well as the autonomic innervation of the bowel and bladder.

Operations on the female reproductive tract can involve cervical stimulation with resultant sensory effects mediated through the autonomic nervous system. Stretching the cervix or anus may produce laryngeal spasm or bradycardia unless drugs such as additional anaesthetic agents or anticholinergic agents (e.g. atropine or glycopyrronium), respectively, are given to block these effects. A regional nerve block of afferent nerve fibres may prevent such reflex activity.

COMPLICATIONS OF GYNAECOLOGICAL OPERATIONS

The major life-threatening complications of gynaecological operations are haemorrhage, sepsis and pulmonary embolism from deep vein thrombosis (DVT). Technical risks for haemorrhage increase where there has been previous pelvic surgery (e.g. caesarean section) or where the anatomy is distorted or cancer is invading or compressing structures, or the patient is obese.

Wound infection from adjacent structures is a risk and bowel preparation may be a requirement as well as prophylactic antibiotics, especially for vaginal hysterectomy. Any additional fluid loss from such a preventive measure should be considered in overall management.

During surgery positioning the unconscious patient requires close supervision because of the danger of pressure (e.g. on exposed nerves). Surgical retractor pressure on the ilioinguinal and genitofemoral nerves is also a factor for nerve damage and the result may be a loss of sensation in the upper anterior thigh or vulva, respectively.

Postoperative nausea and vomiting is common and occurs in over 50% of women if prophylaxis is not given.

Risk of thromboembolism

Deep venous thrombosis occurs in the leg or pelvic veins in up to 17% of patients after gynaecological surgery or up to 26% after major gynaecological surgery.[1] Patients are at an increased risk during gynaecological surgery because of positioning, pelvic instrumentation etc. Pressure effects on the leg veins can impede blood flow (e.g. from stirrups used to elevate the legs or from tissue pressure arising from marked flexion at the groin). In addition, surgical manoeuvres can impede blood flow through the pelvis and the stasis that results can induce DVT. Women more than men also suffer from varicose veins, and these can add to the risks. A DVT can lead to thromboembolism if the thrombus is dislodged, as may occur after surgery and bed rest. This risk increases in obesity because mobility is impaired.

For gynaecological surgery, the risk of thromboembolism is graded into:

- low risk – minor surgery, age less than 40 years;
- intermediate risk – major surgery, surgery lasting over 1 hour, trauma, varicose veins, obesity;
- high risk – previous thromboembolism, pelvic surgery, oral contraceptive pill, factor V Leiden mutation, abdominal malignancy.

Prophylaxis consists of physical methods for low risk, increasing to active pharmaceutical anticoagulation in high-risk groups. Graduated elastic compression stockings are commonly used with early mobilisation and leg exercises. Physical methods avoid tissue pressure by correct positioning and intermittent pressure on the calves to encourage venous blood flow. The risk is best discussed with the woman so that she can actively participate in the preventive measures. For women using hormonal contraception it is not advisable to stop contraception before surgery.[2]

Anticoagulation can begin once the surgical risk of haemorrhage is minimised (i.e. in the postoperative period following close observation for bleeding). Following major surgery subcutaneous low-dose unfractionated heparin (UFH) or subcutaneous low molecular weight heparin (LMWH) can be given. If anticoagulation is planned before surgery adequate time to stop it before a regional nerve block for anaesthesia should be planned (e.g. LMWH is stopped 12 hours before an extradural nerve block).

Positioning

Lithotomy

The lithotomy position is also known as the Lloyd-Davies position, and its hazards can be prevented.

In the elderly woman a history of joint disability or osteoporosis is pertinent, and stretching of hip joints or pelvic girdle during the muscle relaxation of anaesthesia (including inhalational anaesthesia as well as a muscle relaxant technique) should be avoided. The key to avoiding problems while moving the limbs is to have two people, one to hold each leg, to move the limbs symmetrically and to avoid excessive abduction. The stirrups for the feet should allow the calves and legs to hang without pressure external to the stirrup pole. Padding may be necessary to prevent pressure on nerves and to keep the hands and legs away from metal (e.g. to protect from diathermy burns).

Complications

Intraoperative complications of anaesthesia in the lithotomy position include:

- impeded respiratory muscle excursion;
- reflux of stomach contents, especially during light anaesthesia and surgical stimulation;
- lower limb compartment syndrome in prolonged surgery.

Monitoring the anaesthetic agents, respiration and duration of surgery should prevent these. If necessary respiration may have to be controlled, especially in the obese patient, and even a cuffed orotracheal tube placed before surgery. A history of a hiatus hernia may alert the anaesthetist to aspiration risks. Compartment syndrome may require regular leg movement to return the pressures in the legs periodically to normal.

Postoperatively the complications of the lithotomy position include:

- peripheral nerve damage:[3]
  - sciatic nerve by exaggerated knee extension, thigh flexion and external hip rotation;
  - femoral nerve by adduction and rotation of the thigh;
  - common peroneal nerve by compression between the fibula and stirrup;
  - posterior tibial nerve by stirrup compression;
  - saphenous nerve by compression between the stirrups and medial malleolus;
- deep vein thrombosis;
- backache.

Trendelenburg position

A steep Trendelenburg head-down position used to be used with shoulder braces that could cause brachial plexus stretching and damage. For gynaecology a 15° tilt is used that does not require restraint. However, the position should be maintained for as short a time as possible because it induces abnormal pressures in the venous system and increases the pressure in the stomach so that regurgitation can occur, especially in obese women. When the operating table is levelled a slow return to the horizontal position will prevent cardiovascular instability.

ANAESTHESIA FOR GYNAECOLOGICAL OPERATIONS

Women present at all ages, but particularly as young and fit for minor procedures (elective or unplanned) and older and at higher risk for major complex surgery. Thus the choice of anaesthetic technique also varies and little evidence is available to compare technique with outcome. Day-case procedures are common. Propofol is used extensively, mainly because recovery is fast, but where there is a fetus in situ it should be avoided. The response of a pregnant uterus to volatile anaesthetic agents should also be considered (e.g. for termination of pregnancy) because of their potential to relax the uterine muscle and increase blood loss.

SPECIFIC GYNAECOLOGICAL OPERATIONS

Hysteroscopy

Telescopic equipment enables the gynaecologist to inspect the uterine cavity and explore it with accuracy for diagnosis and treatment of intrauterine disease.

The main indication is for anomalous uterine bleeding, so it is important to check the patient's full blood count in case she is anaemic.

Younger women tend to present for intrauterine contraceptive manipulation.

Before hysteroscopy the cervix is dilated, and this carries the risk of stimulating an autonomic response.

The anaesthetic for a hysteroscopy includes induction and maintenance with a selection of drugs relevant to day-case surgery (e.g. propofol for the passage of a laryngeal mask airway, and either total intravenous or inhalational anaesthesia).

Complications include uterine perforation and bleeding, so facilities to manage these risks should be available.

Pain after hysteroscopy requires adequate analgesics, and a combination of a non-steroidal anti-inflammatory analgesic (if not contraindicated) and a codeine and paracetamol combination is usually satisfactory.

Depending on the type of anaesthetic (e.g. opioid) used, prophylactic antiemetics may be indicated.

Endometrial ablation

Endometrial ablation is an alternative to hysterectomy for women who have menorrhagia because it takes less time, recovery is rapid and there is a low morbidity. Postoperative pain from uterine spasms can be severe.

The technique involves infusion of fluid into the uterine cavity and, as with the transurethral resection of prostate (TURP) syndrome, the fluid can be absorbed. The amount of fluid absorbed depends on the infusion pressure (greater for the uterine cavity than for the prostate), vascularity (the uterus can be atrophic in the midproliferative phase or in response to progesterone analogues), number and size of vessels opened, and duration of surgery.[4]

Complications of operative hysteroscopy

In up to 6% of cases symptoms of fluid overload can develop, including hyponatraemia and hypo-osmolality. Other complications include haemorrhage, uterine perforation and embolism of gas or air.

Anaesthetic management

Anaesthesia for hysteroscopy can range from paracervical block with or without sedation, through regional nerve blockade to general anaesthesia. About 5–10% of women who start with local anaesthesia require conversion to general anaesthesia. Postoperatively there is no benefit from local anaesthesia because there appears to be the same incidence of pain and nausea and vomiting. However, for operative hysteroscopy regional anaesthesia has the advantage that central nervous effects from fluid overload can be monitored, and this allows early detection of this risk.

Assisted conception

For transvaginal oocyte retrieval using ultrasound guidance a paracervical block and sedation are usually adequate. For invasive surgical embryo transfer (e.g. gamete intrafallopian transfer [GIFT]), a general anaesthetic is required.

Laparoscopy

Laparoscopy has a history of almost a century. It is used for sterilisation, division of adhesions, investigation of pelvic pain, infertility, and more major surgery such as myomectomy and assisted vaginal hysterectomy.

A rare, but potentially lethal, complication is that of cannulating the aorta. Other life-threatening hazards also occur, so the concept of its being a minor procedure is erroneous.

After trauma by the needle the next hazard is the insufflated gas. This can induce embolism, pressure effects in the gastrointestinal, respiratory and cardiovascular systems, hypercarbia, hypoxia, hypotension and high central venous pressures. Capnographic monitoring can detect many of these problems. The following changes are often observed:

- increase in heart rate;
- increase in peak inspiratory pressures;
- increase in end-tidal carbon dioxide tension.

Protection of the airway with a cuffed endotracheal tube is preferred, and positive-pressure ventilation to prevent hypoventilation and atelectasis. To view the pelvic contents the Trendelenburg position is usual. All these physiological alterations stress the patient. Even if attempts are made to remove all the carbon dioxide the recovery period can be complicated by ventilatory disturbances as an early event and later by severe referred pains.

Methods to reduce these disturbances have been developed without pneumoperitoneum using retraction systems. For these, local anaesthesia with sedation is a reasonable option.

Laparoscopic sterilisation

Most patients have general anaesthesia for laparoscopic sterilisation, but local anaesthesia is possible. The method includes paracervical nerve block and periumbilical and suprapubic injection of 1% lidocaine (lignocaine) plus 4% intrauterine lidocaine (lignocaine). The advantages of local anaesthesia are its safety, rapidity and lower cost.

Postoperative pain relief

The pain experienced after laparoscopy is more severe after instrumental surgery than after diagnostic procedures. It can be reduced by local anaesthetic infiltration of the wound during surgery (e.g. 0.25% levobupivacaine 10 mL) or at the site of surgery (e.g. fallopian tube). The patient often experiences referred pain across the shoulders from peritoneal stretching. The pain should be controlled with regular non-steroidal anti-inflammatory analgesic drugs and a codeine and paracetamol combination (e.g. 1 g paracetamol and 60 mg codeine).

Hysterectomy and myomectomy

An abdominal hysterectomy takes about 20 minutes longer than a vaginal hysterectomy, but may be indicated if the structures are not mobile.

A myomectomy is indicated for the removal of symptomatic fibroids and can be associated with major blood loss.

A surgical manoeuvre that can have a systemic effect is the use of prostaglandins as vasoconstrictors.

Bleeding can also be a problem during hysterectomy, and for this reason the use of ketorolac is no longer indicated because it has a tendency to increase bleeding during this type of surgery.

Prophylaxis for postoperative nausea and vomiting is considered part of the anaesthetic technique.

Vaginal surgery may be performed using extradural nerve block or general anaesthesia. Often a combination is used, so that during the perioperative period the patient can have continuous pain relief available. For example, an extradural nerve block may be used for postoperative pain relief after major surgery. An alternative regimen is patient-controlled analgesia (PCA), for example using morphine as an analgesic. When PCA morphine is used bowel motility is decreased, so lactulose is a suitable adjunct to reduce constipation.

Gynaecological oncology

Hydatidiform mole

Hydatidiform mole is associated with vomiting and bleeding and metastases to lungs. For a uterine evacuation an oxytocin infusion may be required.

Ovarian carcinoma

Preoperative assessment of ovarian carcinoma may reveal potential medical problems, including ascites, liver metastases, pleural effusion, poor nutrition and renal dysfunction.

Radical hysterectomy

The so-called Wertheim's (Ernst Wertheim 1864–1920) abdominal hysterectomy is an extended major surgical procedure, usually for cancer surgery, with an associated morbidity and mortality. High dependency or intensive care will be needed in the recovery period. Often the patients are older than those presenting for hysterectomy and have menorrhagia and are less fit.

Anaesthetic management

The anaesthetic management for a radical hysterectomy should include the following:

- protection from the effects of prolonged surgery (e.g. pressure sores, hypothermia). The woman should be actively warmed using temperature monitoring;
- adequate replacement of fluid and blood losses using large-bore systems with pressurised infusion systems. Bowel preparation before surgery tends to induce dehydration and this, together with preoperative starvation, may induce significant deficits before the operation. Estimation and measurement of fluid and blood losses includes a urinary catheter with half-hourly measures of urine volume;
- invasive monitoring. Arterial and central venous pressure lines are required to monitor pressures as well as the acid–base status of the patient;
- plans for pain relief during and after surgery. These may include a combination of general anaesthesia and regional nerve block;
- consideration of which type of critical care facility may be required after surgery (e.g. elective ventilation may be required to allow cardiovascular stabilisation).

References

1. Nicolaides AN. Prevention of venous thromboembolism. International Consensus Statement. J Vasc Br 2002; 1:133–170.
2. Thromboembolic Risk Factors (THRIFT) Consensus Group. Risk of and prophylaxis for venous thromboembolism in hospital patients. Br Med J 1992; 305:567–574.
3. Irvin W, Andersen W, Taylor P, Rice L. Minimizing the risk of neurologic injury in gynecologic surgery. Obstet Gynecol 2004; 103:374–382.
4. Mushambi MC, Williamson K. Anaesthetic considerations for hysteroscopic surgery. Best Pract Res Clin Anaesthesiol 2002; 16:35–52.

Further reading

Struthers AD, Cuschieri A. Cardiovascular consequences of laparoscopic surgery. Lancet 1998; 352:568–570.

Turnbull D, Farid A, Hutchinson S, Shorthouse A, Mills GH. Calf compartment pressures in the Lloyd-Davies position: a cause for concern? Anaesthesia 2002; 57:905–908.

CHAPTER **5.6**

NEONATAL AND PAEDIATRIC SURGERY

NEONATAL AND INFANT PHYSIOLOGY

Definitions

Definitions relevant to this chapter are:

- preterm – less than 37 weeks' gestation;
- term – 37–42 weeks' gestation;
- post-term – over 42 weeks' gestation;
- low birth weight – ≤2500 g
- infant – 28 days to 1 year;
- child – 1 year to 16 years (dependent on local laws of consent).

Respiratory system

Infants have a larger head, shorter neck and larger tongue than older children and adults.

The neonatal glottic inlet is higher, at C3–C4 compared to C5 in the adult, and the infant epiglottis is longer and curved anteriorly. Before puberty the narrowest part of the larynx is the cricoid ring. At 34 weeks of gestation true alveoli appear, with further reduction in alveolar membrane thickness. Type 2 alveolar cells produce surfactant, which is necessary to reduce surface tension, stabilise alveoli and prevent the respiratory distress of prematurity.

Ribs are more horizontal than in adults and breathing is diaphragmatic rather than intercostal. The rib cage consists of soft cartilage, resulting in paradoxical chest wall movement in conditions associated with airway obstruction (e.g. malacia of the larynx/trachea/bronchi, croup or bronchiolitis).

The neonatal diaphragm has less than 10% fatigue-resistant muscle fibres (25% in adult), increasing the risk of respiratory failure with lung or airway disease.

Functional residual capacity (FRC) lies close to the closing volume (CV) in the infant and the reduction in FRC with anaesthesia or disease can lead to atelectasia and segmental collapse unless positive end-expiratory pressure (PEEP) is applied.

Alveolar ventilation (130 mL/kg/min) and oxygen demand ($\dot{V}O_2$ = 6.4 mL/kg/min) are much higher than in the adult (60 mL/kg/min and 3.5 mL/kg/min, respectively) but the FRC/V_A (alveolar ventilation) is much lower (half), so the reserves of oxygen in the lung of the infant are lower.

Response to hypoxia

Unlike in adults, mild hypoxia in the neonate causes hypoventilation leading to apnoea. Many anaesthetic agents exacerbate this. Normal term neonates up to 52 weeks' post-conceptual age have 'periodic breathing' with intermittent apnoeas of up to 5 seconds duration followed by tachypnoea. This is more pronounced in preterm neonates, with apnoeas of 15 seconds or more, resulting in desaturation and bradycardia.

Cardiovascular system

Oxygen transport

At term red cells contain 70% HbF, which has a higher affinity for oxygen than HbA, with a total Hb of 16–20 mg/dL, increasing oxygen carrying capacity. HbF proportion declines, such that at 6 months 90% is HbA.

Fetal and transitional circulations

Oxygenated blood from the placenta passes from the umbilical vein through the ductus venosus to the inferior vena cava (IVC). It preferentially streams through the foramen ovale to the left atrium and thence to the ascending aorta. Deoxygenated blood from the superior vena cava (SVC) passes through the right atrium and ventricle and pulmonary artery, but is diverted to the descending aorta via the ductus arteriosus.

Three physiological events at birth occur to produce the normal postnatal circulation:

- loss of the placenta with increased vascular resistance and loss of prostaglandin PGE_2;
- reduction in pulmonary vascular resistance (PVR) that occurs with the first breath, mediated by an increase in $P{O_2}$, fall in $P{CO_2}$ and mechanical factors – the resultant increase in pressure in the left atrium shuts the flap-like foramen ovale;
- closure of the ductus arteriosus caused by increased $P{O_2}$, adrenergic stimulation and the loss of PGE_2 from the placenta.

Postnatally, life-threatening 'persistent transitional circulation' can occur in conditions causing reopening of the ductus arteriosus, increased pulmonary resistance and right-to-left shunt through the foramen ovale.

The neonatal heart has less organisation, less increased connective tissue, fewer myofibrils and immature actin/myosin cross-linking. The Frank–Starling curve is flatter and there is consequently less response to volume loading. At term, the left and right ventricles are of equal bulk and there is a rightward axis on the ECG. Gradual thinning of the right ventricle (RV) and hypertrophy of the left ventricle (LV) result from the changes in their outflow impedances, resulting in a 'normal' ECG by 6 months.

Cardiac output in the neonate is 200 mL/kg/min, with a heart rate of 100–180 bpm (adult cardiac output is 80 mL/kg/min, with a heart rate of 55–90 bpm).

Nervous system

Neonatal cerebral blood flow (CBF) is proportionately greater than that in adults (infant CBF = one-third cardiac output). Autoregulation exists, but is better adapted to hypertensive surges rather than to hypotension.

The blood–brain barrier is immature at birth and central nervous system (CNS) depressant drugs such as morphine can cross more easily, leading to increased drug sensitivity. Crossing of unconjugated bilirubin can produce kernicterus.

At birth the parasympathetic nervous system is relatively well developed and tends to dominate the sympathetic nervous system. The neonate has limited responses to cold (vasoconstriction rather than shivering) and there is an increased propensity to bradycardia.

Response to noxious stimuli is characterised by a well-developed appearance of pain (grimace, cry and other motor activity) and stress responses. Appreciation of pain is conjectural, but the pathways are present anatomically by 24 weeks of gestation.

Tendencies to intracranial haemorrhages may be exacerbated by unattenuated stress responses to operation or intubation.

Fluid and electrolytes

Nephrogenesis is complete by 36 weeks of gestation, but the ratio of medullary to cortical nephrons is reduced over the first 6 months after birth, reducing the ability to reabsorb water and solutes. Care must be taken particularly with neonates to ensure adequate sodium and potassium intake, while remembering that electrolyte loads are poorly tolerated. Concentrating ability takes up to a year to become 'mature', although most change occurs within the first 6 months.

Extracellular fluid volume forms 40% of body mass at birth, decreasing to 30% within weeks. This contraction is associated with production of relatively dilute urine. Blood volume at birth is 90–119 mL/kg, decreasing to 75 mL/kg at 6 months.

Water requirements are greater in the neonate than in the older child owing to high urinary and evaporative losses (thin skin, high surface area).

This is exaggerated in any preterm neonate. Typical intravenous requirements are:

- 100 mL/kg/day for the term neonate;
- up to 150 mL/kg/day for preterm infants.

Additional allowances should be made for the effects of radiant heaters and ultraviolet lights. Additional fluid needs to be added for the effect of pyrexia (10 mL/kg/day for each degree over 37°C).

Daily sodium requirement is 3–4 mmol/kg/day for a neonate up to 10 kg, and the daily potassium requirement is 2 mmol/kg/day for a neonate up to 10 kg.

Metabolism and thermoneutrality

Basal metabolic rate is higher in infants and children (neonatal oxygen uptake is 8 mL/kg/min, compared to 3–4 mL/kg/min in adults).

Neonatal caloric requirements are 120 kcal/kg/day (for an adult it is 40 kcal/kg/day). Glycogen stores are relatively low, but brain and myocardium are more glucose dependent (i.e. there is a greater propensity to starvation hypoglycaemia and damage). Calcium homoeostatic mechanisms are less responsive with reduced stores. Transfusion of blood products that contain citrate may require calcium supplementation to prevent hypocalcaemia.

Temperature homoeostasis is aided by the acquisition of subcutaneous fat, which is notably absent in the preterm infant. Babies should be nursed in a thermoneutral environment – a point at which there is minimal metabolic challenge to maintain normal temperature. In the term neonate naked thermoneutrality is 32°C, and clothed it is 24°C. Shivering does occur in the neonate, but is not effective until 3 months. Heat production is reliant on brown fat, but heat loss can rapidly outstrip production.

Drug responses

The neonate is more susceptible than an adult to the effects of CNS drugs. This is due in part to increased drug sensitivity (Fig. 5.6.1), immaturity of the blood–brain barrier and altered pharmacokinetics. In general, however, infants have larger volumes of distribution for most drugs, and even susceptible infants may require larger initial doses of drugs to achieve adequate plasma concentrations.

Drug elimination may be significantly reduced in the newborn owing to immaturity of hepatic elimination (conjugation and oxidative pathways). Enzyme induction develops rapidly after birth. Renal excretion of some drugs (e.g. gentamicin) is related directly to glomerular filtration rate (GFR), and conjugated substances are poorly excreted until proximal tubular function is matured (6 months). This can be delayed until 18 months in preterm infants.

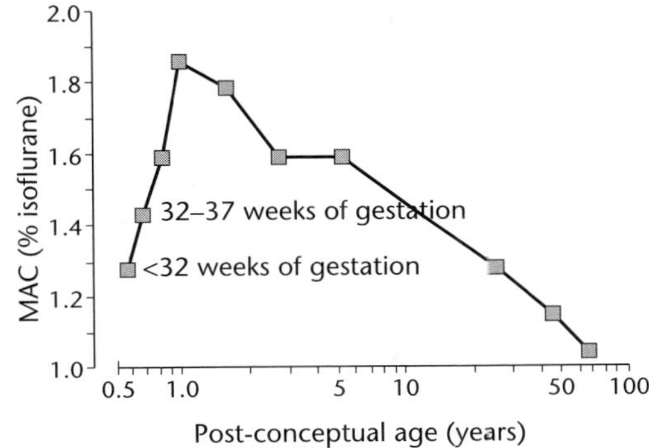

Figure 5.6.1 Effect of age on the Minimum Alveolar Concentration (MAC) of isoflurane. MAC decreases with increasing age from 1 year. However, newborn and preterm infants have increased sensitivity to isoflurane with lower MAC. Reproduced from LeDez and Lerman.[1]

GENERAL ANAESTHETIC CONSIDERATIONS

Pre-anaesthetic clinics

Preoperative screening in preadmission clinics is usually questionnaire based with trained paramedics. They are suitable for up to 80% of elective surgery. Haemoglobin and urine analysis is not usually required, except if sickle cell screening is necessary. Videos or interactive play can be useful for psychological preparation. The assessor needs to understand the home environment (safety and postoperative care) if same-day surgery is planned.

Preoperative visit

Key aims of the preoperative visit are confirmation of fitness for surgery, psychological preparation, and clear explanations of anaesthesia and postoperative pain relief. Many drugs (such as furosemide [frusemide] and captopril) are better avoided on the day of surgery, but others such as anti-asthmatic medication should be prescribed as normal. Patients with endocrine disorders require careful preoperative management.

Psychological preparation is age dependent. Separation anxiety and mistrust of strangers develop at 1 year and can be accompanied later by anger at loss of control. Older children can fear mutilation, pain and death. Individualised plans must be made in conjunction with parents (e.g. if a child refuses to be changed into a theatre gown before surgery, normal clothes should be left on until after induction).

Induction of anaesthesia can be intravenous or gaseous, and many children have a strong preference. If intravenous access is planned, clear surface marking of two preferred vein sites is helpful to place local anaesthetic cream effectively. Regional anaesthesia can provide complete analgesia, but the accompanying paraesthesia, numbness and motor weakness can be frightening without explanation. A visit from a pain nurse is helpful if patient-controlled anaesthesia is planned.

In the UK, written consent for anaesthesia has not been established separately from that for surgery. Consent is usually established with parents if children are less than 16 years old. However, refusal by the child must be taken into consideration, particularly if he or she is fully aware of the consequences of refusal. Common complications relating to anaesthesia and additional procedures (regional blockade) should be fully discussed. Written documentation of the consent process in the medical notes may be invaluable.

Fasting guidelines

Ingestion of a complex meal can take considerable time to clear the stomach, but clear fluids are normally cleared within 2 hours. Neonates and pre-weaned infants will become irritable, dehydrated and hypoglycaemic if starved for extended periods. For elective surgery a widely used scheme is:

- solids – morning case, no solid food overnight; afternoon case, light food at breakfast; no solid food for 6 hours before surgery;
- milk – up to 4 hours before surgery for bottled milk, up to 3 hours before surgery for breast milk;
- clear liquids – up to 2 hours before surgery.

Children with major organ dysfunction, or those acutely ill with infection or trauma, should be treated as though they had a full stomach regardless of fasting interval because these conditions are associated with delayed gastric emptying. Small infants should be scheduled first on an operating list to improve planning, but it may still be necessary to commence intravenous fluids.

Premedication

Premedication was essential for ether anaesthesia to reduce vagal responses, dry secretions and provide 'basal narcosis'. Today, anticholinergics are given intravenously (atropine 20 μg/kg) after induction of anaesthesia for specific cases (bronchoscopy, squint surgery). Preoperative sedation is rarely given for day-stay surgery, and more emphasis is placed on the calming effects of parental presence in the anaesthetic room together with good psychological preparation.

However, older children may request sedation and anxiolysis (benzodiazepines) and it may still be desirable in have significant sedation in active younger children before surgery (chloral hydrate/triclofos). Unfortunately, these agents can have an occasional paradoxical effect, with disinhibition and agitation. Intramuscular preparations are no longer used or sanctioned. Rectal sedation with barbiturates is not commonly used in the UK.

Common premedicant drugs

Sedation

Benzodiazepines are sedative and anxiolytic and provide anterograde amnesia. Midazolam (oral, nasal, sublingual 0.2–0.5 mg/kg up to a maximum of 20 mg) has a very rapid onset of 20 minutes and rapid elimination, making it suitable for day-stay anaesthesia. Its bitter lingering taste is hard to disguise. Diazepam (0.2–0.5 mg/kg orally up to a maximum of 20 mg) tastes better and lasts longer.

Chloral hydrate (oral/rectal 30–50 mg/kg up to a maximum of 1 g) and triclofos (oral 25–30 mg/kg up to 1 g) can provide 'basal narcosis' at high doses and can be useful in the highly active child. Other agents are ketamine 2–5 mg/kg orally and clonidine 2–5 μg/kg orally.

Analgesia

A loading dose of paracetamol (oral 20 mg/kg up to 1 g) and a non-steroidal anti-inflammatory drug (NSAID) such as diclofenac or ibuprofen can be given preoperatively to provide effective co-analgesia with opioids or local blocks. The rectal route can also be used effectively for these drugs. In order to be effective dosing must continue on a regular basis after surgery. Clonidine (oral 0.2–2 μg/kg) provides both sedation and analgesia, but does not induce nausea. Opioids are not usually given before surgery because of vomiting and respiratory side-effects.

Topical local anaesthesia

EMLA® requires 90 minutes to be fully effective, whereas tetracaine (amethocaine) cream is more rapid at 60 minutes. An erythematous rash is quite common with Ametop® (tetracaine (amethocaine) cream) and it can be severe. EMLA® can be used in neonates provided the underlying skin is intact and that excessive doses are avoided. In a busy day-surgery unit, it may be useful to have standing orders to apply the cream immediately on arrival. A promise of pain-free cannulation must be kept if a child's confidence is to be maintained.

EQUIPMENT

Airways

Guedel airways are available in sizes 000, 00, 0, 1, 2, 3 for various sizes of neonate, infant and child. The distance between philtrum and angle of mandible is a guide to size.

Masks

Traditional masks were designed to minimise deadspace (Rendell-Baker Soucek). Modern masks are light, transparent and disposable, but have a larger deadspace. The rim is made of soft plastic or an inflated ring.

Laryngeal mask airway

Laryngeal mask airways (LMAs) are useful in short procedures with spontaneous ventilation. They have less resistance than endotracheal tubes and are of considerable use in difficult upper airway work and for insertion of fibreoptic bronchoscopes. Approximate sizes are:

- 1 for less than 6.5 kg;
- 2 for 6.5–20 kg;
- 2.5 for 20–30 kg;
- 3 for 30 kg and above.

A size 1.5 is also available. The armoured versions have reduced risk of kinking and are longer and narrower. The use of the size 1 has not been widespread because of concerns about secure insertion, increased deadspace and atelectasis. Although it has been used in neonatal resuscitation, it is not yet recommended for controlled ventilation in small children because of the risk of ventilatory impairment from gastric distension.

Breathing systems

Common breathing systems used in paediatric practice include Ayre's T-piece, Bain and circle. The Ayre's T-piece (Mapleson E) with Jackson–Rees modification remains the mainstay of paediatric anaesthesia. It is compact and light, with low deadspace and airway resistance. It can function in spontaneous or controlled ventilation with or without manual continuous positive airway pressure (CPAP). There is no intrinsic heat/humidity conservation and no pressure-relief valve should the bag become occluded. It requires high fresh gas flows for spontaneous ventilation (2.5–3 times calculated minute ventilation). For controlled ventilation high minute ventilation with limited fresh gas flow and rebreathing provides stable end-tidal carbon dioxide concentrations.

The Bain system behaves like a Mapleson E or F circuit and has been used in all age groups (see Ch. 2.1).

The circle system has become popular for controlled ventilation in paediatrics because of heat and moisture conservation as well as cost efficiencies. Care must be taken to compensate for the compression effect of the system (compliance of tubing etc.), with controlled ventilation to ensure that tidal volume is adequate.

Ventilators

Accurate capnography and measurement of airway pressure are particularly important during mechanical ventilation because tidal volume and alveolar ventilation cannot always be measured accurately. Most paediatric ventilators used with T-piece circuits are time cycled and are connected on the expiratory limb as a 'bag squeezer' or 'mechanical thumb'. Neonates may require adapted intensive care ventilators to maintain alveolar recruitment. In circle systems, a bag-in-bottle ventilator is used with paediatric bellows.

Laryngoscopes

For infants and small children, straight blades (Robertshaw, Miller) are more useful to control the epiglottis and visualise the higher laryngeal inlet. The age at which the use of curved blades, such as the Macintosh, comes into play depends on individual choice.

Endotracheal tubes

Endotracheal tubes (ETTs) are made of PVC or polyurethane and marked with both internal diameter (ID) and length graduations in centimetres.

For children over 1 year:

- the appropriate tube (ID) can be approximately estimated by the formula age / 4 + 4;
- the appropriate length for a cut ETT can be approximately estimated by the formula age / 2 + 12 oral (+15 for nasal).

In infants:

- Approximate ID sizes for preterms: <1500 g, 2.5 mm; 1500–3000 g, 3.0 mm; over 3000 g, 3.5mm.
- oral length in cm is given by the formula (6 + weight in kg).

Humidification

Prolonged use of cold dry gases with the Ayres T-piece circuit leads to mucosal damage and mucous plugs. Active heater humidification systems are therefore still used extensively in younger infants undergoing major surgery. Intraluminal heating elements maintain airway temperature distal to the water chamber and prevent condensation ('rainout'). Passive humidification by the use of heat and moisture exchangers (HME) is used in older children combined with microbial filtration. HMEs take up to an hour to develop effective humidification. Commercially available HMEs cover a range of child sizes and appropriate selection will ensure minimal effect on deadspace.

Vascular access

Newer plastic technology not only provides peripheral intravenous or intra-arterial catheters as small as 26 stretched wire gauge (swg), but also provides plastic 'memory' and so is less likely to kink and occlude as the child mobilises. 'Seldinger' kits are available from 24 swg upwards, whereas triple-lumen central venous catheters are available from 4 French Gauge (FG). Intraosseous needles should be available for the shocked child or those with particularly difficult venous access in all acute care areas.

Intravenous fluid administration

Controlled, accurate fluid administration is now practical and reliable owing to the widespread availability of volumetric or syringe pumps. However, appropriately rated pumps must be selected for such use. If large-volume replacement is to take place then infusates should be warmed. Recent devices have achieved this effectively by the use of coaxial heat exchangers.

MONITORING

Apnoea alarms

Apnoea alarms should be used in babies at risk from post-anaesthetic apnoea (e.g all neonates and preterm babies up to 44–60 weeks post-conceptual age). The cut-off for this is contentious and may depend on lingering pathology, such as chronic lung disease or previous nervous system insults.[1]

Gas and vapour analysis

Gas and vapour analysis is standard practice, but the site of the sampling will affect the result, especially in rebreathing circuits. Endotracheal connectors and HMEs are made with side-ports and the closer to the patient the better.

Pulse oximetry

Paediatric probes should be used that do not compress the circulation in the chosen extremity. Longer-term probe application can cause burns. The absorption spectra of HbF and HbA are similar, but meconium on the skin can give a falsely low reading. In the preterm neonate it is important to recognise the significance of a difference between pre- and post-ductal values.

Blood gases

Mild metabolic acidosis is seen in the first weeks of life owing to immature renal acidification of the urine. Plasma standard bicarbonate may be only 20–22 mmol/L.

Normal $Pa{O_2}$ is lower in the newborn (9–10 kPa in air) because of residual atelectasis and extra lung water. New developments emerging include handheld portable gas analysers and 'real-time' intravascular gas analysis using fibreoptic 'optodes'.

Transcutaneous gas measurement

Transcutaneous gas measurement gives continuous readings of blood gases. There are separate oxygen and carbon dioxide electrodes adherent to skin that operate at 43–44°C. This produces the vasodilatation necessary to ensure diffusion of the gases, but thermal injury to the skin will ensue if the electrodes are not moved every 3 hours. The oxygen electrode can be affected by volatile agents (false high). Both electrodes become less accurate as the infant's skin thickens with age.

Noninvasive monitoring of blood pressure

Modern automated oscillometric devices have been shown to be reliable, although there is a tendency to underestimate high systolic and overestimate low diastolic pressures. Cuff size is important – for the arm a cuff should be selected that covers two-thirds of the humerus.

Invasive arterial monitoring

To measure arterial waveform, the tubing connecting the cannula to the transducer should be rigid and as short as possible. This minimises damping and reduces harmonics, which can occur at the higher frequency of infant heart rates (≈3 Hz).

Cardiac output

Reliable and practical cardiac output measurement has proved difficult in paediatrics. It can be estimated using oesophageal or transthoracic Doppler techniques. However, its accuracy depends on assumed aortic cross-sectional area and it may be more useful to track trends rather than absolute values.[2] Other emerging techniques include modified thermodilution, lithium dilution and analysis of the pulse waveform.

Electrocardiography

Electrocardiography can accurately track changes and trends in heart rate and can be a guide to depth of anaesthesia or depletion of intravascular volume. Although there is less emphasis on ECG morphology than in adults it can be important to identify inadvertent intravascular injection of local anaesthetic, or hyperkalaemia after suxamethonium administration.

Temperature

Central temperature should be monitored for all but the very shortest of procedures. Skin temperatures will be affected by the very measures currently employed to raise it. Nasopharynx, oesophagus, tympanic, rectal and bladder sites are all satisfactory. The nasopharyngeal temperature may be affected by leakage of inspired gases.

Neuromuscular monitoring

Neuromuscular monitoring is similar to that in adult practice. However, it must be noted that in the first month of life the fourth twitch is decreased, even in the absence of neuromuscular blockade.

GENERAL ANAESTHESIA TECHNIQUES

Induction

Gas induction has become increasingly popular since the introduction of sevoflurane. Techniques include:

- single maximal breath induction;
- 'blowing up a bag';
- using cupped hands or a blanket;
- a mask held by the child or parents.

Usually 8% sevoflurane is elected from the outset togehter with nitrous oxide and oxygen. Parents need to be aware that during induction a phase of excitement and movement may occur.

Opting for intravenous induction depends on the child's preference, suitability of veins, technical expertise and state of the child. Doses should be titrated to effect: neonates and sick infants may require reduced doses, whereas 3–5-year-olds need relatively larger doses than adults. The pain on induction with propofol (2.5–5 mg/kg) can be reduced by adding 20 mg lidocaine (lignocaine) to 200 mg propofol. Thiopental (2–7 mg/kg) provides a smooth induction but can delay postoperative recovery.

Maintenance

Most simple short procedures require only spontaneous ventilation under a volatile or intravenous anaesthetic agent and analgesia that will extend into the postoperative period. Neonates are usually intubated and ventilated for surgical procedures to ensure adequate gas exchange, and are given local anaesthetic blockade where possible to limit CNS depressant drug usage. In complex procedures where postoperative ventilation is planned, high-dose opioid techniques are often used to minimise stress responses.

Volatile agents

Sevoflurane is expensive and has been associated with delirium and agitation on emergence. Isoflurane remains popular with both circle and T-piece systems. Desflurane, with its irritant properties, is impractical for gas induction. Its low blood gas solubility allows rapid recovery and extubation even after prolonged anaesthesia, making it useful in neonatal anaesthesia. Halothane is arrhythmogenic, particularly in hypercarbia and sympathetic activation, but it is still used extensively worldwide. MAC values are age dependent (see Fig. 5.6.1).

Opioids

Single-dose fentanyl (1–5 μg/kg) has a short clinical effect owing to its rapid redistribution, reducing haemodynamic responses and anaesthetic requirements to surgery and providing some residual analgesia for short procedures. Large doses (25–100 μg/kg) can cause chest wall rigidity and bradycardia.

Morphine given as a loading dose (100–300 μg/kg) followed by a maintenance infusion (10–40 μg/kg/h) provides longlasting analgesia with sedation. Infusion rates are reduced in neonates (5–20 μg/kg/h).

Remifentanil given by infusion (0.1–1 μg/kg/min) provides intense intraoperative opioid anaesthesia. Hydrolysis by cholinesterases causes ultrarapid time-independent elimination and allows rapid extubation, even in newborns. Consequently, to prevent breakthrough pain, alternative analgesia must be effective before the infusion is stopped.

Muscle relaxants

Suxamethonium, although used infrequently in routine paediatric practice, should remain immediately available for rapid emergency airway control. Rocuronium (up to 1 mg/kg) is also used for rapid sequence induction because of its fast onset. Vecuronium (0.1–0.2 mg/kg) remains popular owing to its haemodynamic stability and lack of side-effects.

Total intravenous anaesthesia

Total intravenous anaesthesia (TIVA) is gaining popularity, but requires individualised adjustment of drug doses based on an understanding of age-related pharmacokinetics. Drug combinations include propofol/alfentanil and propofol/remifentanil. They are usually used for longer procedures that require controlled ventilation/muscle relaxation.

Regional analgesia

Regional blocks reduce intraoperative anaesthesia requirements and provide postoperative analgesia and, unlike systemic analgesia, may provide complete analgesia without systemic side-effects, especially in neonates and young infants who have an increased response to opioid side-effects. Simple nerve blocks, which can be extended by the use of indwelling catheters, are useful in orthopaedic surgery and thoracic surgery.

Single-dose caudal anaesthesia is well established for lower body surgery. Less invasive procedures associated with limited postoperative pain (e.g.

hernia repair) can be managed effectively for 6–8 hours with local anaesthesia alone. This duration is insufficient for more invasive procedures (e.g. orchidopexy). Analgesia can be prolonged by adding clonidine (1–2 μg/kg) or ketamine (0.5 mg/kg) to local analgesia. *S*-ketamine may be preferable to racemic ketamine in reducing the risk of hallucinations.

Perioperative analgesia for major abdominal and thoracic procedures can be managed successfully in all age groups with indwelling epidural catheters provided tip placement is appropriate.

Local anaesthesia techniques have an excellent safety record in children, but carry potential risks from both the instrumentation and the drugs. The stereoisomers ropivacaine and levobupivacaine have clinical efficacy similar to that of racemic bupivacaine, but provide an increased margin of safety from systemic absorption or accidental intravascular injection. Clear guidelines relating to dose and duration of the infusion as well as adequate patient surveillance are mandatory with continuous regional anaesthesia.

Postoperative pain management

Acute pain management in children is based on pre-emptive analgesia, multimodal therapy, close monitoring with early intervention, and safety monitoring.

Effective analgesia must be established before the end of anaesthesia. Combinations of drugs or techniques with different modes of action usually improve analgesia and reduce individual side-effects (see below).

Maintaining established analgesia requires identification of early breakthrough pain. Routine monitoring with simple pain tools is useful to alert carers of early analgesia failure. Immediate ward-based treatment must be available, coupled with experienced advice for more difficult issues. Intensive care or high-dependency units need to be considered for patients at increased risk associated with higher risk conditions or with some analgesic techniques.

For major surgery, opioid analgesia remains a cornerstone of postoperative analgesia, with morphine infusions the most popular. Adequate loading with subsequent controlled delivery to optimise analgesia without excessive side-effects is essential. Most schemes, whether patient controlled, nurse controlled or parent controlled, usually combine a background infusion with an additional ‘demanded’ dose. Older children may have less nausea if the background infusion is omitted. Side-effects (ventilatory depression, emesis, constipation and pruritus) can be a problem, but the added sedation from morphine analgesia can be beneficial in younger children.

In specialist medical centres epidural infusions mixtures are used, combining 0.125% bupivacaine with various concentrations of other agents, e.g. fentanyl 0.05–2 μg/kg/h or clonidine 0.1–1 μg/kg/h. Absorption of local anaesthetic agents and toxicity are avoided by limiting duration of infusion to 48 hours and limiting maximum bupivacaine dose to 0.5 mg/kg/h in infants and 0.25 mg/kg/h in neonates.

Paracetamol (acetaminophen) is not potent but can provide useful co-analgesia when given at sufficient dosage to maintain an adequate plasma level.[3] Oral absorption is rapid and less variable than via the rectal route. An intravenous preparation is available. Hepatic dysfunction can occur readily if excess dosage is used.

NSAIDs have a significant opioid-sparing effect and are widely used despite the absence of regulatory data. Early fears about increased bleeding, gastric irritation and renal dysfunction have not been a problem in routine paediatrics. However, theoretical concerns about impaired bone healing have become a relative contraindication for some orthopaedic procedures.[4]

Fluids

Crystalloids

Intraoperative hypoglycaemia can occur in neonates, but is unusual owing to the effects of the stress response on glycolysis and gluconeogenesis. In contrast, excessive perioperative administration of glucose solutions can lead to hyponatraemia, water intoxication and cerebral oedema. Hartmann's solution can be given as a sole agent during surgery, but it is prudent to measure blood glucose hourly during prolonged cases. Alternatively, a fixed maintenance infusion of a glucose-containing solution should be continued throughout, with additional fluid replacement of Hartmann's given independently. A recognised formula for maintenance fluid hourly rates is:

- 10 kg = 4 mL/kg;
- 10–20 kg = 40 + 2 mL/kg;
- over 20 kg = 60 + 1 mL/kg.

It has been shown that a mixture of glucose 2.5% in Ringer's lactate can maintain normal glucose while avoiding hyponatraemia. Increased replacement fluids may be required if the gut remains exposed.

Colloids and blood

The threshold for transfusion will vary with the child's overall condition and associated pathologies. For otherwise healthy children it is acceptable to let Hb drop to 8–9 g/dL, but neonates and children with cardiac or pulmonary conditions may benefit from a Hb raised to 10–13 g/dL. A volume formula for transfusion is:

- (Hb required – Hb actual) × (body weight in kg) × 5 = volume of red cells required (using resuspended SAGM blood).

Fresh frozen plasma and platelets may need replacing earlier than in adults to prevent coagulopathy. These colloids contain citrate and will require additional calcium administration to prevent significant hypocalcaemia if infused quickly.

MANAGEMENT OF COMMON CONDITIONS

Tonsillectomy and adenoidectomy

Techniques with either endotracheal intubation or LMA are used for tonsillectomy and adenoidectomy. Formal intubation secures the airway, while LMA avoids invasion of the subglottis.

Dexamethasone (1 mg/kg, up to 10 mg) significantly reduces postoperative nausea and pain and shortens the time to resumption of feeding.[5] Avoiding volatile agents (e.g. TIVA with propofol) can also reduce postoperative vomiting. Regular administration of NSAIDs and paracetamol can eliminate the need for postoperative morphine and its complications. Perioperative analgesia can be effectively provided by intraoperative fentanyl. Delayed administration of NSAIDs until after surgical haemostasis may reduce the risks of postoperative bleeding.[6]

Adenotonsillectomy can be undertaken in children on a day-case basis, but case selection on clinical and social grounds is essential. Children under the age of 3 years often have upper airway obstruction or other chronic conditions that render the day-case approach unsuitable.[7]

Inguinal herniorrhaphy and orchidopexy

Inguinal herniorrhaphy and orchidopexy are usually day-stay procedures with general anaesthesia and local blockade. Oral analgesia, paracetamol plus an NSAID is given preoperatively. Alternatively, NSAID suppositories can be given after induction.

A popular regional technique for herniorrhaphy is iliohypogastric/ilioinguinal nerve blockade using a total dose of 0.5 mL/kg of 0.25% bupivacaine. Insert a 22 G local anaesthetic (LA) needle one patient's fingerbreadth medial to the anterior superior iliac spine. Pierce the external oblique aponeurosis (palpable click), and deposit one-third to half of the volume. Change the angle inferiorly and laterally to hit the iliac periosteum. Withdraw the needle slowly, depositing another one-third to half of the volume in this track. Any remaining local analgesic can be infiltrated subcutaneously by the surgeon at the end of the procedure.

In orchidopexy, the structures requiring analgesia are more extensive. Afferent nerve supply to testicular structures is as high as T10. Analgesia can be achieved[8] by the use of an adequate volume injected caudally (e.g.1 mL/kg of either 0.125% or 0.25% bupivacaine), which can be supplemented with clonidine 1 μg/kg or preservative-free ketamine 0.5 mg/kg. These agents can double the duration of analgesia. The use of the weaker solutions can minimise postoperative motor blockade. An advantage of caudals is the relative length of postoperative analgesia. Many operators have reported satisfactory results with iliohypogastric and ilioinguinal nerve blockade and local scrotal infiltration for the skin supplied by the pudendal nerve. Some also block the genitofemoral nerve. The total volume used would equate to 0.5 mL/kg of 0.25% bupivacaine, divided in thirds for each nerve. For genitofemoral nerve blockade inject the last one-third volume subcutaneously just lateral to the pubic tubercle. This last volume can also be reserved for preoperative subcutaneous injection of the posterior scrotum or by the surgeon to infiltrate the scrotal wound. Postoperatively, the parents should be instructed to give the child regular oral analgesia for the next 48 hours.

Circumcision

Circumcision is usually performed as a day case with light general anaesthesia and local anaesthetic block. Paracetamol and NSAIDs are given as for herniorrhaphy.

Two types of nerve blockade are commonly employed: A caudal dose of 0.5 mL/kg of 0.25% bupivacaine, with or without clonidine or ketamine (as above). or alternatively, a block of the dorsal nerve of the penis is performed. This has been shown to be as effective as caudal analgesia without the side-effects of urinary retention and motor weakness.[9] A ring block of the penis can be performed using 0.25% plain bupivacaine, using sufficient volume to produce a weal and stay within the maximal dose limit (less than 1 mL/kg), but this is less effective and of shorter duration.

For dorsal nerve block the penis is pulled down and a short-bevel 25 or 22 G needle inserted inferiorly to each pubic ramus, the distance between insertion sites equating to the width of the penis. In each case the needle should follow an inferomedial course at 20° to both the transverse and the sagittal planes until both the superficial and Scarpa's fascia are felt to be sequentially punctured. Then, in each of these two sites, 0.1 mL/kg 0.25% plain bupivacaine should be injected after aspiration. Epinephrine (adrenaline) mixtures are contraindicated.

Pyloromyotomy

Hypertrophic pyloric stenosis occurs in three in every 1000 births, with a ratio of four males to one female. The child will present aged 2–8 weeks with increasing vomiting, which may be projectile and may lead to significant dehydration and a hypochloraemic hypokalaemic alkalosis.

A nasogastric tube should be placed and subsequent gastric losses should be replaced volume for volume by intravenous normal saline (with 20 mmol/L potassium chloride [KCl]). Intravenous maintenance fluids (4 mL/kg/h) should be started, comprising 5% dextrose and 0.45% saline, containing KCl 20 mmol/L, and the estimated fluid deficit is replaced over 24–48 hours with 0.9% saline. The operation should be delayed until there is normal skin turgor and perfusion, urine output of 1 mL/kg/h and a serum chloride over 100 mmol/L and bicarbonate of less than 28 mmol/L.

Methods of intubation vary – some choose rapid sequence induction with the use of cricoid pressure and suxamethonium, whereas others favour the use of non-depolarising blockade or even deep inhalational anaesthesia and intubation. The surgical technique (Ramstedt's, paraumbilical or laparoscopic approaches) and the expected anaesthetic time influence the choice of muscle relaxant. Opioids should be avoided if possible, instead using surgical infiltration of the wound with local analgesic and postoperative paracetamol.[10] Early recovery is enhanced if desflurane is used instead of isoflurane.[11] Surgical practice may require air injection through the nasogastric tube to test mucosal integrity. Feeding is usually commenced soon after surgery, although this is not universal practice.

Strabismus

Key features in relation to strabismus are the oculocardiac reflex in response to surgical movement of the globe, postoperative nausea and vomiting (PONV), and the association of strabismus with occult myopathies and possibly malignant hyperthermia. Surgical conditions are improved by the use of non-depolarising muscle relaxants that abolish extraneous skeletal muscle activity. Suxamethonium can render the 'forced traction test' invalid and should be avoided.

Antiemesis is improved by use of propofol on induction and maintenance[12] and by the pre-emptive use of both 5-hydroxytryptamine inhibitors and dexamethasone, particularly in combination (dexamethasone 150 µg/kg, 50 µg/kg ondansetron).[13] Opioids should be avoided because regular NSAIDs are as effective.[14] Topical NSAIDS (ketorolac 0.5%, diclofenac 1%) have been used with some success.

The incidence of oculocardiac reflex can be reduced by the use of ketamine at induction[15] and by the use of a medial canthal injection of local anaesthetic (2–2.5 mL lidocaine (lignocaine) 1%), which also reduces the need for postoperative analgesia.[16]

If bradycardia occurs, the surgeon should release the globe and intravenous atropine 20 µg/kg should be administered. Glycopyrronium 10 µg/kg can be given prophylactically at induction.

Dental

As a result of deaths in children having outpatient dental anaesthesia the Department of Health recommends that general anaesthesia for dental procedures is only performed in a hospital setting with full facilities.[17]

The vast majority of dental procedures can be performed as day cases. Bacteraemia occurs with dental extractions and all children with known or suspected cardiac lesions should receive antibiotic prophylaxis.

The airway is shared and throat packs are placed by the surgeon to prevent debris and blood entering the airway. In each case the dental surgeon and the anaesthetist must reach a clear understanding that the pack has been removed before the child is allowed to wake. For short procedures a specific nasal mask can be used with spontaneous ventilation using volatile agents. For longer procedures a laryngeal mask can be used, and the reinforced version has a smaller stem and so helps the surgical view. For longer or more extensive operations, nasal intubation and ventilation may be indicated, but care must be taken in patients with hypertrophied adenoids and bleeding tendencies. Analgesia for single extractions can be provided by paracetamol. More extensive surgery requires infiltration of local anaesthesia by the surgeon, supplemented with NSAIDs for at least 24 hours.

The child should be allowed to recover in the left lateral position. Discharge criteria include adequate haemostasis, pain control and toleration of oral fluids. Postoperative nausea and vomiting is not common unless blood has been swallowed.

MANAGEMENT OF SPECIALISED CONDITIONS

Anaesthesia of the preterm infant

Specific preterm pathophysiology must be considered in these high-risk cases. Both brain and lungs are prone to longer-term damage from poorly monitored ventilation. Routine fluid maintenance should continue, but additional replacement fluid should be isotonic (saline or Hartmann's). Hyperoxia must be avoided to prevent retinal damage, and carbon dioxide levels should be kept near awake values. The risks of intraventricular haemorrhage may increase with haemodynamic stress responses to surgery. High-dose fentanyl (25–100 μg/kg) can be used to obtund these.

In the non-ventilated infant, general anaesthesia needs to be precise if extubation is planned. Short-term agents are necessary (desflurane, remifentanil, atracurium), and local anaesthetic techniques should be used instead of opioids where possible. Normothermia must be maintained and ventilatory drive preserved by keeping $P\text{aCO}_2$ within that individual's normal range (often as high as 8 kPa [60 mmHg] in infants with lung disease).

Closure of patent ductus arteriosus

The preterm infant with a widely patent ductus arterious develops cardiac failure and fluid overload. These infants are usually ventilated and surgery is usually carried out in the Neontal Intensive Care Unit (NICU). At least one reliable venous access point must be available. Ventilation should be adjusted after administration of pancuronium (0.1 mg/kg) and fentanyl (5–25 μg/kg slowly, observing blood pressure). During surgery oxygen saturation may drop with lung retraction and surgery may need to be interrupted to restore adequate oxygenation. Blood needs to be available.

Necrotising enterocolitis

These neonates may have a major coagulopathy and interstitial fluid losses. Platelets, blood and coagulation factors of adult proportions may be needed intraoperatively. High-dose fentanyl (up to 100 μg/kg) and muscle relaxant combined with low-dose isoflurane are commonly used. Postoperative ventilation is usually necessary.

Diaphragmatic hernia

Diaphragmatic hernia is not a surgical emergency, the underlying pathology being lung hypoplasia secondary to herniation. The incidence is 1 in 4000, with 75% occurring in the left hemithorax.

Diaphragmatic hernia can be diagnosed antenatally or at birth with respiratory failure and classic radiology. Ventilatory failure may be compounded by severe pulmonary hypertension. Stabilisation with conventional or oscillatory ventilation is necessary and low-dose nitric oxide and surfactant may be beneficial. High-dose opioids may prevent a pulmonary hypertensive crisis in response to interventions. Some centres have elected for extra comporeal membrane oxygenation (ECMO) support and early repair, but the results have not been substantially better than with advanced ventilatory support (60–80% survival). Repair can be carried out on the NICU with high-dose fentanyl/pancuronium anaesthesia.

Tracheoesophageal abnormalities

The commonest variety of tracheoesophageal abnormality is proximal oesophageal atresia with a distal oesophageal fistula into the trachea, but there are several variants, including the less obvious H-type fistula (4%). The overall incidence is about 1 in 4000. It presents with salivation, choking on feeds and occasionally apnoea and bradycardia, and is often associated with other abnormalities (cardiac, skeletal, urogenital), which must be investigated urgently before surgery. A Replogle tube should be left in the proximal pouch on low-flow suction to reduce secretions.

Surgery should be carried out urgently to reduce pneumonitis from gastric contents. Standard neonatal anaesthesia can be used with opioid, volatile agent and muscle relaxant, avoiding nitrous oxide (increasing abdominal gas). Particular care should be taken to avoid insertion of the endotracheal tube through the fistula and inflation of the stomach, which would impair ventilation. Minimal inflation pressures should be continued until the fistula is controlled. Some centres carry out rigid bronchoscopy before thoracotomy. Primary repair is usually possible through a left thoracotomy, but with high atresia and/or a long atretic segment, delayed repair with gastrostomy and cervical oesophagostomy is necessary. After primary repair, the transanastomotic nasogastric tube must remain in situ until the integrity of the repair is confirmed.

Hernia repair in the ex-preterm infant

Hernial sacs are common in ex-preterm infants and require early repair. Such infants may have significant lung pathology and are prone to apnoea, particularly under 60 weeks post-conceptual age. The repair can be carried out awake under spinal anaesthesia.[18] A single injection (0.06 mL/kg + 0.1 mL deadspace (from syringe and needle) of 0.5% bupivacaine) given in a sitting position can produce an adequate block and is well tolerated haemodynamically. However, there is a significant failure rate and the duration of the surgery may outlast the block, particularly for bilateral hernia repair. Adding a caudal block (up to 0.75 mL/kg bupivacaine 0.25%) immediately after the spinal injection augments reliability and duration.[19]

Alternatively, light general anaesthesia with a caudal block may be preferred. After induction (sevoflurane or propofol 2 mg/kg), the infant is intubated (atracurium 0.5 mg/kg) and ventilated, avoiding hypocapnoea. Evanescent volatile agents (sevoflurane, desflurane) are used after induction and opioids are avoided. A standard caudal block (1 mL of 0.25% bupivacaine) is given before surgery.

After surgery, irrespective of technique, apnoea monitoring and close supervision are necessary for 24 hours. Caffeine may reduce the risks of postoperative apnoea.

ACUTE ANAESTHETIC PROBLEMS

Vascular access

Up to 1 week after birth, emergency venous access is easily obtained by cannulation of the umbilical vein using a 5 FG catheter (a sterile feeding tube in an emergency). The stump is trimmed to expose the arteries and vein and a loose ligature is placed around the stump. The catheter is inserted 5 cm and blood is aspirated to confirm its position and flushed with saline. The ligature is tightened. The catheter is further secured with tapes and an abdominal radiograph will confirm the position of the tip.

Venous access can present serious problems in children. Inhalational induction followed by venous cannulation may help, but airway control may require a second anaesthetist. Access routes to be considered by non-specialists are femoral veins, external jugular veins and the intraosseous routes.

For intraosseous access, specially manufactured needles are available. These should be inserted into the marrow of the anteromedial tibia, 1–3 cm (depending on size of child) below the tibial tuberosity or into the inferolateral femur. The bony cortex can only be breached once in each bone as fluids infused through a second successful attempt will escape through the hole caused by the first.

Respiratory tract infections

Runny noses are common in children and not necessarily a contraindication to anaesthesia. However, it is important to establish whether such signs are markers of an active respiratory infection. These include acute changes such as lethargy, insomnia, irritability and anorexia. A pyrexial child (37.5°C) with a new productive cough or with abnormal breath sounds should be postponed. If there is an isolated upper respiratory tract infection then deferment may only be necessary for 2 weeks, but with lower respiratory involvement then an interval of 4 weeks may be indicated to ensure airway oedema and parenchymal infiltrations have resolved.[20]

Airway emergencies

Laryngospasm

Laryngospasm can occur on induction of anaesthesia, with surgical stimulation or on emergence, particularly after airway surgery. In all cases 100% oxygen should be given with positive end-expiratory pressure. During surgery, stimulation should stop and if necessary anaesthesia be increased. If the spasm worsens despite these measures it can be broken with low-dose suxamethonium (0.5–1.0 mg/kg). It may not be necessary to intubate the trachea once the glottis has relaxed if the plane of anaesthesia can be deepened and spontaneous ventilation re-established. Should another dose of suxamethonium be required, this should be preceded by a dose of atropine 20 μg/kg intravenously.

Croup, tracheitis and epiglottitis

Croup, tracheitis and epiglottitis have different aetiologies, but present as acute airway obstruction requiring anaesthetic input. Croup (laryngotracheobronchitis) is usually viral and presents in the first to third years of life. Epiglottitis with *Haemophilus* type b has become rare since vaccination programmes began, but still occurs. Tracheitis is either viral or bacterial (*Staphylococcus* and *Streptococcus* spp.)

Medical interference should be kept to a minimum, particularly in epiglottitis. Radiology can be characteristic, but the child should not be moved to obtain these views. Disturbance of the child with epiglottis may lead to sudden and disastrous loss of the airway. Anaesthesia may be required to make the diagnosis as well as to secure the airway.

The most experienced anaesthetist available should perform the procedure, and in suspected epiglottitis or extreme tracheitis it may be valuable to have an ENT surgeon present with a tracheostomy set ready. Inhalational induction is achieved with oxygen and a non-irritant vapour (halothane or sevoflurane). The induction should take place in the child's preferred posture, at least until consciousness is lost.

Laryngoscopy and oral intubation are carried out in the spontaneously breathing child with deep inhalation anaesthesia alone. After successful oral intubation, the tube can be replaced with an optimal nasal tube. This must be strapped securely so that the child cannot easily self-extubate. Further management will be in the paediatric intensive care unit.

Inhaled foreign body

Rigid bronchoscopy should be performed under inhalational anaesthesia, preserving spontaneous ventilation (positive-pressure ventilation may cause the foreign body to migrate deeper). Halothane or sevoflurane are suitable, the former maintaining more constant depth of anaesthesia where interruptions of anaesthetic administration occur. Premedication with atropine (10–20 μg/kg) prevents bradycardia and excess secretions. The bronchoscope should have a suitable side-arm to attach the anaesthetic breathing system. The larynx can be sprayed with lidocaine (lignocaine) 3–4 mg/kg. Nitrous oxide is contraindicated because air trapping may be present but undetected. The foreign body can be removed by bronchoscopic forceps and suction. Dexamethasone is commonly given (0.25 mg/kg intravenously) to prevent reactive airway oedema, and a chest radiograph should be performed after the procedure to exclude atelectasis, pneumothorax etc.

Bleeding tonsillar bed

The problems are:

- potentially significant hypovolaemia;
- swallowed blood in the stomach;
- a swollen and bleeding pharynx with a difficult view of the airway.

Intravascular volume should be restored before anaesthesia. Classically (in the UK), the child is anaesthetised in a head-down, left lateral position with an inhalational agent before securing the airway. However, this may increase venous congestion and bleeding and is not conducive to rapid control of the airway. Alternatively, the child can be anaesthetised after preoxygenation with rapid sequence induction and cricoid pressure. Ketamine (2 mg/kg) may be useful to maintain haemodynamic stability and either suxamethonium 1–2 mg/kg or rocuronium 1 mg/kg used for rapid relaxation.

Malignant hyperthermia

Malignant hyperthermia (MH)[21] is a rare autosomal dominant condition linked to several chromosomal loci. The crisis is pharmacologically triggered (agents include volatile anaesthetics and suxamethonium), leading to muscle contraction. A hypermetabolic state with respiratory and lactic acidosis ensues, causing hyperthermia, hyperkalaemia and hypercalcaemia. Severe cases have rhabdomyolysis with greatly elevated creatine kinase and myoglobinuria. The condition must be suspected when there is an unexplained rapid rise in expired carbon dioxide and heart rate, possibly associated with supraventricular or ventricular arrhythmias. Hyperthermia is a later sign. Treatment is by immediate cessation of trigger agents, rapid cooling and the administration of dantrolene 1 mg/kg intravenously. Early advice should be sought from a specialised centre for both treatment and later testing.

Latex allergy

Latex allergy is an immediate hypersensitivity reaction to latex products, and is particularly associated with children who undergo operations for spina bifida, possibly owing to repeated latex exposure. Children with a history of food intolerance to vegetables that contain similar proteins (bananas, kiwi fruit, avocado and chestnuts) should also be regarded as at risk. Treatment is initially as for anaphylaxis. Serum should be sent for mast cell tryptase and complement levels (repeated at 6 and 24 hours). To confirm the diagnosis, skin testing and assay for IgE antibodies to latex should be performed 6 weeks after the event.

There should be a trolley with latex-free equipment and the children should be looked after in a latex-free environment in hospital.[22]

References

1. Brennan LJ. Modern day-case anaesthesia for children. Br J Anaesth 1999; 83:91–103.
2. Wodey E, Gai V, Carre F, Ecoffey C. Accuracy and limitations of continuous oesophageal aortic blood flow measurement during general anaesthesia for children: comparison with transcutaneous echography-Doppler. Paediatr Anaesth 2001 11:309–317.
3. Anderson BJ. Comparing the efficacy of NSAIDs and paracetamol in children. Paediatr Anaesth 2004; 14:201–217.
4. Gerstenfeld LC, Thiede M, Seibert K, et al. Differential inhibition of fracture healing by non-selective and cyclooxygenase -2 selective non-steroidal anti-inflammatory drugs. J Orthop Res 2003; 21:670–675.
5. Tom LWC, Templeton JJ, Thompson ME, Marsh RR. Dexamethasone in adenotonsillectomy. Int J Pediatr Otorhinolaryngol 1996; 37:115–120.
6. Dsida R, Cote CJ. Nonsteroidal antiinflammatory drugs and hemorrhage following tonsillectomy: do we have the data? Anesthesiology 2004; 100:749–751,
7. Ross AT, Kazahaya K, Tom LWC. Revisiting outpatient tonsillectomy in young children. Otolaryngol Head Neck Surg 2003: 128:326–331.
8. Verghese S, Hannallah RS, Rice LJ, Belman AB, Patel KM. Caudal analgesia in children: effect of volume versus concentration of bupivacaine on blocking

spermatic cord traction response during orchidopexy. Anesth Analg 2002; 95:1219–1223.

9. Gauntlett I. A comparison between local anaesthetic dorsal nerve block and caudal bupivacaine with ketamine for paediatric circumcision. Paediatr Anaesth 2003; 13:38–42.
10. Habre W, Schwab C, Gollow, I, Johnson C. An audit of postoperative analgesia after pyloromyotomy. Paediatr Anaesth 1999; 9:253–256.
11. Wolf AR, Lawson, RA, Dryden CM, Davis FW. Recovery after desflurane anaesthesia in the infant: comparison with isoflurane. Br J Anaesth 1996; 76:362–364.
12. Reimer EJ, Montgomery CJ, Bevan JC, Merrick PM, Blackstock D, Popovic V. Propofol anaesthesia reduces early postoperative emesis after paediatric strabismus surgery. Can J Anesth 1993; 40:927–933.
13. Splinter WM. Prevention of vomiting after strabismus surgery in children: dexamethasone alone versus dexamethasone plus low-dose ondansetron. Paediatr Anaesth 2001; 11:591–595.
14. Munro HM, Riegger LQ, Reynolds PI, Wilton NC, Lewis IH. Comparison of the analgesic and emetic properties of ketorolac and morphine for paediatric outpatient strabismus surgery. Br J Anaesth 1994; 72:624–628.
15. Hahnenkamp K, Honemann CW, Fischer LG, Durieux ME, Muehlendyck H, Braun U. Effect of different anaesthetic regimes on the oculocardiac reflex during paediatric strabismus surgery. Paediatr Anaesth 2000; 10:601–608.
16. Mather SJ. Anaesthesia for strabismus surgery. In: Stoddart PA, Lauder GR. Problems in anaesthesia; paediatric anaesthesia. London: Martin Dunitz; 2004:153–156.
17. Donaldson L, Wild R. A conscious decision; a review of the use of general anaesthesia and conscious sedation in primary dental care. Report of a Group chaired by the Chief Medical Officer and the Chief Dental Officer. London: Department of Health; 2000. www.doh.gov.uk/dental/conscious.htm.
18. Krane EJ, Haberkern CM, Jacobson LE. Postoperative apnea, bradycardia, and oxygen desaturation in formerly premature infants: prospective comparison of spinal and general anaesthesia. Anesth Analg 1995; 80:7–13.
19. Peutrell JM, Hughes DG. Combined spinal and epidural anaesthesia for inguinal hernia repair in babies. Paediatr Anaesth 1994; 4:221–227.
20. Hannalah RS. Anesthetic considerations for pediatric ambulatory surgery. Ambul Surg 1997; 5:52–59.
21. Wappler F. Malignant hyperthermia. Eur J Anaesth 2001; 18:632–652.
22. Dakin MJ, Yentis SM. Latex allergy: a strategy for management. Anaesthesia 1998; 53:774–781.

CHAPTER **5.7**

NEUROSURGERY

Neurosurgeons operate on lesions in and around the brain, cranial nerves, spinal cord, nerve roots and peripheral nerves. In the past, much of their work involved tumours of the brain and meninges, and aneurysmal disease of the cerebral vessels. Aneurysmal disease is increasingly treated endovascularly by neuroradiologists, and some tumours (acoustic neuromas, meningiomas and pituitary tumours) with radiotherapy (gamma knife). Many surgically treated tumours are first embolised by a neuroradiologist to reduce bleeding.

Advances in computed tomography (CT) and magnetic resonance imaging (MRI), and the development of neuronavigation systems have allowed accurate surgical biopsy or excision of lesions (image-guided surgery). The excision of epileptic foci and placement of stimulating electrodes for the treatment of movement disorders (functional neurosurgery) is now common.

Endoscopic neurosurgical procedures have been devised, largely for the treatment of intraventricular and pituitary lesions. There is increasing interest in 'awake' procedures to guide safe excision margins in tumour surgery and during functional neurosurgery. Trauma provides a substantial caseload, with alcohol intoxication a common precipitating factor.

GENERAL CONSIDERATIONS

Neurological examination

Level of consciousness

The standard measure of global cerebral function, described by the Glasgow Coma Scale (GCS), has a minimum score of three (Table 5.7.1). Patients scoring eight or below are by definition unconscious and should be intubated and ventilated in the acute phase. The GCS is not linear and, because it is calculated from the best response, lateralising signs such as limb deficits and pupil responses should be documented simultaneously.

Cranial nerves

The glossopharyngeal (gag reflex) and vagus (motor and sensory to the glottis for effective cough and speech) nerves are of particular interest to

Eye opening	
Spontaneously	4
To speech	3
To pain	2
None	1
Verbal response	
Orientated	5
Confused	4
Inappropriate	3
Incomprehensible	2
None	1
Motor response	
Obeys commands	6
Localizes pain	5
Withdraws	4
Flexion	3
Extension	2
None	1
Limb movements — the strength of the upper and lower limbs can be scored according to the scale described by the Medical Research Council	
0	No movement
1	A flicker
2	Can move
3	Can resist gravity
4	Can move against resistance
5	Normal power

Table 5.7.1 Glasgow Coma Scale

anaesthetists. The facial and trigeminal nerves are also relevant because the cornea may need protection if they are affected. Pupillary responses are also relevant in the context of raised intracranial pressure and after head injury.

Blood–brain barrier

The pore size in capillary endothelium of tissues such as lung or muscle is about 6.5 nm, which allows the passage of ions but not proteins. The pore size in cerebral capillary endothelium is only 0.7–0.9 nm, which makes it a 'barrier' to even small ions such as sodium ('tight' junctions). This means that, unlike in other tissues, fluid flux across the blood–brain barrier is determined by osmolality rather than oncotic pressure.[1] Thus, if large volumes of isotonic crystalloid fluid are given, there may be peripheral oedema due to dilutional reduction in oncotic pressure, but brain water content is unaffected. However, administration of hypotonic or hypertonic solutions will cause an increase and a decrease in brain water, respectively,[1] although the response is often unpredictable because the integrity of the blood–brain barrier can be degraded by disease (infection, trauma, tumours and epileptic seizures).

Intravenous fluids and neurosurgery

There is no ideal isotonic intravenous fluid for use in neurosurgery. Glucose-containing solutions should be avoided because, after glucose metabolism, the residual free water can worsen cerebral oedema, and hyperglycaemia is associated with poor outcome after head injury (see below, p. 649). Hypotonic fluids such as compound sodium lactate (CSL, Hartmann's solution) have previously been avoided and 0.9% saline considered the crystalloid of choice during neurosurgery (Table 5.7.2). However, infusions of large volumes of 0.9% saline (>3 L) can produce hyperchloraemic metabolic acidosis, and, despite the theoretical objection of relative hypotonicity, many neuroanaesthetists now use CSL for intravenous replacement therapy.[2] A recent study comparing CSL and hypertonic saline (7.5%) as intravenous fluid in traumatic brain injury showed no difference in outcome.[3]

Cerebral blood flow

The cerebral circulation receives about 14% of the cardiac output. Normal cerebral blood flow (CBF) is 50 mL/100 g/min. The normal cerebral metabolic rate for oxygen is about 6 mL/100 g/min for grey matter and 2 mL/100 g/min for white matter (average 3.2 mL/100 g/min). Jugular oxygen saturation is normally 65–70%. Brain energy is derived from oxidative glucose metabolism, with small amounts of lactate metabolism, and

Fluid	Ionic composition mmol/1000 mL					Osmolality
	Na^+	Ca^{++}	K^+	Cl^-	Lactate	
CSL	131	2	5	111	29	278
0.9% saline	154			154		308

Table 5.7.2 Composition of compound sodium lactate (CSL; Hartmann's solution) and 0.9% saline

metabolism of ketones during starvation or hyperglycaemia. The brain has no significant energy stores and ATP levels fall to zero after about 7 minutes of total ischaemia.

CBF is influenced by five factors:

- blood pressure;
- metabolism;
- carbon dioxide;
- oxygen;
- viscosity.

Spinal cord blood flow is believed to behave in a similar way.

Autoregulation

CBF remains constant over a considerable range of mean arterial blood pressures (Fig. 5.7.1). In normal individuals, the limits of this autoregulation are 60 mmHg, below which CBF decreases, and 160 mmHg, above which CBF increases. These limits are approximate and are increased by chronic hypertension. The mechanism of autoregulation is related to an intrinsic characteristic of cerebral vascular smooth muscle whereby reflex contraction or relaxation occurs in responses to changes in intraluminal

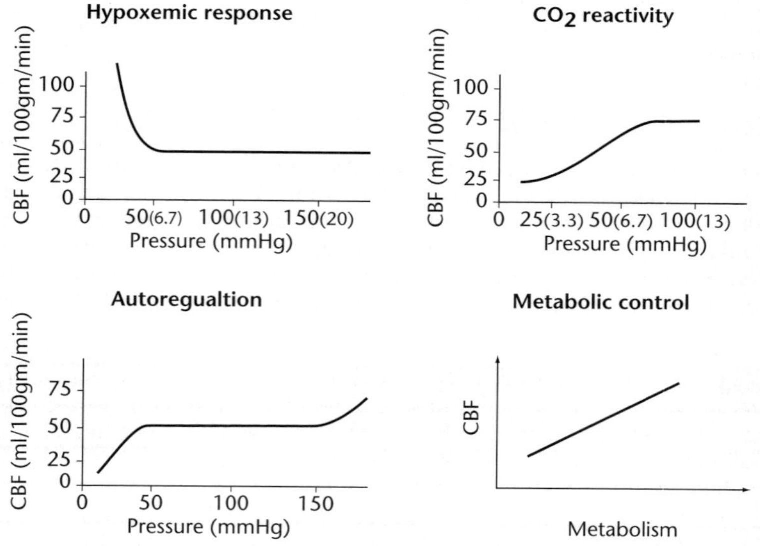

Figure 5.7.1 Factors affecting cerebral blood flow (CBF).

pressure. Autoregulation is impaired by physiological derangements such as hypoxaemia and hypercapnia, by high-dose volatile anaesthetic agents, and by pathophysiological states such as severe head injury, subarachnoid haemorrhage and cerebrovascular disease.

Metabolism

CBF is tightly linked to cerebral metabolism (flow–metabolism coupling). Activation of the cortex results in an immediate focal increase in flow. There is a 10% decrease in CBF during sleep, but rapid eye movement (REM) sleep causes CBF to increase to awake values. Adenosine and nitric oxide may mediate this phenomenon.

Carbon dioxide

CBF increases linearly over the range of 3.3–10 kPa of arterial P_{CO_2} and the change in CBF is complete within 2 minutes of the change in P_{CO_2}. CBF then reverts towards normal within a few hours. Reactivity to carbon dioxide is attenuated in some patients with carotid stenosis, cardiac failure, severe hypotension, and after brain injury. If carbon dioxide reactivity is reduced, a 'steal' may occur in diseased areas as blood is diverted into normally reactive areas when P_{CO_2} rises.

Oxygen

Hyperoxia has little effect on CBF and hypoxia only begins to cause an increase in CBF when arterial P_{O_2} falls below 8 kPa.

Viscosity

Reduced blood viscosity results in increased cerebral microcirculatory flow. Haematocrit is the major determinant of viscosity. A haemoglobin concentration of about 10 g/dL is the best compromise in the cerebral circulation between viscosity and oxygen-carrying capacity.

Intracranial pressure

Because the skull is rigid and its contents (blood, brain and cerebrospinal fluid [CSF]) are essentially incompressible, changes in volume of any of the contents should result in a change in intracranial pressure (ICP). However, if one component of the intracranial contents expands, compensatory mechanisms come into play for a time to maintain a constant ICP. For example, if the brain swells CSF passes into the spinal theca to maintain a constant intracranial volume and hence pressure. This is spatial compensation. However, this compensation readily becomes exhausted and then a small further increase in the volume of one component (e.g. further brain swelling) will cause a large rise in ICP.

Normal ICP is less than 10 mmHg, 15–20 mmHg is high, and over 25 mmHg has a poor prognosis. Raised ICP can be associated with internal herniation of the brain. The forebrain may herniate into the midbrain, causing third-nerve palsy with a large pupil, or the brainstem may herniate through the foramen magnum, causing respiratory arrest.

Because the skull is a rigid container, the driving pressure for blood flow is mean arterial blood pressure minus the ICP, or intraspinal pressure for the spinal cord. For the brain this is called cerebral perfusion pressure (CPP), and is often targeted during head injury management (see below, p. 649).

TECHNICAL CONSIDERATIONS

Anaesthetic agents for neurosurgery

Most anaesthetic agents decrease cerebral metabolic rate. Because CBF is coupled to metabolism, metabolic depression results in a secondary reduction of CBF, which may reduce ICP.

Volatile agents

Most volatile agents are direct cerebral vasodilators as well as depressing cerebral metabolic rate. The overall change in CBF is the balance between these two effects. At low concentrations CBF is reduced with cerebral metabolic rate, but above a certain concentration, typically about 1 MAC, the vasodilator effects predominate. In practice, the vasodilator effects of volatile agents at clinically relevant doses are largely cancelled by mild hyperventilation. Halothane is an exception, in that hyperventilation must be instituted before it is administered, whereas with isoflurane, desflurane, enflurane and sevoflurane the agent can be administered before hyperventilation. Enflurane is associated with seizure activity at high doses and is not used.

Nitrous oxide

Nitrous oxide is also a cerebral vasodilator but, unlike volatile agents, does not decrease cerebral metabolism. In fact, it can increase it. The overall effect is therefore a rise in CBF and ICP. Its presence is also unwelcome when there is a risk of air embolism, which is arguably always present. It is therefore disappearing from neuroanaesthetic practice.

Intravenous agents

Barbiturates, propofol, etomidate and benzodiazepines all decrease cerebral metabolism and CBF. Ketamine is the exception, causing an increase in CBF and little effect on metabolism. Ketamine has been regarded as unsuitable for neurosurgery, but is being reassessed because its haemodynamic properties may be useful in sick patients and it blocks the excitatory *N*-methyl-D-aspartate (NMDA) receptor sites.

Propofol causes movements on induction that can be mistaken for epileptiform phenomena, although it is an effective anticonvulsant. It has been suggested that epileptic patients who are not on treatment and therefore able to drive, should not be given propofol lest they are mistakenly believed to be convulsing.[4]

Muscle relaxants

Suxamethonium causes a brief rise in ICP and can release potassium from denervated muscle. It should be used with caution in neurological disease, but after head injury its ability to allow rapid airway control continues to make it a useful drug.

Analgesics

Opioids have little effect on intracranial dynamics if ventilatory and circulatory parameters are supported. The profound analgesia provided by remifentanil infusion is useful in neurosurgery for periods of intense stimulation, such as insertion of cranial pins for head holding, and when muscle paralysis needs to be avoided to enable monitoring of motor nerve function. If morphine and intravenous paracetamol are given about 40 minutes before the end of surgery, and remifentanil discontinued towards the end, postoperative analgesia is similar and awakening time decreased compared with fentanyl.[5]

The use of non-steroidal anti-inflammatory drugs (NSAIDs) is contentious because of the potential for increased bleeding. Some manufacturers advise against pre- and intraoperative use. Nevertheless, some practitioners use them intraoperatively and the actual risk, although unknown, is probably low.[6] Aspirin is generally considered a contraindication to complex elective neurosurgery.

Volatile or propofol?

Propofol infusion may result in lower ICP and higher CPP than volatile agent anaesthesia,[7] although there is no difference in early postoperative outcome.[8] Overall, choice of agent is relatively unimportant compared to conduct of the anaesthetic.[9]

Practical points

Premedication

Premedication is rarely indicated.

Marking the side

Do not induce anaesthesia without appropriate consent and a skin mark to show the correct side for operation.

Thromboembolic prophylaxis

Heparin is rarely used until the day after surgery, although the risk of postoperative haematoma is unquantified. Calf support stockings and intermittent calf compression provide similar prophylactic efficacy.

Induction

Induction should be smooth. Full doses of hypnotics, analgesics and muscle relaxants should be used to avoid coughing, straining or hypertension. Doses should be chosen to minimise the incidence of hypotension or hypertension, which can cause both brain swelling and increased ICP. This is particularly important when autoregulation might be impaired.

Tracheal tubes

Non-kinking tubes such as the Flexilum® (Mallinkrodt) are traditionally used and there are many ways of securing them. A single sheet of modern adhesive plaster or transparent dressing works well.

Nasogastric tubes and urinary catheters

Consider whether there will be a need for nasogastric drainage or enteral feeding. It is much easier to insert a nasogastric tube at induction than later. If the patient might be difficult to intubate, ask him or her to swallow it before induction. A urinary catheter is probably indicated if surgery is likely to be longer than 5 hours or bloody.

Monitoring

Insert an arterial cannula or central venous catheter if vascular instability is likely (e.g. surgery around the brainstem, or severe blood loss). Modern noninvasive blood pressure monitors are satisfactory for many cases. If evoked potential monitoring for spinal surgery is needed, propofol infusions give the best conditions, although sensory potentials can be successfully recorded with volatile anaesthesia. Motor evoked monitoring (e.g. transcranial stimulation for spinal cord monitoring or facial nerve monitoring during base of skull surgery) requires muscle relaxants to be avoided, although atracurium can be used in full doses for intubation.

Positioning

There are four positions: supine, prone, park bench and sitting. A pin head-holding system is commonly used. Insertion of the pins is very stimulating and requires profound anaesthesia and analgesia. The eyes should be protected with waterproof covering to avoid contamination, and taped shut to prevent hypoxic corneal damage. Precautions to take for the different positions are as follows.

- supine – avoid excessive lateral rotation of the neck and traction on the shoulder, which may cause stretch injury of the brachial plexus;
- prone – ensure no pressure on the eyes. Avoid a horseshoe-type headrest, which is notorious in this respect. Blindness due to ischaemic optic neuropathy or retinal artery thrombosis is a rare complication of the prone position;.[10]
- park bench – place a large pad under the ribs in the dependent axilla to avoid stretching the brachial plexus;

- sitting – the risks of air embolism and hypotension are well known. The head must not be too flexed, which may cause tetraparesis, and venous and lymphatic obstruction can cause severe tongue swelling.

Temperature

Moderate hypothermia does not improve neurological outcome, and is associated with infection and coagulation deficits.[11] Active warming is required to maintain normothermia.

Extubation

Stormy extubation with laryngospasm, coughing and bucking is particularly unwelcome after neurosurgery. It is probably most reliably avoided by deep extubation (e.g. with end-tidal sevoflurane >3%). If recovery is likely to be prolonged, airway management can be assisted by insertion of a laryngeal mask at extubation.

Postoperative analgesia

Some procedures (e.g. posterior fossa surgery, cranioplasty, posterior spinal surgery, ventriculoperitoneal shunt) can be extremely painful. Regular paracetamol, with the first dose given intravenously during surgery, is useful and can be combined with regular oral dihydrocodeine and ibuprofen. Ideally, morphine is given intravenously in 1–3 mg increments, but oral or intramuscular morphine can be given safely and patient-controlled analgesia used if patients are mentally competent. All patients receiving morphine should have added oxygen.

Postoperative haematoma

Postoperative haematoma is often associated with serious morbidity or mortality. The majority occur within 8 hours and virtually all within 24 hours. Aspirin is probably a definite risk factor, and NSAID use is also a possibility. After anterior cervical surgery, swelling causing airway obstruction is not always due to haematoma. Whatever the cause, patients complain of not being able to breathe, but rarely have stridor. Oximetry is not a good guide to airway patency. Complete obstruction can occur suddenly. The priority is to open the wound because release of tissue pressure (or haematoma) may restore the airway.

SPECIFIC OPERATIONS

Neuroradiological embolisation or coiling

The patient must be completely still during imaging and the ventilator should therefore be turned off during runs. Interventional neuroradiological procedures can be lengthy and the contrast medium is hyperosmotic, so a urinary catheter is sometimes required. Blood pressure is conveniently monitored directly using a side-arm of the radiologist's arterial access.

Vascular surgery

A proportion of aneurysms and arteriovenous malformations are unsuitable for radiological treatment. Normothermia and normotension at the patient's preoperative pressure are currently recommended.[11]

Tumour surgery

Glioma, meningioma, pituitary tumour or metastatic carcinoma are the usual pathologies. Sarcoma or chordoma are less frequent. Bleeding is rarely massive, except occasionally with a meningioma, but induced hypotension can sometimes facilitate surgery. Remifentanil infusions are useful for this purpose. Postoperative epilepsy can occur, but the value of phenytoin as a prophylactic anticonvulsant is debated. Dexamethasone decreases ICP by reducing brain swelling associated with tumours, but the hyperglycaemic effect of corticosteroids is unwelcome.[12] Corticosteroids are not currently recommended for swelling associated with head injury.

'Awake' craniotomy is indicated if resection margins impinge on eloquent areas of brain. This can be performed under scalp block only, but more often local infiltration is combined with sedation or general anaesthesia using remifentanil and propofol infusions. Airway control is with a laryngeal mask, which can be removed during the 'awake' phase and re-inserted as necessary.[6]

Pituitary tumours are often approached through the nose (trans-sphenoidal). Dilatation of the nasal passage is extremely stimulating and profound analgesia with remifentanil is required. A throat pack is indicated. Cushing's disease is associated with significant cardiovascular pathology, and acromegaly with glottic stenosis. Severe airway obstruction may occur after extubation in acromegalics, due to the use of too large an endotracheal tube. Postoperative sleep apnoea may also be a problem in these patients, particularly if nasal packs have been inserted.

Spinal surgery

Difficult intubation is common with spinal pathology above the third cervical vertebra, partly because mouth opening is adversely affected.[13] Blood loss from some spinal tumours can be severe. Some thoracic spinal lesions have to be approached through the chest and a double-lumen tube is used. Spinal cord monitoring may be required (see above, p. 646). A weak, hoarse voice and poor cough after anterior cervical surgery can be due to recurrent laryngeal or vagal nerve damage. Postoperative visual loss is a rare complication, and is most common after prone spinal surgery (about 1 in 11 000). Diabetes mellitus, preoperative hypertension, smoking and polycythaemia are risk factors.

Emergency neurosurgery

Emergency neurosurgery is mostly directed towards evacuation of an expanding intracranial extra- or intradural haematoma and relief of raised ICP. The aetiology is often trauma, including intracranial surgery, which may block CSF pathways and cause postoperative acute hydrocephalus requiring drainage. Excision of contused brain and intracerebral haematoma is sometimes indicated. The anaesthetist should maintain CPP without allowing hypertension, which may increase brain swelling, and ensure normal blood gases, glucose and temperature.

Chronic subdural haematoma is rarely urgent, although an acute exacerbation can raise ICP. Many patients can be managed with propofol sedation and local anaesthesia for burr hole drainage. If general anaesthesia is required, return to spontaneous respiration after opening of the dura, which will allow the $P\text{CO}_2$ to rise and the brain to expand again.

HEAD INJURY

Head injury is the leading cause of death in the first four decades of life. The incidence of significant morbidity is high, even in milder forms of injury.

Pathophysiology

Head injury may involve diffuse axonal injury, focal contusions and space-occupying haematomas.

Primary brain injury is the result of physical disruption of neurons or axons due to mechanical trauma at impact and causes variable degrees of irreversible cell damage that cannot be treated.

Secondary brain injury begins from the moment of primary injury and develops during subsequent minutes, hours and days, causing further neuronal damage and worsening of the ultimate neurological deficit. Secondary brain injury arises from both systemic and intracranial changes. Common causes are hypotension, hypoxaemia and raised ICP.

Resuscitation and stabilisation

Consensus guidelines[14,15] for the management of patients with severe head injury focus on prevention, recognition and treatment of conditions known to cause secondary brain injury. This includes surgically remedial compressive lesions and the prevention of secondary systemic insults.

Resuscitation is a key point at which mortality and morbidity can be influenced. The importance of securing the airway and maintaining adequate oxygenation and blood pressure cannot be overemphasised because the risk of secondary brain injury begins and continues from the moment of impact. Initial management is to control the airway, breathing and circulation, followed by a detailed secondary survey to identify other injuries.

Unconscious patients should be intubated and ventilated to maintain PO_2 over 13.5 kPa and PCO_2 at 4.5–5.0 kPa. Systemic blood pressure must be maintained normal or above normal to allow for good neurological outcome,[16] initially by fluid resuscitation. Glucose-containing solutions should be avoided. Blood loss from other injuries should be replaced by blood products as usual. Hypertonic saline solution (7.5%) may improve outcome in patients with multiple trauma because of its effect on ICP. Extracranial injuries that threaten life should be treated before definitive neurosurgical treatment, but otherwise simply stabilised beforehand.

Intensive care management

The aim is to prevent and treat secondary physiological insults. Novel neuroprotective agents may have promise in the future, but are unlikely to affect management strategies in the short and medium term. Although specialist neurocritical care, with therapy guided by ICP and CPP, is likely to benefit patients with severe head injury[17] there is wide variation in practice despite expert consensus guidelines.

Monitoring

General monitoring

Invasive cardiovascular monitoring, ECG and pulse oximetry are mandatory. An oesophageal Doppler monitor or pulmonary artery catheter may assist in directing therapy in those with cardiovascular instability or in whom cardiovascular targets are difficult to achieve. Regular estimation of arterial blood gases, glucose and sodium and monitoring of core temperature are also required to optimise treatment strategies.

Cerebral monitoring

General monitoring will not detect changes in the brain. Cerebral monitors allow measurement of CPP, estimation of CBF and assessment of cerebral oxygenation. Management decisions should not be based on a change in one variable alone. Monitoring of several variables simultaneously – multimodality monitoring – allows cross-validation between monitors, artefact rejection, and greater confidence that treatment is appropriate:

- ICP monitoring using microtransducers placed in the brain tissue via an intracranial access bolt is safe and straightforward. It allows measurement of ICP and CPP. It also detects abnormal ICP waveforms that occur due to phasic increases in ICP triggered by cerebral vasodilatation in response to a reduction in CPP. ICP may also be measured via a catheter placed into the lateral ventricles (external ventricular drain) for therapeutic drainage of CSF;

- transcranial Doppler ultrasonography measures blood flow velocity in the middle cerebral artery, which is an indirect measure of CBF. It can also demonstrate the loss of pressure autoregulation and carbon dioxide reactivity, which are indicators of poor prognosis;
- jugular venous bulb oximetry ($SjvO_2$) is a global measure of cerebral oxygenation and assesses the balance between cerebral oxygen supply and demand. A catheter placed in the jugular bulb, a dilatation of the internal jugular vein, allows sampling of venous blood draining from the brain. Oxygen saturation can be measured by intermittent sampling or continuously using a fibreoptic catheter. A reduction in $SjvO_2$, or an increase in arteriojugular difference in oxygen content, provides a useful indicator of inadequate CBF. A fall in $SjvO_2$ below 50% is associated with an adverse neurological outcome. Although rises in $SjvO_2$ suggest cerebral hyperaemia, regional ischaemia cannot be excluded because $SjvO_2$ is a flow-weighted global measure. Newer techniques for measuring the adequacy of cerebral oxygenation include near-infrared spectroscopy, brain tissue $P\text{O}_2$ microprobes and cerebral microdialysis.

General aspects of care

Ventilatory support is vital to ensure adequate oxygenation, with $P\text{O}_2$ higher than 13.5 kPa and normal $P\text{CO}_2$. Respiratory complications are common and many patients soon require advanced ventilatory support. The importance of maintaining a normal or above-normal blood pressure has already been discussed. Following adequate volume resuscitation, the hypotensive effect of sedative agents may require additional support with modest doses of vasopressors or inotropes. Aiming for normoxia, normocarbia, normotension, normoglycaemia and normothermia is a good rule of thumb.

There is a high calorific requirement after head injury. Early feeding has been associated with an improved neurological outcome. Despite delayed gastric emptying after head injury, enteral feeding is possible in most patients and is associated with a lower incidence of hyperglycaemia than parenteral nutrition. Hyperglycaemia should be avoided[18] with a normal blood glucose maintained by an insulin infusion. Early mobilisation is crucial for the best outcome. Skilled neurophysiotherapists must be part of the multidisciplinary team to ensure early rehabilitation.

Maintenance of cerebral perfusion pressure

Conventional approaches to the management of head injury have concentrated on a reduction in ICP, but it has never been shown that lowering ICP in patients with intracranial hypertension improves outcome. A definitive study is now unlikely on ethical grounds. ICP above 20 mmHg is a powerful predictor of adverse outcome and treatment should be initiated if the ICP is above 20–25 mmHg. However, there has been a recent change in emphasis to maintain an adequate CPP rather than just a reduction in ICP. CPP should be maintained at higher than 60 mmHg,[19] but there is debate on the best means of doing so. One approach recommends aggressive fluid replacement and cardiovascular support with vasopressors and inotropes to increase arterial pressure and induce secondary reductions in ICP.[20] Although this strategy is associated with a reduction in secondary cerebral ischaemia, mortality and morbidity are similar to those of other treatment strategies because of a high incidence of systemic (particularly respiratory) complications.[21] Alternatively, CPP can be maintained by control of ICP using carefully controlled hyperventilation guided by $SjvO_2$ monitoring ('optimised hyperventilation').[22] Both strategies have a role if appropriately applied and carefully monitored.

Control of intracranial pressure

Sedation and analgesia

Intravenous anaesthetic agents are routinely used to reduce ICP in patients with serious head injury by a dose-dependent reduction in cerebral metabolism and CBF while maintaining pressure autoregulation and carbon dioxide reactivity. Barbiturates have largely been replaced by propofol, which is the sedative of choice on the neurointensive care unit. Care must be taken to avoid hypotension. Adjunct analgesic infusions are often used. Muscle relaxants have no direct effect on ICP, but may prevent rises produced by coughing and straining on the endotracheal tube. They may also facilitate mechanical ventilation and maintenance of oxygenation in the presence of pulmonary injury.

Posture

A neutral position of the head and neck with moderate head-up tilt (15–20°) is best to facilitate cerebral venous drainage and reduce ICP. Care must be taken to ensure there is no reduction in blood pressure.

Osmotherapy

Although 0.5 g/kg mannitol effectively reduces cerebral oedema and ICP in acute settings, chronic mannitol therapy in intensive care is not associated with improved neurological outcome.[23] It should only be administered when needed for specific indications, and discontinued if significant and sustained reductions in ICP are not achieved. Plasma osmolality should be regularly monitored during mannitol therapy. There has been recent interest in the use of hypertonic saline solutions for ICP reduction.

Hyperventilation

Hyperventilation was once the mainstay of treatment to reduce ICP by reducing cerebral blood volume. However, this is achieved by cerebral vasoconstriction and there is a risk of worsening cerebral ischaemia. Focal reductions in CBF probably occur more frequently than previously imagined, and focal ischaemia, often undetectable with conventional monitoring, might be common even during modest hyperventilation. A prospective randomised study of empirical hyperventilation after serious head injury demonstrated an adverse effect on outcome,[24] although the target $P\text{CO}_2$ (3.3 kPa) was excessively low. A target $P\text{CO}_2$ below 4.5 kPa is not recommended for blind therapy, but in cases of intractable intracranial hypertension responsive to hyperventilation, reduction below 4.5 kPa should be guided by SjvO_2 monitoring to minimise the risk of additional ischaemia.[22]

Other

CSF drainage via a ventriculostomy and decompressive craniectomy is increasingly used to reduce ICP.

Temperature

Moderate hypothermia (32–34°C) reduces neuronal damage in animal models of serious head injury, and several small clinical studies over the past decade have demonstrated benefit from early and late therapeutic hypothermia. However, a recent randomised multicentre study found no difference in neurological outcome when treated with 48 hours of moderate hypothermia compared to those maintained at normal temperature. However, it did suggest that rapid rewarming of patients who present with hypothermia may be deleterious.[25] Moderate hypothermia remains an effective adjunct to controlling elevated ICP in some patients and part of treatment protocols in many neurointensive care units. Pyrexia is common and an independent predictor of poor outcome. Although the effect of controlling pyrexia on clinical outcome has not been tested, it should probably be treated aggressively.

Systemic complications

Acute lung injury (ALI) is common after serious head injury, secondary to direct pulmonary injury, aspiration, neurogenic pulmonary oedema,[26] and as a complication of treatment.[21] Pneumonia occurs in over 40% of patients and usually presents some days after injury.

Significant cardiovascular complications may also occur and include cardiac arrhythmias, T- wave and ST segment changes, and neurogenic hypertension. Myocardial ischaemia occurs in about 50% of patients, probably related to excessive stimulation of the sympathetic nervous system. This acute, usually reversible, cardiac injury ranges from hypokinesis with normal cardiac output to low-output cardiac failure. Anterior and posterior pituitary insufficiency may contribute to cardiovascular instability in some patients.

Management of systemic complications presents a significant challenge because established ventilatory strategies for ALI may be inappropriate after head injury. The prone position and permissive hypercarbia are both contraindicated in the presence of raised ICP, and fluid restriction to reduce alveolar oedema conflicts with the requirement to maintain cerebral perfusion. Positive end-expiratory pressure (PEEP) has traditionally been avoided in head injury to prevent rises in ICP, but ventilation without PEEP often fails to correct hypoxaemia in ALI. With proper volume resuscitation, PEEP up to 10 cmH_2O does not increase ICP and may even result in a decrease because of improved cerebral oxygenation.

Haemodynamic instability is common after severe head injury. The initial hyperdynamic phase is often followed by hypotension refractory to fluid resuscitation and catecholamine vasopressors. Such patients may respond to a low-dose vasopressin infusion. Good neurological outcome depends upon the prevention of hypoxaemia and hypotension at all stages of management. Timely and appropriate intervention to optimise cardiorespiratory function minimises the risk of secondary brain injury.

References

1. Zornow MH, Todd MM, Moore SS. The acute cerebral effects of changes in plasma osmolality and oncotic pressure. Anesthesiol 1987; 67:936–941.
2. Tommasino C. Fluids and the neurosurgical patient. Anesthesiol Clin North Am 2002; 20:329–346.
3. Cooper DJ, Myles PS, McDermott FT, et al. Prehospital hypertonic saline resuscitation of patients with hypotension and severe traumatic brain injury: a randomized controlled trial. JAMA 2004; 291:1350–1357.
4. Sneyd JR. Propofol and epilepsy. Br J Anaesth 1999; 82:168–169.
5. Gelb AW, Salevsky F, Chung F, Ringaert K, et al. Remifentanil with morphine transitional analgesia shortens neurological recovery compared to fentanyl for supratentorial recovery. Can J Anaesth 2003; 50:946–952.
6. Sarang A, Dinsmore J. Anaesthesia for awake craniotomy. Br J Anaesth 2003; 90:161–165.
7. Petersen KD, Landsfeldt U, Cold GE, et al. Intracranial pressure and cerebral hemodynamic in patients with cerebral tumors: a randomized prospective study of patients subjected to craniotomy in propofol–fentanyl, isoflurane–fentanyl, or sevoflurane–fentanyl anesthesia. Anesthesiol 2003; 98:329–336.
8. Talke P, Caldwell JE, Brown R, Dodson B, Howley J, Richardson C. A comparison of three anesthetic techniques in patients undergoing craniotomy for supratentorial intracranial surgery. Anesth Analg 2002; 95:430–435.
9. Todd MM, Warner DS, Sokell MD, et al. A prospective comparative trial of three anesthetics for elective supratentorial craniotomy. Anesthesiol 1993; 78:1005–1020.
10. Hunt K, Bajekal R, Calder I, Meacher R, O'Sullivan C, Acheson J. Changes in intraocular pressure in anesthetized prone patients. J Neurosurg Anesthesiol 2004; 16:287–290.

11. Cottrell JE, Hartung J. Cool it on cooling – at least during aneurysm surgery. J Neurosurg Anesthesiol 2004; 16:113–114.

12. Pasternak JJ, McGregor DG, Lanier WL. Effect of single dose dexamethasone on blood glucose concentration in patients undergoing craniotomy. J Neurosurg Anesthesiol 2004; 16:122–125.

13. Calder I, Picard J, Chapman M, O'Sullivan C, Crockard HA. Mouth opening – a new angle. Anesthesiol 2003; 99:799–801.

14. The Brain Trauma Foundation. Guidelines for the management of severe head injury. American Association of Neurological Surgeons, Joint Section on Neurotrauma and Critical Care. J Neurotrauma 1996; 13:641–734.

15. Maas AI, Dearden M, Teasdale GM, et al. European Brain Injury Consortium – Guidelines for management of severe head injury in adults. Acta Neurochir (Wien) 1997; 139:286–294.

16. Chesnut RM. Avoidance of hypotension: conditio sine qua non of successful severe head injury management. J Trauma 1997; 42:S4–S9.

17. Patel HC, Menon DK, Tebbs S, Hawker R, Hutchinson PJ, Kirkpatrick PJ. Specialist neurocritical care and outcome from head injury. Intens Care Med 2002; 28:547–553.

18. Lam AM, Winn HR, Cullen BF, et al. Hyperglycaemia and neurological outcome in patients with head injury. J Neurosurg 1991; 75:545–551.

19. Robertson CS. Management of cerebral perfusion pressure after traumatic brain injury. Anesthesiol 2001; 95:1513–1517.

20. Rosner MJ, Rosner SD, Johnson AH. Cerebral perfusion pressure: management protocol and clinical results. J Neurosurg 1995; 83:949–962.

21. Robertson CS, Valadka AB, Hannay HJ, et al. Prevention of secondary ischemic insults after severe head injury. Crit Care Med 1999; 27:2086–2095.

22. Cruz J. The first decade of continuous monitoring of jugular bulb oxyhemoglobin saturation: management strategies and clinical outcome. Crit Care Med 1998; 26:344–351.

23. Roberts I, Schierhout G, Wakai A. Mannitol for acute traumatic brain injury. Cochrane Database Syst Rev 2003; 2:CD001049.

24. Muizelaar JP, Marmarou A, Ward JD, et al. Adverse effects of prolonged hyperventilation in patients with severe head injury. A randomized clinical trial. J Neurosurg 1991; 75:731–739.

25. Clifton GL, Miller ER, Choi SC, et al. Lack of effect of induction of hypothermia after acute brain injury. N Engl J Med 2001; 344:566–563.

26. Bratton SL, Davis RL. Acute lung injury in isolated traumatic brain injury. Neurosurg 1997; 40:707–712.

CHAPTER **5.8**

OBSTETRICS

PREGNANCY: ANATOMY AND PHYSIOLOGY

Parturition produces major physiological changes in the mother as a result of the effects of placental and pituitary hormones and the enlarged tissue mass (breasts, uterus and fetus).

The enlarged uterus pushes the diaphragm and heart upwards, resulting in ECG changes of right axis deviation (large Q and inverted T waves in lead III) and decreasing the vertical depth of the thorax, thereby reducing the functional residual capacity from the 20th week and potentiating airway closure. Minute ventilation increases by up to 50%, with a reduction in end-tidal carbon dioxide. Peak expiratory flow rate is unchanged. Cardiac output reaches a peak at term, an increase of about 30–50% normal, mainly by an increase in heart rate, vasodilation and increased blood volume. These changes stress a diseased heart in the third trimester.

Haematological investigations include a reduced haematocrit (because the percentage increase in red blood cells is less than the increase in plasma volume) and a hypercoagulable state.

Mechanisms for pain during parturition

Autonomic nerves that originate in the uterus pass through the hypogastric sympathetic plexuses into the spinal cord in segments T10–L1 and thence are relayed to the thalamus and cortex. The pelvic floor has a somatic innervation through the pudendal nerves to sacral segments. Hence the pain of labour is mediated by both visceral and somatic nociceptors, partly depending on the stage of labour, and is experienced predominantly in the lower abdomen (as referred pain) and perineum. Visceral pain is often accompanied by autonomic symptoms such as nausea and vomiting. The fetus, when presenting in the posterior position, may alter pain patterns because of constant pressure on tissues.

Some of the drugs used for pain relief have altered pharmacokinetics and pharmacodynamics during parturition as a result of hormonal and cardiovascular effects. For example, lidocaine (lignocaine) is less protein bound and nerves are more sensitive to local anaesthetic drugs. Lower doses of local anaesthetic agents are used in pregnant than in non-pregnant women.

Neuraxial nerve blocks in pregnant women may extend higher than in a non-pregnant person.

Placental transfer of drugs occurs to some extent with all agents, especially those with a high lipid solubility and minimal ionisation. Occasionally drugs are altered or destroyed in their passage across the placenta.

Summary of anatomical and physiological changes

The anatomical and physiological changes of pregnancy (with risks for anaesthesia summarised in brackets) are:

- increased basal metabolic rate (hypoxia occurs faster);
- enlarging abdominal mass and decreased sphincter tone (regurgitation, aspiration);
- reduced functional residual capacity (reduced oxygen reserve on pre-oxygenation);
- altered airway anatomy (failure to intubate);
- increased blood flow to uterus/placenta (potential for haemorrhage);
- enlarged uterus (uterine atony and bleeding; aortocaval occlusion/supine hypotension).

Aortocaval occlusion (supine hypotensive) syndrome

When the enlarging uterus presses on the major vessels in the abdomen, starting at about 20 weeks of gestation, the degree of occlusion will depend on the pressure within the vessel (e.g. a higher pressure is needed to occlude the aorta than the inferior vena cava [IVC]), and on the position of the vessel in relation to the uterus (e.g. the aorta is left of the IVC). Hence it is rational to position a woman in the left tilted position to avoid IVC occlusion. However, aortic occlusion may compromise uterine blood flow.

If the IVC is occluded, venous return to the heart may be reduced. However, compensation is usual through vasoconstriction and diverted blood flow through the azygos system via the paravertebral and extradural veins. Once this venous compensation is removed (e.g. by sympathetic nerve paralysis induced by extradural analgesia) then IVC occlusion becomes more hazardous for both mother and fetus.

MATERNAL MORTALITY

The commonest causes of maternal death[1] are hypertensive states, haemorrhage and pulmonary embolism. General anaesthetic deaths are mainly associated with aspiration of stomach contents (e.g. women not starved) or hypoxia (e.g. with difficult intubation) and regional anaesthesia with hypotension from any cause complicated by sympathetic nerve block.

Critical care for women at risk may be required in intensive care units in up to 1% of women and in high-dependency units for at least those women who have caesarean section. Coexisting morbidities can add to the risk.

General anaesthetic risks

Aspiration of stomach contents

Regurgitation (passive) and vomiting (active) may result in aspiration of liquids or solids. Preparation for anaesthesia begins with:

- a policy of nil by mouth for at least 4 hours, if not longer – prior use of opioids can delay stomach emptying;
- reduction in gastric acid production (e.g. H_2-blockers, plus antacids).

For the past decade a non-solids oral regimen during labour is considered to have maintained a reduced frequency of inhalation. The plan of prophylactic management includes:

- restriction of food;
- reduction of acid production (e.g. oral ranitidine 150 mg twice daily – started the night before anaesthesia, or intravenous ranitidine 50 mg slowly, preferably 2 hours before anaesthesia);
- neutralisation of any acid produced (e.g. clear alkaline solution such as 0.3 mmol/L sodium citrate 30 mL given just before anaesthesia);
- increasing lower oesophageal sphincter tone (e.g. prokinetic drugs such as metoclopramide 10 mg intravenously).

With these preparations, physically emptying the stomach using a large-bore gastric tube is rarely contemplated. However, use of equipment for such procedures may prevent aspiration if a woman presents unprepared for general anaesthesia following a large meal.

Further preparations perioperatively (i.e. on induction and extubation) include the rapid availability of a functioning wide-bore suction tube, a tilting table and facilities to protect the larynx using a cuffed tracheal tube. Tracheal suction may also be required.

The clinical features of aspiration may take hours to start after the event and include bronchospasm, dyspnoea, oxygen desaturation, tachycardia, hypotension, hypoxia and metabolic acidosis. Investigations may show radiographic changes, and the differential diagnosis includes pulmonary embolism and asthma. A diagnosis may be made by checking the pH of tracheal aspirate or by observing solids in the trachea. The symptoms and signs may be severe and respiratory support in an ITU may be required.

Failed intubation

Pregnancy is a contributing factor to failed intubation because it results in an increase in breast size, which impedes laryngoscopy, an increase in soft tissue mass around the airway making it more difficult to visualise the larynx, and an increase in metabolic rate and decrease in the reservoir of oxygen in the functional residual capacity after preoxygenation, thus increasing the risk of hypoxia if the lungs are not ventilated. See Chapter 2.6 for a plan of management.

At caesarean section, if intubation fails the mother is awakened and a regional nerve block is considered. Because of the risk of total spinal anaesthesia an extradural block is also contraindicated, so that a spinal nerve block is the best option.

Anaesthetic outpatient clinic

To prevent morbidity and mortality, weekly clinics have developed where women with potential anaesthetic problems can be reviewed before anaesthetic intervention or where women who have suffered complications have time for follow-up and debriefing. Combined clinics for cardiac and diabetic patients also have a risk management role. The types of patient referred to such clinics include those with previous back surgery, back pain or previous unacceptably painful labours, and patients with coagulation disorders.

PAIN RELIEF DURING LABOUR AND DELIVERY

Non-pharmacological

Drugs may cross the placenta to the fetus and any method that avoids this or restricts their use is potentially attractive. In the 1950s Grantly Dick Read taught so-called 'natural childbirth' with a focus on the woman's control of breathing and relaxation. The Cochrane collaboration has established that water immersion can reduce analgesic requirements in the first stage of labour,[2] and hypnosis warrants further investigation as a suitable method.[3] Transcutaneous electrical nerve stimulation (TENS) can be used, but the evidence for its effectiveness is inadequate.[4]

Pharmacological methods

The acute pain of labour can be inhibited through the activation of a number of neurotransmitter systems, for example opioids and γ-aminobutyric acid (GABA) or the inhibition of excitatory systems (e.g. *N*-methyl-D-aspartate [NMDA] and sodium channels).

Inhalational agents

Volatile anaesthetics (isoflurane, sevoflurane, desflurane) can be used in subanaesthetic concentrations (to avoid uterine relaxation effects) with or without nitrous oxide. Usually a draw-over breathing system is used, but these are not widely available and are not approved for independent midwifery practice. Cumulative effects on the mother and neonate have been recorded following use.

Nitrous oxide is safe for the mother and fetus in pre-mixed concentrations of 50:50 with oxygen (Entonox).[5] At higher concentrations pain relief increases, but safety is compromised by an increased risk of sedation and loss of the airway. For optimal results with Entonox, inhalation is encouraged to begin at the start of a contraction.

Parenteral agents

Opioids (e.g. diacetyl morphine [heroin, diamorphine], pethidine [meperidine], buprenorphine, meptazinol) have been used during labour. In the UK, independent midwives can use pethidine in divided doses up to 200 mg.

After maternal administration placental transfer occurs for all opioids and their effects depend on dose, perfusion (placenta and fetal circulation) and time since administration. In the neonate the adverse central nervous system depressant effects of μ opioids (MOP) may be reversed using naloxone.

Patient-controlled analgesia (PCA) is an alternative to a regional nerve block during labour, e.g. when women have bleeding disorders. Fentanyl and remifentanil have been used.[6] The dose for fentanyl is a bolus of 10–25 μg with a lockout of 3–5 minutes and no background infusion. The paediatrician should be warned that the baby may need an opioid antagonist (e.g. naloxone).

Neuraxial agents

For the use of extradural blockade in labour, the midwife managing the mother must be trained and competent in the delivery of analgesia by this technique. It is a usual policy that extradural opioids are to be avoided if a mother has had intramuscular pethidine within 4 hours to avoid maternal respiratory depression.

Before an extradural nerve block is sited the stage of labour is assessed, fetal heart rate is monitored, and the maternal blood pressure is measured. The anaesthetist must be aware of the full obstetric and medical history of the woman and discuss the risks and benefits to her before extradural catheter insertion. A witnessed verbal consent is essential.

Once the catheter is in place the anaesthetist can give the first dose of the analgesic mixture, and subsequent doses are prescribed or given directly by the anaesthetist if there is a particular indication (e.g. dural tap).

Monitoring of maternal blood pressure, pulse and fetal heart rate is essential following a top-up dose because of adverse drug effects.

Following all neuraxial nerve blocks in labour a postnatal ward round to check for satisfaction and complications is part of normal patient care. No patient should be discharged less than 6 hours after their last top-up extradural injection.

The opioid receptor agonists fentanyl, diamorphine, sufentanil and pethidine have all been used via the neuraxial route to manage labour pain and are usually combined with sodium channel blockers (e.g. local anaesthetics).

Pethidine acts not only at the opioid receptors, but also at sodium channels, and a local anaesthetic type nerve blockade when given neuraxially can provide analgesia.

Opioid drugs are used off licence for intrathecal indications and so neurotoxic constituents should be avoided.

The opioids can induce synergistic effects on the quality of nerve blockade and this property is valuable in obstetric analgesia and anaesthesia. Side-effects of opioids may be troublesome. Pruritus is common and an opioid antagonist, naloxone, titrated to effect or chlorphenamine (chlorpheniramine) can be used as treatment. Gastric stasis and frank vomiting are other common problems.

Paracervical block

Local anaesthetic drug effects on the fetus often complicate paracervical block.

Differences between parenteral opioids and regional nerve block.

Large randomised controlled studies of regional nerve block or comparisons with systemic opioid analgesia have not shown any major detrimental effects of regional nerve block.[7,8]

REGIONAL NERVE BLOCK DURING LABOUR AND DELIVERY

All regional nerve blocks require sterile precautions, intravenous access, resuscitation drugs and appropriate staff (anaesthetists and midwives) available. A low-dose extradural block (LDE) is designed to achieve minimal motor nerve block and avoid other adverse effects by combining a local anaesthetic agent with an opioid.

Managing general risks

To reduce the risks of regional nerve blockade during labour and delivery it is necessary to:

- use an aseptic technique;
- have resuscitation facilities available;
- prevent accidental intravenous injection by aspiration before injection;
- test with an adequate dose to induce motor nerve block for inadvertent intrathecal injection – for example 15 mL of 0.1% bupivacaine =

15 mg = 3 mL of 0.5% bupivacaine or 3 mL of 2% lidocaine (lignocaine);

- manage the various causes of hypotension – supine position, bleeding, sympathetic nerve blockade etc.;
- be aware that opioids are associated with gastric stasis and hence pose potential airway aspiration problems;
- provide support for mothers when they are mobile because motor control can be slightly impaired;
- be aware that sepsis (chorioamnionitis) can increase maternal temperature and hence the fetal temperature, precipitating fetal tachycardia during prolonged extradural analgesia.

Finally, resuscitation of the fetus for severe fetal distress may be necessary.

Techniques of regional nerve blockade

The fastest onset of analgesia is obtained by using a spinal injection, but longer-term pain relief is only realistic if an extradural catheter is in position. The time to effective analgesia with extradural analgesia is about 20 minutes, but pain relief starts sooner.

If the combined spinal extradural (CSE) or LDE mixtures fail and the mother has pain there are a number of options. If the pain is unilateral an additional top-up dose with the painful side dependent may be sufficient; a stronger concentration can be used with the same positioning; or if these fail then the catheter may be pulled out 1 cm in case it has migrated to one side.

If there is no block after the block has been successful, either another top-up is needed or the catheter may have come out of the space. A repeat insertion may be required or conversion to a CSE because labour has progressed.

Drugs can be delivered into an extradural catheter by different methods – patient-controlled extradural analgesia (PCEA),[9] top-ups and infusions.

Drugs for pain relief

Bupivacaine

Bupivacaine plain (a racemic mixture of L- and D-bupivacaine) is used in concentrations from 0.0625 to 0.25% for labour analgesia, though the weaker solutions (e.g. 0.1%) require support from added opioid, such as fentanyl 2 μg/mL. Premixed solutions are preferred to reduce drug administration errors. Doses can range from 10–15 mL and are used as an LDE regimen. The advantages are smaller dose, therefore safer; minimal effect on muscle strength, thus preserving movement; bladder sensation may be retained. It is the advantage of mobility that has given rise to the term 'mobile extradural'; however, the term has also been applied to a CSE technique.

For the spinal component of a CSE a suitable dose is 0.25% bupivacaine 1 mL and 15–25 μg fentanyl, or if there is a premixed 0.1% solution of bupivacaine with 2 μg/mL of fentanyl then 3–5 mL of this solution can be administered. This dose can be injected through a 27 G spinal needle positioned within the extradural needle before inserting the extradural catheter.

Ropivacaine

Ropivacaine (structural isomer of bupivacaine) has been used in concentrations of 0.2% for labour analgesia,

L-Bupivacaine

L-Bupivacaine (levobupivacaine) demonstrates less motor block and cardiotoxicity than the stereoisomer D-bupivacaine (in the racemic bupivacaine mixture).[10]

Lidocaine (lignocaine)

Lidocaine (lignocaine), from 0.5 to 1.0%, has a duration of action of 1–2 hours, and over time tachyphylaxis occurs.

Others

Neostigmine induces nausea and vomiting and α_2-adrenergic blocking drugs may demonstrate hypotensive side-effects.

Vasopressors

Ephedrine is an indirectly acting vasopressor with mixed action at adrenoreceptors, and is given in doses from 3–6 mg or as a 30 mg infusion. Ephedrine can cause tachycardia, exhibits tachyphylaxis, and is associated with fetal acidosis, unlike methoxamine and phenylephrine, which are both α-adrenergic agonists. Phenylephrine is potentially the drug of choice in a dose of 100 μg as required.[11] Its direct action may speed its onset and the lack of heart rate increase (often accompanied by bradycardia) makes it appropriate where tachycardia is a presenting feature of hypotension.

Extradural (extradural) anaesthesia

Lumbar extradural blockade

Lumbar extradural nerve block has been established as an effective analgesic in most situations during childbirth. Previous caesarean section is not a contraindication, and with a low-dose technique pain (from scar or uterus) or fetal bradycardia can indicate impending uterine rupture, sometimes together with cardiovascular instability.

Contraindications

Contraindications of lumbar extradural nerve block are few, but relate to serious complications, including:

- patient refusal (but, consider the risks of general anaesthesia);
- infection (e.g. local sepsis);
- potential for trauma to the spinal cord (e.g. coagulation defect [pre-eclampsia, coagulation therapy, pre-existing disorder], increasing the risk of pressure effects from a haematoma);
- potential for hypovolaemia and hypotension (e.g. haemorrhage, vasodilation).

The relative contraindications for which a risk–benefit ratio has to be determined and optimised are best approached electively through referrals to an anaesthetic antenatal clinic.

A coagulation screen is required at least 3 hours before regional analgesia in antepartum haemorrhage, placental abruption, anticoagulant therapy, major sepsis, liver disease, and for pre-eclampsia (see below, p. 673). A coagulation screen is not required if aspirin or non-steroidal anti-inflammatory drugs (NSAIDs) have been taken.

Managing maternal complications

The risks of extradural anaesthesia to be discussed with women include:

- failure (unilateral, unblocked segment, catheter falls out) – to be managed by a change in position or the catheter pulled out a little (aseptically) or repeat insertion;
- hypotension with avoidance of IVC occlusion (have in place intravenous line, fluids and vasopressors);
- motor blockade preventing ambulation and loss of sensation to bladder distension (by promoting regular checks to prevent bladder distension);
- post-dural puncture headache (PDPH) – prevent dural tap by using fluid for extradural space identification, and avoid movement during insertion.

The relative risks, ranked from common to rare, are itching = non-ambulation > failure > headache = transient numbness = reactions to skin preparation > nerve palsy = accidental injection (life-threatening).

Nerve damage is more common from pressure effects delivered by the fetus or obstetrician than related to nerve block.[12]

Technique

During extradural catheter insertion the fetus should be continuously monitored. The mother can sit on the bed or lie on her side. The best position is one in which she flexes her lumbar spine and does not rotate the spine.

Pillows can support her to achieve this.

The extradural space is located by a loss of resistance technique that varies with operator experience. At all times the anaesthetist has visual identification as to how far the Tuohy needle is in from the skin by the 1 cm markings on the needle.

On siting the needle check that no fluid is aspirated and for easy loss of resistance.

After passing the extradural catheter allow it to hang below the insertion so that fluid (if any) can drain down the catheter. Such fluid may be blood, saline (from the loss of resistance technique) or cerebrospinal fluid (CSF).

After 20 minutes the anaesthetist checks the nerve blockade. The mother should have warm feet, be able to raise her legs against resistance, and a reduced sensation to ethyl chloride spray should be demonstrated on both sides of her body.

During the extradural analgesia, a midwife who is adequately trained should be able to check the nerve block and call the anaesthetist if the block extends above the abdomen.

Accidental dural puncture and autologous blood patch

A dural puncture (DP) is accidental during planned extradural nerve block, in contrast to a deliberate DP during intrathecal nerve block. Any DP can result in headache, and the pain severity is influenced by the size of the hole in the dura, which in turn depends on needle size, number of punctures and bevel orientation.

Confirmation of a CSF tap is made by testing the fluid aspirated from needle or catheter, which will be:

- positive for glucose;
- warm;
- positive for protein;
- turbid when thiopental is mixed with CSF (a pH test).

If DP is diagnosed with an extradural needle in situ, conversion to spinal analgesia may be considered; however, the extradural catheter is firm and has the potential to damage the spinal cord if close by. Consideration of this approach should include the indications for regional nerve block and the ease of the technique.

In the event of the decision to site an extradural catheter intrathecally, then no more than 2 cm of the catheter should be passed into the CSF. A standard low-dose extradural of 0.1% bupivacaine and 2 μg/mL fentanyl 3–5 mL can be used as top-up doses. The catheter should be clearly marked.

An alternative approach is to site an extradural catheter in another space and explain what has happened to the patient, with discussion about management. An anaesthetist should give all doses of local anaesthetic, with full resuscitation facilities available.

Not all patients will complain of a headache (about four out of five).

Methods to prevent a headache include adequate fluids (oral, intravenous and possibly extradural) and analgesia, plus an extradural blood patch the day after delivery. A repeat patch should also be discussed with the patient, and follow-up of the woman until she is pain free is essential.

There is no evidence basis for DP management other than blood patch. A day's rest only delays the appearance of the symptoms. Caffeine 200 mg orally up to three times a day has been advocated. It has a role as a short-acting analgesic. Other, longer-acting analgesics are preferable.

Where there has been no identified DP, as occurs in about half of the patients, an alternative diagnosis should be sought. The most common is migraine. Often symptoms of DP refer to the neck and shoulder, and a muscular origin may be identified for these pains. Other more sinister diagnoses may be excluded by history, examination and investigation. Fever may indicate a febrile origin (e.g. meningitis, though chemical meningism may not demonstrate a fever). A cerebral thrombosis may complicate pregnancy more than the non-pregnant state, and cerebral pathology may be more frequent in obstetrics because of conditions such as pre-eclampsia.

There is no restriction on the mode of delivery after accidental DP with an extradural needle because there is no evidence of increasing adverse effects with expulsive manoeuvres.

A blood patch is indicated if the headache is severe and preventing normal function, and other diagnoses have been excluded. A blood patch is contraindicated if the woman is septic. Fresh maternal blood is obtained from her arm aseptically and immediately injected through a Tuohy needle. Up to 20 mL may be delivered unless the woman complains of backache or other pain. Once the decision to stop injecting has been made the needle should be flushed with saline to avoid spilling the blood into other tissues and initiating a painful inflammatory response or acting as a conduit for infection. Occasional bradycardia, for which atropine is required as treatment, has been reported. Blood cultures taken at the time of the blood patch can be useful if the woman develops pyrexia. Follow-up of the woman with a letter to her general practitioner is part of normal patient care.

Sacral (caudal) extradural blockade

For forceps delivery or episiotomy when the lumbar route is not available, a caudal approach may provide pain relief. Apart from the risks and complications mentioned above injection into the fetal head is an additional complication. Neither can it be assumed that the dural sac ends at the second sacral vertebra because there is always a small percentage of patients with abnormal anatomy.

Intradural (spinal) and combined spinal extradural (CSE) anaesthesia

The elements of the CSE technique are described above. It is useful when a woman is in the late stage of labour and experiencing severe pain. Analgesia should begin within 5 minutes, but there is a greater risk of pruritus and post-spinal headache after breaching the dura. When the spinal needle is passed, if the woman experiences paraesthesia the needle should be withdrawn and the spinal component abandoned.

Occasionally the position of the vertebral spaces is not accurate, and in at least 10% of people the spinal cord extends below the first lumbar vertebra segment, so there is a chance that the needle has touched the nerves in the intrathecal space. Further damage must be avoided. An injection of local anaesthetic solution may take away the pain, but it may also be injected into the nerve, causing traumatic pressure effects and subsequent nerve damage.

After a successful spinal injection has worn off, the next dose of local anaesthetic for the CSE will be into the extradural space and is given by an anaesthetist to check catheter placement.

OPERATIVE OBSTETRIC PROCEDURES

For all operative procedures with the fetus in situ a lateral tilt is essential to protect the mother from aortocaval occlusion and subsequent hypotension.

For any type of anaesthesia, monitoring should include blood pressure, pulse rate, electrocardiography (ECG) and oxygen saturation.

Routine checks include anaesthetic and resuscitative drugs, monitors, anaesthetic equipment and machines.[13]

Any obstetric procedure where a concentrated solution of local anaesthetic is used requires an anaesthetist to be present and an operating theatre with adequate facilities and anaesthetic assistance.

All patients for anaesthesia, whether general or regional, should be seen preoperatively. At this time information can be given about the intended procedure and its risks. A routine assessment would include a drug and allergy history, previous anaesthetics, general symptom enquiry and specific questions, such as the indications for the obstetric emergency. An examination of the airway is essential (teeth, neck and jaw movement, pharyngeal and anatomical measures) as well as the back, if a regional nerve block is the anaesthetic of choice for both mother and anaesthetist.

In the preoperative preparation the risks of surgery should be assessed in case further investigations or treatments are appropriate (e.g. blood ordered, coagulation screen).

Lithotomy position

Anaesthesia must not be induced in the lithotomy position because the pressure on the stomach can force gastric contents into the pharynx and lungs and access to the airway is more difficult. When a patient is put into this position the following risks should be minimised:

- regurgitation and aspiration of stomach contents (use a cuffed oral endotracheal tube and suck out the nasal passages before extubation);
- pressure on calf muscles inducing deep vein thrombosis (use correct position);
- limited respiratory muscle excursion (monitor and ventilate if necessary);
- pressure on peripheral nerves such as the sciatic, femoral, common fibular, posterior tibia, saphenous and brachial plexus (avoid by careful positioning and padding);
- backache from moving legs independently (always move legs together).

Instrumental and complex vaginal delivery

Anaesthesia may be required for instrumental (forceps/ventouse) and for complex vaginal (breech/twin) delivery. Where an extradural catheter is in situ the existing nerve block is assessed by an anaesthetist and extended with a top-up as far as T6 (lower sternum). If there is uncertainty about the vaginal route of delivery when a top-up is given, then a higher nerve block is indicated (to T_4 – the nipples) to be ready for a caesarean delivery. For example, for a twin delivery the assumption has to be made that a top-up is for caesarean section.

In the absence of an extradural nerve block a number of options are suitable. If caesarean section is not contemplated the possibilities are low spinal, extradural sacral block, bilateral pudendal nerve block, or general anaesthesia with a cuffed oral tracheal tube. A nerve block to T10 (umbilicus) may be adequate only if the operator limits their activity to the pelvic region.

Retained placenta

In some women there may be a state of shock or compensated hypovolaemia associated with severe blood loss or there may be a contraction ring in the uterus causing the situation, and tocolytics (such as volatile anaesthetics) are required to reverse the smooth muscle spasm, but with the likelihood of increased bleeding from the placental bed. In all cases (from minor to major blood loss) the estimated and expected blood loss needs careful assessment.

Maternal resuscitation includes oxygen, fluids (via large-bore cannulae), blood and monitoring, including urine output and coagulation. If resuscitation is incomplete then a general anaesthetic with precautions against aspiration (including rapid sequence induction) should be the method of choice. A regional anaesthetic has to aim to block to T6 (lower sternum).

Caesarean section

The operation

The obstetrician requires access through the non-muscular lower uterine segment, which is retracted once the baby is delivered. If the baby is premature and the lower segment is not formed then the main body of the uterus is incised. This approach loses more blood than normal and in future pregnancies the scar formed may dehisce. At the time of opening the abdomen, usually the bladder overlies the uterus; however, routinely a catheter is passed into the bladder to reduce distension and protect it from trauma.

Grades of urgency for caesarean section

Agreement between the obstetrician and anaesthetist determines to some extent the type of anaesthesia. Outcome may be influenced by the grade of urgency,[14] and the following definitions without a time base have been agreed:

- grade 1 – immediate threat to life of mother or fetus;
- grade 2 – maternal or fetal compromise that is not immediately life-threatening;
- grade 3 – needing early delivery, but no maternal or fetal compromise;
- grade 4 – at a time to suit the patient and maternity team.

Caesarean section is a common operation and the rate in England increased from 11% in 1990 to 22% (only about a half are grade 4) in 2002. In the US in 2002 the rate was 26%. The World Health Organization in 1985 recommended a rate of up to 15%, but its relevance to modern obstetric practice, with changes in the frequency of maternal and fetal disorders, is debatable.

What should be considered is the overall risk of maternal mortality from caesarean section being higher than that of a vaginal delivery (about 1 in 10 000). The risks of an emergency caesarean section are related to previous caesarean section, trial of labour, abnormal presentation, multiple gestations, haemorrhage, pre-eclampsia, premature labour, intrauterine growth retardation, augmented labour and medical diseases.

Anaesthetic technique

For all types of anaesthesia for caesarean section the technique includes:

- prophylaxis to prevent aspiration;
- blood sent for group and save;

- trained anaesthetic assistance;
- at least a 16 G cannula connected to intravenous fluid;
- pelvic and abdominal tilt;
- vasopressor and anticholinergic drugs available;
- oxygen (not mandatory for regional nerve block, but should be given if indicated e.g. caesarean section for fetal distress);
- oxytocin after delivery in a dose of 5 units given slowly (hypotension can result from rapid administration) – if requested an oxytocin infusion can be set up of 40 units/500 ml 0.9% saline at 125 ml/h;
- antibiotic administration as prophylaxis for sepsis (e.g. co-amoxiclav 1.2 g);
- admission to a high-dependency recovery area for at least 6 hours;
- adequate pain relief;
- adherence to thromboembolism guidelines after surgery.

Regional nerve blockade

Extradural, spinal or CSE techniques may be used. A single-shot spinal has no back-up if surgery is not finished by the time the block wears off. However, it is a popular method because of its speed. A CSE can prolong a nerve block if surgical complications are expected (e.g. slow dissection at repeat caesarean section) and also provide postoperative pain relief. The pencil-point spinal needle for a single shot may be 25 or 27 G; for a CSE a 27 G is used.

Useful doses for regional nerve block are as follows:

- extradural – 20 mL levobupivacaine 0.5% plus fentanyl 75 μg as a bolus;
- spinal – 2–3 mL heavy bupivacaine 0.5% with diamorphine 300 μg or fentanyl 20 μg. The hyperbaric solution is aimed to locate in the thoracic intrathecal space within 5 minutes; if the woman sits up for a long period the hyperbaric solution may track caudally and not rise over the pelvic brim when she is tilted on the operating table;
- CSE – a smaller dose is given than for a spinal, with a top-up through the extradural catheter of either saline or local anaesthetic.

Hypotension is common soon after a spinal nerve block because the majority of sympathetic tone in the lower part of the body is lost. A fluid preload with up to 1 L of electrolyte solution is advised, and the mother should be asked about symptoms of nausea and vomiting. Nausea often precedes hypotension. Blood pressure should be measured every minute while the nerve block is developing, and prompt treatment of deviations lower than 100 mmHg (or greater than 20% decrease) with a vasopressor is essential. If the pulse rate also decreases an anticholinergic drug should also be administered, especially if an α-adrenergic agonist is used.

The extent of the nerve block for both upper and lower (especially for an extradural nerve block) limits is measured and documented. A block to T_4 (nipples) and S5 (anal canal) is required. The type of sensation blocked is also recorded, and more than one type of sensation, especially those relating to pain sensation (thermal, prick) is advised. The sensation of touch can also relate to adequacy of block. It is not possible to block total sensation, however. Parasympathetic stimulation and visceral afferents may relay through cranial nerves, thus bypassing the spinal cord. Thus the mother requires information about the type of feelings she may experience.

If the mother complains of pain she should be believed and reassured that treatment is in hand, with rapid attempts made to relieve the pain, stopping the surgery if necessary. Various alternatives may be available – an extradural top-up, Entonox via a facemask, extradural opioids, local anaesthetic infiltration by the surgeon, and rarely intravenous boluses of fentanyl, alfentanil or ketamine may be given (with monitoring to avoid respiratory depression). The choice may depend on the time of the pain, the fetus in situ and surgical complications. General anaesthesia may be the best option if surgery has recently started, and a maternal request for general anaesthesia should not go unheeded. Records of all manoeuvres, drugs given, explanations and responses should be made in the patient's notes.

Combinations of analgesics can relieve pain after surgery. If intrathecal fentanyl has been used and an extradural catheter is in place diamorphine 2.5 mg in 10 mL can be injected for longlasting pain relief. No systemic opioids should then be given for 6 hours. Rectal paracetamol and/or diclofenac are available if not contraindicated (e.g. because of peptic ulcer, asthma, and impaired renal function, as may occur with pre-eclampsia). Morphine in boluses can be given and a PCA or oral codeine/dihydrocodeine prescribed. The opioids and NSAIDs are best given regularly.

In addition, regular antiemetics and laxatives are vital to return the mother to normal function.

General anaesthesia

A rapid sequence induction is required with thiopental and suxamethonium, cricoid pressure applied before induction of anaesthesia, a functioning suction, and equipment at hand for a difficult intubation. A smaller cuffed endotracheal tube may be appropriate, but no less than 6.0 mm because of airway resistance effects.

Anaesthesia should be monitored and maintained with an adequate amount of anaesthetic agents to prevent awareness. Nitrous oxide can be used with isoflurane and atracurium or vecuronium for neuromuscular paralysis. Monitoring the effects of a neuromuscular blocking agent with a nerve stimulator and checking for reversal of paralysis before awakening is essential. Occasionally women are sensitive to the effects of neuromuscular blocking agents (e.g. because of abnormal pseudocholinesterase levels) and a prolonged neuromuscular block is experienced. Pain relief should be considered intraoperatively and be in place before the end of surgery (e.g. intravenous morphine followed by PCA morphine, bilateral ilioinguinal nerve blocks).

On completion of the caesarean section the mother is moved on to her side to prevent aspiration and extubated when awake and responding to commands to open her mouth.

Awareness and general anaesthesia

This hazard complicates inadequate anaesthesia. It can result from enthusiasm to limit fetal sedation or from drug or equipment error. The medicolegal consequences demand an adequate record, especially of the volatile anaesthetic agents used and any cerebral monitoring. Signs of awareness are not reliable and the only sure way to know if it has happened is a direct question on postoperative follow-up. A satisfactory explanation should be given if the patient has memory for events.

Cervical suture

All types of anaesthesia have been used for cervical suture. New drugs are to be avoided because of their potential effects on the fetus. Safe drugs for general anaesthesia include thiopental and isoflurane. Nitrous oxide is to be avoided. For regional anaesthesia an adequate block is required with good pain relief after the procedure.

When an intra-abdominal suture is used early in pregnancy general anaesthesia is preferred. Later in pregnancy regional anaesthesia is the method of choice because of the potential for a 20+ week gestation to have effects on the gastrointestinal tract that could lead to aspiration of stomach contents. However, control of the cardiovascular system with prevention of hypotension that could stress the fetus is an important goal. Return home more than 6 hours after such a regional procedure is reasonable if the woman is able to walk, has passed urine, and has no pain and her vital signs are stable.

CRITICAL CARE IN OBSTETRICS

Pre-eclampsia and eclampsia

Pre-eclampsia is thought to be a multisystem disorder of blood vessels and commonly associated with placental mechanisms of implantation after about 20 weeks of gestation. Both pre-eclampsia and eclampsia can occur days after delivery. The diagnosis is made on a constellation of features as follows:

- mild pre-eclampsia is defined as a diastolic blood pressure above 90 mmHg and 1+ proteinuria (>0.3 g/24 h);

- severe pre-eclampsia is defined when systolic blood pressure is over 160 mmHg or the diastolic blood pressure is over 110 mmHg on two occasions more than 4 hours apart with 3+ proteinuria (>3 g/24 h). Oedema is not essential. Additional symptoms include hypogastric tenderness (from liver involvement), visual disturbance, headache and nausea and vomiting;
- eclampsia is manifest if convulsions occur;
- haemolysis, elevated liver enzymes and low platelets (HELLP) syndrome may be another form of presentation with elevated lactate dehydrogenase (LDH) and aspartate aminotransferase (AST);
- trends in investigations include full blood count (FBC), urea and electrolytes (U & E), urate and liver function tests (LFTs) every 12 hours can be used to support the diagnosis;
- trends in clinical signs as well as blood pressure (quarter-hourly) and urine output (hourly), including muscle tone (clonus, hyperreflexia), and fetal Doppler measurements for reduced blood flow, are used in diagnosis and monitoring. There is no single investigation or clinical sign that is diagnostic of pre-eclampsia; other medical conditions, e.g. epilepsy may have to be excluded.

Specific anaesthetic problems

Specific anaesthetic problems of pre-eclampsia and eclampsia are as follows:

- laryngeal oedema;
- coagulation abnormalities contraindicating regional anaesthesia (e.g. platelets $<80 \times 10^9$/L and with the potential for bleeding during surgery);
- pulmonary oedema from leaking endothelium – potentiated by sepsis, fluid overload, corticosteroids for a premature fetus etc;
- risk of convulsions (during regional nerve block);
- exaggerated hypertensive response to laryngoscopy (opioids are often used to overcome this, but they can potentially induce neonatal respiratory depression and the paediatrician should be alerted to this problem) or drugs having sympathomimetic properties (e.g. epinephrine (adrenaline) added to local anaesthetic solutions;
- use of magnesium sulphate ($MgSO_4$) can induce prolonged neuromuscular block, dysrrhythmias;
- close monitoring of renal function to prevent deterioration;
- eclampsia is not an emergency and pressure for an immediate general anaesthetic can add extra risk;

- risk of placental abruption. Bleeding from this cause may manifest as hypotension during labour extradural but not be recognised.

All obstetric units are expected to have guidelines for the management of pre-eclampsia and eclampsia. There is no curative treatment, but therapy can slow progress and allow a successful outcome. Overtreatment can induce hypotension that can precipitate maternal cerebral ischaemia and acute placental insufficiency. The following points have been included in recent guidelines for management on a high dependency unit:

- target blood pressure is 140/90 mmHg;
- use parenteral drugs for easy titration and immediate cessation;
- continuous fetal cardiotocograph monitoring;
- fluids to maintain plasma volume unless there is significant renal impairment or pulmonary oedema with a central venous pressure over 10 cmH_2O;
- drugs – labetalol before hydralazine before nifedipine (slow-release tablets 20 mg). Hydralazine used to be first choice, but it can cause tachycardia and headache and is more likely to induce maternal hypotension.

Specific anaesthetic management

Specific anaesthetic management for delivery of a treated pre-eclamptic woman is as follows:

- recent blood results (full blood count, urea and electrolytes, liver function tests);
- coagulation tests within 3 hours of anaesthesia (if the recent platelet count is $>100 \times 10^9$/L a coagulation screen is not essential);
- nil by mouth;
- antacid prophylaxis – ranitidine, sodium citrate;
- withhold low molecular weight heparin (LMWH), ideally for 12 hours.

Magnesium sulphate

The MAGPIE trial[15] was designed for women with pre-eclampsia who were randomised to either control or $MgSO_4$. It showed that with $MgSO_4$, out of 1000 pre-eclamptic women eleven fewer would progress to eclampsia, compared with no $MgSO_4$. The women most at risk are Afro-Caribbean, and it may be in this group that $MgSO_4$ should be used. The effects of $MgSO_4$ have to be closely monitored and clinical signs of toxicity include slow respiration, loss of muscle reflexes, drowsiness, paralysis and cardiorespiratory arrest. The antidote for magnesium toxicity is 10 mL calcium gluconate 10% injection. The therapeutic range is 2–4 mmol/L measured 4–6 hours after the loading dose. Levels should be checked if toxic effects or a convulsion occur. $MgSO_4$ is contraindicated in acute renal or cardiac failure.

Amniotic fluid embolism

A dramatic change in cardiorespiratory status at the time of membrane rupture (e.g. at caesarean section) may indicate the passage of amniotic fluid into the general circulation. Collapse, desaturation, respiratory distress and coma suddenly present and death is common. The resultant haematological effects of the amniotic fluid are to induce disseminated intravascular coagulation (DIC) with hypofibrinaemia and excessive bleeding. These signs may be the first indication of the condition. The diagnosis may be confirmed if quantities of fetal tissues are present in maternal fluids or tissues. If the mother is resuscitated her ECG may show signs of right heart strain because the pulmonary circulation may be blocked by fibrin deposits.

Disseminated intravascular coagulation

The diagnosis of DIC is made by a coagulation screen, and widespread abnormalities are measured, often with fibrin degradation products. DIC is associated with major haemorrhage, intrauterine fetal death, amniotic fluid embolism and hydatidiform mole. Continuing bleeding may be the first sign as fibrin and fibrinogen are destroyed by fibrinolysins or products in the amniotic fluid stop the conversion of prothrombin to thrombin. A fibrinogen less than 150 mg/100 mL is characteristic. Specialist advice from haematology is valuable and products such as fresh frozen plasma and fibrinogen may be required.

Convulsions

The differential diagnosis for convulsions is from the following:

- local anaesthetic toxicity;
- eclampsia;
- amniotic fluid embolism;
- total spinal anaesthesia;
- hypoxia (e.g. from pulmonary embolism);
- poor control of epilepsy (not unusual because the normal doses of antiepileptic drugs have to be increased in line with the increase in plasma volume).

SUDDEN COLLAPSE IN OBSTETRICS

Although the maternal death rate is low in developed countries, women still suffer the complications of pregnancy and may need resuscitation and often prolonged critical care.

The differential diagnosis includes:

- haemorrhage;
- sepsis;

- aortocaval occlusion;
- anaphylaxis (increasing frequency, especially from latex);
- shock from acute inversion of the uterus (with associated bradycardia from autonomic activity);
- amniotic fluid embolism;
- cerebrovascular event.

Specific maternal resuscitation activities include positioning the woman to avoid IVC occlusion (manually lift the uterus or use a human wedge), consider help in intubation, check cervical dilation and consider urgent fetal delivery. Cardiopulmonary resuscitation is unlikely to be successful with a gravid uterus.

Haemorrhage

Blood loss is common during delivery, but can occur ante- and postnatally. During delivery the uterus contracts and this releases blood into the systemic circulation. Thus on average an autotransfusion of about 500 mL occurs. This volume may not contain many red blood cells if the woman has been anaemic.

Antenatal blood loss can compromise the fetus either through a poor maternal blood supply or from direct loss of blood (e.g. placental abruption). Antepartum haemorrhage occurs from placenta praevia, placental abruption (associated with pre-eclampsia, cocaine use) or other causes. Postnatal blood loss from the reproductive tract may be less dramatic and the origin can be hard to find without surgery.

Maternity units all require a protocol for major obstetric haemorrhage and drills are now established to test the process. All maternity units should have O-negative blood available for use in an emergency, but group-specific blood is preferred.

General guidance (not in specific order) is as follows:

- an emergency call is logged into the operator;
- two large-bore intravenous cannulae are sited;
- blood is removed for crossmatch and coagulation screen and sent urgently to the laboratory;
- fluids are delivered intravenously by pressurised systems;
- fluids are warmed to body temperature;
- urine output is measured (catheter);
- monitoring of blood pressure, heart rate, respiration, temperature, fetal heart rate and contractions if applicable;
- arterial cannula is sited for monitoring and blood sampling (e.g. blood gases, acidosis);

- central venous pressure measurement – if no clotting problems access to neck may be possible; consider a long line through the antecubital fossa;
- consider drugs such as oxytocin or prostaglandin;
- longer-term management in ICU or possible radiological embolisation.

Placenta praevia

Placenta praevia is usually diagnosed on ultrasound near to term because the placenta can move away from the os during the last trimester. If the placenta lies in the path of the surgeon at caesarean section blood loss before delivery of the baby is expected. If the woman has had a previous caesarean section and has diagnosed placenta praevia the chances of a placenta accreta have to be considered.

It is before the delivery that discussions are best conducted about the potential for a hysterectomy should the bleeding be life-threatening. The type of anaesthetic selected will depend on the experience of the anaesthetist, the mother's preferences and the expected pathology. In all cases blood loss is expected, and precautions such as two large-bore intravenous lines are never misplaced. Questions arise as to whether to place an arterial line electively. A pressurised and warmed system for delivering blood is mandatory.

THROMBOEMBOLISM RISK MANAGEMENT IN PREGNANCY AND DELIVERY

Thromboembolism prophylaxis for caesarean section depends on the risk category of the woman. In the low-risk category (i.e. patients without risk), thromboembolic deterrent (TED) stockings and low molecular weight heparin (LMWH) such as enoxaparin 40 mg subcutaneously once daily after surgery are routine.

For higher-risk patients, such as those with a previous deep vein thrombosis (DVT), thrombophilia or pulmonary embolism, enoxaparin antenatally may be prescribed, in which case appropriate timing of a regional nerve block is advised.

In very high-risk women, such as those with prosthetic valves, individual regimens will be in place and a window in the use of heparin will be sought. An extradural or spinal nerve block should not be sited within 6 hours of subcutaneous heparin or 12 hours of LMWH unless there are special circumstances. Heparin should not be administered within 2 hours of an extradural or spinal injection or catheter manipulation.[16] After removal of an extradural catheter, LMWH can be given 1–2 hours later as the first dose in normal patients, and thereafter once daily. For a single-shot spinal the LMWH can be given 1–2 hours after spinal needle removal.

SEVERE FETAL DISTRESS

In severe fetal distress[17] resuscitation with the fetus in situ should be considered in all cases and may convert a 'crash' caesarean section into a more controlled situation. Steps to take are as follows.

- Full lateral position for the mother (to the opposite side if already full lateral and no fetal response).
- Oxygen – at least 6L/min by mask.
- Stop oxytocin infusion (if applicable).
- Site large-bore intravenous cannula and give fluids.
- Measure maternal blood pressure and if less than original give ephedrine 3–6 mg intravenously slowly.
- Prepare for emergency caesarean section and top-up extradural if present; consider spinal or, if no clear maternal contraindications, a general anaesthetic.
- A top-up extradural requires anaesthetic monitoring. Moving a patient onto an operating table with a full spinal block may cause cardiovascular instability as well as problems in positioning if adequate personnel are not available.

References

1. Thomas TA, Cooper GM. Editorial Board of the Confidential Enquiries into Maternal Deaths in the United Kingdom. Maternal deaths from anaesthesia. An extract from 'Why Mothers Die 1997–1999, the Confidential Enquiries into Maternal Deaths in the United Kingdom'. Br J Anaesth 2002; 89:499–508.
2. Cluett ER, Nikodem V, McCandlish R, Burns E. Immersion in water in pregnancy, labour and birth. Cochrane Database Syst Rev 2004; 2:CD000111.
3. Smith CA, Collins CT, Cyna AM, Crowther CA. Complementary and alternative therapies for pain management in labour. Cochrane Database Syst Rev 2003;2:CD003521.
4. Carroll D, Tramer M, McQuay H, Nye B, Moore A. Transcutaneous electrical nerve stimulation in labour pain: a systematic review. Br J Obstet Gynaecol 1997; 104:169–175.
5. Rosen MA. Nitrous oxide for relief of labor pain: a systematic review. Am J Obstet Gynecol 2002; 186(suppl 5):S110–S126.
6. Thurlow JA, Laxton CH, Dick A, Waterhouse P, Sherman L, Goodman NW. Remifentanil by patient-controlled analgesia compared with intramuscular meperidine for pain relief in labour. Br J Anaesth 2002; 88:374–378.
7. Wilson MJ, Cooper G, MacArthur C, Shennan A, Comparative Obstetric Mobile Extradural Trial (COMET) Study Group UK. Randomized controlled trial

comparing traditional with two "mobile" extradural techniques: anesthetic and analgesic efficacy. Anesthesiology 2002; 97:1567–1575.

8. Loughnan BA, Carli F, Romney M, Dore CJ, Gordon H. Randomized controlled comparison of extradural bupivacaine versus pethidine for analgesia in labour. Br J Anaesth 2000; 84:715–719.
9. Paech MJ. Patient-controlled extradural analgesia in obstetrics. Int J Obstet Anesth 1996; 5:115–125.
10. Bardsley H, Gristwood R, Baker H, Watson N, Nimmo W. A comparison of the cardiovascular effects of levobupivacaine and rac-bupivacaine following intravenous administration to healthy volunteers. Br J Clin Pharmacol 1998; 46:245–249.
11. Cooper DW, Carpenter M, Mowbray P, Desira WR, Ryall DM, Kokri MS. Fetal and maternal effects of phenylephrine and ephedrine during spinal anesthesia for cesarean delivery. Anesthesiology 2002; 97:1582–1590.
12. Loo CC, Dahlgren G, Irestedt L. Neurological complications in obstetric regional anaesthesia. Int J Obstet Anesth 2000; 9:99–124.
13. The Association of Anaesthetists of Great Britain and Ireland and the Obstetric Anaesthetists' Association. Guidelines for obstetric anaesthesia services. London: The Association of Anaesthetists of Great Britain and Ireland and the Obstetric Anaesthetists' Association; 1998.
14. Lucas DN, Yentis SM, Kinsella SM, et al. Urgency of caesarean section: a new classification. J Roy Soc Med 2000; 93:346–350.
15. The MAGPIE trial Collaborative group. Do women with pre-eclampsia, and their babies, benefit from magnesium sulphate? The Magpie Trial: a randomised placebo-controlled trial. Lancet 2002; 359:1877–1890.
16. Horlocker TT, Wedel DJ, Benzon H, et al. Regional anesthesia in the anticoagulated patient: defining the risks (The second ASRA Consensus conference on neuroaxial anesthesia and anticoagulation). Reg Anesth Pain Med 2003;28:172–197.
17. Thurlow JA, Kinsella SM. Intrauterine resuscitation: active management of fetal distress. Int J Obstet Anesth 2002; 11:105–116.

CHAPTER **5.9**

OPHTHALMIC SURGERY

GENERAL CONSIDERATIONS

Anaesthesia for ophthalmic surgery has changed dramatically in recent years. Much cataract surgery is now performed under topical anaesthesia only, and much vitreoretinal surgery under local anaesthetic nerve block. When general anaesthesia is used the laryngeal mask airway has generally replaced endotracheal tubes.

Anatomy of the eye and orbit

The sclera is the tough outer coat of the eye, with the transparent cornea at the front. The sclera is surrounded by Tenon's capsule, an avascular membrane. The cornea is oxygenated through both surfaces — from aqueous humour and air. Aqueous humour fills the space between the cornea and the lens, which is divided by the iris into anterior and posterior chambers.

The lens is attached to the ciliary body by the suspensory ligament. Between the ciliary body and the front edge of the retina is the pars plana, the entry point for vitreoretinal surgery. The retina and the choroid behind it are very vascular.

Six extraocular muscles move the eye (Fig. 5.9 1). There are two obliques (superior and inferior). The four rectus muscles (lateral, medial, superior and inferior) form a cone behind the eye which contains all the sensory nerves to the eye, as well as the motor nerves and the ciliary ganglion. All these muscles are extremely sensitive to muscle relaxants because of their high level of innervation.

The eye is not in the centre of the orbit, being more superior than inferior. The inferior margin of the orbit is an obvious and easily palpable landmark and drops away from the eye as it goes laterally.

Innervation

Motor innervation

Motor innervation is as follows:

- superior oblique muscle from the fourth cranial nerve (trochlear nerve);
- lateral rectus from the sixth cranial nerve (abducens nerve);

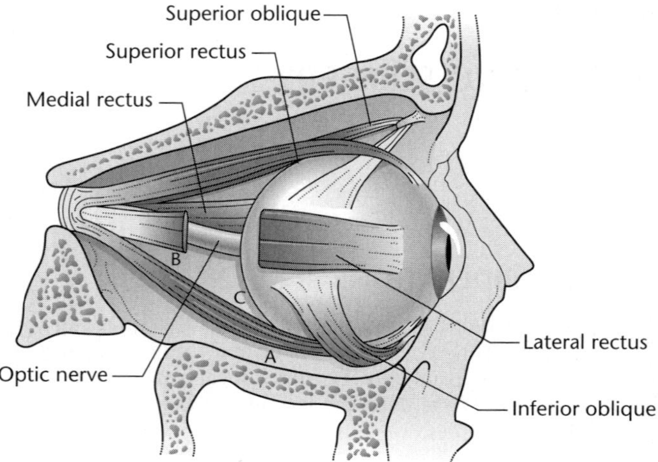

Figure 5.9.1 Diagram of the superolateral aspect of the right eye. The extraocular muscle cone is shown surrounding the optic nerve. The lateral rectus is partially excised for clarity. The intraconal structures (not shown) include the third, fourth and sixth cranial nerves supplying the extraocular muscles, the ophthalmic branch of the fifth cranial nerve (V1, sensory to the sclera and cornea), ciliary ganglion (transmitting sensory fibres to V1 and both sympathetic and parasympathetic fibres to the eye) and the retinal vessels (from the ophthalmic vessels). A and C are extra- and intraconal sites for peribulbar injections. Local anaesthetic must diffuse from site A into the cone to reach the sensory and motor neurones. B indicates the target site for a true retrobulbar injection.

- all other extraocular muscles, including levator palpebrae superioris, from the third cranial nerve (oculomotor nerve);
- orbicularis oculis by the seventh cranial nerve (facial nerve).

Sensory innervation

The optic nerve conveys vision only.

The conjunctiva is innervated superiorly from the supraorbital, supratrochlear and infratrochlear nerves and laterally from the lacrimal nerve, and the circumcorneal area from the long ciliary nerves. The sclera and cornea are innervated by the long and short ciliary nerves. All these are derived from the ophthalmic division of the fifth cranial nerve (trigeminal nerve).

The conjunctiva is innervated inferiorly from the infraorbital nerve, the terminal branch of the maxillary division of the fifth cranial nerve.

Parasympathetic innervation

Fibres from the Edinger–Westphal nucleus (parasympathetic part of the third nerve nucleus in the midbrain) run with the third cranial nerve, synapse in the ciliary ganglion, then pass via the short ciliary nerves. Stimulation causes constriction of the pupil and contraction of the ciliary muscle.

Sympathetic innervation

Fibres from T1 synapse in the superior cervical ganglion and pass via the carotid plexus to join the long ciliary nerves. Stimulation causes dilatation of the pupil.

Intraocular pressure

Normally intraocular pressure is 10–20 mmHg. It is determined by the production of aqueous humour in the ciliary body (normally 0.1 mL/h) and its absorption at the canal of Schlemm, venous sinuses at the junction of the iris and cornea.

It may be lowered by:

- intravenous anaesthetics;
- inhalational anaesthetics;
- hypotension;
- hypocapnia;
- reduction in venous pressure, including head-up tilt;
- mannitol and acetazolamide;
- mechanical pressure on the eye to increase absorption of aqueous humour.

It may be raised by:

- hypertension;
- hypercapnia;
- raised venous pressure, including head-down tilt;
- suxamethonium (transient effect);
- local anaesthetic block.

Ketamine has little effect.

LOCAL ANAESTHETIC TECHNIQUES

Topical

Local anaesthetic techniques are increasingly used for cataract surgery. Proxymetacaine 0.5%, oxybuprocaine 0.4% or tetracaine (amethocaine) 0.5%. Tetracaine (amethocaine) is an ester-linked drug and so may damage the cornea if used in excess. There is no akinesia. The iris remains sensitive. It is usually administered by the surgeon, without the help of an anaesthetist.

Sub-Tenon block

Sub-Tenon block is increasingly used for cataract surgery where a stationary eye is required. It is often unsatisfactory for vitreoretinal surgery. A blunt cannula is passed into the plane between Tenon's capsule and the sclera, and used to inject 3–5 mL of local anaesthetic. It is often administered by the surgeon without the help of an anaesthetist.

Retrobulbar block

Retrobulbar block is achieved by injection into the muscle cone behind the eye. It has been used since the mid-1930s, but is increasingly regarded as out of date and unsafe because there is a significant incidence of perforation of the globe, haemorrhage, and intradural injection through the sheath of the optic nerve.

Peribulbar block

Peribulbar block can be a true extraconal injection, allowing the local anaesthetic to diffuse into the muscle cone, or a peribulbar approach to the intraconal space. The terminology is confusing. A true retrobulbar injection implies the use of a special needle over 31 mm long and a relatively straight trajectory, whereas the peribulbar approach uses a standard 25 mm needle and a curved approach, usually through the conjunctiva.

Peribulbar block is increasingly used for vitreoretinal surgery and other forms where a greater level of akinesia and analgesia is needed. An anaesthetist should always be available.

Drugs commonly used

Drugs commonly used for nerve blocks in ophthalmic surgery are as follows:

- lidocaine (lignocaine) — usually 2%;
- bupivacaine — 0.5 or 0.75%;
- prilocaine — 2–4%;
- hyaluronidase — 7.5–15 units/mL. This improves spread of local anaesthetic solutions. Higher concentrations do not enhance its effect;
- sodium bicarbonate — 8.4%. This neutralises the acidity of the local anaesthetic solution. In ophthalmic surgery it does not seem to increase the rate of onset, but reduces the sting on injection. It also improves the activity of hyaluronidase, which is most effective at a neutral pH;

- epinephrine (adrenaline) – 1 in 200 000 solution. It is used to reduce orbital perfusion and extend the duration of the block. As the retinal arteries are end-arteries this adds unnecessary risk for minimal gain, which may be achieved by using longer-acting drugs;
- vecuronium – a small dose (0.5 mg) has been suggested to reduce the mobility of the eye but has not gained wide acceptance.

For peribulbar block the preferred solution is an equal mixture of 2% lidocaine (lignocaine) and either 0.5% or 0.75% bupivacaine, to which is added 7.5–15 units/mL of hyaluronidase. Luer-lock syringes should always be used. Caution is needed if the axial length of the globe is over 26 mm because perforation of the globe is more likely.

Technique

Inferolateral block

The commonest approach for an inferolateral block is through the conjunctiva, to which topical local anaesthesia, such as proxymetacaine, has been applied. An alternative used by some is a percutaneous approach with a subcutaneous weal.

The old point of entry (junction between the medial, and lateral third of the lower orbital margin) should be abandoned in favour of a more lateral point about 5 mm below the lateral canthus, where the orbital rim is at its lowest. A standard 25 mm orange needle (25 G) is used.

With the conjunctival approach, the tip of the needle travels around the globe with the syringe moving through 90° in a plane in a line between the needle entry point and the centre of the pupil. In a normal-sized eye (22–25 mm axial length) the length of the needle is equal to or greater than the diameter, so that when the hub of the needle is level with the cornea, the tip is beyond the globe. Thus an extra 30° drop of the syringe is possible, allowing the needle tip to enter the cone at the front. The bevel of the needle must be toward the sclera. The syringe should always be held very gently so that it travels mostly under its own weight. Normally 5 mL of solution are injected.

Medial block

Medial block has been used as the sole block, but is more commonly used in conjunction with an inferolateral block to improve akinesia.

Entry is made either superficial to the caruncle, through the caruncle or under the plica semilunaris. The angle of the needle is as flat as possible without the shaft touching the cornea. The bevel must be toward the globe.

The syringe is advanced at 90° to the midline until bone is touched. The syringe is withdrawn 1–2 mm to keep out of the periosteum and then moved parallel to the medial orbital wall, but with the syringe angled so that the needle is going away from the superonasal quadrant where the blood vessels are situated. Up to 4 mL of solution is injected, provided there is no rise in orbital pressure.

Superior block

Superior blocks should be avoided. The superonasal quadrant contains most of the blood vessels, and in the superotemporal quadrant the eye is close up under the bone with minimal space between eye and bone.

Complications

Globe perforation

Globe perforation is the most serious complication. Signs are a soft eye, blood in the eye, and loss of red reflex. If it is suspected, the patient should be referred to a vitreoretinal unit without delay.[1]

Retrobulbar haemorrhage

Retrobulbar haemorrhage is an acute haemorrhage caused by puncture of an artery. The bleeding will not stop until the area is tamponaded. It is important therefore to apply pressure as soon as possible to minimise the volume at which it tamponades to reduce the principal problem, which is the inability of the eyelids to close, leading to corneal dehydration.

Intradural injection

Intradural injection may occur if long needles are used. As for a retrobulbar block this may affect the brainstem and cause respiratory arrest.

Minor complications

Minor complications include venous bleeding which causes bruising but no rise in pressure, chemosis, and muscle weakness after return of sensation.

GENERAL ANAESTHESIA

Indications

Indications for general anaesthesia are:

- potential failure of cooperation by the patient, especially those with learning difficulties;
- patient phobias, especially severe claustrophobia;
- children;
- a lengthy operation – it is unreasonable to expect a patient to lie still for more than about 1.5 hours;
- various technical surgical problems.

Common problems

Common problems encountered by the anaesthetist are as follows:

- diabetes mellitus – many patients presenting for vitreoretinal surgery have experienced poor control of diabetes for many years, and may have impaired function of other organs such as the kidneys and heart, even at a relatively young age;
- old age – often with severe respiratory disease and cardiac disease that may be asymptomatic;
- other medical diseases – such as rheumatoid arthritis, Down's syndrome, Marfan's syndrome and a number of rarer congenital diseases, such as dystrophia myotonica, in which strabismus may occur;
- associated trauma – in cases of perforating eye injury.

Drugs used in general anaesthesia

Premedication

Premedication may be omitted. Avoid opioids because they contribute to postoperative vomiting. Antiemetics may be given routinely. Benzodiazepines are often given.

Intravenous agents

Propofol, thiopental and etomidate all reduce the pressure in normal and glaucomatous eyes.

Suxamethonium

Suxamethonium increases intraocular pressure by 7–8 mmHg on average. This rise is smaller than the fall caused by an intravenous induction agent followed by an inhalation agent, and is no reason to avoid suxamethonium when needed for intubation. The rise starts 30 seconds after administration, is maximal at 2 minutes, and has disappeared by 6 minutes. The mechanism is not fully understood. Contraction of the extraocular muscles may cause about 20% of the rise, but 80% still occurs in a curarised patient. These effects can be reduced by the prior injection of a small dose of a non-depolarising relaxant or acetazolamide 500 mg.

Non-depolarising relaxants

Non-depolarising relaxants may be used to allow intermittent positive-pressure ventilation (IPPV), which has the advantage that $P\text{CO}_2$ can be controlled.

Volatile agents

Volatile agents facilitate IPPV, and also allow quiet spontaneous respiration. They provide good conditions and cause minimal postoperative nausea.

Nitrous oxide

Nitrous oxide should be avoided when intraocular gases such as sulphur hexafluoride SF_6 or perfluoropropane C_3F_8 are used. Nitrous oxide diffuses into and enlarges any gas bubble, and must never be used if there is gas in the eye.

Non-steroidal anti-inflammatory drugs

Non-steroidal anti-inflammatory drugs (NSAIDs) are excellent for post-operative analgesia. Other simple analgesics such as paracetamol may also be used.

Suitable general anaesthetic techniques

The main priority is to avoid rises of intraocular pressure because of the risk of iris or vitreous prolapse. Ideally the eye should be soft before the anterior chamber is opened. This is particularly true for corneal graft surgery, where the eye is completely open.

Endotracheal tubes are rarely needed. The laryngeal mask usually provides an excellent airway, is less likely to cause coughing during the operation or in recovery, and less likely to cause a sore throat. In any operation where the eye is effectively open, such as corneal grafting, coughing may cause vitreous loss or expulsive haemorrhage. Where general anaesthesia is combined with local analgesia, the patient should be kept deep enough so that he or she does not move if a painful stimulus overcomes the nerve block.

Spontaneous respiration via a laryngeal mask is suitable, with enough volatile agent to prevent coughing. If ventilation is inadequate, then IPPV may be instituted with or without muscle relaxants. Alternatively, muscle relaxation (monitored with a nerve stimulator), endotracheal intubation and IPPV may be used, supplemented by intravenous or inhalation agents. This technique is more likely to cause postoperative coughing, but is necessary if the stomach may be full. It allows optimal control of $P\text{CO}_2$.

SPECIFIC OPERATIONS

Vitrectomy (including retinal detachment)

Avoid nitrous oxide because it is likely that either SF_6 or C_3F_8 gas will be used. Nitrous oxide will diffuse into the gas in the vitreous, causing an acute rise in pressure. If it has been given, it should be turned off for at least 15 minutes to allow sufficient elimination before intravitreal gas is used.

It is particularly important to avoid postoperative vomiting or coughing after retinal detachment surgery because it may cause further detachment. Posturing of the patient may be required as soon as the operation is finished. This is made easier if local anaesthesia has been used.

The addition of a scleral buckle for repair of retinal detachment is much more traumatic and may be a relative indication for general anaesthesia. It will cause more postoperative pain, best treated by combining local and general anaesthesia. NSAIDs are useful postoperatively.

Perforating eye injury

Other injuries should be considered. Induction of anaesthesia must avoid coughing and straining, which cause an acute rise in intraocular pressure with the danger of loss of vitreous. Surgery is often not urgent and the optimal time of operation must be discussed with the surgeon. Each case must be judged on its merits, attention being paid to urgency, likelihood of a full stomach and possible difficulty in tracheal intubation.

Opinions vary as to the use of suxamethonium. As it causes a rise in intraocular pressure which is less than the drop caused by the intravenous induction agent and inhalation agent, its use is justified if there is a full stomach and the need for rapid sequence induction.

If surgery is urgent, a suitable technique is preoxygenation, propofol induction, a small dose of non-depolarising relaxant to limit the rise in intraocular pressure, followed by suxamethonium and the use of cricoid pressure. Some anaesthetists prefer a generous dose of a rapid-onset non-depolarising relaxant such as rocuronium.

Squint correction

Induction with propofol followed by inhalation anaesthesia with spontaneous respiration through a laryngeal mask is usually suitable for squint correction. As the patient is often a child, gas induction may be more appropriate.

Various stimuli arising in or near the eye, especially traction on the rectus muscles or pressure on the eyeball, may cause bradycardia and arrhythmias. This is the oculocardiac reflex. It is more pronounced in the young, and may rarely cause cardiac arrest. Prophylactic use of glycopyrrolate or atropine is recommended. As always, adequate cardiac monitoring is essential. Immediate management is to ask the surgeon to relax the eye muscles, and to give intravenous atropine.

Dacrocystorhinostomy

Small amounts of blood completely occlude the surgeon's field in dacrocystorhinostomy. A nasal cocaine pack is used to cause vasoconstriction of the adjacent nasal mucosa. Head-up tilt is useful.

Dacrocystorhinostomy may be performed using local anaesthesia and sedation.

Tonometry in neonates

Tonometry in neonates may be performed using ketamine because it is the only anaesthetic agent that does not lower the intraocular pressure.

References

1. Duker JS et al. Inadvertent globe perforation during retrobulbar and peribulbar anesthesia. Patient characteristics, surgical management, and visual outcome. Ophthalmology 1991; 98:519–526.

Further reading

Kumar C, Dodds C, Fanning G. Ophthalmic anaesthesia. Liss (NL): Swets & Zeitlinger; 2002.

CHAPTER **5.10**

ORAL, DENTAL AND MAXILLOFACIAL SURGERY

Dental surgery includes simple extractions (exodontia), usually carried out for caries, but also in older children for orthodontic reasons, and restorative procedures such as conservation (filling) or crowning of teeth.

Oral surgery is more invasive such as excision of bone cysts, and the removal of third molar or supernumerary teeth involving the raising of gum flaps or the removal of bone.

Maxillofacial surgery includes operations to correct congenital deformities of the facial bones to give a normal appearance (orthognathic surgery) and operations to treat cancer.

DENTAL SURGERY

The first general anaesthetic (GA) administered in England was for the extraction of a molar tooth in a dental surgery in 1846. James Robinson, a dentist, gave the anaesthetic and performed the operation. Over the next 150 years large numbers of GAs were performed in dental surgeries, for example as many as 2.5 million in 1952. They were often administered by dentists who could act as both operator and anaesthetist until this practice was stopped by the General Dental Council (GDC) in 1981. The 'Poswillo Report' published in 1990 recommended that standards of staffing and equipment should be the same wherever an anaesthetic was given – hospital, dental clinic or dental surgery – and that GA should be avoided wherever possible. In 1998 the GDC stated that only accredited anaesthetists should be responsible for dental anaesthetics. This markedly reduced dental surgery anaesthetic numbers. In 2000 the Department of Health effectively restricted dental anaesthesia to hospitals, thus bringing it into line with anaesthesia for other surgical specialties for the first time after more than 150 years.

GENERAL CONSIDERATIONS

Indications for use of general anaesthesia in dentistry

For some patients the provision of GA to carry out simple extractions remains the technique of choice. Indications for GA for dentistry include:

- inability (mainly in children) to tolerate dental treatment using local anaesthesia (LA);
- failure of previous attempt to treat under LA;
- patients with special needs, or whose medical disability may make it impossible to sit still (e.g. uncontrolled movements);
- acute infection when LA may not be effective because of the local change in pH and there is a risk of spreading infection;
- true allergy to LA, which is very rare.

Dental surgery is usually carried out on an outpatient basis and most of the patients are children who, for unknown reasons, are more likely to have GA for dental treatment in the UK than in any other European country.

TECHNICAL CONSIDERATIONS

Preparation for dental anaesthesia

Preoperative instructions

Written preoperative instructions must be given. Patients should be advised to make arrangements for an appropriate escort and means of transport home. Excessive starvation periods should be avoided – 6 hours for food and 2 hours for clear fluids is adequate.

History, examination and investigations

General health should be assessed using a questionnaire checked by the anaesthetist. Children with special health problems are not uncommon, and it is important to ascertain the exact nature of their illness, preferably by contacting the specialist looking after them. Sometimes anaesthetic risk has to be weighed against the benefit of dental surgery. Children often have colds or minor upper respiratory tract infections. Cancellation of the operation is not necessary if they are otherwise well and afebrile. Patients with chest infections or those who are unwell should be postponed. Recent immunisation is not a reason for cancellation.

Haemoglobin estimation is not necessary unless otherwise indicated. Sickle screening is needed for Afro-Caribbean or African patients, and has been recommended for those of Mediterranean or Middle Eastern origin.

Consent

For children, consent from the parent or legal guardian is needed for operation and insertion of suppository, if appropriate. However, because of the nature of the surgery, not uncommonly paediatric patients are 'in care', and carers may not be eligible to give consent.

Premedication

Local anaesthetic cream may be applied over a suitable vein in the antecubital fossa. Premedication is not usual in dental surgery, but is sometimes used in children whose behaviour is especially challenging. Midazolam either orally in a dose of 0.25–0.5 mg/kg or intranasally 0.2–0.3 mg/kg has been used, with a maximum dose recommendation of 20 mg/kg. Children need a trained paediatric recovery nurse.

Anaesthetic technique

Induction of anaesthesia

There are a number of issues to consider, as follows:

- children are often very frightened and may prefer to sit in the parent's lap;
- ECG and pulse oximetry should be monitored during induction;
- induction may be gaseous or intravenous. Single-breath induction using sevoflurane is quite popular with older children, who enjoy the challenge of having their breath-holding ability timed. In younger children 30% oxygen in nitrous oxide with sevoflurane gives faster induction than oxygen and sevoflurane alone. It is mandatory to establish intravenous access before or immediately after induction for all but the very shortest operations;
- propofol should be given via an antecubital vein to decrease the risk of pain on injection, which can cause behavioural problems in future anaesthetics. Antibiotic prophylaxis can be given intravenously at induction if indicated (see below). The eyes should be taped.

Airway management

Communication with the dentist is essential. The type of airway management will depend on the type and difficulty of the proposed surgery.

Nasal mask

For many years nasal masks such as the Goldman or McKesson were used with a purely inhalational anaesthetic technique. When both surgeon and anaesthetist are familiar with the technique it is still used for brief operations on children. The mouth is kept open with a prop and the anaesthetist holds the mask over the nose while supporting the jaw in order to maintain the airway and provide counterpressure for the surgeon.

Packing from buccal sulcus to buccal sulcus so as not to obstruct the airway is done by the dentist. This prevents excessive mouth breathing and aspiration of foreign material or blood. There is always some mouth breathing and high gas flows are needed.

Using a nasal mask demands an exceptional degree of vigilance. Adequate self-ventilation can be detected only be a combination of looking at chest movement, observing the reservoir bag and listening to the airway. Enlarged adenoids may make nasal anaesthesia impossible. Scavenging is difficult, but pollution is generally calculated on a time-weighted average, and because of short exposures in brief operations is unlikely to be significant. It is not a technique to be used by the occasional dental anaesthetist or in difficult airways, and has been largely superseded by the laryngeal mask airway (LMA).

Laryngeal mask airway

Use of the LMA is associated with better oxygenation than a nasal mask. Soiling of the airways is not seen, but some anaesthetists like to place a pack on top of the LMA. The reinforced LMA is recommended because the tube is narrower and more pliable. Even so, LMAs have to be held firmly because they tend to become displaced. They are now widely used in dental anaesthesia.[1]

Endotracheal tube

Nasal intubation is indicated when more room is needed in the mouth (e.g. for conservation). Pre-formed nasal tubes can be used and tubes can be softened by warming in sterile water. Small children (under 5 years) may be intubated orally. Care should be taken in intubating children who have had cleft palate repair. Even with a cuffed tube, a pack must be inserted. Many dental drills spray large volumes of water into the mouth, and suction by the assistant is important. Most dental operations are short and patients breathe spontaneously, but if the patient is to be intubated with a non-depolarising muscle relaxant, he or she may be ventilated.

Nasopharyngeal airways

Use of nasopharyngeal airways has been associated with a high incidence of epistaxis, which tends to make airway maintenance more, not less, problematical.

Maintenance of anaesthesia with inhalational agents

Sevoflurane

Sevoflurane is useful as an induction agent. With a nasal mask, the high flows needed make it an expensive option.

Isoflurane

Isoflurane is widely used in contemporary practice, but it is not recommended for dental surgery in spontaneously breathing patients. It is irritant and is associated with coughing, salivation and desaturation.

Halothane

Halothane was the mainstay of dental anesthesia for many years, but in 1999 the Committee on Safety of Medicines restricted its use in dental anaesthesia to hospitals because of the high incidence of arrhythmias (see below).

Enflurane

Enflurane has been said to be the most suitable inhalational agent for dental anaesthesia, with fewer irritant properties than isoflurane and a short recovery time.

Postoperative management

Oxygen therapy

In the recovery phase, oxygen is given and saturation closely monitored: 30% of dental deaths were found to occur in the recovery phase, probably because of unrecognised respiratory obstruction. Laryngeal mask airways or endotracheal tubes should be removed after vital reflexes have returned. The patient is placed in the lateral position without a pillow so that the head is down. Anaesthetists should not leave until they are satisfied that the airway is safe.

Nausea and vomiting

Encourage patients to spit out blood rather than swallowing it because this tends to make them sick.

Analgesia

Analgesia is more effective if it is given preoperatively and may be given on admission. Paracetamol can be given in a loading dose of 20 mg/kg and non-steroidal anti-inflammatory drugs (NSAIDs) can also be given (e.g. diclofenac 1 mg/kg). Asthmatic children should be asked whether they have had NSAIDs with no problems.

Local anaesthetic blockade

Local blocks given under GA are effective in older children, but those under about 5 years of age tend to find numbness more distressing than pain.

Opiates

Opiates are seldom needed in dental surgery.

Discharge criteria

Patients should be able to walk and drink before leaving. They should have written postoperative instructions and contact details for advice if necessary.

ADDITIONAL POINTS

Monitoring

Standards of monitoring are the same as for any other GA. Pulse oximetry, ECG and blood pressure cuff are mandatory. Capnography should be used with endotracheal tubes or laryngeal masks. It rarely registers in cases using a nasal mask unless the gas flow through the nose is large and the seal around the nose and the pack is very effective.

Position of patient

Position of the patient has been a contentious issue. Traditionally dental patients were anaesthetised sitting up with an occipital support so that the head was erect and the jaw sloped down, thus enabling blood to dribble out forwards rather than back into the pharynx. In the supine position, protection of the airway is more difficult using a nasal mask. Advocates of the lying position pointed to the risks of supine hypotension in sitting patients, postulating that it was a cause of mortality in dental anaesthesia, although in a study comparing the two groups blood pressure was not found to be different. Patients are now usually flat or semi-recumbent.

Antibiotic prophylaxis

Given the nature of the patient population, congenital cardiac abnormalities are common. Operations needing cover are extractions, scaling and gum surgery. Patients needing cover are those with valve lesions, most congenital heart defects apart from isolated secundum atrial septal defects, and those with a history of endocarditis. Prophylaxis is with amoxicillin at induction and a further dose 6 hours later. If the patient is penicillin allergic, vancomycin or teicoplanin with gentamicin, or clindamycin may be given. High-risk patients receive amoxicillin and gentamicin.[2]

Patients with Down's syndrome

Patients with Down's syndrome may have heart defects, and are also at risk of cervical spine instability. There is no screening procedure that predicts those at risk of neurological problems caused by this condition.[3] Cervical spine radiographs in children have no predictive validity for subsequent acute subluxation/dislocation at the atlantoaxial joint. However, care must be taken while manipulating the head and neck in the unconscious patient.

Arrhythmias

Stimulation of the trigeminal nerve during dental surgery leads to increased sympathetic discharge. Together with high circulating catecholamine levels in frightened patients under halothane anaesthesia, there was a high rate

(18–75%) of arrhythmias, especially tachyarrhythmias such as multifocal ventricular ectopics and even runs of ventricular tachycardia. It is possible that a number of dental anaesthetic deaths resulted from unrecognised or untreated arrhythmias. They can be prevented by preoperative use of LA blockade and β-blockers, and intraoperatively stopping surgery or lidocaine (lignocaine) intravenously will terminate them. Pre-treatment with atropine tends to increase their incidence. With enflurane and isoflurane the occurrence rate is much lower – about 10%. Bradycardias are uncommon.

Sedation

Dental surgeries which treat paediatric patients may call upon anaesthetists to administer sedation. The only sedation approved for children by The Scottish Intercollegiate Guidelines Network Report on Paediatric Sedation is nitrous oxide, which is used as part of the 'relative analgesia' technique and involves breathing 40–70% nitrous oxide in oxygen.

Intravenous sedation can be used for adult patients with the purpose of diminishing anxiety and apprehension without obtunding protective reflexes. The patient should remain conscious and appropriately responsive to questions or commands. Titration of a single drug such as diazepam or midazolam is preferred to the use of multiple drugs. Monitoring of vital signs, including pulse oximetry, should be employed.

ORAL SURGERY

Oral surgery is more invasive than dental surgery and involves the raising of gum flaps and sometimes the removal of bone, but seldom results in significant blood loss. Few types of oral surgery are performed on small children. Like dental surgery, oral surgery is often performed on a day-case basis and the procedure is essentially the same.

TECHNICAL CONSIDERATIONS

Airway management

For reasons of access the use of an oral endotracheal tube or LMA is often inappropriate and in most cases a cuffed nasal endotracheal tube should be used. The airway should be protected with a pack, even in the presence of a cuffed tube. Patients are often ventilated, partly because surgical access means that the surgeon tends to lean on the patient's chest.

Postoperative management

NSAIDs are of more use than opiates, and dexamethasone has been shown to decrease the pain and swelling after third molar extractions. Preoperative administration of analgesics is more effective than intra- or postoperative administration.

MAXILLOFACIAL SURGERY

Maxillofacial surgery is surgery involving the bones and soft tissues of the face. It demands a high degree of expertise from both the surgeon and the anaesthetist. Maxillofacial surgical procedures are generally performed to treat the results of trauma, congenital abnormalities or cancer.

TRAUMA

Minor injuries

Relatively minor injuries with little soft tissue damage, such as an isolated arch fracture of the zygoma, are seldom operated on as an emergency. Management is as for oral surgery and intubation is oral or nasal depending on the operation.

Major injuries

In major injuries to the face the airway is the first priority. There may be airway obstruction caused by haematoma, oedema, foreign bodies or loss of tongue support in bilateral mandibular fractures. Nursing the patient prone may be helpful. Intubation is indicated with any degree of airway compromise. Progressive worsening of the airway must be anticipated, and input from an experienced faciomaxillary surgeon as to the likely course of events can be helpful. Oral intubation can be used in the emergency situation, although nasal intubation may be performed provided there is no possibility of cerebrospinal fluid (CSF) leak.

Rapid sequence induction is necessary because the stomach may be full of blood or food, and equipment for emergency tracheostomy or cricothyrotomy must be available in case intubation is impossible.

Intubation may be difficult. Oedema limiting mouth opening may follow mandibular fractures, and mobile maxillary fractures make laryngoscopy difficult. Fibreoptic intubation may not be possible because of the presence of blood. Patients with poor mouth opening may need tracheostomy under LA.

There may be associated head, chest or abdominal injuries, and up to 10% of patients with major facial trauma have cervical spine injuries. This possibility must be remembered during intubation. Maxillary fractures are classified into the three le Fort groups according to the lines of fracture. There is a 25% incidence of CSF leak with le Fort II and III fractures.

Other life-threatening injuries are treated first. Facial fractures are usually treated after comprehensive imaging and diagnosis, and may sometimes be delayed to let swelling subside. Nasal intubation is then usually needed and fibreoptic intubation may be useful. If it is impossible, tracheostomy may have to be performed. Jaws are seldom wired together at the end of surgery, but close liaison with the surgeon to establish which surgical approach is to be used is essential.

There may be considerable operative blood loss and invasive monitoring is needed.

Postoperatively, high-dependency unit care is needed for major facial injuries, and the patient should not be extubated until his or her airway is deemed safe and he or she is alert enough to maintain it. If the jaws are wired together, wire cutters must be kept at the bedside.

ORTHOGNATHIC SURGERY

Orthognathic surgery is usually carried out in late teenage or early adulthood when the facial bones have stopped growing. Patients may be difficult to intubate and it should not be assumed that once they are paralysed they can be ventilated. Awake fibreoptic intubation may be the safest and easiest technique in an obviously difficult airway. Otherwise, provided the airway is checked for ease of inflation, any one of the techniques to help a difficult intubation may be tried, such as bougies and the McCoy laryngoscope. Preoperative tracheostomy is rarely needed. The operations are long and blood loss may be considerable.

SURGERY FOR CANCER

Patients having surgery for cancer are often older than those described above, and the association between oral cancer and smoking implies that many have coexisting medical conditions.

Careful preoperative airway assessment is essential because the tumour may compromise the airway or make intubation difficult. Consultation with the surgeon must take place as to the route of intubation or even whether elective preoperative tracheostomy is needed. A history of previous successful intubation does not mean that it will be possible subsequently. The ability to ventilate by facemask must be checked before spontaneous ventilation is lost. Intubation is usually via the nose. Equipment to deal with difficult intubation and to perform cricothyrotomy in an emergency must be available. Awake fibreoptic intubation may be appropriate, depending on the tumour site.

Invasive monitoring is needed because blood loss can be large. If a flap is to be part of the technique the patient and theatre need to be kept warm, fluids heated, and hypotension avoided.

Postoperatively, these patients usually need to be nursed in an intensive care unit and must be carefully assessed before they are extubated.

References

1. Brimacombe J, Berry A The laryngeal mask for dental surgery – a review. Aust Dent J 1995; 40:10–14.
2. British National Formulary 47. London: British Medical Association and Royal Pharmaceutical Society of Great Britain; 2004:257.
3. Morton RE, Khan MA, Murray-Leslie C, Elliott S. Atlantoaxial instability in Down's syndrome: a five year follow up study. Arch Dis Child 1995; 72:115–119.

CHAPTER **5.11**

ORTHOPAEDIC AND TRAUMA SURGERY

GENERAL CONSIDERATIONS

Pre-assessment

Pre-assessment clinics are particularly valuable in orthopaedics. Major elective surgery is increasingly offered to a frail elderly population with considerable co-morbidity. The anaesthetist can assess fitness, but also patients benefit from full discussion of the recommended anaesthetic technique. Where several techniques may be offered, as in lower limb surgery, it is helpful for both parties to agree the final choice.

Blood conservation

New policies for blood transfusion have raised the cost and reduced the supply of donor blood. Modern transfusion practice should therefore focus on blood conservation. In addition, blood transfusion is immunosuppressive and may increase the infection rate, an important consideration when implants are used. The following points should be noted:

- routine transfusion for total hip replacement or total knee replacement is no longer appropriate. The author gives blood for about every third hip replacement, in a population that includes complex primary and revision hip surgery;
- preoperative optimisation of the haemoglobin level, using iron supplementation or erythropoietin if indicated, is only possible if pre-assessment takes place at least 4 weeks before surgery;
- strict application of transfusion thresholds is a powerful tool for conserving the blood supply. Good evidence on suitable transfusion thresholds[1] comes almost exclusively from critical care patients. Typical practice is to transfuse only if the haemoglobin is less than 8 g/dL, or 10 g/dL if there is known coronary artery disease. However, if rehabilitation is delayed by anaemia, it may be wise to give blood;
- anaesthetic technique influences blood loss, being less with regional analgesia. Other techniques include isovolaemic haemodilution, autologous predonation and cell salvage (see Ch. 2.7).

Tourniquets

Arterial tourniquets[2] on the upper or lower limb give a bloodless surgical field. The tourniquet should be:

- wider than half the limb's diameter – the widest possible tourniquet reduces direct pressure under the cuff while maintaining arterial occlusion;
- placed over the widest part of the limb – this also reduces direct pressure;
- padded carefully and not twisted round after application – friction burns and skin abrasions can occur;
- free of any cleaning solutions that can damage the skin under the tourniquet;
- inflated to a maximum pressure of 250 mmHg for the lower limb (or 100 mmHg above systolic pressure) and 200 mmHg for the upper limb (or 50 mmHg above systolic pressure) – ischaemic time should not exceed 2 hours – for longer operations, deflate for 10 minutes before inflating again;
- attached to an automatic gas control system – the commonest cause of tourniquet injury is accidental over-pressurisation.

Exsanguination

- Exsanguination is contraindicated if there is tumour, deep venous thrombosis (DVT) or frank sepsis in the limb;
- esmarch bandage exsanguination is not recommended. This stretchy rubber bandage gives uncontrolled and sometimes very high pressures. The Rhys-Davies exsanguinator is safe on normal-sized limbs. When rolled onto the limb, it gives a controlled and evenly spread pressure;
- maximum exsanguination can also be achieved by elevating the arm to 90° or the leg to 45° for 5 minutes;
- for the leg, approximately 800 mL blood may pass into the remaining circulation as exsanguination occurs. This may not be tolerated by patients with cardiac failure, especially if there is a tourniquet on the other leg.

Tourniquet inflation

- Tourniquet pain develops over 30–60 minutes, causes a raised heart rate and blood pressure, and may be difficult to control with opioids or increased depth of anaesthesia. Circulatory changes may occur with regional analgesia, even with adequate sensory block, but resolve on deflation;
- tourniquet pain and surgical stimulation cause a systemic hypercoagulable state due to catecholamine release. Platelet aggregation is increased;

- antibiotics must be administered 5 minutes before inflation for full penetration into the tissues.

Tourniquet deflation

- $P\text{CO}_2$ may increase by 2.5 kPa, causing a critical rise in intracranial pressure in a patient with head injury. It may be necessary to increase minute volume by 50% for 5 minutes in a ventilated patient to control this rise;
- potassium may rise by 0.3 mmol/L and lactate to 2.3 mmol/L. The resulting acidosis causes a fall in peripheral vascular resistance and blood pressure. In addition, the limb fills with blood and filling pressures are reduced, exacerbating the hypotension;
- core temperature falls as cool venous blood from the occluded limb enters the circulation;
- tissue ischaemia causes the release of tissue plasminogen activators, which result in thrombolysis and increased surgical bleeding after the tourniquet is deflated.

Other dangers of tourniquets

- Nerve injury may occur at the point of compression. The radial nerve is most at risk in the arm and the sciatic nerve in the leg. Paralysis has been described, usually related to high inflation pressures;
- muscle damage may occur in the whole limb, related to long ischaemic time and to high pressures;
- vascular disease and sickle cell disease are relative contraindications to tourniquets. Although tourniquets have been used successfully in patients with sickle cell disease, there is a risk of sickle cell crisis. Patients with sickle cell trait have also been reported to develop sickle cell crisis associated with tourniquet use;
- pulmonary embolism, which may occasionally be massive and/or fatal, may occur at exsanguination if there is a DVT. Exsanguination should therefore be avoided if there is a DVT. Emboli have also been shown on transoesophageal echocardiography when the tourniquet is deflated after knee replacement, but these are not usually clinically significant.

Cement

Cement is commonly used in joint replacement surgery. The quality of the interface between bone and cement is important to prevent future loosening, which is more likely at this interface than at the cement-prosthesis interface. Modern techniques include pressurised cementing, which forces cement into bone canaliculi. This is especially important in cemented hip replacement surgery.

A dry operating field improves cement penetration into bone. Regional analgesia is the commonest strategy to help achieve this. Some surgeons use a warm prosthesis to shorten the setting time of the cement.

Hypotension and hypoxia may occur during cementing, especially if pressurised, and are clinically significant in about 10% of patients. This is no longer thought to be a direct effect of the methyl methacrylate monomer in cement entering the circulation, but rather due to showers of microemboli of platelets, red cells and fat. These have a systemic inflammatory effect causing vasodilatation, ventilation–perfusion mismatch in the lungs, and pulmonary vasoconstriction. There may be alveolar collapse and local haemorrhage. Circulatory collapse and death may occur.

The anaesthetist may use hypotension to achieve a dry operating field, but significant hypovolaemia should be avoided because this predisposes to a severe reaction to pressurised cementing. The surgeon should warn the anaesthetist as cementing begins. Intravenous fluid, vasopressors, increased inspired oxygen concentration, and occasionally inotropic support may be required. A transient severe episode may precipitate myocardial infarction. Cement reactions are less common in knee replacement because pressure is not used to the same degree.

Thromboembolic disease

Deep venous thrombosis is very common after major lower limb joint surgery. Without prophylaxis, the approximately quoted incidence is as shown in Table 5.11.1.

Two extensive papers[3,4] describe current opinion on prophylaxis in a wide range of surgical patients, including detailed reviews of evidence in orthopaedic patients. For the individual patient, the decision is 'best made by combining knowledge of the literature, including group recommendations, with clinical judgement, including that patient's unique risk for thrombosis and the potential for adverse consequences'.[3]

Operation	DVT seen on venography (%)	Clinical DVT (%)	Non-fatal pulmonary embolism (%)	Fatal pulmonary embolism (%)
Total hip replacement	55	4	1.2	0.3
Total knee replacement	65	10	1.9	0.4
Fractured neck of femur	65	5	8	2

Table 5.11.1 Approximately quoted incidence of deep venous thrombosis after major lower limb joint surgery without prophylaxis. From Nicolaides and Gillespie[5]

The following points are relevant in orthopaedic surgery:

- prophylaxis with warfarin or heparin is associated with bleeding. Any haematoma increases the risk of infection in the prosthetic joint, which may then need further surgery;
- the data available are complex and sometimes conflicting. Data from other surgical specialties cannot be extrapolated to orthopaedics. Some trials do not stratify for individual risk factors, which makes interpretation difficult;
- it may not be appropriate to use the incidence of DVT on venography rather than the clinical incidence;
- knee replacement has a higher incidence of DVT than hip replacement, but less commonly in proximal veins. Proximal DVT is more likely to result in significant pulmonary embolism;
- the risk of fatal pulmonary embolus risk is very low. An extremely large study would be required to compare methods of prophylaxis;
- symptomatic DVT should be prevented for its own sake, not just to prevent pulmonary embolus. It may lead to venous ulceration and considerable morbidity.

All orthopaedic units should have an agreed protocol for prophylaxis. The anaesthetist should ensure patients are identified as low, medium or high risk, and that appropriate prophylaxis is prescribed. The following strategies are used in orthopaedics:

- early mobilisation and good hydration;
- compression stockings;
- pneumatic foot pumps or intermittent calf compression devices. These reduce the incidence of DVT rate by 50%,[3] which is similar to warfarin, but without the risk of bleeding. Some patients find them uncomfortable. In healthy volunteers, compression stockings reduce the venous blood volume in the leg which reduces peak velocity in the popliteal vein when the foot pumps inflate. This suggests that compression stockings and foot pumps should not be used together;
- low molecular weight heparin (LMWH), starting either postoperatively or 12 hours preoperatively. There is strong evidence that the extended use of LMWH reduces the incidence of clinical DVT after hip replacement.[3,4] However, practice varies between different orthopaedic units. The standard dose is 40 mg once daily.[4] This does not prevent the use of spinal or epidural anaesthesia[3,4,7] provided LMWH is not given within 12 hours either side of the spinal injection or the epidural catheter insertion or removal;
- extended prophylaxis with LMWH or warfarin for 6–12 weeks postoperatively may be used for high-risk patients, especially after hip

replacement because 2% of these patients develop DVT more than 10 days after surgery;[4]

- melagatran is a direct thrombin inhibitor. It appears to be as effective as LMWH and work is under way to assess the risk of bleeding;
- fondaparinux, a selective inhibitor of factor Xa, is the first of a new class of antithrombotic drugs, the synthetic pentasaccharides.[6] They are twice as effective as LMWH in reducing DVT after major hip or knee surgery. A subcutaneous dose has a half life of 17 hours. There does not appear to be an increase in clinically relevant bleeding,[6] and they are recommended prophylaxis in orthopaedic surgery;[3]
- low-dose aspirin probably has little benefit over other methods and is not widely recommended;
- a vena caval filter may be considered, but this is controversial and used only for highly selected cases.[4]

Other emboli

Air embolism

Air embolism occurs when large veins are open to air, particularly when venous pressure is low. It classically occurs during shoulder surgery in the sitting position when the open veins are higher than the right atrium. It can also occur during pelvic surgery. A large bolus of air in the right heart prevents forward flow of blood. If it breaks up and flows to the lungs there is severe ventilation–perfusion mismatch. The main clinical features are an abrupt reduction in expired carbon dioxide, loss of blood pressure, hypoxaemia and possible cardiac arrest.

The surgeon should immediately flood the site with saline to prevent further air entry. Nitrous oxide should be discontinued to prevent enlargement of air bubbles in the blood. The patient should be laid flat or tilted head-down to reduce air entry. If a central venous line is in place, air may be aspirated from the right atrium. External cardiac massage may help break up the air bolus in the heart.

Prevention is principally by good surgical technique. Ventilation with positive end-expiratory pressure (PEEP) raises intrathoracic pressure and makes air embolism less likely.

Fat embolism

Fat emboli[8] can almost always be demonstrated with fractures of the femur, tibia and pelvis. However, the incidence of the fat embolism clinical syndrome is less than 1% of such fractures. The syndrome may arise spontaneously if high-risk fractures are not fixed, and so fixation should be within 24 hours or sooner unless head or chest injury prevents this. The syndrome is also seen in major soft tissue injury, bone marrow harvesting, liposuction, hepatic failure, acute pancreatitis and severe burns. Its principal features are:

- respiratory – tachypnoea, haemoptysis, crepitations, hypoxaemia, and patchy shadows or 'snowstorm' on the chest radiograph;
- petechial rash – classically over the upper body and mucous membranes;
- neurological – confusion, decreased conscious level, decerebrate posturing and coma;
- thrombocytopenia – probably due to platelet consumption;
- tachycardia and pyrexia over 39°C;
- jaundice, acute renal failure, unexplained anaemia.

Fat emboli always occur to some extent during reaming of long bones before nailing. Surgeons therefore avoid intramedullary fixation when other modes of fixation are feasible. The clinical signs may be noted during or after surgery. Treatment is supportive, usually in intensive care. Small prospective randomised trials suggest steroids are helpful, but there is a risk of overwhelming sepsis.

Tumour embolism

Patients with disseminated malignancy may present with pathological fractures. Fixation, or prevention of an imminent fracture, may improve the quality of the life that remains. However, reaming a long bone full of tumour carries a very high risk (up to 50%) of significant or fatal tumour embolus. Massive pulmonary embolus may occur. Prolonged resuscitation may then not be appropriate, although advanced life support should be instituted at first. This information should be discussed frankly in advance with the patient so that they can make an informed choice about their care.

Anti-inflammatory drugs in orthopaedics

Non-steroidal anti-inflammatory drugs (NSAIDs) are very useful agents for bony pain. Many patients control their arthritic symptoms with NSAIDs, and many tolerate them without unwanted effects on the stomach, the kidney or on asthma. However, in the perioperative setting of starvation, possible dehydration and general anaesthesia, their tolerance may be different. For this reason, together with their antiplatelet effects, few of these drugs are licensed for acute postoperative pain, although they are effective and widely used.

NSAIDs inhibit osteocyte activity and therefore reduce the formation of new bone. Where bone healing is critical or delayed the surgeon may wish to avoid or restrict the use of NSAIDs. Conversely, where there is a risk of heterotopic ossification (unwanted bone formation in soft tissue around joints, most commonly around the hip), NSAIDs may be used to prevent this, often indomethacin 75 mg/day together with a proton pump inhibitor to protect the stomach.

Infection in orthopaedics

Infection around a prosthesis is a disastrous complication. The infection often cannot be cleared without removal of the prosthesis and staged revision surgery may be required. A Girdlestone hip or fused knee joint may be the final outcome. Prophylactic antibiotics are used for all operations involving a prosthesis, guided by local microbiologists.

Urinary catheters may introduce infection. Common practice has been to avoid them where possible. However, when a catheter is required, it is preferable to insert it in the clean theatre environment before the prosthesis is inserted, rather than postoperatively on the ward. In many centres a catheter is routinely inserted before all lower limb joint replacements, and is not associated with increased infections.[9] Insertion is covered with an appropriate additional antibiotic, such as 120 mg gentamicin intravenously.

A great advance in preventing infection has come from the use of filtered air flow systems.[10] Orthopaedic theatres should be fitted with systems to provide up to 500 changes of air per hour. Strategies to maximise the benefits of these systems are as follows:

- some systems focus laminar air flow on a central square containing the operating table. A screen of sterile drapes in line with the border of this square optimises air flow past the patient;
- the anaesthetist should avoid leaving the door to the anaesthetic room open because this disturbs air flow;
- the number of people in theatre should be kept to a minimum because each person introduces a fresh load of organisms to the air;
- extra strategies to conserve heat and warm the patient are required.

The literature does not provide evidence that wearing a surgical mask reduces wound infection.[10] More bacteria are shed from skin and clothing than are expelled from the nose and mouth. Masks increase the shedding of squames due to friction on the skin of the face and neck, so orthopaedic surgeons often wear hoods tucked in around the neck with a facemask on top. However, on surfaces directly opposite the face bacterial counts are increased, and these are reduced for a short period of time by a suitable surgical mask.[10] Orthopaedic surgeons often ask the circulating team, including the anaesthetist, to wear a facemask despite the lack of evidence. Anaesthetists should also avoid hairstyles that increase shedding of organisms into the air.

A plastic visor will protect the anaesthetist from blood when power tools or mechanical washing devices are being used.

TECHNICAL CONSIDERATIONS

Regional techniques

Orthopaedic surgery provides many opportunities for regional and peripheral nerve blocks. The following should be considered:

- is there a clinical reason to offer a regional block (e.g. spinal anaesthesia reduces blood loss in hip surgery) or a contraindication (e.g. clotting defect)?
- would a regional block provide helpful postoperative analgesia (e.g. interscalene block for shoulder surgery)?
- could the patient be managed satisfactorily without the nerve block? Any tendency to offer a block because it provides an opportunity to acquire new skills rather than for the benefit of the patient should be resisted.
- would a catheter placed for continuous nerve blockade be helpful? This is increasingly widespread, but requires experience, skill and regular practice. Should the assistance of a more experienced anaesthetist be sought?
- will a numb limb be a hazard to the patient postoperatively? Will it interfere with rehabilitation (e.g. patients after knee hemiarthroplasty may wish to walk on the first day)? Can the patient look after a numb and weak limb? With careful selection and instruction patients may be discharged home in this state, but they have suffered disastrous burns after, for example, falling asleep against a hot radiator;
- will the block be the sole anaesthetic, or will sedation or a general anaesthetic be necessary too?
- finally, but importantly, is the patient willing to receive the block either awake or asleep? The anaesthetist should explain the risks, benefits and alternatives. If a patient declines a nerve block without an apparently sound reason, their wishes must be respected;

The following regional blocks are useful for orthopaedic surgery;

- spinal and epidural anaesthesia – the addition of opioids improves the analgesia but also increases postoperative nausea, vomiting, itch and urinary retention;
- femoral and sciatic nerve blocks – these may be used in combination for knee or more distal surgery. Analgesia may last 18–24 hours;
- femoral 3-in-1 block as described by Winnie in 1973[11] is useful as an adjunct to general anaesthesia for hip surgery, including fractured neck of femur and hip replacement. This blocks the lumbar plexus as local anaesthetic injected into the femoral sheath in the inguinal region

tracks proximally, by means of distal digital pressure and massage. Large volumes of solution are required. The three nerves blocked are the femoral nerve, lateral cutaneous nerve of the thigh and obturator nerve. Block of the obturator nerve is least reliable. It supplies sensory fibres to the hip joint;

- lumbar plexus block by the posterior approach[12,13] is more reliable than the three-in-one block for hip surgery, but is not effective as the sole anaesthetic. Hypotension and urinary retention are less common than with epidural analgesia. Patients with fractured neck of femur who cannot have a spinal anaesthetic should have a lumbar plexus block, by either the three-in-one or the posterior approach;
- popliteal nerve block[14] is useful for foot or ankle surgery. Posterior and lateral approaches are described. The lateral approach is useful in trauma patients when raising the leg in a plaster cast or turning prone may be difficult. The saphenous nerve, coming from the femoral nerve, may supply part of the great toe and therefore popliteal block alone is not reliable for surgery in this area;
- ankle block is a ring block useful for postoperative analgesia in the foot. Five separate nerves are blocked and only the injections appropriate for the operation need be done. In skilled hands it can be effective, but occasional practitioners have a lower success rate;
- brachial plexus block – the interscalene approach is commonly used for postoperative analgesia in shoulder surgery. The axillary approach, used for elbow, forearm and hand surgery, gives less reliable cover of the lateral aspect of the arm and supplementary distal blocks may be required for full anaesthesia. Patients with arthritis or after trauma sometimes cannot be positioned for an axillary block. The supra- and infraclavicular approaches (see Ch. 4.2) are reliable blocks for forearm and hand surgery, but carry a risk of pneumothorax;
- peripheral nerve blocks in the forearm or wrist are helpful for minor procedures or as adjuncts for partially effective brachial plexus blocks. The tourniquet area is not covered, which limits their usefulness;
- Bier's block is most useful in a patient unfit for general anaesthesia when brachial plexus blockade has failed. Hand surgeons notice an excessive ooze of blood. A double cuff must be used to allow anaesthesia of the tourniquet area.

Continuous infusion techniques using a catheter

This practice is increasingly common in the UK and Europe.[9] Catheters are mainly used for:

- femoral nerve block;
- psoas compartment catheter for lumbar plexus block;

- interscalene, infraclavicular and axillary approaches to the brachial plexus.

Before or after induction of general anaesthesia?

Orthopaedic patients may present particular difficulties for performing blocks awake. Arthritis or injury may prevent optimal positioning and patients with fractures cannot usually tolerate twitches from nerve stimulation. The anaesthetist should discuss risks, benefits and alternatives with the patient and then decide whether to perform the block with the patient awake, asleep or anaesthetised. There is a body of established opinion[15] that peripheral nerve blocks may be conducted in anaesthetised patients, assuming a meticulous technique. Ultrasound may be used to guide nerve blocks, especially for identifying vessels and other hazards.[16] This is not widely practised and requires education, training and resources to buy machines.

Sedation techniques

A fear of being awake in the operating theatre is a barrier for many patients to accepting a regional technique for major orthopaedic surgery. Drilling into bone is noisy, and simple conversation to distract the patient may be ineffective. The use of sedation can sometimes lead to a confused and uncooperative patient. There should always be a plan for airway management, if either control is lost or the procedure unexpectedly lasts longer than the duration of the regional block. This can happen in any major joint surgery. Placing a laryngeal mask may be easy, but intubation of a patient in the lateral position under a sterile screen may be difficult. Unless intubation is likely to be very straightforward, definitive airway control from the outset should be considered.

A range of sedation techniques or light levels of general anaesthesia can be offered. The following are suggested:

- intermittent boluses of 0.5–1 mg midazolam. The level of consciousness is likely to fluctuate with this technique. It is useful where the aim is anxiolysis rather than sedation. Disinhibition may also occur. Oxygen should usually be given;
- continuous infusion of propofol, using a standard syringe driver (1–3 mg/kg/h titrated to effect) or a target-controlled infusion pump (3–5 μg/mL). Stable sedation is usually achieved. Amnesia is usual, but not guaranteed. Airway control may be a problem, especially if the patient is supine. Oxygen should usually be given and breathing monitored. The author uses capnograph tubing taped into a hole in the oxygen face mask;
- general anaesthesia, using spontaneous respiration through a laryngeal mask airway and a volatile anaesthetic agent. There will usually be more hypotension.

SPECIFIC OPERATIONS

Hip replacement and revision hip surgery

Around 50 000 hip replacements are performed annually in the UK. The impact on quality of life is profound and an increasingly frail patient population is requesting hip replacement. Revision surgery is a major procedure, and patients tend to be older and frailer than for primary hip surgery. The orthopaedic anaesthetist must consider, with the surgeon and the patient and their family, whether the risk–benefit analysis is in the patient's favour.

The overall death rate after hip or knee replacement is probably between 0.1 and 0.5%.[4] The incidence of significant complications after hip replacement is about 4–5%. This includes dislocation, infection, DVT and non-fatal pulmonary embolus. Many patients simply say that they would 'rather be dead' than live in pain. Providing the anaesthetist believes that the patient is adequately informed, then the decision to proceed should be made by the patient.

Use of regional techniques

Regional anaesthesia is recommended as the technique of choice by the British Orthopaedic Association. It has the following benefits:

- reduced risk of DVT and pulmonary embolus;
- reduced blood loss and less frequent need for blood transfusion;
- a drier surgical field, which may give better conditions for cementing;
- there may be less confusion in recovery, when lack of cooperation can lead to early dislocation.

Sedation or general anaesthesia should be offered in addition to the regional technique, but some patients prefer to be awake. A common dose for spinal anaesthesia is 2.5–3 mL 0.5% bupivacaine with or without 250–300 μg diamorphine in 0.5 mL normal saline.

Patients may not tolerate the lateral position for more than about 2 hours. Many patients have arthritis in other joints and become very uncomfortable after this. A general anaesthetic may become necessary. This may be given if and when the patient becomes uncomfortable, but is difficult in the lateral position during surgery. It should not be undertaken lightly. An alternative is to combine the regional technique with a general anaesthetic from the outset. More hypotension is expected with this combination, which can be managed with vasopressors and fluids.

Specific hip procedures

There are several different kinds of hip prosthesis. The acetabular and femoral components may be cemented or uncemented. If an uncemented component is used then there is less benefit from a dry field during the period of insertion. There is also a hip resurfacing procedure, most commonly the Birmingham operation. The articular surface of the femoral head is removed and a metal cap placed over its remains. This is generally offered to younger, more active patients because the components are less likely to wear or dislocate. It avoids pressurised cementing within the femoral shaft with its associated risk of emboli, but there is more blood loss (500–700 mL) because a circumferential capsulotomy is required. It should be considered carefully in patients for whom blood transfusion may not be possible, such as Jehovah's Witnesses. It may be appropriate to aim for moderate hypotension in selected patients to reduce blood loss.

Complex primary hip replacement and revision hip surgery are becoming more common. The anaesthetist should ask the surgeon for an estimated time and expected blood loss. Bone grafting, using donor or native femoral head, adds an extra 2 hours. The surgeon may change the planned procedure if difficulties arise. Invasive monitoring should be considered.

Practical points

Most surgeons use the lateral position. Some use the supine position with a sandbag under the hip. There should always be good venous access and warming devices. Many centres opt for a urinary catheter in all patients, covered with antibiotic such as 120–160 mg gentamicin. Expected measured blood loss is 300–500 mL, but a similar amount is lost postoperatively into the tissues and the drain, if used. Blood transfusion should not be routine. In revision surgery blood loss may be 1–2 L and cell salvage should be considered. If the hip is infected blood loss is greater and at times may be brisk.

After surgery great care should be taken to avoid early dislocation. When the patient is moved or turned the surgeon should supervise the hip personally. Internal rotation must be avoided and the legs kept abducted using a wedge-shaped pillow between the ankles.

There is a range of options for postoperative analgesia: intrathecal diamorphine, but this may cause nausea, itch and urinary retention; a weaker opioid such as codeine, with oral or intramuscular morphine if needed; or patient-controlled intravenous morphine. Constipation should be anticipated. NSAIDs and regular paracetamol are helpful.

Knee replacement surgery

Total knee replacement is a markedly painful operation, much more so than hip replacement. Revision knee surgery is variable and should be discussed with the surgeon beforehand. Postoperative pain can be severe.

Hemiarthroplasty or Oxford knee replacement is sometimes performed in patients with single-compartment arthritic changes. This occurs when a varus or valgus knee develops arthritic changes confined to the compartment taking the main load. The surgeon uses a small anterior incision, it takes less time than a total knee replacement, and blood loss is less. It is considerably less painful afterwards, and patients may be mobilised on the day of surgery and discharged after just 3 days. A femoral nerve block may be unhelpful because rehabilitation is delayed.

Use of regional techniques

A variety of anaesthetic techniques are used. Postoperative pain management is a prime consideration. Early mobilisation may be planned using a passive movement machine, which flexes the knee to a prescribed degree and is painful without nerve blockade. Anaesthetic and analgesic techniques available include the following:

- epidural analgesia may be combined with a general anaesthetic, and extended postoperatively;
- femoral and sciatic nerve blocks used alone or combined with general anaesthesia. These blocks give good analgesia, have a lower incidence of urinary retention than epidural analgesia, and the patient is more mobile. They are time consuming and take 30 minutes to become effective;
- a femoral nerve block alone provides useful postoperative analgesia;
- a spinal anaesthetic alone does not provide postoperative analgesia, but may be combined with epidural analgesia or with a femoral or sciatic nerve block or both.

Opioid analgesia after general anaesthesia is an option, but significant doses will be needed. Patient-controlled analgesia gives greater patient satisfaction, but has little advantage in efficacy or safety over intermittent intramuscular morphine. NSAIDs are a useful supplement.

Patient preference and other diseases should partly determine the choice of technique. The incidence of DVT is reduced by regional anaesthesia. Blood loss is controlled by the tourniquet during surgery, but regional analgesia, including femoral and sciatic nerve blocks, gives good control of blood pressure during the early recovery phase and reduces bleeding.

Practical points

The patient is supine for knee replacement surgery and airway control under sedation can be a problem. The operation takes 60–90 minutes. The tourniquet is released after application of a firm compression bandage and there may be 500–700 mL blood loss in the first few minutes. The surgeon may wish to clamp the drain for a period. The use of a reperfusion drainage system, by which drained blood is transfused back into the patient, is well established. However, returning unwashed blood to the patient in this way is associated with increased febrile episodes and is not necessarily recommended. Hidden loss in the tissues may equal the visible loss. Regular haemoglobin checks are advised, but strict transfusion thresholds should be observed. Blood transfusion is required infrequently. Aprotinin may be useful.

Other knee operations

Knee arthroscopy is a common short procedure (15–60 minutes) performed as a day case under tourniquet. NSAIDs provide adequate postoperative analgesia, and the surgeon may place local anaesthetic into the knee joint and portal sites (20 mL 0.5% bupivacaine).

Cruciate ligament reconstruction is a 2-hour, mainly arthroscopic, procedure performed in the supine position. There is a small incision below the knee to secure the reconstructed tendon. Postoperative pain is variable, but generally moderate. NSAIDs with a medium-strength opioid such as codeine may be given, and the patient is then likely to require one or two doses of intramuscular morphine. Some anaesthetists offer a femoral nerve block with weaker local anaesthetic solution (e.g. 0.25% bupivacaine) to allow earlier mobilisation.

Ankle and foot surgery

Operations on the metatarsals and toes are common. Other procedures are ankle arthrodesis, tendon transfers, ankle arthroscopy or ankle replacement in specialist centres. The patients often have diabetes mellitus, vasculopathy and peripheral neuropathy and need careful preoperative assessment.

Postoperative pain is significant. Osteotomy, bunion surgery, ankle arthrodesis and replacement are particularly painful. A nerve block is desirable, such as ankle, popliteal or sciatic block. Compartment syndrome of the foot is an important consideration and it is wise to discuss this possibility with the surgeon before any nerve block. Patient-controlled intravenous morphine may be needed after the block wears off. This may prevent same-day discharge, even after limited surgery. NSAIDs should be used with care because they impair bone healing. Wound healing is a particular problem in the foot, owing to the lack of soft tissue volume to accommodate swelling and possible vascular compromise.

Shoulder surgery

Patients requiring shoulder surgery vary from fit sports players with recurrent injuries to patients with severe rheumatoid arthritis, an unstable neck and other morbidity. Apart from diagnostic arthroscopy, all shoulder surgery is extremely painful and a plan to manage postoperative pain is a high priority.

Specific procedures

The commonest shoulder surgery procedures are rotator cuff repairs and operations on the acromioclavicular joint. These take 1–2 hours and are either arthroscopic or open. Blood loss is minimal. Shoulder replacement is a 2–3-hour procedure and blood loss is usually less than 500 mL.

Practical points

For shoulder surgery the patient is usually placed in the 'deckchair' position with the feet adjacent to the anaesthetic machine. Practical considerations include the following:

- there is restricted or no access to the head. The patient should usually be intubated. Patients with rheumatoid arthritis affecting the neck may need an awake intubation. A south- facing pre-formed or armoured tube is most convenient;
- long ventilator tubes and intravenous connecting lines are needed. Alternatively, a venous cannula is placed in the foot;
- the head must be carefully secured to the support;
- the head-up position should be reached slowly, checking the blood pressure as the tilt is increased. Vasopressors may be needed as well as fluids;
- the brain is significantly above the arm. This must be taken into account when deciding the target blood pressure;
- for long procedures, warming devices should be used and body temperature monitored. If the patient is completely covered by a waterproof sterile drape, heat loss may be less than anticipated.
- air embolism may occur;
- at the end of surgery the patient should not be allowed to wake until safely placed on a trolley or bed. The head support may not prove adequate as the patient starts to move about.

Postoperative analgesia usually includes an interscalene brachial plexus block. If this was by a single injection, there must be a robust plan for when the block wears off. Inpatients can receive patient-controlled intravenous opioid, although there may be an unacceptable time delay until this provides adequate analgesia. Patients discharged with a working block often have severe pain at home.[17] Instructions on the use of multiple oral analgesics are often misunderstood. Some centres now provide patient-controlled regional analgesia via an interscalene catheter, even allowing this at home in selected patients.[18]

Elbow surgery

Elbow replacement

Elbow replacement is most commonly performed in patients with rheumatoid arthritis, who may have significant other morbidity, including an unstable neck. It takes about 2 hours. A tourniquet is used. The procedure is as follows:

- the patient is usually in the lateral position with the operated arm uppermost and 'draped' over a padded support with the hand hanging down. The prone position may also be used, with the arm over the edge of the table, but this presents difficulties, especially in patients with unstable necks;

- an endotracheal tube or laryngeal mask may be used. If intubated, patients with rheumatoid arthritis affecting the neck may require awake intubation;
- brachial plexus block is not adequate as the sole anaesthetic, but is extremely useful for postoperative pain. The axillary block is the route of choice. Early mobilisation is important, and a continuous passive movement machine may be used, which is greatly facilitated by brachial plexus block. A single injection of local anaesthetic may provide analgesia for up to 24 hours, but this may be prolonged by the use of an axillary catheter.

Elbow arthrolysis

Elbow arthrolysis is performed to correct stiffness in the elbow. An axillary block with a catheter is ideal to facilitate postoperative continuous passive movement.

Hand surgery

Operations on the hand are frequently suitable for local or regional analgesia, which must extend to the tourniquet area unless the operation lasts less than 10 minutes (e.g. carpal tunnel release). Brachial plexus blocks and more distal blocks are useful. A Bier's block gives less good conditions for hand surgery owing to venous engorgement, but can be useful when all else fails. Brachial plexus block is useful where sympathectomy is required, as for finger reimplantation or free flap surgery, and may be prolonged by the use of a catheter.

Spinal surgery

Over 25 000 spinal operations are carried out annually in the UK.[19] These range from short operations such as microdiscectomy to major and lengthy procedures with massive blood loss and additional anterior access through the chest or abdomen. These major procedures require anaesthetists experienced in this area. Successful results depend on close cooperation between surgeon and anaesthetist.

Pre-assessment

Five principal pathologies present for spinal surgery:

- trauma;
- infection;
- malignancy with vertebral collapse;

- idiopathic or congenital problems, usually scoliosis;
- degenerative disease of the bones or the discs.

Pre-existing neurological deficit should be documented. The anaesthetist should discuss the stability of the spine with the surgeon. A full range of aids to intubation, including equipment for awake intubation, may be needed. Radiographic screening time is sometimes prolonged, so pregnancy should be excluded in women of childbearing age.

Particular care with pre-assessment is needed for scoliosis and extensive malignancy.

Scoliosis

Patients with scoliosis now tend to undergo a single major procedure instead of the multiple procedures of the past. Untreated idiopathic scoliosis may progress rapidly, causing a restrictive respiratory defect, pulmonary hypertension, right heart failure, respiratory failure and death in the fourth or fifth decade. Duchenne muscular dystrophy, cerebral palsy and von Recklinghausen's disease (neurofibromatosis) are important causes of scoliosis and these patients may have other associated pathologies. Respiratory and cardiac function must be carefully assessed and the risks of surgery fully explained to the patient and family. Postoperative high-dependency or intensive care should be considered. Scoliosis surgery improves respiratory function, quality of life and life expectancy.

Duchenne muscular dystrophy Patients with Duchenne muscular dystrophy are an exceptionally high-risk group. The mortality is especially high over the age of 12 years. Difficulties include lack of venous access, higher blood loss, cardiac involvement and severe respiratory compromise.

Metastatic cancer

Patients with metastatic cancer are increasingly being offered surgery to stabilise the spine. They may have respiratory or circulatory complications of their disease or its treatment, and be poorly nourished with acute and chronic pain.

Positioning

Correct positioning for spinal surgery helps lower the venous pressure which may reduce blood loss and provide a clear operating field. If prone, the legs should be lowered and the abdomen should hang freely to avoid raised pressure in the inferior vena cava. This can be achieved by using a Montreal mattress, (a full-length curved mattress with a hole in the middle for the abdomen), or a Wilson frame. Some surgeons use a knee–chest position with special supports. This gives a horizontal lumbar spine. Face and head supports designed to protect pressure points are available. Alternatively, a skull clamp (with pins into bone) will avoid pressure on the face.

If the spine is unstable, positioning should be supervised by the surgeon. At least five people are needed, who all understand the principles of a log roll.

The anaesthetist should check that the brachial plexus is not stretched or compressed in the axilla by the spinal mattress. These may occur if the arms are placed on supports beside the head. An alternative is to place the arms by the sides of the patient but this reduces access to the arms. The neck should not be extended. Care should be taken with the following pressure points:

- the superior orbital nerve as it passes over the rim of the orbit;
- the eyes must be protected to prevent retinal detachment and the eyelids should be fully closed to avoid the cornea becoming dry and sticking to the lid – an abrasion occurs when the eye opens;[20]
- the skin over the maxilla.

Access to the arms is limited if placed by the side. Excellent venous access and extension tubing will be needed.

Conduct of anaesthesia

The basic requirement for spinal surgery is for slight hypotension with low venous pressures. A mean arterial pressure of 60 mmHg is required to maintain spinal cord perfusion in normotensive patients. There is no evidence to support any particular technique. Invasive monitoring may be appropriate.

An armoured endotracheal tube is useful because it cannot be easily kinked. Radiographic imaging of the upper cervical spine may be obscured by a metallic tube. Access to the airway is very poor and fixation of the tube must be totally secure. If an anterior approach is used to the thoracic spine, a double-lumen tube or bronchial blocker allows collapse of one lung, although if using a single-lumen tube, simple lung retraction may achieve satisfactory operating conditions. Discussion with the surgeon is needed.

Blood loss

Blood conservation should be a priority. Complete avoidance of blood transfusion is possible in major spinal surgery. Simple measures include preoperative optimisation of the haemoglobin, modest hypotension and control of coagulation. Thromboelastography conducted in theatre gives rapid information about clotting. Laboratory investigations, such as the international normalised ratio (INR) and platelet count, should be available. Cell salvage is beneficial. There is additional benefit from antifibrinolytic agents such as aprotinin.[19] Warming devices for fluids and the whole patient should be used, and body temperature monitored.

Spinal cord monitoring

Spinal cord monitoring is used when significant alterations to spinal curvature are made, usually during scoliosis surgery. Direct cord injury or interruption of its blood supply may occur. Spinal cord monitoring may reduce the incidence of neurological damage from 3.7–6.9% to 0.5%.[19] Cord function used to be checked by waking the patient up during the operation. This required considerable anaesthetic skill, and does not provide continuous monitoring of spinal cord integrity. It has been replaced by somatosensory evoked potential (SSEP) monitoring, where a sensory nerve in the leg (e.g. posterior tibial nerve) is stimulated and activity is sensed by an epidural electrode placed above the level of surgery by the surgeon. If surgical placement is not possible the sensing electrode may be placed beforehand by the anaesthetist using an awake cervical epidural injection.

A neurophysiologist interprets the data during the operation. Neural transmission is affected by deep anaesthesia. Nitrous oxide 60% with isoflurane 0.5 MAC has little effect, but higher levels of isoflurane can abolish the SSEP altogether. Intravenous agents and opioids also affect the SSEP. A constant depth of anaesthesia allows interpretation of subtle changes in the SSEP.

Some centres use motor evoked potentials, where the stimulus is applied to the cord above the level of surgery and electrical activity sensed in the appropriate muscles. Muscle relaxant is avoided. An infusion of propofol and remifentanil may be used.

Postoperative considerations

Pain can be severe for around 4 days after major spinal surgery. Intravenous opioids are most useful, either continuous infusion or patient-controlled, but ileus may occur. Respiratory depression is a particular hazard because there may already be respiratory compromise. High-dependency care should be considered. Intrathecal opioids given by the surgeon may be useful. Epidural analgesia, via a catheter placed by the surgeon, has been successful, but risks masking neurological sequelae of the surgery. The risk of abscess or haematoma is very low. Extrapleural catheters and paravertebral blocks are also used.

Thromboembolism is common. Without prophylaxis the incidence of DVT is 15% and of symptomatic pulmonary embolus 2.2%.[19] Compression stockings or pneumatic leg pumps should be used, but the use of heparin or warfarin is controversial because of the risk of bleeding.

Paediatric elective orthopaedic surgery

Children presenting for elective orthopaedic surgery commonly have conditions such as cerebral palsy, muscular dystrophy or arthrogryposis (a group of congenital conditions characterised by multiple joint contractures). Staged or multiple procedures are common, and every effort should be made, especially at the first anaesthetic, to make it free of stress for the child. If fear of the anaesthetic room can be avoided, this will greatly ease the difficulties at subsequent – sometimes dozens return visits.

ANAESTHESIA FOR TRAUMA SURGERY

Trauma is the leading cause of death in the first four decades of life in the UK and USA. Significant disability after trauma is about three times the death rate. Death within minutes of the injury is mostly due to injury to the head, high spinal cord, or heart and great vessels. Late deaths are often due to sepsis and multiorgan failure. In between these two groups, the deaths within hours of the injury may be preventable with assessment and an early management process that accurately identify all significant injuries.

Assessment of the multiply injured patient

In February 1976, a plane carrying a trauma surgeon and his family crashed in rural Nebraska, USA. Although he survived the crash, some of his family did not, and he witnessed the deficiencies of a non-specialised remote hospital dealing with multiply injured patients. On his recovery he set up a scheme to care for trauma patients, now practised in more than 50 countries. The Advanced Trauma Life Support (ATLS) programme describes a simple protocol for rapid assessment and early management of patients with multiple injuries. All anaesthetists should be familiar with its basic elements.[21]

The first three steps are:

- establish an adequate airway with cervical spine control;
- breathing – is it adequate?
- circulation – is it adequate?

Emergency treatment of these three components is instituted as necessary. A rapid assessment of disability (neurological status) is performed, together with three basic radiographs of the chest, lateral cervical spine and pelvis. This whole sequence is the primary survey and should identify all immediately life-threatening injuries. Treatment or resuscitation is started without delay. This may include taking the patient to theatre for laparotomy or thoracotomy.

When circumstances permit, the secondary survey is performed. This is a full head-to-toe assessment and seeks to identify all remaining injuries. It includes a log roll to assess the posterior surface of the patient, look for evidence of spinal injury and assess anal tone or injury. Many centres include a trauma computed tomography (CT) scan in their protocol, which replaces diagnostic peritoneal lavage and more reliably detects significant intra-abdominal injury. CT assessment can also include the spine, brain and thoracic structures as indicated. Definitive management of all injuries is then planned. The ATLS manual[21] gives details of the full assessment process, management of specific injuries and guidelines for fluid resuscitation.

Further points to consider are as follows:

- the mechanism of injury should be known to the early management team, which predicts likely injuries. For example, a high-velocity impact in a restrained patient may lead to injuries of the great vessels, including those not immediately apparent, such as pulmonary vein injuries;
- conversely, certain injuries indicate the degree of the impact. For example, first rib fracture is a high-impact injury and suggests other intrathoracic injuries, such as significant lung contusion;
- some physical signs suggest underlying injury. For example, seat belt marks may indicate injury to the spleen or pancreas;
- hypothermia occurs as a result of exposure both before hospital and during initial assessment. Temperature should be monitored and the patient kept covered as much as possible. Warming devices should be used;
- major trauma causes coagulopathy, which must be monitored and aggressively treated. Antifibrinolytic drugs such as aprotinin may be useful.

General considerations for trauma anaesthesia

- Secure intravenous access and ensure crossmatched blood and efficient warming devices for blood and the whole patient;
- patients with significant trauma have delayed gastric emptying. This is mediated by muscarinic cholinergic receptors and is caused by pain, fear, anxiety, shock, disgust (e.g. amputated finger) and opioids, and also acute grief reactions due to injuries in other people. The anaesthetist should assess the individual status of the patient and plan rapid sequence induction as needed;
- nerve blocks are very useful for analgesia in certain circumstances. Femoral nerve blocks are widely used for fractures of the proximal femur, but distal third fractures are innervated by the sciatic nerve. Ring blocks are useful for fractured digits. Positioning may be difficult in patients with fractures. They may not tolerate the use of a nerve stimulator while awake. If nerve damage already exists, it should be documented and a nerve block used only with caution.

Compartment syndrome

Compartment syndrome may occur in any limb injury, not only fractures. Haemorrhage and oedema within a restricted fascial compartment cause a rise in pressure and prevent normal perfusion of the muscles and other structures. If untreated, muscle necrosis may occur with later nerve and vessel damage, contractures, and sometimes loss of the limb.

There should be a high index of suspicion in tibial shaft fractures, displaced tibial plateau fractures and forearm fractures. When planning anaesthesia for these injuries, nerve blockade and epidural analgesia are relatively contraindicated. If in doubt, discuss with the surgeon. If anaesthetic factors strongly indicate regional analgesia, compartment pressure monitoring should be established.

Compartment syndrome can also occur in the foot, particularly after crush injury or a fall causing calcaneal fracture. It is not uncommonly missed, and the patient presents several weeks later with contractures of the foot due to undiagnosed muscle necrosis in one compartment and the unopposed action of muscles in other compartments.

Signs and symptoms of compartment syndrome are:

- pain worsened by passive stretching – this is the earliest sign. Classically, pain is disproportionate to the degree of injury or surgery;
- the limb is pale and cool;
- paraesthesia in the distribution of nerves that cross the compartment;
- the distal pulse may be preserved and does not exclude compartment syndrome – loss of the distal pulse is a late sign;
- muscle weakness – this is also a late finding.

If there is clinical suspicion, compartment pressure should be measured by inserting a needle attached to a pressure monitoring line. The diagnosis is confirmed if the pressure is within 30 mmHg of diastolic blood pressure.

Management of compartment syndrome includes:

- release tight bandages or plaster;
- avoid elevation because this further reduces perfusion;
- rapid sequence induction of anaesthesia for urgent surgical decompression and debridement of necrotic muscle;
- splinting of the limb to prevent contracture.

Specific fractures and their management

Head and chest injury are discussed elsewhere (Chs 5.7 and 5.14, respectively).

Pelvic fractures

Bleeding from pelvic fractures can be massive, unrecognised and cause rapid death.

Anterior–posterior fracture dislocation of the ilium on the sacrum may occur, often bilaterally, after compression injury. This 'open book' injury tears posteriorly placed veins within the pelvis. It also considerably increases the capacity of the pelvis, which impairs or delays tamponade.

Vertical shear pattern fractures, where the ilium moves superiorly on the sacrum, are also associated with massive blood loss.

If pelvic fractures are unstable, emergency external fixation may be required, bringing the pelvis together and improving tamponade. This may be performed under local anaesthesia in the resuscitation room. It should take priority over an emergency laparotomy because circulatory collapse may occur as the abdomen is opened and any tamponade provided by the abdominal wall is lost. Laparotomy is possible working around an external fixator. Injuries of the urethra, bladder, vagina and rectum should also be considered with any fractured pelvis.

Definitive fixation of the pelvic fracture can occur later, and may require transfer to a specialist centre. Anaesthetic considerations are as follows:

- fixation may require plating via several different approaches. Prior discussion with the surgeon is required;
- epidural analgesia is useful for postoperative pain, which may be considerable due to extnsive muscle stripping and multiple incisions. The surgeon must confirm that the pelvis is stable for turning. The author anaesthetises the patient before inserting the epidural as the turn cannot be tolerated awake. The epidural 4 block is only established when the risk of massive blood loss has passed;
- there may be considerable blood loss. This varies with the approach. The posterior approach risks injury to the superior gluteal artery, which may be very difficult to control. Both anterior and posterior approaches may involve considerable dissection and muscle stripping, which can be associated with prolonged oozing. Cell salvage should be considered. Rapid massive blood loss is also possible. At least two large cannulae and efficient blood warming should be used;
- if there is co-morbidity, invasive monitoring may be useful but is not essential in a healthy patient with an isolated injury;
- air embolism may occur.

Spinal fractures

If the paramedics consider spinal injury is a possibility, the patient will be transferred to hospital on a spinal board with 'triple immobilisation' of the neck. This means use of a cervical collar, sandbags and tape to prevent turning of the head. The patient should be moved off the board within 1 hour of arrival to protect pressure areas. Spinal injury precautions require log rolling by at least five trained personnel and is described in detail in the ATLS manual.[21]

Full spinal injury precautions must continue until the whole spine is cleared in two respects. It should be radiologically normal and clinically normal with no pain, because ligamentous injury alone can lead to spinal cord injury. To make this assessment, the patient must be conscious and without neurological injury, the influence of alcohol or drugs, or severe pain elsewhere distracting him or her from back or neck pain. In practice, this may be difficult to achieve.

Nursing care is greatly complicated if the spine cannot be cleared. However, spinal cord injury is so serious that only a senior clinician should authorise discontinuation of spinal injury precautions.

Other considerations include the following:

- if there is cord transection there is loss of sympathetic tone below the level of transection. Hypotension ('spinal shock') responds to fluid and vasopressor therapy. If there is a significant cord injury without transection, some recovery is possible. Perfusion pressures must be kept high, hypoxia avoided, and high-dose methylprednisolone given as soon as possible;
- the neck must be stabilised in-line during intubation. Awake fibreoptic intubation may be necessary;
- suxamethonium should not be given to patients with spinal cord injuries except in the first 12 hours. It may cause massive and fatal potassium efflux from denervated muscle cells. If rapid sequence induction is required, a modified technique using rocuronium should be used.

Fractured neck of femur

There are about 50 000 isolated fractured necks of femur each year in England. In 1998–1999, the patients were elderly (mean 80 years) and their hospital stays lengthy (mean 21 days). In one audit, hospital mortality rate was 5–24%.[22]

The main considerations for fractured neck of femur are as follows:

- senior anaesthetists should be involved. Assessment should take place early to ensure that the patient is appropriately resuscitated and investigated. Early management should include fluid resuscitation and analgesia. Opioids should be prescribed in adequate doses. Excessive concern about cardiac failure and respiratory depression may lead to inadequate fluid administration and analgesia. The patients may not be able to express the degree of their pain;
- although co-morbidity is common, investigations should only be requested urgently before surgery if they will influence management;
- a nerve block is useful for post-operative analgesia, most commonly the three-in-one lumbar plexus block. Psoas compartment, lateral cutaneous and subcostal blocks may be used as alternatives;[23]
- the fracture should be fixed on the next available daytime trauma list after investigations have been completed. Mortality at 1 year may be over 10% greater if surgery is delayed more than 24 hours.[24] Delay causes rapid deterioration due to chest infection, electrolyte imbalance, thromboembolism, pressure sores and urinary infection;
- regional anaesthesia may be advantageous. Meta-analysis showed a reduced incidence of DVT and mortality at 1 month, although this was

not sustained.[25] There may also be less myocardial infarction and less postoperative confusion or hypoxia. Regional anaesthesia is recommended by the Scottish Intercollegiate Guidelines Network;[26]

- achieving a position for spinal injection in patients with fractured neck of femur is difficult because of pain, often compounded by arthritis and kyphoscoliosis. Some anaesthetists sedate the patient for turning, using boluses of 0.5–2.0 mg midazolam, 10–30 mg propofol or 10 mg ketamine. Sedation may lead to confusion and lack of cooperation. Other anaesthetists perform a femoral nerve block, but this takes 30 minutes to work. Some patients will tolerate a careful turn without sedation provided there is a full explanation, a soft bed, some light anxiolysis and a swift spinal injection after the turn;
- there are two types of operation. If the fracture is extracapsular (intertrochanteric), the blood supply to the femoral head is preserved. Screw fixation is performed, most commonly a dynamic hip screw, with the patient supine raised on a high table to facilitate X-ray screening. If the fracture is intracapsular (subcapital), avascular necrosis of the femoral head occurs in about 6% of cases, particularly if the fracture is displaced, and a cemented hemiarthroplasty is usually performed. If there is great concern over the cardiovascular stability of the patient, the surgeon may be willing to consider an uncemented prosthesis (Austin–Moore hemiarthroplasty). However, these have an increased incidence of early thigh pain, even with minimal activity, and a cemented prosthesis should be used where possible. For all these operations operating time is about 1 hour and blood loss is 200–400 mL.

Amputation

The unwelcome procedure of amputation may be an option in the early management of severe crush or impact injuries, or it may follow a long series of interventions aimed at saving the limb. For example, it may be the final consequence of compartment syndrome, perhaps after a relatively minor fracture.

General anaesthesia with or without epidural analgesia is commonly used. Spinal anaesthesia is also used, in which case most patients request sedation also. In orthopaedics and trauma, unlike vascular surgery, the circulation is usually excellent and blood loss may be massive. A tourniquet should be used where possible. Regional techniques exacerbate the effects of hypovolaemia, which must be managed aggressively.

There is no evidence that pre-emptive epidural analgesia started 24 hours beforehand reduces the incidence of phantom limb pain.

Paediatric trauma

Trauma is the leading cause of death in the UK in children under 14 years.[27] Over half relate to road traffic accidents. Staff at the receiving hospital may not be fully experienced in paediatric trauma, but all anaesthetists should be competent in the initial management and stabilisation of an injured child, before transfer to a paediatric centre if necessary (see Ch. 5.6).

Some key principles are as follows:

- initial management follows the same pattern as in adults – airway with cervical spine control, breathing, circulation, rapid assessment of disability, primary radiographs and secondary survey. Knowledge of the normal range of vital signs in small children is essential;
- the cervical spine of children is highly mobile and the head is relatively large. This makes serious neck injury more likely. Spinal cord damage without bony injury is more likely than in adults. Cervical spine radiographs need expert interpretation because 'pseudosubluxation' (a normal variant) may occur;
- blood pressure is a notoriously poor indicator of hypovolaemia in children. Peripheral vasoconstriction, tachycardia and drowsiness are better indicators. If hypovolaemic, 20 mL/kg of intravenous fluid should be given initially, repeated once if necessary, after which blood should be considered. Intraosseous access to the circulation is useful in small children. Brain injury is not a reason to withhold intravenous fluid. More damage will be done by failing to restore blood volume than by giving excess fluid;
- Head injury causes more than 50% of trauma deaths in children. Children are more likely to have diffuse brain injury with cerebral oedema, and less likely to have intracerebral haemmorhage requiring surgical treatment. Children are more likely than adults to have a fit after relatively minor head injury, and so need anticonvulsant treatment;
- the ribs are incompletely ossified in children and cartilaginous joints are more elastic, so the thoracic cage is much more flexible than in adults. Rib fractures are rare, but severe underlying thoracic trauma may still be present;
- the abdomen is also poorly protected because the thoracic cage is short and flexible. The liver, spleen and kidneys are at risk from minor impacts. Paediatric surgeons are more likely to attempt conservative management of injured solid organs than in adults, but possible perforation of the bowel will always be explored. It is especially important to try to conserve the spleen because of the lifelong risk of sepsis;
- children are prone to aerophagia (air swallowing) when distressed. Extreme gastric distension may occur, which gives a risk of vomiting and may confuse clinical findings in the abdomen. A gastric tube should be used;
- parents and other family members also require the care of the admitting trauma team. There will be anxiety and fear, and there may be overwhelming guilt, even if the accident was not predictable or preventable. Parental presence with the child should be considered at all stages, and the family cared for by expert personnel.

References

1. Hebert PC, Wells G, Blajchman MA, et al. A multicenter, randomised, controlled clinical trial of transfusion requirements in critical care. N Engl J Med 1999; 340:409–417.
2. Kam PCA, Kavanaugh R, Yoong FFY. The arterial tourniquet: pathological consequences and anaesthetic implications. Anaesthesia 2001; 56:534–545.
3. Geerts WH, Pineo GF, Heit JA, et al. Prevention of venous thromboembolism. The seventh American College of Chest Physicians conference on antithrombotic and thrombolytic therapy. Chest 2004; 126:3385–4005.
4. Nicolaides AN. Prevention of venous thromboembolism: international consensus statement guidelines complied in accordance with the scientific evidence. Int Angiol 2001; 20:1–37.
5. Gillespie W, Murray D, Gregg PJ, Warwick D. Risks and benefits of prophylaxis against venous thromboembolism in orthopaedic surgery. Journal of Bone and Joint Surgery 2000; 82:475–80.
6. Turpie AGG, Eriksson BI, Bauer KA, Lassen MR. New pentasaccharides for the prevention of venous thromboembolism. Chest 2003; 124:371–376.
7. Checketts MR, Wildsmith JAW. Central nerve block and thromboprophylaxis – is there a problem? Br J Anaesth 1999; 82:164–167.
8. Mellor A, Soni N. Fat embolism. Anaesthesia 2001; 56:145–154.
9. Connolly D. Orthopaedic anaesthesia. Anaesthesia 2003; 58:1189–1193.
10. Skinner MW, Sutton BA. Do anaesthetists need to wear surgical masks in the operating theatre? A literature review with evidence based recommendations. Anaesth Intens Care 2001; 29:331–338.
11. Winnie A, Ramamurphy S, Durrani Z. The inguinal paravascular technique of lumbar plexus anaesthesia: the 3 in 1 block. Anesth Analg 1973; 52:989–996.
12. Sim IW, Webb T. Anatomy and anaesthesia of the lumbar somatic plexus. Anaesth Intens Care 2004; 32:178–187.
13. Chayen D, Nathan H, Chayen M. The psoas compartment block. Anesthesiology 1976; 45:95–99.
14. Vloka JD, Hadzic A. Sciatic nerve blocks – lateral popliteal approach. In: Chelly JE, ed. Peripheral nerve blocks: a colour atlas. Philadelphia: Lippincott Williams & Williams; 1999:87–88.
15. Fischer HBJ. Regional anaesthesia – before or after general anaesthesia? Editorial. Anaesthesia 1998; 53:727–729.
16. Peterson MK, Millar FA, Sheppard DG. Ultrasound guided nerve blocks. Br J Anaesthesia 2002; 88:621–623.
17. Wilson AT, Nicholson E, Burton L, Wild C. Analgesia for day case shoulder surgery. Br J Anaesth 2004; 92:414–415.

18. Klein SM. Beyond the hospital. Continuous peripheral nerve blocks at home. Anesthesiology 2002; 96:1283–1285.

19. Raw DA, Beattie JK, Hunter JM. Anaesthesia for spinal surgery in adults. Br J Anaesth 2003; 91:886–904.

20. White E, Crosse MM. The aetiology and prevention of perioperative corneal abrasions. Anaesthesia 1998; 53:157–161.

21. American College of Surgeons. Advanced trauma life support student manual. Chicago: American College of Surgeons; 1997.

22. Jandziol AK, Griffiths R. The anaesthetic management of patients with hip fractures. Br J Anaesth CEPD Rev 2001; 1:52–55.

23. Parker MJ, Griffiths R, Appadu BN. Nerve blocks (subcostal, lateral cutaneous, femoral, psoas) for hip fractures. (Cochrane review). Cochrane Database Syst Rev 2002; Issue 1.

24. Casaletto JA, Gatt R. Post-operative mortality related to waiting time for hip fracture surgery. Injury 2004; 35:114–120.

25. Urwin SC, Parker MJ, Griffiths R. General vs regional anaesthesia for hip fracture surgery: meta-analysis of randomised trials. Br J Anaesth 2000; 84:450–455.

26. Scottish Intercollegiate Guidelines Network. Prevention and management of hip fracture in older people – a national clinical guideline. Edinburgh: Scottish Intercollegiate Guidelines Network; 2002.

27. Dykes H. Paediatric Trauma. Br J Anaesth 1999; 83:130–138.

CHAPTER **5.12**

OTORHINOLARYNGOLOGY

GENERAL CONSIDERATIONS

Otorhinolaryngology operations range from short day-case procedures, such as grommet insertion or endoscopy, to complex head and neck resections lasting many hours. Patient age ranges from neonate to the elderly. The boundaries with dental surgery and skull base neurosurgery (e.g. translabyrinthine removal of acoustic neuroma) are becoming increasingly blurred.

The shared airway

The surgeon and anaesthetist desire simultaneous access to the airway, may be compromised by disease. The vocal cords must be immobile if they are the site of surgery.

Tracheal intubation may not be possible if it interferes with surgical access. Ventilation may be maintained with the supraglottic Sanders injector technique.

Intravenous anaesthesia is particularly useful. Short-acting opioids allow control of cardiovascular reflexes and rapid awakening.

Breath-holding and laryngospasm on emergence may be severe.

TECHNICAL CONSIDERATIONS

If surgery is carried out in the throat or nose, the anaesthetist must preserve a clear airway while optimising surgical access, and prevent soiling of the trachea and bronchi with blood and debris. The anaesthetist should be prepared to deal with failure of any of these. Although general anaesthesia is commonly employed, it is worth remembering that many operations can be undertaken under local anaesthesia.

Local anaesthesia

One report[1] describes major resections carried out under local anaesthesia, such as laryngectomy with neck dissection, with good results. Lack of anaesthetic equipment or expertise, patient or surgical preference, patient co-morbidity, faster recovery and low morbidity are the usual driving forces.

A certain amount of fortitude is desirable. In middle ear surgery, vestibular activation may produce nausea. It is difficult for an awake patient to sustain the immobility required for microscope-directed surgery for more than 1 hour.

Techniques

Oral or nasal mucosa

Oral or nasal mucosa may be anaesthetised for minor surgery with topical 4–10% lidocaine (lignocaine), supplemented by further injection. Dental cartridges are commonly used, containing 3% prilocaine with 1:80 000 epinephrine (adrenaline) (12.5 μg/mL). Cocaine 5% is a useful analgesic and vasoconstrictor, but is subject to legal restrictions. Idiosyncratic reactions have been reported.

Maxillary branch of the trigeminal nerve

The maxillary branch of the trigeminal nerve passes through the foramen rotundum and may be blocked at the sphenopalatine ganglion at the back of the nasal cavity by local anaesthetic instilled into the nose.

A traditional anaesthetic and vasoconstrictor solution described initially by a Birmingham surgeon in 1947 has undergone some modification. Moffett's solution now contains 1 mL 1:1000 epinephrine (adrenaline) (1 mg), 2 mL 5% cocaine (100 mg) and 1–2 mL 8.4% sodium bicarbonate diluted to 10 mL with 0.9% saline.

The patient is positioned supine over a shoulder roll with the neck and head extended. The anaesthetic solution is dribbled into the dependent roof of the nasal cavity. The patient should spit out excess solution rather than swallow it. Cotton wool buds dipped in solution may be passed into the nasal cavity, or the cavity packed with gauze soaked in solution.

Supraorbital nerve

The supraorbital nerve supplies sensation to the ipsilateral forehead and scalp up to the vertex. It may be blocked at the supraorbital notch.

Trigeminal nerve

The trigeminal nerve supplies sensation to the face through its mandibular, maxillary and ophthalmic divisions. Each division, or the terminal branches, may be blocked (see Ch. 4.2).

Greater auricular nerve

The greater auricular nerve (C2, C3), a branch of the superficial cervical plexus, is blocked to provide analgesia after tympanomastoid surgery through a postauricular incision. A needle is inserted in front of the lower anterior border of the mastoid process, and advanced first between the mastoid process and meatus, infiltrating 3–5 mL local anaesthetic. The needle is then withdrawn and redirected subcutaneously posterior to the meatus and ear canal until the needle tip is cranial to the canal, infiltrating 4–6 mL of anaesthetic solution.

Cervical plexus block

Cervical plexus block is useful for operations in the neck (see Ch. 4.2).

Tympanic membrane

The tympanic membrane may be anaesthetised for myringotomy with 0.1–0.2 mL of lidocaine (lignocaine)/prilocaine cream (EMLA®), applied for 15 minutes. It may be toxic to the middle ear and should be used sparingly.

General anaesthesia

Preoperative assessment and consent

A number of operations are suitable for day surgery (e.g. myringoplasty, grommets).

The airway should be carefully evaluated to anticipate problems. Magnetic resonance imaging (MRI) or computed tomography (CT) is useful when the airway is affected by disease. Obstructive sleep apnoea should be recognised.

Assess the risks and benefits if controlled hypotension is to be used.

The patient should be informed of the use of intravenous fluids, nasogastric tube, nasal packs, urinary catheter or spinal drain, and warned of postoperative nausea and cranial nerve damage if appropriate. Postoperative analgesia should be discussed and consent obtained for analgesic suppositories. Some patients will have impaired hearing.

Heparin, for deep vein thrombosis prophylaxis, should probably be avoided for middle ear or skull-base surgery.

Major cases are likely to need high-dependency postoperative care.

Premedication

No premedication is required for short or day-case procedures, or if not desired by the patient. Apply EMLA® cream or tetracaine (amethocaine) gel over marked veins in children or anxious adults.

The dose of oral benzodiazepine for sedation is:

- in children – up to 0.5 mg/kg midazolam (maximum 20 mg), perhaps with 20 mg/kg paracetamol for analgesia;
- in adults – 20–30 mg temazepam or 10–15 mg diazepam.

Intramuscular opioid – 10 mg morphine with 0.2–0.4 mg hyoscine – provides sedation and antisialogogue activity. Further antiemetic may be needed.

Antisialogogue alone is 0.6 mg atropine or 0.4 mg glycopyrrolate intramuscularly.

Sedation should be avoided if there is a compromised airway or obstructive sleep apnoea.

Monitoring

In addition to standard monitoring, consider the following:

- arterial cannula to monitor blood pressure and assess acid–base status in procedures with controlled hypotension, neck surgery around the vagus or carotid sinus, or affecting the internal carotid artery or internal jugular vein, and extensive head and neck resections with flaps or free grafts;
- central venous pressure if there is cardiac disease or if blood loss is likely to be excessive;
- facial nerve monitoring;
- recurrent laryngeal nerve monitoring;
- body temperature and urine output for longer procedures (over 3–4 hours).

Technique

Conventional intravenous agents such as thiopental 3–5 mg/kg or propofol 1–3 mg/kg are used for induction, followed by maintenance with a target-controlled infusion of propofol (initial blood level 4–8 μg/mL) or inhalation agent. Analgesia is with opioid infusion or boluses (e.g. fentanyl 1–2 μg/kg, alfentanil 10–20 μg/kg or remifentanil 1–2 μg/kg).

Airway maintenance with laryngeal mask or tracheal intubation is aided by deep anaesthesia, suxamethonium 1.5 mg/kg (avoid in children) or non-depolarising agent.

Throat pack is used for oral, nasal, dental or sinus surgery to prevent airway soiling.

Protect the eyes with tape and pads. A head ring, shoulder roll and head-up tilt are often required. Use a warming blanket for operations long than 30–45 minutes.

Emergence

Remove any throat pack and suction the pharynx under direct vision. If airway soiling is possible, position the patient on their side until awake.

Deep extubation will give a smooth emergence, but consider awake extubation if airway control is of prime importance. Consider extubation while the patient is still paralysed and inserting a laryngeal mask airway to provide a smoother emergence.

SPECIFIC OPERATIONS

Intranasal operations

Intranasal operations are polypectomy, septoplasty, rhinoplasty and functional endoscopic sinus surgery. Either a laryngeal mask or a cuffed endotracheal tube may be used with a throat pack, depending on the anaesthetist's confidence, the surgeon, the amount of blood loss and the duration of surgery. A flexible laryngeal mask or a south-facing preformed tube allows the airway to be secured away from the nose.

Topical nasal vasoconstriction is extremely useful and may be applied by the anaesthetist or surgeon. Commonly used vasoconstrictors include 5–10% cocaine, cocaine paste, xylometazoline or ephedrine drops or spray, Moffett's solution, or dental cartridge injection of local anaesthetic with epinephrine (adrenaline) 1:80 000. Vasoconstriction by block of the sphenopalatine ganglion, which carries the vasodilator fibres to the nasal blood vessels, has also been described.

The surgeon may wish the eyes to be uncovered, otherwise they should be taped shut.

Surgery is easier with controlled hypotension. Profuse bleeding may cause the operation to be abandoned. The gown should be loose around the neck and the patient positioned head-up. Opioids should be short acting, such as alfentanil or remifentanil, because postoperative pain is not marked.

After the throat pack is removed, pharyngeal suction should include an attempt to remove blood clots from behind the soft palate. With an endotracheal tube this can be done using a laryngoscope. With a laryngeal mask, suction is applied to the upper surface of the mask at the back of the pharynx. It is usual to leave the laryngeal mask in place until awakening. Nasal packs are likely to be placed by the surgeon and may stay in overnight. These occlude the nasal airway, which is uncomfortable, and may be hazardous in patients with obstructive sleep apnoea.

Postoperative analgesia is usually provided by simple oral agents. If opioids are required, patients with obstructive sleep apnoea will require oxygen and careful observation.

Manipulation of fractured nasal bones

Minor manipulation of fractured nasal bones can sometimes be carried out under intravenous anaesthesia in the head-down position or using a laryngeal mask. If the fracture is more than 2 weeks old, vigorous surgical manipulation may be required. The safe technique involves tracheal intubation and throat pack to prevent aspiration of blood should bleeding occur. The anaesthetic agents should permit rapid return of protective reflexes (e.g. propofol, remifentanil, alfentanil). If plaster of Paris is applied, the closed eyes may be protected with adhesive tape. If there is unfortunate brisk haemorrhage with only a laryngeal mask in place, it is reasonable to suction continuously at the back of the pharynx for a few minutes and pack the nose, hoping it will abate, but it must be possible to intubate rapidly to protect the airway.

Tonsillectomy

If tonsillectomy is conducted in a child with a genuine cold, there is a risk of intraoperative laryngeal spasm, bronchospasm and hypoxia. There is also a risk of profuse bleeding, postoperative chest infection, and even cardiac arrest up to 4–6 weeks afterwards.

For children, the right psychological atmosphere is of greatest value in obtaining smooth induction of anaesthesia without tears, requiring rapport with the child, the parent and even the child's toys. Preoperative crying and tachycardia increase surgical bleeding. Suitable premedication, especially for fractious children, is 0.5 mg/kg temazepam or 0.2–0.5 mg/kg midazolam syrup. Some advocate oral analgesia preoperatively.

Tetracaine (amethocaine) gel or EMLA® cream provide painless venepuncture. Marking the best veins helps nurses locate the patch correctly. Sevoflurane may be used for induction in the sizeable minority of children who have needle phobia. Parents are warned that either approach may be needed.

A south-facing preformed oral endotracheal tube may be kept clear of the operative field by a Doughty blade on a Boyle–Davis gag, and also allows uninterrupted access to the adenoids. When the gag is inserted, the anaesthetist should ensure that the airway is patent by seeing and feeling appropriate chest movement, bag movement and capnography. The tube may kink at the teeth or at the back of the tongue where the gag ends. Either spontaneous breathing or intermittent positive-pressure ventilation (IPPV) is acceptable. Removal of the gag can sometimes causes accidental extubation, so facilities for reintubation including suxamethonium should always be available. In teenagers and adults, a nasal tube can be used. Some anaesthetists use a reinforced laryngeal mask, claiming this provides a smoother emergence.

Concern has been raised that the tonsillar bed may contain the abnormal prion protein implicated in variant Creutzfeldt–Jakob disease. Recommendations are for the use of single-use airway equipment, including laryngoscope, if patient safety is not compromised. Single-use surgical equipment of poor design was associated with an increased incidence of serious postoperative haemorrhage.

The patient is normally supine with a shoulder roll. The eyes must be taped. Intravenous fluid (Hartmann's not dextrose) is helpful, giving at least 4 hours of maintenance requirement. Blood loss may easily reach 10% of blood volume in small children. If this happens blood should be taken during surgery for haemoglobin and group and save or crossmatch. The cannula should remain in place postoperatively, but fluids are not normally required.

Extubation should be either deliberately deep or awake. There is no clear consensus. Laryngospasm is common. Deep extubation should be in the tonsil position (pillow under the shoulders, semiprone, prevented from rolling onto the face by the pillow and by flexed knees and hips), and this position maintained under the anaesthetist's supervision until full consciousness is regained. If awake extubation is chosen an oral airway should be positioned alongside the tracheal tube to prevent occlusion through biting. A 'no-touch' technique, in which no stimulation is given until awakening, appears successful.[2]

Analgesia by suppository is useful, but needs parental permission. Paracetamol 40 mg/kg is more effective than 20 mg/kg, but total daily dose should not exceed 90 mg/kg. Non-steroidal anti-inflammatory drugs (NSAIDs) also provide good analgesia (e.g. 0.5–1 mg/kg diclofenac, total maximum daily dose 2 mg/kg). NSAIDs impair platelet function and a meta-analysis[3] indicated more frequent significant postoperative primary and secondary haemorrhage. However, they are commonly used in the UK.[4]

Dexamethasone (0.1–0.2 mg/kg, up to 4–8 mg total dose) reduces the incidence of nausea and vomiting and may aid analgesia. Topical application or injection of local anaesthetic in the tonsillar fossae has been described, but not always with benefit.

Anaesthesia for post-tonsillectomy haemorrhage

Postoperative primary or secondary haemorrhage occurs in 2–10% of cases. Surgical intervention is required in 1–5%. This is a grave responsibility and senior assistance is desirable.

Assessment Assessment is usually on the ward as follows:

- estimate blood loss (often underestimated), insert a larger intravenous cannula if necessary, start resuscitation with crystalloid or colloid (20–40 mL/kg initially) and obtain crossmatched blood (transfusion is used earlier in children);
- consider the advisability of immediate surgery or leave time for resuscitation;
- check previous anaesthetic chart for tube size used and any problems.

Problems The problems associated with post-tonsillectomy haemorrhage are hypovolaemia and a stomach likely to be full of blood clot.

Visible blood loss is only a fraction of the total. If a child is shocked the deficit is at least 20% of blood volume, rising to probably 50% when the child is close to circulatory collapse. A reduced dose of anaesthetic is required. A rapid sequence induction may be used, although some prefer inhalation induction with the patient initially in the lateral position. In either case, cricoid pressure and tracheal intubation are used.

The blood pressure is checked frequently during induction.

Gastric aspiration while the patient is still intubated may be advisable to reduce the risk of postoperative regurgitation.

Awake extubation is usual.

Upper airway obstruction

Upper airway obstruction may be acute or chronic.

Acute obstruction develops over minutes, hours or a few days, whereas chronic obstruction develops over weeks, months or years. In acute obstruction, the respiratory muscles are untrained and symptoms and signs of respiratory difficulty are prominent. In chronic obstruction, when airway narrowing has developed over a number of months, adult patients with a surprisingly narrow airway (about 3.5 mm diameter) may be asymptomatic at rest.

Acute obstruction

Causes

Causes of acute obstruction are:

- infections in the upper airway (retropharynx, floor of the mouth, epiglottis), including diphtheria;
- oedema due to anaphylaxis, angiotensin-converting enzyme (ACE) inhibitors, angioedema, trauma or burns;
- presence of foreign body or blood clot or haemorrhage (postoperative or into a cyst).

Presentation

Acute obstruction presents with dyspnoea, anxiety, restlessness, feeling of impending doom and inability to lie flat, possibly associated with sore throat, dysphagia or dysphonia.

There may be obvious swelling of the lips, tongue, floor of the mouth or neck, stridor (noisy breathing), increased work of breathing as judged by a high respiratory rate, dilating alae nasi, rib and intercostal retraction, use of accessory muscles, sitting upright holding on to trolley, cyanosis, sweating and tachycardia.

The patient may be pyrexial if the cause is infective.

Inspiratory stridor indicates extrathoracic pathology. Expiratory stridor indicates intrathoracic narrowing.

Management

It may be dangerous to send the patient to a normal radiography suite, and safer to perform a portable X-ray in a high-dependency unit, or flexible nasendoscopy by the surgeon. Foreign bodies are often radiolucent, but bronchial obstruction is revealed by paired inspiratory and expiratory films where one lung fails to empty in expiration.

Treatment

Acute obstruction is treated with 60–100% inspired oxygen by mask with saturation monitoring. Consider heliox (helium 70–79% oxygen 21%), judging whether this is beneficial by improved work of breathing and oxygenation. Give nebulised or parenteral epinephrine (adrenaline) if there is anaphylaxis. It may be necessary to proceed to emergency cricothyrotomy (needle or surgical) or secure the airway by intubation or tracheostomy.

Anaesthesia for securing the airway Anaesthesia for securing the airway may be needed for removal of a foreign body or to drain pus or a haematoma. A typical case would be Ludwig's angina (angina is from the Greek word for 'strangulation'). This progressive infection of the submandibular and sublingual spaces, first described by Wilhelm von Ludwig in 1836, was usually fatal. A senior surgeon and anaesthetist are needed. It is generally advised to maintain spontaneous respiration until the airway is secured. The options are as follows:

- inhalation induction with 100% oxygen and volatile agent (sevoflurane or halothane), maintaining spontaneous respiration, and intubation when deep. This is conducted in theatre with the surgeon scrubbed and ready to undertake rapid tracheostomy;
- awake fibreoptic intubation, which is likely to be very difficult and is also conducted in theatre with the surgeon ready to undertake rapid tracheostomy;
- tracheostomy under local anaesthesia.

In circumstances where there is no surgeon available to undertake a rapid tracheostomy, consider insertion of a cricothyrotomy needle before induction of anaesthesia or a surgical cricothyrotomy.

Chronic obstruction

Causes

Causes of chronic obstruction are benign or malignant tumours, inflammatory conditions such as Wegener's granulomatosis, and progressive scarring secondary to surgery or radiotherapy.

Assessment

There is time available to perform CT or MRI of the entire airway and flexible nasendoscopy to identify the degree and site of narrowing. The surgeon and anaesthetist should jointly review the findings, and discuss whether surgery is required for biopsy, debulking or securing the airway.

Airway management

Options for airway management include:

- inhalation induction (with the surgeon ready to perform a tracheostomy);
- intravenous induction, paralysis and direct laryngoscopy;
- awake fibreoptic intubation;
- tracheostomy under local anaesthesia.

Surgical tracheostomy

Surgical tracheostomy was first described in the second century AD, and was first reported in Britain by Martine (1730). Percutaneous and translaryngeal tracheostomy are considered in Chapter 2.6.

Indications

Surgical tracheostomy is indicated for:

- relief of acute upper airway obstruction;
- management of chronic airway obstruction (including obstructive sleep apnoea);
- management of airway trauma;
- planned secure airway following head and neck surgery;
- if tracheal intubation is needed for longer than 7–10 days.

Anaesthesia for surgical tracheostomy

Surgical tracheostomy may be undertaken under local or general anaesthesia. It is prudent to check the size of the planned tracheostomy tube and all connectors with the surgeon and scrub nurse.

If general anaesthesia is selected, airway management may be difficult owing to the underlying condition. Ideally a nasal or oral tracheal tube is placed, but the operation may be accomplished with a facemask or laryngeal mask. Anaesthesia may be intravenous or inhalational, but 100% oxygen should be given for several minutes before tube changeover. At changeover, the anaesthetist withdraws the tube slowly (guided by the surgeon) until only its tip is visible in the trachea and the surgeon attempts to insert the tracheostomy tube. The anaesthetist must confirm correct placement of the tracheostomy tube by bag movement, chest movement and capnography before removing the nasal or oral tube.

Particular problems in trauma to the larynx and trachea

Particular problems in trauma to the larynx and trachea are:

- airway obstruction requiring emergency intubation, which is often difficult, especially if due to a damaged epiglottis;
- massive carotid haemorrhage with cerebral ischaemia;
- pneumothorax;
- concomitant injury to the head, cervical spine or oesophagus;
- air embolism – the patient should be nursed in a head-down position to prevent air being sucked into an open vein;
- a full stomach.

Obstructive sleep apnoea

The criteria for a diagnosis of obstructive sleep apnoea are apnoea occurring repeatedly during sleep due to complete obstruction to the airway (with continued diaphragm movement) for more than 10 seconds, leading to a reduction in oxygen saturation of more than 4%. Most patients are overweight males with a large collar size, but the condition exists in children.

Symptoms of obstructive sleep apnoea include snoring, choking during sleep, altered personality and poor sleep quality. Daytime sleepiness is common and is assessed by the Epworth Sleepiness Scale, which scores the likelihood of falling asleep in eight situations: sitting and reading, watching TV, sitting in a meeting, sitting after lunch, car passenger for an hour, lying down in the afternoon, talking to someone, and stopped for a few minutes in a car. For each situation the score ranges from 0 (none) to 3 (high chance). A score over 15 is significant when due to obstructive sleep apnoea. Patients with previously unrecognised obstructive sleep apnoea should be referred to a sleep specialist before undertaking elective surgery.

Obstructive sleep apnoea is a far from benign condition. Patients may present for surgery to improve the upper airway (septoplasty, tonsillectomy, palatoplasty) or for an unrelated condition. Problems include difficult airway management, preoperative and postoperative hypoxia, carbon dioxide narcosis, and excessive respiratory sensitivity to opioids. Particular problems occur if the nasal airway is occluded by packs.

Patients should be nursed postoperatively in a high-dependency unit with oxygen saturation monitoring. Oxygen should be given by mask when opioids are required for postoperative analgesia and continued for at least 24 hours after the opioid is stopped. Patients who are managed with home continuous positive airway pressure (CPAP) should bring the device into hospital and use it postoperatively. In children undergoing urgent adenotonsillectomy there is a high chance of early postoperative medical intervention, including reintubation.[5]

Laryngoscopy and microsurgery of the larynx

Problems with laryngoscopy and microsurgery of the larynx include the following:

- the jaw and cords need to be relaxed. The vocal cords normally need to be immobile for surgery, but the surgeon may sometimes need to observe cord movement. The view may be impaired by secretions, so always give an antisialogogue;
- laryngoscopy causes reflex hypertension and tachycardia;
- there may be lesions that obstruct the airway;
- the patient must be oxygenated and ventilated, avoiding airway soiling by blood, debris or smoke;
- postoperative recovery of airway control should be rapid and without laryngospasm.

Options in adults

Microlaryngeal tube

The trachea is intubated with a cuffed microlaryngeal tube (5.0–6.0 mm inner diameter) through the nose or mouth (consult with the surgeon). The tube lies posteriorly, enabling most of the cords to be seen. The muscle relaxant used depends on the expected duration of surgery. Inhalational or intravenous anaesthesia may be used. There is good control of the airway during surgery, with secure ventilation, vocal cord immobility and prevention of airway soiling. Topical lidocaine (lignocaine) 3 mg/kg on the cords reduces emergence laryngospasm and facilitates awake extubation.

Supraglottic injector

A 16 G Sanders (USA anaesthetist, 1967) injector needle is attached to the surgeon's suspension laryngoscope. The laryngoscope must be pointing at the larynx and the cords adequately paralysed. Ventilation is by the traditional manual injector technique – the needle is connected to a 400 kPa oxygen supply, activated by a manual lever or button. Adequate inspiration and expiration should both be confirmed by inspection of chest movement. A special jet ventilator may also be used. Intravenous anaesthesia is required.

Transglottic injector

A Hunsaker tube is placed transglottically with ventilation using a manual Sanders or jet ventilator. Expiration must be assured to prevent barotrauma. Some jet ventilators have the safety feature of not providing a positive pressure burst until the tracheal pressure has fallen to baseline.

Subglottic injector

A transtracheal jet ventilation needle is inserted through the cricothyroid membrane or trachea. Barotrauma must be avoided.

Laser surgery to the larynx

Carbon dioxide laser (light amplification by stimulated emission of radiation) was first produced in 1965 with 10.6 μm wavelength. Argon, yttrium-aluminium-garnet (YAG) and potassium titanyl phosphate (KTP) lasers are also used. The surgeon, using the operating microscope, guides the laser beam to excise laryngeal lesions. Formal protocols ensure safety of the patient and staff.

Anaesthesia is as for laryngoscopy, but includes the added danger of potentially fatal airway fires, the laser energy igniting the tracheal tube with oxygen or nitrous oxide as the oxidant. If fire develops, immediately stop ventilation and remove the burning tube before dousing any remaining burning material with saline.

Laser-induced fires are avoided by using a metal tube or a commercial laser-proof tube. Even with the latter, it is wise to reduce the oxidant source by avoiding nitrous oxide and using the lowest possible inspired oxygen. Alternatively, avoid a tube altogether and use supraglottic ventilation with a Sanders injector attached to the surgeon's laryngoscope.

Removal of foreign bodies

Ingested

An ingested foreign body may lodge in the oesophagus at points of physiological or pathological narrowing, such as the cricopharyngeus (15 cm from incisors), aortic arch (23 cm), left main stem bronchus (27 cm) or diaphragmatic hiatus (40 cm). Ingested coins, toys, nails and safety pins are commonly found in children or in high-risk adults such as prisoners, alcoholics, and those with psychiatric illness or mental retardation. They may be retained for decades and present with a fistulous connection between the oesophagus and respiratory or vascular systems. Food bolus impaction is commonest in elderly edentulous adults, and 80–95% of these have organic oesophageal narrowing.

Points for the anaesthetist

- give preoperative intravenous fluids if a theatre delay is likely. An antisialogogue is useful (e.g. glycopyrronium) intravenously or intramuscularly;
- use intravenous induction, short-acting opioid, paralysis and intubation. Avoid cricoid pressure if the foreign body is sharp or in the upper oesophagus;
- keep the patient paralysed while the rigid endoscope is in the mediastinum;
- postoperatively, maintain intravenous fluids if there is any doubt about oesophageal or pharyngeal perforation and observe for the triad of mediastinal pain, pyrexia and surgical emphysema. If present, start antibiotics immediately (or at surgery if suspicious). Patients can be very sore, and analgesia by suppository is useful.

Inhaled

Mortality due to an inhaled foreign body has two peaks – under 1 year (mortality 1:100 000) and over 75 years (mortality 1:10 000). It is the sixth commonest cause of accidental death in children. Non-fatal episodes are commonest in children (85% are under 15 years), particularly 3–5 years. Early signs and symptoms are coughing, choking, cyanosis, respiratory distress, noisy or laboured breathing, and unequal chest movement or air entry. The foreign body is often radiolucent (e.g. plastic, food items), but chest radiography may show obstructive emphysema where paired inspiratory and expiratory films show failure of one lung to empty, indicating ball-valve obstruction in that bronchus. Presentation can be late, with unresolving pneumonia, consolidation or collapse.

Immediate management of an inhaled foreign body causing respiratory obstruction is the Heimlich manoeuvre, or inversion and back-slapping in babies or small children. Tracheostomy or cricothyrotomy may be life-saving. Definitive treatment is removal, either by rigid bronchoscopy under general anaesthesia[6] or by flexible bronchoscopy under sedation and topical anaesthesia in adults.[7]

Anaesthetic management of a child with an inhaled foreign body is as follows:

- the senior anaesthetist and surgeon should confirm the diagnosis and assess the urgency and starvation status;
- in extremis give 100% oxygen and intubate, or consider cricothyrotomy or tracheostomy;
- consider trial of heliox, guided by respiratory work and oxygen saturation;
- induction with sevoflurane or halothane in oxygen, insert intravenous cannula (if not sited already), give 20 μg/kg atropine intravenously, and tape eyes. When a deep level of anaesthesia is established, insert a laryngoscope and spray the cords and trachea with lidocaine (lignocaine) 3 mg/kg. Any response to lidocaine (lignocaine) administration indicates the anaesthesia is not deep enough;
- when depth of anaesthesia is sufficient, the rigid bronchoscope is inserted and the breathing system attached to its side-arm. Anaesthesia is maintained with spontaneous respiration of volatile agent in oxygen. Alternatively, the child may be paralysed and ventilated through the bronchoscope;
- the operation may be lengthy – give intravenous fluids and maintain body temperature. Anaesthesia must be deep enough to keep the vocal cords relaxed when the foreign body is withdrawn through them.

Excision of pharyngeal pouch

Pharyngeal pouch was first described by Ludlow of Bristol in 1764. The patient may have recurrent chest infections due to aspiration of the pouch contents. The commonest operation is endoscopic stapling, but resection through an external neck incision is sometimes necessary. Tracheal intubation is required for any surgical approach. There is a risk of pouch contents discharging at intubation. Cricoid pressure cannot prevent this, and indeed handling of the neck should be avoided at this time. If an external approach is necessary, after intubation the pouch is packed by the surgeon, who may also place a nasogastric tube. Intravenous fluids are required postoperatively, but recovery after uncomplicated endoscopic stapling is rapid.

Laryngectomy

The first laryngectomy (excluding upper epiglottis) was by Billroth on New Year's Eve 1873. In 1887, 103 total laryngectomies were reported and only nine patients survived 1 year.

Preoperative assessment

The patients are usually men over 50 years, and respiratory and cardiovascular co-morbidity are common as the risk factors for laryngeal cancer and cardiorespiratory disease are similar. The patient must be prepared for a period without speech postoperatively (e.g. mouthing requests, prepared cards, writing equipment).

Assess any narrowing of the laryngeal aperture – look for signs or symptoms of upper airway obstruction, review the anaesthetic record from the previous biopsy, repeat flexible nasendoscopy, and review CT and MRI.

Discuss the need for possible blood transfusion, arterial line, nasogastric tube and possible urinary catheter. A central venous line should not be placed in the internal jugular vein, and is not needed routinely for simple laryngectomy.

Anaesthetic technique

If there is laryngeal obstruction plan the intubation carefully, with a back-up plan if the first fails.

Surgeons are not usually keen to start with tracheostomy under local anaesthesia, but this may be necessary.

Use a shoulder roll and head ring, place padded arms by the side, and tape and pad eyes. Protect against pressure sores. Insert an arterial cannula and nasogastric tube. Ensure DVT prophylaxis. Monitor and maintain body temperature. Use a large-bore intravenous cannula. Blood loss can be significant, so crossmatch 4 units and intermittently check the haemoglobin.

The airway is interrupted when the larynx is divided from the upper trachea. Give 100% oxygen prior to changeover for several minutes or until end-tidal oxygen is about 90%. Check the scrub nurse has the correct tube and connectors. The oral tracheal tube is removed and another is placed directly into the upper trachea, and the circuit tubing is moved from the head to the chest. Use of a special J-shaped Montando tube or an armoured tube, making certain that the intubation depth line is clearly visible external to the tracheostome, prevents inadvertent endobronchial intubation.

At the end of surgery, a cuffed tracheostomy tube with a standard 15 mm connector is inserted to allow inspired gas to be warmed and humidified and to protect against soiling of the respiratory tract by blood.

Watch for vascular reflexes from retraction of the carotid sinus giving an unstable arterial pressure and bradycardia. Atropine and a vasoconstrictor should be readily available.

Watch for air embolism.

Recover in a high-dependency environment. Postoperative IPPV is not needed. Substantial analgesia is required because a new tracheostomy often causes great discomfort for the first few days. Infusion of 1–5 mg/h morphine intravenously is appropriate. There is no risk of upper airway obstruction or aspiration.

Care of the tracheostome should include humidification and aseptic suction.

Nasoenteral nutrition may be required while the wound heals.

Pharyngolaryngectomy

Cancer of the hypopharynx may be treated by simple pharyngolaryngectomy followed by multiple plastic operations. It causes similar anaesthetic problems to laryngectomy, but one-stage operations using colon or stomach as replacement are very lengthy and pose additional problems:

- blood loss is greater. Crossmatch 6 units of blood. Ensure DVT prophylaxis. Insert arterial and central venous cannulae (the latter is usually subclavian), urinary catheter and nasogastric tube. Protect eyes and pressure areas;
- space around the patient is restricted. The anaesthetist must have adequate access. Bradycardia, hypotension and arrhythmias may occur during mobilisation of the oesophagus and transfer of stomach or colon to the neck;
- use inhalation or intravenous anaesthesia, avoiding nitrous oxide because the operation is lengthy;
- mediastinal contents may be damaged. Tracheal rupture has occurred, which requires immediate endobronchial intubation;
- total thyroidectomy is also performed. Postoperative thyroxine is required. Parathyroidectomy may cause postoperative hypocalcaemia with tetany;
- analgesic requirements are considerable. Consider epidural analgesia for the abdominal incision. Postoperative IPPV may be needed until the patient is warm and stable. Consider a feeding jejunostomy for postoperative nutrition.

Operations on the middle and inner ear

The main problems of operations on the middle and inner ear are as follows:

- patients may have preoperative hearing loss. They should be assessed in a quiet, well-lit room. The anaesthetist should sit close, speak clearly and slowly, and allow lip reading.;

- the theatre is often darkened (the anaesthetist should not work in total darkness);
- nitrous oxide will diffuse into the middle ear, raise the pressure and may interfere with tympanic membrane reconstruction;
- facial nerve monitoring may be required during skull-base, middle ear, mastoid or parotid surgery;
- airway protection is not required and a laryngeal mask may be suitable for some shorter operations;
- some operations take several hours. Positioning and DVT prophylaxis are important;
- controlled hypotension is valued by the surgeon for middle ear surgery;
- quiet emergence is desirable. There is a strong tendency for postoperative vomiting. Nystagmus may also be a problem postoperatively.

Myringotomy

General anaesthesia is usual for children with glue ear. About 1 million procedures are performed annually in the USA. Although facemask anaesthesia is possible, surgical and anaesthetic conditions are better with a laryngeal mask. Some advocate avoiding nitrous oxide until insertion of the grommet. Incision of the tympanic membrane is stimulating and anaesthetic depth must be adequate, generally including a short-acting opioid such as alfentanil or fentanyl.[8]

Bradycardia or cardiac arrest may occur if the surgeon incises the area of tympanic membrane supplied by the auricular branch of the vagus nerve, but may be prevented by atropine.

Postoperative analgesia is conveniently managed by giving a suppository of NSAID or 20 mg/kg paracetamol during anaesthesia, assuming there is consent.

Middle ear and mastoid surgery

Airway

The airway may be managed by laryngeal mask or intubation, but it is extremely inconvenient to have to adjust a poorly placed laryngeal mask during surgery. Tracheal intubation provides a more secure airway at the expense of greater difficulty in providing calm emergence. The tracheal tube may be replaced by a laryngeal mask at the end of surgery before emergence starts.

Facial nerve monitoring

Facial nerve monitoring is often employed when this nerve is at risk. Needle electrodes placed in the muscles around the mouth and eye monitor the electromyogram, giving an audible and visual alert when there is mechanical or electrical stimulation of the nerve. Suitable stimulation currents are 1–5 mA. Correct functioning of the monitor should be tested before surgery by tetanic stimulation with a peripheral nerve stimulator placed over the facial nerve just in front of the ear to elicit these audible and visual alerts. Muscle relaxants are not used during the operation, and the airway may be managed by:

- laryngeal mask;
- using suxamethonium or mivacurium to facilitate intubation, and ensuring the relaxant has worn off before surgery;
- intubation under deep inhalation or intravenous anaesthesia, aided by an opioid such as 20 μg/kg alfentanil or 1–3 μg/kg remifentanil and 3 mg/kg topical lidocaine (lignocaine) to the larynx;
- intubation under target-controlled or manual infusions of propofol and remifentanil, using the same drugs for maintenance of anaesthesia.

Nitrous oxide

Nitrous oxide increases middle ear pressure by diffusion.[9] The rise peaks at 30–60 minutes when the pressure may reach 180 mmH_2O, the pressure at which passive ventilation occurs through the eustachian tube. This rise may be greater when the eustachian tube is blocked, and in this situation there may be excessive negative pressures in the recovery phase. Increased middle ear pressure has been implicated in hearing impairment, stapes disarticulation, tympanic membrane rupture and displacement of tympanic membrane graft. These problems are prevented by using air/oxygen mixtures throughout surgery, or withdrawing nitrous oxide 10–30 minutes before grafting. Middle ear pressure changes may contribute to postoperative nausea and vomiting. Intravenous anaesthesia appears to give better conditions than a balanced inhalation anaesthetic.[10]

Minimise bleeding

The surgeon appreciates all attempts to facilitate his view through the operating microscope. Calmness in the preoperative period and a stable cardiovascular system during induction and maintenance of anaesthesia are helpful. The gown should not be tight around the neck. Head-up tilt should be used. Levels of anaesthesia must be adequate and incorporate sufficient analgesia. An infusion of 10–20 μg/kg/h remifentanil is useful,[11] providing stable conditions with a relative bradycardia. A common first choice of drug to induce additional hypotension is 0.25–1.0 mg/kg labetalol.

Intra-arterial blood pressure monitoring is not usually required when these techniques achieve modest levels of hypotension (systolic about 80 mmHg), but should be used when potent hypotensive agents are given by infusion, or in selected patients in whom the risks of hypotension are greater than normal.

Duration of surgery

Mastoid surgery may take 2–3 hours. Positioning and temperature control are important. Tape and pad the eyes because instruments are passed over the head towel. In the absence of thrombophilia, DVT prophylaxis is usually by compression stockings and pneumatic leg cuffs only rather than by using heparin, because even minor bleeding under the operative microscope is unwelcome.

Postoperative analgesia

Morphine 0.1 mg/kg provides reasonable analgesia for the early postoperative period following mastoid surgery, but oral analgesia such as paracetamol or NSAIDs is usually sufficient thereafter. A greater auricular nerve block with 0.5% bupivacaine at the end of surgery helps reduce the requirement for analgesia and hence opioid-induced vomiting.[12]

Nausea and vomiting

Nausea and vomiting often result from labyrinthine disturbance during middle ear surgery and opioid administration. They are less frequent if nitrous oxide and opioids are avoided, and may respond to 12.5 mg prochlorperazine intramuscularly. Intravenous fluids should be continued.

Skull-base surgery

Neurosurgical considerations (see Ch. 5.7) apply for these lengthy operations. Facial nerve (7th, stylomastoid foramen) monitoring may be required. The glossopharyngeal, vagus and accessory nerves (9th, 10th and 11th, jugular foramen), and the hypoglossal nerve (12th, hypoglossal canal) also may be damaged. Both the jugular vein and carotid artery may be removed at surgery. A lumbar spinal drain may be used. Overnight high-dependency care is required.

References

1. Prasad KC, Shanmugam VU. Major surgeries under regional anesthesia. Am J Otolaryngol 1998; 19:163–169.
2. Tsui BCH, Wagner A, Cave D, Elliott C, El-Hakim H, Malherbe S. The incidence of laryngospasm with a 'no touch' extubation technique after tonsillectomy and adenoidectomy. Anesth Analg 2004; 98:327–329.
3. Marret E, Flahault A, Samama C-M, Bonnet F. Effects of postoperative, nonsteroidal, antiinflammatory drugs on bleeding risk after tonsillectomy. Anesthesiology 2003; 98:1497–1502.
4. Homer JJ, Swallow J, Semple P. Audit of pain management at home following tonsillectomy in children. J Laryngol Otol 2001; 115:205–208.

5. Brown KA, Morin I, Hickey C, Manoukian JJ, Nixon GM, Brouillette RT. Urgent adenotonsillectomy. An analysis of risk factors associated with postoperative respiratory morbidity. Anesthesiology 2003; 99:586–595.
6. Farrell PT. Rigid bronchoscopy for foreign body removal: anaesthesia and ventilation. Paediatr Anaesth 2004; 14:84–89.
7. Rafanan AL, Mehta AC. Adult airway foreign body removal: what's new? Clin Chest Med 2001; 22:319–330.
8. Kinkel JC, Cohen IT, Hannallah RS, et al. The effect of intranasal fentanyl on the emergence characteristics after sevoflurane anesthesia in children undergoing surgery for bilateral myringotomy tube placement. Anesth Analg 2001; 92:1164–1168.
9. Karabiyik L, Bozkirli F, Celebi H, Goksu N. Effect of nitrous oxide on middle ear pressure: a comparison between inhalational anaesthesia with nitrous oxide and TIVA. Eur J Anaesth 1996; 13:27–32.
10. Mukherjee K, Seavell C, Rawlings E, Weiss A. A comparison of total intravenous with balanced anaesthesia for middle ear surgery: effects on postoperative nausea and vomiting, pain and conditions of surgery. Anaesthesia 2003; 58:176–180.
11. Degoute C-S, Ray M-J, Manchon M, Dubreuil C, Banssillon V. Remifentanil and controlled hypotension; comparison with nitroprusside or esmolol during tympanoplasty. Can J Anesth 2001; 48:20–27.
12. Suresh S, Barcelona SL, Young NM, Seligman I, Heffner CL, Coté CJ. Postoperative pain relief in children undergoing tympanomastoid surgery: is a regional block better than opioids? Anesth Analg 2002; 94:859–862.

CHAPTER **5.13**

PLASTIC SURGERY AND THE CARE OF BURNS

PLASTIC SURGERY

Plastic surgery involves the body wall rather than body cavities and viscera. Procedures are widely varied in site and complexity, from excision of minor skin lesions to extensive and prolonged reconstructive procedures following trauma or excision of malignancy. Plastic surgeons are increasingly subspecialised to deal with the main areas of interest. These include skin malignancy, reconstruction following breast or head and neck malignancy, reconstruction following trauma, hand and upper limb surgery following trauma or congenital abnormalities, cleft lip and palate surgery, burns surgery and aesthetic surgery. Patients may be referred for tissue cover of exposed viscera or fracture sites following primary surgery elsewhere or following necrotising fasciitis.

The anaesthetist is therefore required to provide operating conditions for a wide variety of procedures. Patients may be very young, as for cleft lip and palate surgery, or elderly with significant coexisting pathology.

GENERAL ANAESTHESIA

Breast, abdominal wall, and head and neck reconstruction will normally require general anaesthesia. Reconstructive procedures include tissue transfer (flap) surgery:

- pedicled flaps comprise locally raised skin, fascia and muscle flaps, which remain attached to their blood supply and are translated locally to replace nearby destroyed or excised tissue;
- free flaps involve raising tissue in a similar way, but dividing it from its blood supply and transferring it to a distant site, re-providing arterial and venous connections by microanastomosis to convenient nearby vessels.

Prolonged procedures

Reconstructive surgery may be prolonged, sometimes exceeding 12 hours in duration. The choice of anaesthetic technique should therefore enable timely recovery, with a total intravenous technique employing propofol and a rapidly acting opiate being an ideal choice. Where appropriate, a suitable regional technique enables a combined approach with lighter anaesthesia, and provides excellent postoperative analgesia. Artificial ventilation will normally be preferred.

Meticulous attention to patient positioning, pressure area care, and maintenance of body temperature is essential.

Invasive monitoring of arterial and central venous pressure enables management of blood loss and monitoring of haemoglobin, acid–base balance and blood gases. A urethral catheter enables monitoring of urine output and fluid balance.

Tissue transfer and replantation

For pedicled and free flap surgery, the aim should be to produce a warm, well-perfused and well-oxygenated patient, particularly at the end of surgery, with a haemoglobin concentration of 8–10 g/dL for optimal flap oxygenation.

Depending on the duration of surgery and the ASA classification of the patient, a period of postoperative ventilation and rewarming may be required to stabilise the patient and the flap.

Replantation of traumatically amputated digits or even hands and forearms require, similar techniques to free flap surgery.

Hypotensive anaesthesia

Surgeons may request hypotension to reduce blood loss and provide a clear field for fine dissection, particularly for head and neck surgery. Induced hypotension should be employed cautiously, with particular regard to the cardiovascular condition of the patient and always ensuring adequate cerebral and coronary blood flow. A smooth technique, with a minimal degree of hypotension, avoidance of hypertensive episodes, tachycardia and hypercapnia, and good patient positioning will usually provide a satisfactory operative field without compromising patient safety.

Cleft lip and palate

Primary cleft lip and palate surgery is performed early in the first year of life to optimise feeding and speech development. Anaesthesia should only be provided by an experienced paediatric anaesthetist who is competent in the management of the possible airway problems associated with cleft disease. Recovery and ward staff should also be experienced with these patients.

REGIONAL AND LOCAL ANAESTHESIA

Wherever possible regional techniques should be combined with general anaesthesia to provide optimal operative and recovery conditions.

Spinal and/or epidural anaesthesia provides excellent conditions for lower limb reconstructive surgery, and postoperative analgesia.

Thoracic epidural anaesthesia can be employed for abdominal reconstruction or breast reconstruction using an abdominally sourced tissue graft.

Brachial plexus block provides excellent anaesthesia for hand and upper limb surgery, either as a sole technique or combined with sedation or general anaesthesia. A catheter can be sited at the time of blockade to provide continuous analgesia following digital replant surgery.

BURNS

THE BURN WOUND

Burns are usually thermal injuries to the skin and subcutaneous tissues, but may also be eletrical or chemical. Frequent presentations include flame burns in adults, and scalds in children.

The cutaneous burn wound may be complicated by injury to the airway, associated smoke inhalation, or associated trauma. Electrical burns may be associated with cardiac arrhythmias.

Burns requiring hospital admission occur most frequently in the extremes of age, among socioeconomically deprived groups, and in those suffering from debilitating or psychiatric illness.

Mortality increases with increasing burn size, with increasing age, and with associated inhalation injury.

Burn wound severity is described by percent body surface area (BSA) affected, and depth (i.e. superficial [first degree], partial thickness [second degree] or full thickness [third degree]). The deeper partial-thickness and full-thickness burns will normally require excision and grafting to heal.

The burn wound releases local mediators (histamine, prostaglandins, bradykinin, nitric oxide, serotonin, substance P), which cause local inflammation and burn wound oedema. In major burns the release of circulating mediators (cytokines, endotoxin, nitric oxide) triggers a systemic inflammatory response, immune suppression and hypermetabolism.[1]

RESUSCITATION AND INITIAL MANAGEMENT OF THE PATIENT WITH A BURN INJURY

First aid

At the scene, first aid for a patient with a burn injury should include copious application of cool (not ice-cold) water to cool thermal injuries and dilute chemical agents. Application of plastic kitchen film will improve comfort and reduce contamination.

Assessment

On arrival at hospital, the time of injury and the causative agent should be ascertained. High-flow oxygen should be administered. Assessment of the airway, breathing and circulation (ABC etc.) should be systematic.

An initial assessment of body surface area burned should be made using 'the rule of nines', a more detailed burn chart if available, or by estimation using the palm of the patient's hand as representing 1% of their body surface area (BSA). The depth of burn is of less importance for initial resuscitation. An adequate assessment can only be made with full exposure of the body surface.

Active steps must be taken to maintain body temperature because these patients will lose heat rapidly. Warm airflow blankets and radiant heaters are effective.

It is important to remember that burns can be associated with other major trauma, particularly where the history includes an explosion, a road traffic accident, or escape from an elevated position.

Analgesia

Analgesia should be provided as soon as possible. Patients will be in pain and distress following significant injuries. For all except minor injuries, an intravenous opiate should be titrated against observed effect. Care will need to be taken where the airway is at risk. Although full-thickness burn areas may be insensate to pinprick, areas of painful partial-thickness burn will also be present, and the patient will undoubtedly be in distress.

Analgesia for minor injuries will be required for examination and dressing, and may be adequately provided by oral opiate preparations.

Airway

The burned airway is threatened by oedema, which develops during the first hours following injury; therefore the airway may deteriorate.

Features suggesting a threat to the airway include a facial burn, singed nasal hair, a hoarse voice, damage to the oropharyngeal mucosa and developing stridor. A circumferential burn to the neck may threaten the airway as subcutaneous oedema develops. Aerosolised epinephrine (adrenaline) and an erect posture may reduce airway oedema and improve airway patency.[2]

If there is any doubt as to airway stability, the airway should be secured earlier rather than later, because intubation is likely to become more difficult.[3]

Intubation should be performed by an experienced anaesthetist, with trained assistance, in a well-equipped facility. The chosen technique will depend on the operator's expertise, but conventional orotracheal intubation performed early and employing a rapid sequence induction will normally be safe.

Should the airway have already deteriorated then consideration should be given to an inhalation induction technique or awake fibreoptic intubation under local anaesthesia. Where the upper airway is severely compromised, emergency cricothyroidotomy or tracheostomy under local anaesthesia should be considered, though these are rarely needed in practice.

Suxamethonium, though recognised to cause rapid rises in serum potassium in major burns, threatening cardiac arrest, is safe to use during the first 24 hours post burn. High doses of non-depolarising relaxants are a safe alternative.

Endotracheal tubes should be left uncut, or cut 4–5 cm long, to allow for the development of orofacial oedema.

Patients who are to be transferred by ambulance to a burns service should either have no risk to the airway, or their airway secured before transfer.

Breathing

Ventilation can be compromised by a near or fully circumferential burn of the chest or abdominal wall. Inevitable oedema developing beneath a non-compliant burn wound (or eschar) may greatly reduce chest compliance or diaphragmatic movement. In this situation deep incision of the burn wound (escharotomy) should be performed at the earliest opportunity.

Any burn incident that occurs as a result of combustion within a confined space (e.g. house, shed, garage, car, boat) will result in an inhalation injury until proved otherwise.

Smoke inhalation increases the mortality of cutaneous burns by at least a factor of two. Patients often present with no apparent respiratory distress, with normal saturation and blood gases. Auscultation and chest radiography may also be normal initially. Respiratory function deteriorates over the first 24 hours. Injury is due to the toxic effects of smoke on the upper and lower respiratory tract. In the absence of a clear history, soot around the face and airway and carbonaceous sputum suggest the diagnosis.

Inhalation of the products of combustion may lead to systemic poisoning (carbon monoxide, cyanide), which can lead to death at the scene. Carbon monoxide has 250 times greater affinity for haemoglobin than oxygen, thereby displacing oxygen and reducing oxygen carrying capacity. It shifts the oxygen dissociation curve to the left, reducing tissue oxygenation, and binds to cytochrome oxidase, inhibiting several intracellular enzymes. Poisoning can be detected by measuring carboxyhaemoglobin levels, where any reading above 15% is significant. Survivors may develop cardiac and neurological sequelae. Administration of 100% oxygen reduces the half-life of carboxyhaemoglobin by a factor of four.

Circulation

Secure wide-bore venous access should be achieved as soon as possible after arrival at hospital, through unburned skin if possible. Developing oedema and hypovolaemia will make venepuncture more difficult with time.

In patients with minor burns, hydration can be maintained by the oral route with venous access being maintained with a slow infusion.

Patients with major burns (>10% Body Surface Area [BSA] in children; >15% BSA in adults) or any complicated burns (inhalation injury, other trauma) will require formal intravenous fluid resuscitation. An infusion of warmed Ringer's lactate solution should be commenced immediately and not be delayed while detailed calculations of burn size are made.

The capillary leak associated with burns is proportional to the BSA burned, and has led to the use of formulae to calculate fluid requirements. These formulae should be recognised as estimates based on population studies, and do not predict the exact requirements for an individual patient.

The most commonly used regimen is the Parkland formula, which uses warmed Ringer's lactate solution. It requires 4 mL/kg body weight per percent BSA burned to be given over the first 24 hours post burn, with half of this volume given in the first 8 hours and the remainder over the next 16 hours. For example, a 70 kg man with a 50% burn would require 7000 mL of fluid in the first 8 hours, and 7000 mL over the ensuing 16 hours. Any delay in beginning the infusion should be made up by the end of the first 8 hours.

Patients receiving intravenous resuscitation should have a urinary catheter inserted. The Parkland formula will provide adequate salt and water for adults and older children. Smaller children weighing less than 20 kg require further free water, and in these patients the resuscitation volume should be added to a calculated basal daily fluid requirement.[4]

The circulation must be monitored to assess the adequacy of resuscitation. Simple noninvasive observation of pulse rate, blood pressure and capillary refill should be monitored, along with urine output and core peripheral temperature difference to give an estimate of adequacy of tissue perfusion. Urine output should exceed 0.5 mL/kg/h, with a minimum of 10 mL/h in children.

Invasive haemodynamic monitoring may predispose to infection and should be reserved for patients likely to require intensive care.

Fluid requirements in excess of predictions are seen in association with inhalation injury.[5]

TRANSFER OF THE PATIENT WITH A BURN INJURY

Patients with significant burn injuries will normally be referred to a specialist burns service. Published referral criteria include burns with inhalation injury, larger burns of resuscitation size, complex injuries and extremes of age. Anaesthetists will be asked to accompany patients for transfer, and should have experience in the transfer of critically ill patients. Prior to transfer, the patient should be stabilised with particular regard to the airway, breathing and circulation, appropriate monitoring should be available during the journey, and a means of conserving body temperature should be employed. Advice from the receiving unit should be sought as to any specific requirements in particular injury scenarios.

CONTINUING CARE OF THE PATIENT WITH A BURN INJURY

Escharotomy

Circumferential burns affecting limbs, the neck, thorax or abdomen may require urgent surgical release of the constricting eschar to ensure adequate blood flow and venous return in distal tissues, and to facilitate adequate ventilation. These are surgical procedures and require the attendance of an anaesthetist and provision of anaesthesia. Ketamine or propofol can be employed as part of an intravenous technique, or an inhalational technique can be employed. Effective escharotomy should extend the length of the burn and reach undamaged tissue deep to the burn. Significant blood loss is therefore to be anticipated.

Monitoring

Patients with major injuries should be observed in a high-dependency area for the initial 24–36 hours. During this time particular attention should be paid to adequacy of fluid resuscitation, development of oedema, the airway and adequacy of ventilation.

Nutrition

Burned patients become profoundly catabolic and have high nutritional requirements if they are to recover. Enteral nutrition should be fully established for all patients with significant burns during the first 24 hours and supervision by a dietician is usual. Insulin by sliding scale is commonly required to maintain blood glucose below 6 mmol/L.

Intensive care

Intubated patients and those with significant inhalational injury or complex major injuries will require a period of intensive care, including artificial ventilation. Central venous and arterial cannulation will be required. Monitoring may include the use of the oesophageal Doppler device as a relatively noninvasive means of estimating key haemodynamic parameters without increasing the risk of sepsis.

Patients with burns in excess of 50% BSA or involving inhalation injury may have higher fluid requirements in the first 24 hours than predicted by formulae.

Following the initial 24–36-hours period of resuscitation, major cases, in excess of 20–25% BSA, will develop a systemic inflammatory response syndrome, with immune suppression and a high risk of sepsis. Multisystem failure may require support as for other critically ill patients. Repeated visits to the operating theatre will be required, which is likely to prolong the intensive care stay. Tracheostomy is considered where patients remain intubated for 7 days or more. A percutaneous technique is employed unless there is a burn or significant oedema over the neck, when a formal surgical technique is preferred.

Inhalation injury

Inhalation injury should be confirmed by bronchoscopy in intubated patients. Respiratory mucosa and small airways will be damaged by carbonaceous particles, and by a cocktail of compounds produced by combustion, including aldehydes and acid radicals.

The lung injury develops over the first 24–36 hours, and will require a period of artificial ventilation, regular physiotherapy and bronchial lavage.[2]

Regular inhalation of nebulised bronchodilators, 0.18% sodium bicarbonate, heparin, and n-acetyl cysteine (3), have been employed to limit the lung injury and facilitate lavage. Such a regimen will normally continue until carbonaceous sputum is no longer produced. Prophylactic antibiotics are not recommended.

Infection control

Meticulous infection control procedures must be applied in all areas where patients with burns are nursed. Despite topical antimicrobial preparations, a burn wound will invariably become contaminated, and patients with burns are susceptible to generalised sepsis. Antibiotics should be used in response to positive cultures and where there are clinical signs of sepsis. Doses may need to be increased, with blood levels being monitored where appropriate.

ANAESTHESIA FOLLOWING BURN INJURIES

Major burns require repeated visits to the operating theatre for dressing changes, escharectomy, and harvest and application of split-skin autograft.

Alternative covering of the excised burn with cadaveric skin or artificial skin substitutes will allow time for donor sites to heal before reharvesting.

There is a trend towards early complete burn excision, which requires prolonged surgery and teams of anaesthetists and surgeons, and may involve major blood loss. An alternative approach is to perform serial interval burn excisions following completion of the resuscitation period. Changes in patient position require enough personnel, with lifting equipment for safety and to avoid disturbing grafted areas.

Preoperative assessment

A full assessment should be repeated at each surgical episode. Particular attention should be paid to the possible difficult airway and intubation. Clotting abnormalities are common with major burns, and platelets and fresh frozen plasma may need to be transfused before surgery. Ensure that crossmatched blood is available.

General anaesthesia

General anaesthesia will normally be the method of choice for major burns. Whichever technique is chosen, requirements for induction and maintenance agents may be increased in the catabolic patient with a large volume of distribution who has become tolerant of intravenous opiates and repeated anaesthetic episodes.

Intubation is preferred in patients on continuous enteral feeds and long-term opiate medication, and in whom changes in posture will be required intraoperatively. Where burns of the face and neck are involved, laryngoscopy and intubation may become progressively difficult with repeated visits to theatre.

Surgical episodes may be prolonged. Maintenance of body temperature will require warming blankets, radiant overhead heaters, warmed intravenous fluids, and temperature monitoring.

Extensive excision may result in major blood loss. This can be minimised by subcutaneous infiltration of a dilute epinephrine (adrenaline) solution (1:500 000–1:1 000 000) before escharectomy. Estimation of blood loss is difficult, and intraoperative haemoglobin estimation, along with blood gases and other parameters, is recommended.

Effective monitoring of the ECG and pulse oximetry may be technically difficult with extensively burned patients.

Local and regional anaesthesia

Minor burns procedures can be performed under local infiltration anaesthesia. Topical local anaesthetic creams can allow small areas of split-skin graft to be harvested. For procedures involving the lower extremities, epidural or intrathecal anaesthesia is used either alone or with sedation or general anaesthesia. Care should be taken to avoid neuroaxial blockade where a burned, and possibly contaminated, area occurs near to the injection site. Brachial plexus blockade is suitable for smaller procedures on the distal upper limb.

References

1. Maclennan N, Heimbach D, Cullen B. Anaesthesia for major thermal injury. Anaesthesiology 1998; 89:749–770.
2. Demling RH. Pulmonary problems in the burn patient (a leading cause of morbidity and mortality). J Burns Surg Wound Care 2004; 3:5.
3. Sheridan R. Airway management and respiratory care of the burn patient. Int Anaesthesiol Clin 2000; 38;129–145.
4. Sheridan R. Burns. Crit Care Med 2002; 30 (suppl):S500–S514.
5. Cancio L, Chavez S, Alvarado-Ortega M, et al. Predicting increased fluid requirements during resuscitation of thermally injured patients. J Trauma 2004; 56;404–414.

Further reading

Settle JAD. Principles and practice of burns management. Edinburgh: Churchill Livingstone; 1996.

CHAPTER **5.14**

THORACIC SURGERY

In the UK specific thoracic operations are performed with the following frequencies (as a percentage of total thoracic procedures):

- open pneumonectomy 3%;
- open partial lung resection 14%;
- mediastinoscopy 9%;
- video-assisted thoroscopic surgery (VATS), including lung resections 12%;
- oesophageal resection and other upper gastrointestinal surgery 4%;
- a variety of bronchoscopic and gastroscopic procedures (41%).[1]

Most procedures are for the diagnosis and treatment of malignancy, although some benign but incapacitating conditions such as emphysema may benefit from surgery.

Patients may suffer severe respiratory insufficiency, which can be further compromised by the procedure itself, and smoking-related cardiovascular disease. Preoperative assessment will frequently include interpretation of lung function tests, which may help predict the adequacy of postoperative respiratory function. A decision to deny surgery on the basis of lung function tests cannot be made lightly. Equally, surgery that results in a patient with insufficient respiratory capacity is not desirable. Preserving the ability to cough and clear secretions postoperatively is paramount.

Many operations on structures within the pleural cavity are facilitated by isolation of the lung on the nonoperative side. This allows ventilation while the lung of the operative side is collapsed to improve operative exposure. Purulent secretions may also be prevented from soiling a healthy lung and an air leak through a bronchopleural fistula may be controlled. Many procedures, including major lung resection, may be accomplished with the aid of a thoracoscope (VATS).

ASSESSMENT OF PULMONARY FUNCTION

Patients in whom lung resection is proposed should have lung function tests. These may be performed in a laboratory or at the bedside.

Spirometry measures dynamic lung volumes and provides information about airway resistance. Common measurements obtained are forced vital capacity (FVC) and forced expired volume in 1 second (FEV_1). If the FVC is reduced but the ratio of FEV_1/FVC is preserved (>70%), the pattern is said to be restrictive. If this ratio is reduced, the pattern is obstructive.

Maximum breathing capacity can also be measured, as can the diffusion capacity of the alveolar membrane using carbon monoxide (CO) as a marker gas (DLCO). A DLCO less than 40% predicted is associated with a markedly increased mortality rate.[2]

Measurements are usually given as a percentage of values predicted for normals of equivalent height and sex.

Little difficulty is presented by patients who have an FEV_1 over 2 L and maximum breathing capacity of more than 50% predicted. Those who do not achieve this need further testing. Poorer pulmonary function test measurements can be tolerated in patients in whom surgery less than pneumonectomy is proposed or in whom an improvement can be expected following surgery (e.g. if airway obstruction by tumour is to be relieved).

Arterial blood gases are measured on room air as a baseline. $PaCO_2$ values over 6.0 kPa or oxygen saturation less than 90% signal greater peri-operative risk.

Assessment of patients in whom surgery for emphysema or bullous lung disease is considered should have their exercise capacity measured using a standard walk test.

ANAESTHETIC CONSIDERATIONS

Open pneumothorax and lung collapse

The lungs are normally kept inflated by the difference between atmospheric pressure in the alveoli and the negative pressure (about –5 cmH_2O) in the potential space between the two layers of pleura. This balances the elastic recoil of the lung and the tendency of the chest wall to spring outwards.

When the chest is opened, the negative pressure is lost and the elastic recoil causes collapse of the lung on that side. The mediastinum, unless fixed by adhesions, shifts towards the other side, compresses the healthy lung and interferes with cardiac function. If the lung is adherent to the chest wall, these effects may not be marked. The lung collapse causes ventilation–perfusion ($\dot{V}/\dot{Q}$) mismatch, shunting, hypoxia and a high pulmonary vascular resistance. Spontaneous respiration is possible with an open hemithorax, but it is inefficient because only the lung on the nonoperative side expands with diaphragmatic contraction. The inspired gas for this lung comes partly from the trachea and partly from the lung on the operative side (effectively increasing deadspace). This transfer of gas from one lung to the other is known as *pendelluft* and can be lethal.

These problems are overcome with intermittent positive-pressure ventilation (IPPV).

Pulmonary secretions

Excessive secretions are uncommon, but occur in lung abscess, bronchiectasis, bronchopleural fistula and tumours, when infected secretions lie distal to an obstructed bronchus. Improvement may be obtained by preoperative postural drainage and antibiotics.

Methods for preventing the spread of secretions into healthy parts of the lungs during surgery include the following:

- regional or local analgesia and preserving the cough reflex (e.g. for drainage of empyema);
- regular tracheal suction, especially after the position is changed or the lungs manipulated;
- surgical clamping of a bronchus as soon as the chest is open;
- posture – a drainage or an antidrainage posture may be employed. The patient can be positioned so that secretions from the diseased lung will flow into the trachea for suction and not contaminate the healthy lung. Alternatively, secretions can be retained in the diseased lobe (e.g. sitting for lower lobectomy in bronchiectasis). An empyema is often drained with the patient sitting, especially if there is any chance of bronchopleural fistula;
- endobronchial intubation (the most usual solution) where the healthy lung is isolated with inflatable cuffs.

Endobronchial instrumentation/intubation

In adults double-lumen endobronchial tubes are routinely used if isolation of one lung is required. A single-lumen tracheal tube with a bronchial blocker or a long single-lumen endobronchial tube are alternatives. The use of a fibreoptic bronchoscope greatly improves the accuracy of the placement of these devices. Double-lumen tubes are not generally available for paediatric use.

Double-lumen endobronchial tubes

A variety of tubes have been developed to allow isolation of one lung and independent ventilation of either. They all have the essential feature of having two separate tubes, bonded together, one of which extends beyond the distal end of the other. The longer tube has a cuff which, when it is correctly placed in one or other main bronchus, can be inflated to isolate that lung. This cuff is slotted to allow ventilation of the right upper lobe in most right-sided tubes. The shorter tube is designed to open just above the carina. A cuff proximal to the opening of the shorter tube is inflated to seal the trachea.

Tubes are designed to align with normal anatomy and are specifically designated for either right or left endobronchial intubation because the angle at which the right main bronchus continues from the carina is steeper than that of the left. The design also takes into account the usual shorter distance from the carina at which the upper lobe bronchus branches from the main bronchus on the right. Tubes are manufactured in a range of sizes suitable for small to large adults.

Anatomical limitations to satisfactory placement of double-lumen tubes include the laryngeal inlet (limits the diameter of tube), angulation of the carina, and distance from the carina and orientation of the origin of the upper lobe bronchus. Correct placement may be checked bronchoscopically by visualising the endobronchial cuff at the origin of the main bronchus.

Paediatric flexible fibreoptic instruments allow visualisation through the endobronchial lumen and may be useful if ventilation of the upper lobe is in doubt.

A double-lumen tube is inserted through the laryngeal inlet under direct vision with the aid of a laryngoscope. Holding the tube so that the endobronchial part curves upwards facilitates this. Once the tip of the tube is through the cords it is rotated approximately 120° towards the side of proposed endobronchial intubation while the patient's head is turned in the opposite direction. A sequence for checking correct placement clinically is as follows:

- step 1 – the tracheal cuff is inflated slowly until a seal is obtained while both lumina are employed to inflate the lungs. Bilateral breath sounds at the apices are auscultated;
- step 2 – the tracheal catheter mount is occluded or clamped, its lumen opened to air and the endobronchial side ventilated. The endobronchial cuff is slowly inflated until no gas is heard escaping via the endotracheal lumen. Unilateral breath sounds are auscultated on the appropriate side, including the apices;
- step 3 – step 2 is repeated, except that the endobronchial side is occluded and the endotracheal lumen ventilated.

Unilateral breath sounds and high inflation pressures at step 1 usually indicate that the tube is inserted too far and both lumina are in a main bronchus. Absent apical breath sounds and high inflation pressure at step 2 suggest that the endobronchial cuff is distal to or occluding the upper lobe bronchus. It is arguable that correct positioning of an endobronchial tube should be checked routinely with a flexible bronchoscope.[3]

Most operations other than left pneumonectomy can be performed using a left-sided double-lumen tube, which is easier to place correctly. Although some anaesthetists prefer to use a double-lumen tube on the nonoperative side others advocate the use of left-sided tubes in all except where there is a contraindication.[4]

Single-lumen endobronchial tubes

Specifically designed single-lumen endobronchial tubes are occasionally used in specialised centres. These generally have tracheal and bronchial cuffs and sometimes a carinal hook. Deflation of the tracheal cuff when the bronchial cuff is inflated allows one-lung ventilation and deflation of the non-ventilated lung. Soiling from spillage of gastric contents into the non-ventilated lung is a risk. Uncut standard endotracheal tubes may be employed in an emergency or in difficult cases. Appropriate positioning usually requires a rigid or fibreoptic bronchoscope.

Endobronchial blockers

One or other lung may be isolated by the positioning of a balloon-tipped catheter into the origin of a main bronchus. Fogarty catheters are most frequently employed in paediatric practice and may be useful where laryngeal or tracheal narrowing prevents the use of a double-lumen tube in adults.[5]

Specifically designed bronchial blockers are now available and are either incorporated into a specialised single-lumen endotracheal tube or require an adapted catheter mount with a port for a fibreoptic bronchoscope and a fixation device for the blocking catheter. These blockers have a lumen that allows the application of suction, but are too small for the passage of a suction catheter. Positioning requires the use of a bronchoscope. Balloon inflation is observed directly with the bronchoscope and the apex and base of the lung to be isolated are auscultated for the absence of breath sounds. Intraoperative collapse of the lung on the operative side is best achieved by opening the breathing circuit to air on opening of the chest with the patient paralysed. The balloon is then inflated either under direct vision with a bronchoscope or with the volume of air required to seal the main bronchus on initial positioning.

Endobronchial intubation in infants

An uncuffed tube, 1 cm longer than the distance from mouth to carina measured on the lateral chest radiograph, will tend to enter the bronchus on the opposite side to the bevel. The bevel is cut for the desired side and the tube is passed into the bronchus and rotated through 180° so that the upper lobe orifice is not obstructed. The bevel should be extended with a slit for right endobronchial intubation to allow for the more proximal position of the right upper lobe orifice.[6]

One-lung ventilation

Traditionally, the same minute volume used in two-lung ventilation is applied to the single lung. However, a smaller tidal volume or pressure-controlled ventilation may reduce stretch-related lung injury.[7]

Problems with endobronchial tubes and one-lung ventilation

- Difficulty with insertion – especially if the anatomy is abnormal or distorted. Double-lumen tubes are larger in diameter and of a different conformation than conventional endotracheal tubes. Laceration of endobronchial or tracheal cuffs by the patient's teeth during intubation is common, particularly with plastic tubes;
- dislodgement – during positioning of the patient, and movement of the head and neck;
- trauma – to the larynx and airways;
- kinking – of thin-walled single-lumen endobronchial tubes;
- hypercapnia, which is seldom a problem in practice;
- arterial hypoxaemia during one-lung anaesthesia – a higher fractional inspired concentration of oxygen ($F_{I}O_2$) is generally employed. Collapse of the upper lung and hypoxic pulmonary vasoconstriction increase its vascular resistance. Nonetheless, blood does flow through this collapsed lung and the shunt causes hypoxaemia, which is little improved by ventilation with 100% oxygen. The lower lung will be at a disadvantage too because its FRC will be reduced, with some atelectasis. The problem can be helped by the following:
    - encouraging collapse of the non-ventilated lung with suction or surgical manipulation;
    - cautious application of positive end-expiratory pressure (PEEP), which can improve oxygenation in severe hypoxaemia[8] (but may divert blood to the upper lung and reduce cardiac output so worsening hypoxaemia);
    - insufflating, intermittently inflating, applying continuous positive airway pressure (CPAP) or using high-frequency jet ventilation (HFJV) in the collapsed lung with 100% oxygen. In some cases, relative hypoxia may have to be tolerated because frequent reinflation of the lung on the operative side may prolong and hinder surgery, which may present a greater risk to the patient;
    - clamping the pulmonary artery when a pneumonectomy is performed.

PRINCIPLES OF ANAESTHESIA FOR THORACOTOMY

Median sternotomy is used for access to the thymus, retrosternal goitres and anterior mediastinum; lateral thoracotomy is used for most other thoracic operations.

Endobronchial intubation, which allows isolation and deflation of the lung on the operative side is, usual for operations on other than mid-line structures. However, many procedures (including lung resection) can be performed without this, but this requires a degree of surgical cooperation and experience. High-frequency ventilation (using oscillation or a jet) has its enthusiasts and may be useful in experienced hands for difficult cases such as bronchial rupture or fistula.[9]

Preoperative considerations

Premedication is not necessary for thoracotomy. An opiate or anxiolytic may be used, but care must be taken to avoid postoperative respiratory depression. A vagolytic may be useful to avoid bradycardia if a thoracic epidural is employed preoperatively[10] or where vagal reflexes are likely to be a problem.

Patients with coexisting cardiovascular disease will require careful monitoring, but for patients undergoing open thoracotomy, invasive arterial and central venous pressure monitoring is usual anyway. Placing a radial arterial line and large-bore venous cannula in the forearm of the operative side avoids the problems of compression in the lateral position. A central venous catheter is normally inserted into the internal jugular vein of the operative side.

There is little evidence for increased efficacy of 'pre-emptive' analgesia. A thoracic epidural (with the catheter tip positioned between the level of the fourth to sixth thoracic vertebrae and infusate of local anaesthetic mixed with a lipid-soluble opioid such as fentanyl) and adjuvant non-steroidal analgesic is considered by many to be best practice for the provision of postoperative analgesia.[11] However, local anaesthetic infusion via a catheter placed behind the posterior parietal pleura during surgery may be as effective,[12] particularly if used in combination with patient-controlled analgesia (PCA).

Intraoperative considerations

Positioning

Most lung resections are performed in the lateral position. Occasionally, an approach via a median sternotomy with the patient supine is used. Care must be taken to avoid injuries due to pressure or to the brachial plexus by traction on the upper arm.

Bronchial stapling/suturing

Bronchial stapling/suturing is usually performed with the bronchus clamped. Use of a double-lumen tube gives control of the opposite lung, and helps the anaesthetist test the bronchial stump for leaks.

Blood loss

Blood loss may be extensive. At least one large-bore cannula is essential. A central venous catheter allows venous pressure monitoring and more rapid drug delivery.

Closure of the chest

The lungs should be fully expanded before closure. Residual air in the pleural cavity can be removed by an intrapleural drain connected to an underwater seal or a Heimlich disposable flutter valve.

Accidental pneumothorax

A contralateral pneumothorax during thoracotomy can be caused during mediastinal dissection or during bilateral procedures. On the operative side, it may occur if chest drainage is occluded after chest closure in the presence of a continuing air leak from the lung. It is a risk during any operation near the pleura or where local blocks are performed in the region of the thorax (brachial plexus block, intercostal nerves). It may be a cause of cardiovascular collapse and be difficult to diagnose. Radiography may be useful, but presents a logistical challenge. Drainage should ensue as a matter of urgency. Puncture of the lung itself will usually close spontaneously, but chest drains are usually required as a precaution.

Postoperative considerations

Postoperative hypoxaemia

Atelectasis, sputum retention, poor pain relief and fluid overload may all contribute to postoperative hypoxaemia. Patients who have undergone a thoracotomy will require oxygen in the immediate postoperative period for up to 24 hours and chest physiotherapy. Pneumothorax should be excluded. A chest radiograph is routinely obtained in recovery after all thoracotomies.

Cardiac arrhythmias

The most common cardiac arrhythmia after thoracotomy is atrial fibrillation.[13]

Torsion of remaining lobe

Torsion of the remaining lobe may occur after lobectomy. The presentation may be insidious and up to 2 weeks postoperatively. Chest radiography shows increased density of the affected lobe, which is engorged. Resection of the affected lobe is usual.[14]

Herniation of the heart

Removal of pericardium together with lung resection, particularly on the right, may allow the heart to be displaced from the mediastinum. Cardiovascular collapse is usually profound. Chest radiography may be diagnostic. Emergency re-exploration is required.[13]

SPECIFIC OPERATIONS

Diagnostic procedures

Bronchoscopy

Rigid bronchoscopy

The principles of anaesthesia for rigid bronchoscopy are:

- to maintain oxygenation and carbon dioxide removal during the procedure;
- hypnosis and reduction of autonomic response;
- muscle relaxation to allow passage of the scope and to facilitate the conduct of endotracheal and endobronchial manipulations.

Total intravenous anaesthesia is commonly employed, but inhalational techniques can be used, either by using a ventilating bronchoscope (which has the proximal end sealed by a removable eyepiece and a side-arm that connects to an anaesthetic breathing system) or, less ideally, by using intermittent ventilation via a tube inserted into the open proximal end of a conventional rigid bronchoscope.

Muscle relaxation is obtained with either a short-acting, non-depolarising muscle relaxant or suxamethonium. A prophylactic antimuscarinic may be appropriate, particularly if repeated doses of suxamethonium are required. An infusion of the ultrashort-acting opioid remifentanil may reduce the cardiovascular response to the procedure, but particularly in the event of unexpected hypoxia, severe bradycardia may occur.

Ventilation is normally maintained by using a high-pressure (4 bar) gas injector via a cannula attached to the proximal end of the bronchoscope, which is directed distally. This creates a venturi, which entrains air into the bronchoscope. The anaesthetist stands beside the patient, intermittently releasing the high-pressure gas. The chest and abdomen are observed as a monitor of adequate tidal volume. Care must be taken that the tubing is firmly attached to the injecting cannula because high-pressure gas flow can cause whipping, and injury can occur if the injector tubing comes adrift.

At the end of the procedure, the bronchoscope is removed and the pharynx carefully suctioned. Ventilation is maintained with a bag and face or laryngeal mask, anaesthesia is discontinued and muscle relaxation reversed if a non-depolarising agent has been used. The patient is normally recovered in a sitting position. Nebulised epinephrine (adrenaline) (2 mL, 1:1000 solution),[15] intravenous dexamethasone (8 mg) and CPAP via a tight-fitting mask may help alleviate post-procedure laryngospasm, which may be an occasional complication.

Fibreoptic bronchoscopy

Commonly, fibreoptic bronchoscopy is performed under topical anaesthesia and sedation with midazolam or diazepam. Opioids may be used in addition, but apnoea must be avoided. Local anaesthetic agents may inhibit bacterial growth in microbiological cultures.[16]

A flexible fibreoptic scope may be passed via an endotracheal tube or laryngeal mask airway under general anaesthesia. The diameter of the tube must be great enough to provide adequate ventilation as well as smooth passage of the instrument, and should be checked before induction. The bronchoscope will partially occlude the endotracheal tube and impair ventilation, which may be a particular problem in children. A 3.6 mm diameter paediatric scope will reduce the cross-sectional area of a 5 mm internal diameter tube by almost 50%.[17]

Removal of an inhaled foreign body

Removal of an inhaled foreign body is most common in children and from the right lung. An inhaled foreign body is usually removed via a rigid bronchoscope under inhalation or total intravenous anaesthesia. Respiratory obstruction may be present and can act as a valve so that a segment of lung becomes hyperinflated. These cases can be dangerous and need experience.

Oesophagoscopy

Relaxation of the postcricoid sphincter is needed for rigid oesophagoscopy, and is achieved using muscle relaxants or deep anaesthesia. In obstructive lesions, regurgitation may occur from a dilated oesophagus above the lesion. Rapid sequence induction and intubation should be used. Suction should always be available. The technique should allow rapid return of reflexes.

At the end of the procedure the pharynx must be sucked clear of blood etc. and the patient turned on the inside.

Oesophagoscopy may cause trauma, perforation and bleeding after biopsy or with oesophageal varices.

Intermittent propofol and suxamethonium or a short-acting non-depolarising muscle relaxant, using IPPV with oxygen and nitrous oxide, or spontaneous respiration using a volatile agent, are both satisfactory techniques. Short- or ultrashort-acting opioids will reduce the response to stimulation.

The flexible fibreoptic instrument usually requires light sedation only.

Mediastinoscopy

Mediastinoscopy is performed in the supine position with a single-lumen endotracheal tube. If a mediastinoscopy is planned to precede a thoracotomy, a single-lumen tube should be employed first and then changed because a double-lumen tube may reduce the surgical access. These patients may have obstruction of the superior vena cava and the trachea. An armoured endotracheal tube may be considered. The anaesthetist should be prepared for haemorrhage, which may be considerable and may necessitate sternotomy.

Intrathoracic surgery

Pneumonectomy

A right pneumonectomy removes 55% of the patient's lung tissue and if the function of the remaining lung is compromised, the patient is in a precarious position postoperatively. The major problems are pulmonary hypertension worsened by hypoxia, and oedema of the remaining lung from mechanical damage, reduced lymph drainage and left ventricular failure.

A lateral approach is usual, but the prone or supine position may be used. A double-lumen tube is usual, but a single-lumen tube may be adequate (with or without a bronchial blocker) in some circumstances. If problems are encountered inserting a right-sided double-lumen tube, a left-sided tube may be used for a left pneumonectomy, by withdrawing it slightly for the bronchial suture.

Suction should not be applied postoperatively to pleural drains, which should be clamped. Intermittent transient release of the clamp (e.g. no more than 1 minute every 1 hour) reduces the risk of mediastinal shift, which should be suspected in the event of postoperative cardiovascular instability. Some surgeons prefer not to employ pleural drains after pneumonectomy to avoid this complication.

Postpneumonectomy pulmonary oedema carries a high mortality rate. It appears to be related to the perioperative use of blood products and higher ventilatory inflation pressures, but not postoperative fluid balance.[18] Treatment is with ventilation and diuretics.

The uncommon 'postpneumonectomy syndrome' is caused by excessive lateral shift of the mediastinum into the empty hemithorax, most commonly after right pneumonectomy. It presents with dyspnoea and recurrent respiratory infection, which may occur weeks or even years following surgery. It may be treated by the insertion of a stabilising prosthesis.[19]

Lobectomy

One or (in the case of the right lung) two lobes may be resected. Upper lobectomy is sometimes carried out for carcinoma, along with a segment of the main bronchus (sleeve resection). There will be a large air leak and difficulty with ventilation unless one-lung anaesthesia is used. Lower lobectomy is usually for tumour, but may be for bronchiectasis in children, and the volume of sputum may be large. In older children a Magill blocker may be useful. In young children with copious sputum the sitting position may be considered.

There may be considerable alveolar air leak afterwards, which decreases when IPPV is stopped. Low-pressure suction (–5 cmH_2O) should be applied postoperatively to pleural drains to keep the lungs expanded. If the volume of air leak is very large, it may be greater than the capacity of the suction system and tension pneumothorax may result.

Lung volume reduction surgery

The principle is to reduce lung volume by resecting the worst-functioning lung tissue, allowing better function from remaining lung tissue and improved pulmonary and diaphragmatic mechanics. The procedure is probably only justifiable for patients with both predominantly upper lobe emphysema and low baseline exercise capacity.[20] Any degree of sedation postoperatively is undesirable, and interpleural or epidural analgesia is preferable to opioid analgesia. The surgical approach may be via lateral thoracotomy, or median sternotomy if bilateral. Thorascopy is frequently employed. Bilateral procedures are accomplished sequentially but care must be taken to avoid kinking of the dependent chest drain during the resection of the second side.

Lung cysts and bullae

Large cysts compress surrounding lung tissue and may have a valvular communication with a bronchus, allowing gas to pass in more easily than out. Intermittent positive-pressure ventilation and coughing may therefore cause further distension or even a tension pneumothorax. Early isolation of the cyst from ventilation with a double-lumen tube or bronchial clamp is desirable. If the cysts are bilateral, high frequency jet ventilation (HFJV) may be considered to minimise barotrauma.[19] Nitrous oxide may distend lung cysts because of its much greater solubility than nitrogen and should be avoided. Care is required to distinguish between a tension pneumothorax and distension of a cyst.

Pulmonary hydatid cysts are common in sheep-rearing communities.[21] They can be bilateral and multiple, and need excision if they become large. They may erode the bronchial wall and become infected. Accidental rupture of the cyst into the bronchi during surgery risks dissemination of the disease. Endobronchial intubation is indicated.

Bronchopleural fistula

An abnormal communication between the intrathoracic respiratory system and the pleural cavity may be caused by trauma, neoplasm or infection or arise congenitally (e.g. bullae, tracheo-oesophageal fistula). Most present after pneumonectomy, especially if right-sided. This produces two consequences:

- a gas leak from the lung, which may make ventilation impossible (but which is usually small);
- a collection of fluid in the pleural cavity or post-pneumonectomy space may flood the bronchial tree.

If surgical repair is contemplated, isolation of the remaining lung is preferable. A bronchial blocker in the bronchial stump may easily be pushed through the weakened suture line. Ideally a double-lumen tube is used to isolate the opposite lung, maintaining spontaneous respiration until this is achieved. This has been done using only a propofol infusion.[22] The experienced anaesthetist, however, may simply use suxamethonium to perform a bronchoscopy and then pass an endobronchial tube. An uncut single-lumen tube, positioned with the aid of a fibreoptic bronchoscope, may be suitable, but the cuff may occlude the upper lobe bronchus. Awake endobronchial intubation may also be considered. High-frequency oscillation or jet ventilation may be valuable in compensating for a large volume gas leak.[23].

Formation of a pleurocutaneous fistula (Clagett window) may control a chronically infected post-pneumonectomy space.[24]

Lung abscess and drainage of empyema

Lung abscesses may be caused by aspiration, obstruction by tumour or spread from elsewhere. The vast majority respond to antibiotics alone. Radiologically guided drainage may be required. Surgery is occasionally necessary.[25] Preoperative postural drainage, positioning so that the affected part of the lung is dependent at induction, and rapid isolation of the lung on the unaffected side may protect it from soiling with infected material.

Operations more extensive than simple drainage, such as rib resection for empyema, and those in children require general anaesthesia. The presence of a possible bronchopleural fistula will normally require a double-lumen tube. Awake intubation under local analgesia in the sitting position should be considered with a large fistula or empyema.

Other intrathoracic operations

Thoracoscopy

Video-assisted thoracoscopic surgery (VATS) can be used for many thoracic operations, including lung resection. It is particularly useful for diagnostic procedures. It is associated with less postoperative respiratory dysfunction than open thoracotomy. Surgical difficulty, inadequate exposure of the operative site or haemorrhage may precipitate conversion to an open procedure. Local anaesthetic infiltration of the port sites or multilevel intercostal blocks will greatly assist immediate postoperative analgesia.

Mediastinotomy (left anterior thoracotomy)

The mediastinum may be approached lateral to the sternum through the second left intercostal space with the patient supine for biopsy of lymph nodes in the aortopulmonary window. The pleural cavity is opened and therefore endobronchial intubation will allow collapse of the lung on the operative side. Adjacent vascular structures have the potential to bleed catastrophically.

Segmental lung resection, open lung biopsy

Isolation of the lung on the operative side greatly facilitates segmental lung resection and open lung biopsy. Thoracotomy is required where the procedure cannot be performed thorascopically.

Pleuradhesis, pleurectomy

Pleuradhesis and pleurectomy may be performed by the instillation of talc or other irritant into the pleural cavity after drainage of a recurrent (frequently malignant) pleural effusion during thoracoscopy. Recurrent pneumothoraces are more frequently treated by performing pleurectomy with or without excision of the apical bleb. Whether performed thorascopically or as an open procedure, lung isolation is preferred. Postoperative analgesia is important and may be provided by a combination of local anaesthetic blocks, regular simple analgesics and PCA. Non-steroidal analgesics should be avoided.

Decortication

Haemorrhage may be a problem. For decortication, keeping the lung inflated can aid surgery. This is frequently a difficult and bloody procedure carried out on a patient who may be compromised by chronic infection. Postoperative ventilation may be necessary, but as a significant postoperative air leak is common, it is best avoided. Observation in an intensive care unit setting may be appropriate.

Retrosternal goitre

Surgery for a retrosternal goitre is performed through an upper median sternotomy. Postoperative tracheal collapse with respiratory embarrassment is treated with CPAP, helium–oxygen or, if severe, tracheal intubation.

Tracheal, oesophageal and chest wall surgery

Tracheal stenosis and tracheal perforation

Preoperative dilatation may allow passage of a tracheal tube with inflation of the cuff beyond the operation site. Difficulties are more likely in children. Rare complete tracheal rings present a considerable challenge, and homograft replacement of the segment may be considered. Cardiopulmonary bypass may be necessary in some cases.[26]

Insertion of tracheal stents has been managed with a rigid bronchoscope and a Sanders injector or HFJV. A bronchoscope can be used to place catheters for HFJV beyond an obstruction, although a free outflow for the gas must be provided to prevent lung distension.

The use of the neodymium yttrium-aluminium-garnet (Nd-YAG) laser is associated with the risk of airway fire and special precautions must be taken. This includes limiting F_{IO_2}, using low-ignition tubes (or avoiding them altogether by jetting through a rigid bronchoscope) and filling tracheal tube cuffs with saline.[27] Posterior tracheal wall perforation has been successfully treated by the use of covered stents.[28]

Oesophagectomy

The patient's general condition is often poor owing to lack of nutrition. Assessment and treatment to correct nutritional and electrolyte deficiencies are therefore important. A short period of enteral nutrition (or parenteral if needed) preoperatively may be of great benefit (see Ch. 2.8). The operation may be long and bloody, and may involve opening the abdomen as well as the thorax. Postoperative analgesia may be best provided by a preoperatively sited thoracic epidural.[29]

Thymectomy

Thymectomy for myasthenia gravis

The approach for thymectomy for myasthenia gravis is transcervical or by splitting the sternum, when one or both pleural cavities may be opened. For preoperative and anaesthetic management of myasthenia, see Chapter 1.2. A single-lumen endotracheal tube is required. Haemorrhage may be significant and large-bore venous access is essential.

Pectus correction

A relatively small proportion of patients with pectus excavatum undergo surgical correction. Surgery is undertaken towards the end of the pubertal growth spurt. Lung function should be assessed preoperatively. Intraoperative blood loss may be dramatic. Postoperative pain control may be difficult. The metal bar is removed after 6 months or so. A minimally invasive approach is now widely employed.[30]

Transplantation

Lung transplantation

Survival after lung transplantation is disappointing compared to that following heart transplantation – 3-year survival in the UK for adults was between 48 and 59% in the period 1995–1999.[31] In the USA for the year 2000, 1-year survival for both adult and paediatric patients was 77%; 31% of paediatric recipients were alive 9 years after transplantation and only 24% of adults survived 11 years.[32] The majority of transplants are of single lungs, but double-lung (either single lungs sequentially, or as a block) and heart–lung block procedures are performed. There is a growing interest in live donation of lung tissue, but as yet this is confined to a few centres.

Anterolateral thoracotomy in the lateral position is the standard approach for single lung transplantation. Bilateral procedures are normally performed via a median (occasionally transverse) sternotomy. En-bloc procedures and, often, the second of sequential single-lung transplantations are performed using cardiopulmonary bypass.

The transplanted lung has neither normal lymphatic drainage nor autonomic innervation and postoperative pulmonary oedema is a risk. The lowest left ventricular filling pressure compatible with adequate tissue perfusion is the target for fluid replacement.

Lung transplant recipients frequently require endobronchial or tracheal procedures to treat stenoses and tracheo- or bronchomalacia related to the airway anastomosis.

Indications

Emphysema and pulmonary fibrosis account for 60% of transplants and the remaining indications include sarcoid, α_1-antitrypsin deficiency and primary pulmonary hypertension.

Anaesthetic technique

Assessment of potential lung transplant recipients necessarily involves a multidisciplinary team. Of particular importance are the assessment of right ventricular function and the detection of pulmonary hypertension. Severe emphysema dictates that care be taken to avoid postoperative overdistension of the remaining lung in single lung recipients. Nitrous oxide is avoided because air may remain in the graft vasculature after anastomosis.

Full invasive monitoring is established before induction, with strict attention to asepsis. A pulmonary artery catheter is normally placed before induction, but may need to be withdrawn into its sheath before pneumonectomy. Patients may be haemodynamically unstable and difficult to ventilate adequately. Large-volume blood loss should be anticipated because pleural adhesions are common. Antifibrinolytics may be employed.

Problems

Problems of lung transplantation include:

- haemorrhage as adhesions are separated;
- pulmonary hypertension when the pulmonary artery is clamped, in which case cardiopulmonary bypass will be needed;
- postoperative accumulation of lung water (due to ischaemia before implantation, denervation and section of lymphatic drainage in new lung). Postoperative fluid restriction is usual. Obliterative bronchiolitis is a frequent late complication.[33]

PNEUMOTHORAX

Spontaneous pneumothorax

Spontaneous pneumothorax is common in two age groups – young adults and elderly patients with emphysema. Indications for surgery for spontaneous pneumothorax are:[34]

- persistent air leak;
- recurrent pneumothorax;
- contralateral spontaneous pneumothorax;
- first pneumothorax in a high-risk patient.

Tension pneumothorax

Thoracic trauma (see below, p. 778), rib fractures, ruptured bullae and central venous pressure line insertion may all cause a tension pneumothorax. Signs suggestive of a tension pneumothorax include:

- cyanosis;
- rapid deterioration in vital signs;
- decreased or absent breath sounds;
- decreased pulmonary compliance during anaesthesia.

Tension pneumothorax is treated with urgent thoracocentesis.

THORACIC AORTIC ANEURYSM AND DISSECTION

Thoracic aortic aneurysm and dissection result from degeneration of the intima and are associated with hypertension and connective tissue diseases. Occasionally dissection presents in pregnancy.[35]

Classification of dissection is according to either Debakey (who carried out the first repair in 1955, and described types I, II and III according to the location of the intimal tear) or the Stanford criteria (type A – all types that include the ascending aorta; and type B – confined to the back).

The mortality rate without surgery of type A (I and II) is said to be 50% in 48 hours and 90% in 3 months. Perioperative mortality rate for type B (III) is, at best, about the same as that for conservative treatment (5–20%).[36]

Dissection frequently presents with characteristic pain (sudden onset, radiating through to the back). Pericardial tamponade, coronary occlusion and aortic regurgitation may all occur with proximal dissection. Distal dissection may involve other arteries, including the carotids and renals.

Any rise in preoperative arterial pressure must be aggressively controlled and frequently requires the use of intravenous β-antagonists and vasodilators such as sodium nitroprusside.

Aneurysms may be asymptomatic or cause symptoms because of pressure on other structures. The risk of rupture is proportional to the diameter. The development of endovascular stenting techniques is likely to radically change the traditional approach to thoracic aortic disease.[37]

The surgical strategy is to replace the diseased section of aorta to prevent rupture or further dissection. Cardiopulmonary bypass and deep circulatory arrest may be used to facilitate the formation of the proximal anastomosis, but does not appear to influence outcome.[38] The approach may be via a left thoracotomy or median sternotomy depending on the anatomy.

Endobronchial intubation allows collapse of the left lung to improve surgical access, but positioning of a standard tube may be difficult if there is distortion of the tracheobronchial anatomy. Extensive thoracoabdominal aneurysms may require very large incisions.

The right radial artery is used to monitor proximal aortic pressure. A femoral arterial cannula is useful for monitoring distal pressures. If one or both kidneys are supplied from the false lumen of a dissection, postoperative fenestration from the true lumen may be required and can be accomplished radiologically.[39]

Recovery may be prolonged.

THORACIC TRAUMA

Chest trauma is often associated with multiple other injuries (head injury, abdominal injury, bony injury etc.). The mortality rate from chest trauma is 30% when associated with a head injury. Flail chest is associated with an increased mortality rate.[40]

Thoracic injuries can be classified as:

- penetrating – stab, gunshot etc.;
- non-penetrating – blunt chest trauma, deceleration injury, barotrauma and blast injury.

Non-penetrating injuries may be associated with contusions of the myocardium, rupture of the thoracic aorta, tracheal and bronchial rupture, pulmonary contusions, oesophageal injury (rare) and diaphragmatic rupture (loops of bowel in the chest on radiography).

Haemothorax

A diagnosis of haemothorax is based on the history and clinical examination. The origin of the bleeding includes punctured lung, tears of the internal mammary artery, injury to the great vessels and injury to the intercostal vessels.

Initial treatment of haemothorax is oxygen, a chest drain and analgesia. This may be the only surgical treatment in over 80% of patients.[41] The decision to proceed to thoracotomy is based on an assessment of rate and total volume of bleeding associated with injury, as follows:[42]

- shock or arrest with suspected correctable intrathoracic lesion;
- specific diagnosis (e.g. penetrating cardiac or blunt aortic injury);
- evidence of ongoing thoracic haemorrhage (drainage of 1000–1500 mL initially, >500 mL in the first hour or >1500 mL in first 24 hours after insertion of chest drain).

Cardiac tamponade

Cardiac tamponade should be suspected in a patient with a raised systemic venous pressure (which may be difficult to interpret in hypovolaemia), hypotension, pulsus paradoxus (a reduction of >10 mmHg of systolic pressure in inspiration without change in diastolic pressure), tachycardia (usually >100) or respiratory distress and a history of:

- recent cardiac surgery;
- cardiac instrumentation;
- blunt or penetrating chest trauma;
- malignancy;
- connective tissue disease;
- renal failure;
- septicaemia;
- treatment with ciclosporin, anticoagulants or thrombolytics.

Electrical alternans or nonspecific ST–T wave changes may be seen on the ECG. A chest radiograph may show an enlarged heart shadow with clear lung fields.

Echocardiography may be diagnostic, but posterior tamponade can be missed on transthoracic views. Characteristic diastolic collapse of the right ventricular free wall, right atrium, left atrium or, rarely, ventricle may be absent in the presence of raised right ventricular pressure, right ventricular hypertrophy or infarction.[43] If in doubt, transoesophageal echocardiography is indicated.

Pericardiocentesis is necessary to relieve tamponade in the rapidly deteriorating patient, but surgery (formation of a pericardial window, either thorascopically or as an open procedure) is the definitive treatment (see Ch. 5.2).

Rupture of descending thoracic aorta

Traumatic rupture of the descending thoracic aorta usually occurs at the level of the ligamentum arteriosum. The adventitia holds the aorta in place; consequently, control of arterial pressure is critical. Invasive arterial monitoring (right radial will normally reflect the pressure in the aorta proximal to the injury) and administration of hypotensive agents may delay complete rupture. A CT scan, transoesophageal echography or an arch aortogram is necessary to define the extent of the injury.[44] Surgical access is greatly facilitated by isolation and collapse of the left lung. Patients frequently have other serious injuries.

References

1. The United Kingdom Thoracic Surgical Register 1999–2000 Annual Report. Available on www.ctsnet.org/section/outcome/.
2. Burke JR, Duarte IG, Thourani VH, Miller JI Jr. Preoperative risk assessment for marginal patients requiring pulmonary resection. Ann Thorac Surg 2003; 76:1767–1773.
3. Klein U, Karzai W, Bloos F, et al. Role of fiberoptic bronchoscopy in conjunction with the use of double-lumen tubes for thoracic anesthesia: a prospective study. Anesthesiology 1998; 88:346–350.
4. Campos JH. Lung isolation techniques. Anesthesiol Clin North Am 2001; 19:455–474.
5. Park HP, Bahk JH, Park JH, Oh YS. Use of a Fogarty catheter as a bronchial blocker through a single-lumen endotracheal tube in patients with subglottic stenosis. Anaesth Intens Care 2003; 31:214–216.
6. Vas L, Naregal F, Nobre S, Dongre H. Anaesthetic management for a left pneumonectomy in a child with bronchopleural fistula. Paediatr Anaesth 2000; 10:210–214
7. Tugrul M, Camci E, Karadeniz H, Senturk M, Pembeci K, Akpir K. Comparison of volume controlled with pressure controlled ventilation during one-lung anaesthesia. Br J Anaesth 1997; 79:306–310
8. Klingstedt C, Hedenstierna G, Baehrendtz S, et al. Ventilation–perfusion relationships and atelectasis formation in the supine and lateral positions during conventional mechanical and differential ventilation. Acta Anaesth Scand 1990; 34:421–429.
9. Ihra G, Gockner G, Kashanipour A, Aloy A. High-frequency jet ventilation in European and North American institutions: developments and clinical practice. Eur J Anaesthesiol 2000; 17:418–430.
10. Kawamoto M, Matsumoto C, Yuge O. Atropine premedication attenuates heart rate variability during high thoracic epidural anesthesia. Acta Anaesthesiol Scand 1996; 40:1132–1137.
11. Vaughan RS. Pain relief after thoracotomy. Br J Anaesth 2000; 87:681–683.
12. Richardson J. Epidural analgesia for postoperative pain relief. Bulletin 4. London: The Royal College of Anaesthesists, November 2000; 174.
13. Reed CE. Physiologic consequences of pneumonectomy. Consequences on the pulmonary function. Chest Surg Clin North Am 1999; 9:449–457.

14. Cable DG, Deschamps C, Allen MS, et al. Lobar torsion after pulmonary resection: presentation and outcome. J Thorac Cardiovasc Surg 2001; 122:1091–1093.

15. Scott PV. Nebulised adrenaline in adults with upper airway obstruction. Anaesthesia 1995; 50:476.

16. Olsen KM, Peddicord TE, Campbell GD, Rupp ME. Antimicrobial effects of lidocaine in bronchoalveolar lavage fluid. J Antimicrob Chemother 2000; 45:217–219.

17. Jeffery P, Holgate S, Wenzel S, Endobronchial Biopsy Workshop. Methods for the assessment of endobronchial biopsies in clinical research: application to studies of pathogenesis and the effects of treatment. Am J Respir Crit Care Med 2003; 168:S1–S17.

18. van der Werff YD, van der Houwen HK, Heijmans PJM, et al. Postpneumonectomy pulmonary edema: a retrospective analysis of incidence and possible risk factors. Chest 1997; 111:1278–1284

19. Valji AM, Maziak DE, Shamji FM, Matzinger FR. Postpneumonectomy syndrome: recognition and management. Chest 1998; 114:1766–1769.

20. National Emphysema Treatment Trial Research Group. A randomized trial comparing lung-volume-reduction surgery with medical therapy for severe emphysema. N Engl J Med 348:2059–2073.

21. Safioleas M, Misiakos EP, Dosios T, Manti C, Lambrou P, Skalkeas G. Surgical treatment for lung hydatid disease. World J Surg 1999; 23:1181–1185.

22. Donnelly JA, Webster RE. Computer-controlled anaesthesia in the management of bronchopleural fistula. Anaesthesia 1991; 46:383–384.

23. Ha DV, Johnson D. High frequency oscillatory ventilation in the management of a high output bronchopleural fistula: a case report. Can J Anaesth 2004; 51:78–83.

24. Galvin IF, Gibbons JR, Maghout MH. Bronchopleural fistula. A novel type of window thoracostomy. J Thorac Cardiovasc Surg 1988; 96:433–435.

25. Mansharamani NG, Koziel H. Chronic lung sepsis: lung abscess, bronchiectasis, and empyema. Curr Opin Pulm Med 2003; 9:181–185.

26. Elliott M, Roebuck D, Noctor C, et al. The management of congenital tracheal stenosis. Int J Pediatr Otorhinolaryngol 2003; 67(suppl 1):S183–S192.

27. Scherer TA. Nd-YAG laser ignition of silicone endobronchial stents. Chest 2000; 117:1449–1454

28. Madden BP, Sheth A, Ho TB, McAnulty G. Novel approach to management of a posterior tracheal tear complicating percutaneous tracheostomy. Br J Anaesth 2004; 92:437–439

29. Watson A, Allen PR. Influence of thoracic epidural analgesia on outcome after resection for esophageal cancer. Surgery 1994; 115:429–432.

30. Park HJ, Lee SY, Lee CS, Youm W, Lee KR. The Nuss procedure for pectus excavatum: evolution of techniques and early results on 322 patients. Ann Thorac Surg 2004; 77:289–295.

31. Anyanwu AC, Rogers CA, Murday AJ, Steering Group. Intrathoracic organ transplantation in the United Kingdom 1995–99: results from the UK cardiothoracic transplant audit. Heart 2002; 87:449–454.
32. Edwards LB, Keck BM. Thoracic organ transplantation in the US. Clin Transpl 2002; 29–40.
33. Bracken CA, Gurkowski MA, Naples JJ. Lung transplantation: historical perspective, current concepts, and anesthetic considerations. J Cardiothorac Vasc Anesth 1997; 11:220–241.
34. Waller DA, Forty J, Morritt GN. Video-assisted thoracoscopic surgery versus thoracotomy for spontaneous pneumothorax. Ann Thorac Surg 1994; 58:372–376.
35. Immer FF, Bansi AG, Immer-Bansi AS, et al. Aortic dissection in pregnancy: analysis of risk factors and outcome. Ann Thorac Surg 2003; 76:309–314.
36. Karmy-Jones R, Aldea G, Boyle EM Jr. The continuing evolution in the management of thoracic aortic dissection. Chest 2000; 117:1221–1223.
37. Gowda RM, Misra D, Tranbaugh RF, Ohki T, Khan IA. Endovascular stent grafting of descending thoracic aortic aneurysms. Chest 2003; 124:714–719.
38. Lai DT, Robbins RC, Mitchell RS, et al. Does profound hypothermic circulatory arrest improve survival in patients with acute type a aortic dissection. Circulation 2002; 106(suppl 1):I218–I228.
39. Chavan A, Lotz J, Oelert F, Galanski M, Haverich A, Karck M. Endoluminal treatment of aortic dissection. Eur Radiol 2003; 13:2521–2534.
40. Liman ST, Kuzucu A, Tastepe AI, Ulasan GN, Topcu S. Chest injury due to blunt trauma. Eur J Cardiothorac Surg 2003; 23:374–378.
41. Kalyanaraman R, De Mello WF, Ravishankar M. Management of chest injuries – a 5 year retrospective survey. Injury 1998; 29:443–446.
42. Karmy-Jones R, Jurkovich GJ, Nathens AB, et al. Timing of urgent thoracotomy for hemorrhage after trauma: a multicenter study. Arch Surg 2001; 136:513–518.
43. Maisch B, Ristic AD. Practical aspects of the management of pericardial disease. Heart 2003; 89:1096–1103.
44. Feliciano DV, Rozycki GS. Advances in the diagnosis and treatment of thoracic trauma. Surg Clin North Am 1999; 79:1417–1429.

Further reading

Gosh S, Latimer RD. Thoracic anaesthesia: principles and practice. Oxford: Butterworth–Heinemann; 1999.

Kaplan JA. Thoracic anesthesia. 3rd edn. New York: Churchill Livingstone; 2003.

CHAPTER **5.15**

ANAESTHESIA IN UNUSUAL ENVIRONMENTS

ABNORMAL AMBIENT PRESSURE

Low ambient pressure — altitude

Barometric pressure (PB) is measured in millibars (mbar) by pilots, millimetres of mercury (mmHg) by meteorologists and kilopascals (kPa) by physiologists. The pascal is the SI unit for pressure (N/m^2). One atmosphere at sea level is approximately 1000 mbar (or 1 bar, identical to 100 kPa). The 'standard' atmosphere is 101.325 kPa. This is the same as 760 mmHg, the height to which mercury rises in the evacuated capillary column of a barometer at sea level due to atmospheric pressure acting on the reservoir at its base. Barometric pressure decreases exponentially with altitude, halving every 5.5 km (18 000 feet).

Temperature decreases linearly by 2°C per 300 m (1000 feet) up to 12.2 km (40 000 feet), where it is approximately −60°C. An aircraft flying at this altitude has its interior pressure at the equivalent of 1.5–2.4 km (5000–8000 feet) and its temperature 19–24°C. There is therefore a large difference in pressure and temperature between the cabin and the exterior. Aircraft without internal pressure and temperature control systems do not fly above 3.6 km (12 000 ft, Table 5.15.1).

Altitude (low ambient pressure) can be simulated in a hypobaric decompression chamber, and depth (high pressure) in a hyperbaric compression chamber. Most pressure chambers can be used for either.

Problems of anaesthesia at altitude

More than 10 million people live at altitudes over 3000 m (10 000 feet), and some hospitals in the Andes are above 5000 m. At altitude it is appropriate to quantify anaesthetic potency using partial pressure of inhaled anaesthetic agents rather than concentration. Minimum alveolar partial pressure (MAPP) is more useful than minimum alveolar concentration (MAC).[1] The following should also be considered.

Oxygen

Oxygen 30% has the same partial pressure at 3000 m (10 000 feet) as 20% oxygen at sea level. At least 40% oxygen should be given during anaesthesia

Altitude (m)	PB (mmHg)	PIO2 (mmHg)	FIO2 for PIO2 to be 150 mmHg (%)	Notes
19 200	47	0	–	
12 200	141	20	–	Upper level for airliners
8 848	236[b]	40	79	Everest summit
6 100	349	63	50	Consciousness may be lost without oxygen enrichment
5 500	380	70	45	Barometric pressure halved
3 000	523	100	32	
1 800	609	118	27	
0	760	150	21	
Depth underwater (m)	**PB (mmHg)**	**PIO2 (mmHg)**	**FIO2 for PIO2 to be 150 mmHg (%)**	**Notes**
10	1520	309	10	
50	4560	945	3.3	Lower limit of air diving
200	15 960	–	0.9	
500	38 760	–	0.4	Deeper diving prevented by severe high-pressure nervous syndrome

[a]Note that partial pressure of alveolar water vapour is always 47 mmHg
[b]PB on Mount Everest's summit is probably slightly higher, and has been measured at 253 mmHg[1]

Table 5.15.1 Barometric pressure P_B and moist inspired oxygen partial pressure PiO_2 in mmHg, and the inspired oxygen concentration FiO_2 needed to make PiO_2 its sea-level value of 150 mmHg (20 kPa) at various altitudes and depths[a]

and recovery at altitude. A high-airflow oxygen enrichment (HAFOE) mask provides higher than expected oxygen concentrations and a lower flow rate (oxygen flow plus entrained air) than at sea level. This is because of the lower pressure difference between the atmosphere and the negative pressure created by the jet of oxygen issuing from the nozzle. The overall effect is to reduce inspired PO_2 (PB × inspired oxygen concentration). However, HAFOE masks may safely be used at altitude if allowance is made for this.

Nitrous oxide

The efficacy of nitrous oxide is reduced as PB decreases. The analgesic effect of 50% nitrous oxide at 3000 m (10 000 feet) is minimal. In addition, no more than 60% may be given, to allow for the recommended 40% inspired oxygen. Consequently, the preferred carrier gas for inhalation anaesthesia at altitude is oxygen-enriched air.

Cylinder pressure gauges

Cylinder pressure gauges are reliable at altitude because the reduction of PB is so small compared to cylinder gas pressure.

Flowmeters

Flowmeters (rotameters) underestimate the actual gas flow delivered. Gas density is proportional to PB, and so is reduced at altitude. At high flow rates the space around the bobbin acts like an orifice, through which flow is inversely proportional to the square root of the gas density, and hence of PB.[1] The error is about 20% at 3000 m. It should affect all gases equally, but this may not be true at lower flows, where laminar flow around the bobbin is governed by viscosity. Inspired oxygen monitoring is essential.

Vaporisers

Saturated vapour pressure (SVP) changes with temperature, but not with PB. Therefore, at a given dial setting, the partial pressure (and mass) of vapour delivered is the same whatever the altitude. However, because the density of the carrier gas is reduced at altitude, the vapour concentration is increased. Splitting ratio is minimally affected by changes in PB. Hence the clinical anaesthetic effect from a given dial setting is similar for all altitudes, assuming ambient temperature is maintained constant.

Gas and vapour analysers

Gas and vapour analysers respond to specific properties of the gas or vapour being monitored, and measure the number of its molecules, which is its partial pressure. Calibration is conventionally in percentage units, in line with clinical practice at sea level. Care must be taken to interpret concentrations correctly at altitude. For example at 5500 m, where PB is half its sea level value, concentration of oxygen in dry air is 20.9% (as at sea level) but its partial pressure is only 10.6 kPa (79 mmHg or 0.209 × 380 mmHg). The analyser would read 10.5% oxygen if it did not compensate for the reduced PB. Similar confusion may arise with carbon dioxide and vapour analysers if they have been calibrated in percentage at sea level.

Low temperatures

Low temperatures are associated with altitude. It is important that ambient temperature is adjusted to as near normal working temperature (19–24°C) as possible. Separation may occur in Entonox cylinders below –7°C, and liquid nitrous oxide may settle in the bottom of the cylinder. If this happened, initially a high concentration of oxygen would be breathed, providing inadequate analgesia. Later a dangerously low concentration of oxygen would be breathed, when the cylinder was nearly empty with only pure nitrous oxide remaining.

Pathophysiology

Changes in both acclimatised and unacclimatised persons include:

- hyperventilation resulting from the hypoxic stimulus;
- respiratory alkalosis, which gradually becomes compensated by excretion of bicarbonate;
- polycythaemia;
- pulmonary hypertension and fluid retention.

In addition, pulmonary and cerebral oedema are often associated with rapid ascent to high altitude. Descent of a few hundred metres can result in a dramatic improvement. A lightweight portable hyperbaric chamber (Gamow bag) weighing 8 kg can be used at altitude for emergency treatment. It can be pressurised to approximately 100 mmHg above ambient pressure and includes a rebreathing system.

Anaesthesia

Hypoxic respiratory drive at altitude is vital, and so respiratory depression from anaesthetic agents and opioids is more serious than at sea level. Where possible, patients who are not fully acclimatised should be transferred to a lower altitude. A higher incidence of post-dural puncture headache was reported before the introduction of pencil-point spinal needles.

High ambient pressure – depth

Pressure underwater is the force of the weight of water (mass × acceleration due to gravity) acting on unit area. As water is incompressible its density does not vary with depth, so pressure increases linearly with depth. It may be assumed that

10 m of water = 1 atmosphere = 100 kPa = 760 mmHg.

As a diver descends to depth, gas partial pressures increase along with ambient pressure. At 40 m depth the pressure is 5 atmospheres absolute (ATA)

– four water plus one for the atmosphere above. This is 3800 mmHg. Inspired PO_2 is 760 mmHg if breathing air, the equivalent of 100% oxygen at sea level.

At 40 m the high PN_2 causes narcosis, 15% loss of cognitive skills and 5% loss of manual dexterity. Sports divers breathe compressed air to a depth limit of 50 m using self-contained underwater breathing apparatus (SCUBA). Deeper than 50 m nitrogen (air) should be avoided and replaced with a helium–oxygen mix.

Saturation diving

Saturation diving is when nitrogen is washed out of the body and equilibrium with helium is reached in the blood and tissues. This is used for commercial purposes, often to depths of 200–300 m. Such divers live in a pressure chamber for weeks at a time, entering and exiting the chamber via a hatch into a diving bell, which can be winched down to the sea bed or their working depth.

Saturation divers may become ill or injured. As decompression to one atmosphere may require several days or more to allow helium excretion without bubble formation, doctors may need to undergo compression and enter the chamber. Surgery could be performed in a large compression chamber with the medical team equilibrated at high pressure. The logistical problems of transporting a sick diver in a portable pressure chamber to a medical pressure chamber are extremely challenging.

Problems of anaesthesia in a compression chamber

Oxygen toxicity

Acute cerebral toxicity may cause convulsions if inspired PO_2 exceeds 200 kPa (2 ATA). Chronic pulmonary oxygen toxicity may occur in saturation diving. Inspired PO_2 should not exceed 0.5 ATA, which limits inspired oxygen concentration to less than 2% at 250 m. Safety regulations dictate the use of 98% helium and 2% oxygen at this depth. The diving supervisor who controls the pressure chamber and its atmosphere in some ways assumes the responsibility of an anaesthetist.

High-pressure nervous syndrome

Tremor, loss of fine movement control and disorientation can occur at 500 m, but may occur at lesser depths, especially if compression is rapid (>1 m/min). It is probably caused by pressure on neuronal membranes and altered enzyme function. The risk may be reduced by the use of small fractions of nitrogen mixed with heliox.

Thermal balance

Pressure increase raises temperature and rapid ascent (decompression) lowers temperature. The gas breathed at depth is at ambient pressure, of increased density, increases the work of breathing and has a high heat capacity. If the diving bell is immersed or the diver is free swimming his body loses heat because of conduction and respiratory convection. Body surface warming using hot water immersion suits and warming inspired heliox are important diving routines.

Pressure reversal of anaesthesia

Pressure reversal of anaesthesia affects all general anaesthetics, with around 30% loss of potency at 31 ATA. Most research has been on rodents in bench top compression chambers. Clinical research into hyperbaric anaesthesia is rare. Studies of anaesthetic potency in volunteers during saturation diving are unlikely.

Inflatable cuffs

Cuffs on tracheal tubes and Foley catheters should be filled with water.

Voice communication

Breathing helium distorts speech. Sophisticated unscrambling devices are widely used.

Glass containers

Drug ampoules may implode on compression, but opening them beforehand may make them unsterile.

Bubble formation

Decompression cause gas, especially nitrogen, to come out of solution and increase in volume by Boyle's law. This occurs in fatty tissues, joints, brain etc. and is called decompression sickness. Bubbles might also appear in local anaesthetic solution after injection into the body.

Colonisation of the skin and external auditory canal

Colonisation of the skin and external auditory canal with Gram-negative organisms such as *Proteus* and *Pseudomonas* spp. occurs in saturation divers working in a warm humid environment.

Anaesthetic techniques

Only life-saving operations should be considered, adopting conservative treatment during decompression. Ketamine is the anaesthetic agent least affected by pressure reversal. Propofol infusion with opioids is an option, though an increased dose requirement should be expected. Intravenous regional analgesia is useful for limb injuries. For major procedures, use morphine 2–3 mg/kg with paralysis and intermittent positive-pressure ventilation (IPPV) using ambient atmospheric gas. Manual IPPV with a self-inflating bag and non-rebreathing valve is probably safest, although a ventilator powered by, and delivering, the same mixture of gas as in the chamber atmosphere is feasible. Inhalation agents are not used because the chamber atmosphere is recycled.

Hyperbaric oxygen therapy

When breathing 100% oxygen at sea level the dissolved oxygen concentration in blood is about 2.1 mL/dL. At 3 ATA this increases to 6.2 mL/dL, which exceeds the arteriovenous difference at rest (5 mL/dL) and therefore satisfies tissue oxygen demand. This enhancement of dissolved oxygen can be of therapeutic value. However, the theoretical possibility of oxygen transport entirely without red cells is unrealistic because of obligatory haemoglobin involvement in carbon dioxide transport.

Hyperbaric oxygen is of proven value in anaerobic infections, and in selected patients with tissue hypoxia, such as osteoradionecrosis, osteomyelitis and compartment syndrome. It is of value in carbonmonoxide poisoning if treatment is started within 30 minutes. There is a debate about its value in multiple sclerosis. It can be lifesaving in decompression sickness, but because hyperbaric facilities only exist in certain centres, patients who have suspected symptoms and signs may require to be transferred to the nearest facility by air. The flight path should be planned to be low altitude so that gas expansion within the embolising bubbles is minimised.

UNUSUAL CIRCUMSTANCES

Anaesthesia may have to be administered in unpredictable conditions in the field:

- following major disasters (earthquake, nuclear explosion, mining and other industrial accidents);
- in remote regions such as Antarctica;
- in war zones, where there may also be weapons of mass destruction.[2]

Apparatus for field use

Apparatus for intravenous anaesthesia is portable, unlike medical gas cylinders, which are heavy and need refilling. Volatile agents may be vaporised in air or oxygen-enriched air using portable draw-over apparatus. Essential features include the following:

- a calibrated vaporiser, such as the Oxford Miniature Vaporiser (OMV) or Ohmeda Universal Portable Anaesthesia Complete Vaporiser (PAC), with sufficiently low resistance to allow spontaneous ventilation;
- equipment to provide IPPV, such as a self-inflating bag between the vaporiser and the airway. There must be a one-way valve to prevent reverse flow of gas back to the vaporiser, and a non-rebreathing valve (Ambu E) at the airway to direct expired gas into the atmosphere;[3]
- a source of oxygen to enrich inspired air. Oxygen can be fed into an open-ended length of reservoir tubing upstream from the vaporiser.

This was the concept of the military Triservice anaesthesia apparatus, which included two OMV50s in series giving a mixture of two vapours (trichloroethylene and halothane). Various modifications have since been developed:

- Oxford inflating bellows (OIB) for manual IPPV or a portable automatic ventilator;
- oxygen concentrator;
- air compressor likely to be integral with the oxygen concentrator;
- switch to allow draw-over or plenum mode gas flow;[4]
- use of isoflurane or sevoflurane – the inspired sevoflurane concentration can be increased, especially in spontaneous ventilation, if carrier gas (air) is drawn over two sevoflurane vaporisers in series.

These systems have been introduced in mission hospitals around the world with guidance from the Societies of the World Federation of Anaesthesiologists. Because anaesthetists in these hospitals are not usually medically qualified and the hospitals are permanent buildings, equipment design features should concentrate on safety and simplicity without the limitation of lightweight and compact construction. The anaesthetic in these circumstances is most likely to be halothane, which is one-tenth the price of sevoflurane. The Glostavent is the most recent example of an anaesthetic machine designed for use in remote regions.[5]

However, for anaesthesia in the field, portability of apparatus is essential.[6] Infusion and syringe pumps, airway equipment, various anaesthetic drugs and self-inflating bags are all portable. Oxygen availability is restricted by cylinder size and weight. An alternative source is an oxygen concentrator, which produces a continuous supply of oxygen but needs a reliable source of electricity. In the event of a power failure, cylinder oxygen should be available.

Anaesthesia techniques in the field

General anaesthesia

A common technique is the use of thiopental or propofol, muscle relaxant, tracheal intubation, IPPV with air (preferably oxygen-enriched) using a Laerdal self-inflating bag or OIB, supplemented with halothane, isoflurane or sevoflurane from an Oxford Miniature or PAC vaporiser. IPPV rather than spontaneous ventilation has been shown to improve oxygenation when using air as carrier gas.[6]

Ketamine

Intravenous or intramuscular ketamine may be useful for analgesia in patients trapped following accidents who may be hypovolaemic and have restricted access to their airway. Ketamine and midazolam, maintaining general anaesthesia with neuromuscular blockade and low-dose isoflurane, have been shown to be safe and effective.

Regional analgesia

Regional analgesia may be useful for limb surgery or some elective abdominal operations.[7]

Where assistance is limited and there are multiple casualties, general anaesthesia with a secured airway using a tracheal tube is likely to be the safest option in a field hospital or combat support unit.

Intensive care in the field has been made available for injured servicemen and women on operational military service,[8] following political influence to promote worldwide the same standard of care in a British field hospital, or naval equivalent, as in the UK. This is linked with repatriation of appropriately stabilised critically ill patients by military aeromedical transportation. In recent years this combination has proved to be effective.

References

1. Stoneham MD. Anaesthesia and resuscitation at altitude. Eur J Anaesth 1995; 12:249–257.
2. Baker DJ. Management of casualties from terrorist chemical and biological attack: a key role for the anaesthetist. Br J Anaesth 2002; 89:211–214.
3. Eltringham RJ, Varvinski A. The Oxyvent. An anaesthetic machine designed to be used in developing countries and difficult situations. Anaesthesia 1997; 52:668–672.
4. Perndt HKS. The ULCO anaesthetic suitcase. Anaesth Intens Care 2002; 30:800–803.
5. Eltringham RJ, Wei FQ, Thomas W. Experience with the Glostavent anaesthetic machine. Update Anaesth 2003; 16:31–35.
6. Lunn DV, Young PC. The Ohmeda Universal PAC drawover apparatus. Anaesthesia 1995; 50:870–874.
7. Buckenmaier CC, Lee EH, Shields CH, Sampson JB, Chiles JH. Regional anesthesia in austere environments. Regi Anesth Pain Med 2003; 28:321–327.
8. Roberts MJ, Fox MA, Hamilton-Davies C, Dowson S. The experience of the intensive care unit in a British army field hospital during the 2003 Gulf conflict. J Roy Army Med Corps 2003; 149:284–290.

CHAPTER **5.16**

UROLOGICAL AND RENAL SURGERY

GENERAL CONSIDERATIONS

For anaesthesia in patients with impaired renal function, see Chapter 1.2.

Age

Patients presenting for urological surgery are frequently at the extremes of age. It is well recognised that children have particular needs (see Ch. 5.6); however, elderly patients, particularly those over 80, also need special consideration.[1]

Preoperative care

Many elderly patients will be ASA 2 or greater with cardiovascular disease. Long-term medication should usually be continued throughout the hospital stay. The elderly are at particular risk of confusion if anticholinergic drugs that cross the blood–brain barrier, such as hyoscine, are used for premedication. Most elderly patients require no premedication. If they are particularly anxious a small dose of an oral benzodiazepine such as temazepam may be used.

Heroic surgery may be unwise in some patients. Most urological procedures are elective. The consultant should recommend treatment after full discussion with the patient, and if necessary the family and other team members involved in care.

Intraoperative care

Anaesthetic techniques that are appropriate for young fit adults may be unsafe in the elderly.

Fluid balance

Fluid balance is more difficult in the elderly. Excess fluid with borderline or overt renal failure can cause acute cardiac failure and pulmonary oedema. Dehydration can precipitate further renal impairment. Central venous pressure monitoring is useful in major surgery.

Temperature

The elderly cannot increase their metabolic rate to counteract heat loss. Shivering may increase oxygen demand above the capacity for supply.

Conservation of heat by active warm air systems, warming intravenous fluids and operating whenever possible in a warm environment all help maintain body temperature and aid recovery.[2] Active warming techniques should be continued in recovery.

Postoperative care

Many problems of pre- and intraoperative care extend into the postoperative period, such as maintenance of temperature, deep venous thrombosis (DVT) prophylaxis and fluid management, especially in relation to renal disease. The elderly are also prone to confusion and pain management can be difficult.

Pressure areas

Most pressure sores develop within the first 24 hours following surgery. They may be compounded by periods of hypotension with poor skin perfusion. They prolong hospital stay, delay rehabilitation and may produce fatal sepsis. Preventive measures are especially important during prolonged operations.

Pain management

Good-quality pain assessment is the key to success.

Opioids, when given in the correct doses by the most appropriate route of administration, work well. Care must be taken with non-steroidal anti-inflammatory drugs (NSAIDs), including COX-2 inhibitors, particularly with the risk of renal failure in those with existing renal disease. Hypovolaemia adds greatly to the risk of NSAID.

Extra- or intradural anaesthesia can be useful (see below and Ch. 4.3). There may be improved survival owing to a reduction in venous thromboembolism, myocardial infarction, haemorrhage, pneumonia and respiratory failure. The benefits include altered coagulation, improved blood flow and improved analgesia.[3]

Extradural infusions using a mixture of local anaesthetic and opioid can provide good quality postoperative analgesia, but there can be a significant incidence of technical problems and systems must be in place to ensure safe nursing care. In some hospitals this can be provided on the general ward, in others the patient will require admission to a high-dependency unit.

Rehabilitation

Early mobilisation is extremely important. Physiotherapists and occupational therapists need to be involved.

Variety of surgery

Urological procedures fall into a number of categories:

- paediatric reconstructive surgery for congenital abnormalities, performed in specialised centres and not considered in this chapter;

- minor surgery on the genitalia, such as circumcision and vasectomy;
- minimally invasive surgery, including cystoscopy and transurethral resection of the prostate (TURP);
- major surgery such as cystectomy, nephrectomy and renal transplantation.

Patients with bladder cancer may present for repeated 'check' cystoscopies. These are often performed under topical anaesthesia and do not involve the anaesthetist. If there is a need for extensive examination or biopsy, general anaesthesia may be required. These patients can be old and frail. The fact that they have had a recent general anaesthetic without problems should not result in a false sense of complacency. Appropriate preoperative assessment is always necessary.

TECHNICAL CONSIDERATIONS

General anaesthesia

Spontaneous breathing through a laryngeal mask is commonly used for minor surgery. More major surgery frequently requires the use of muscle relaxants and intermittent positive-pressure ventilation (IPPV).

Regional analgesia

Regional techniques are frequently used for urological procedures, either as the sole anaesthetic or in combination with general anaesthesia. They provide useful postoperative analgesia.

Topical anaesthesia is usually all that is required for flexible cystoscopy and is given by the surgeon.

Intradural (spinal) anaesthesia is frequently used as the sole anaesthetic for operations such as TURP.

A single-shot caudal extradural injection of local anaesthetic through the sacral hiatus can aid analgesia for procedures such as circumcision.

A lumbar extradural catheter is often appropriate for major urological surgery, often in combination with a general anaesthetic. Extradural anaesthesia has the particular advantages of helping to reduce blood loss and potentially providing excellent postoperative analgesia.

An understanding of the nerve supply is important. Afferent fibres providing pain sensation generally run with the autonomic nerves.

Nerve supplies

Kidney

Afferent fibres run through the coeliac, renal and superior hypogastric plexuses and continue in the thoracic and lumbar splanchnic nerves, T10 to L1. Some afferents may run with vagal fibres, explaining the nausea and vomiting that can accompany renal pain.

Ureter

Afferents follow a similar path to the kidney, ending in T10 to L2.

Bladder and urethra

Sympathetic fibres from L1 and L2 through the hypogastric and pelvic plexuses are motor to the bladder. Pain from the dome of the bladder reaches the spinal cord in segments T11 to L2, following a similar path to the nerves from the ureter. Pain from the bladder neck and urethra goes with the pelvic splanchnic nerves, S2 to S4.

Prostate

Afferents run in T11 to L2 and S2 to S4 following the same pathways as above.

Testis

Afferents run with the sympathetic nerves through the coeliac plexus and lesser splanchnic nerve, T10 to L1.

Penis, scrotum and distal urethra

Penis, scrotum and distal urethra are supplied by the pudendal nerve, S2 to S4. The skin at the base of the penis and some skin on the anterior aspect of the scrotum is supplied by the ilioinguinal (L1) and genitofemoral (L1, L2) nerves.

Somatic nerves of lower abdominal wall

Afferents are T11 to L1.

SPECIFIC OPERATIONS

Cystoscopy and bladder tumours

Bladder cancer shows a strong association with smoking. Close attention must be paid to other smoking-related diseases in the preoperative assessment. These operations are performed as day-case procedures (see Ch. 5.3).

Topical analgesia

Lidocaine (lignocaine) 1 or 2% urethral gel may be satisfactory, especially in women, or if a flexible fibreoptic cystoscope is used in men. Severe cystitis makes local analgesia unsuitable because bladder distension with irrigating fluid causes painful spasm.

General anaesthesia

If general anaesthesia is used, there must be:

- complete loss of sensation;
- relaxation of the bladder sphincters and abdominal wall;
- no straining, coughing or respiratory obstruction.

These points can be difficult to accomplish smoothly, especially in the elderly with heart and lung disease. General anaesthesia should never be undertaken lightly, and may rarely even require tracheal intubation. Spontaneous respiration using oxygen, nitrous oxide and a volatile agent with a small dose of intravenous opioid is a common technique.

A patient with bladder cancer may present for cystoscopy at regular intervals. Anaemia (sometimes severe) is common. If resection of tumour is performed there is no significant absorption of the irrigation fluid. Bladder perforation may occur. Stimulation of the obturator nerve passing near the ureteric orifice may cause violent adduction of the leg, but can be prevented by obturator nerve block or a muscle relaxant. Suxamethonium is suitable. Irrigation with normal saline is used postoperatively to prevent clot retention.

All instrumentation of the lower urinary tract is likely to cause significant bacteraemia. Prophylactic antibiotics are used, commonly a single dose of 120 mg gentamicin. If the patient is at risk of endocarditis, this must be combined with 1.0 g amoxicillin, and a further oral dose of 500 mg 6 hours afterwards.

Transurethral resection of the prostate

General anaesthesia, either with spontaneous respiration or IPPV, may be supplemented by caudal extradural block to reduce bleeding and postoperative pain. Intradural block is also very satisfactory, commonly with 2–3 mL heavy or plain 0.5% bupivacaine. The block must reach T10. Blood loss during this operation is difficult to measure, but is usually about 7–20 mL per gram of prostate resected. It is increased by raising venous pressure (straining, excessive transfusion, excessive absorption of irrigant), prolonged operation time and release of plasminogen activators from the prostate. An antifibrinolytic drug such as 0.5–1.0 g tranexamic acid may be useful. Blood loss is usually less with regional than with general anaesthesia.

Irrigation

Glycine 1.5%, at a pressure of less than 70 cmH_2O, is widely used for irrigation. Although slightly hypotonic (2.1% is isotonic) it has good optical properties, is non-electrolytic and prevents dissipation of diathermy current during resection. Glycine has a half-life of 85 minutes. Metabolic products include oxalate, which may precipitate in the renal tubules if urine flow is low during the first 10 postoperative days, and ammonia which is a cerebral depressant. Glycine is an inhibitory neurotransmitter and may cause transient blindness. The amount absorbed via the prostatic veins is typically around 700 mL or 20 mL/min, but can reach several litres, depending on surgical skill, pressure of irrigant and duration of operation. Cold irrigating solutions may cause hypothermia.

TURP syndrome

Glycine absorption can result in water intoxication, cerebral oedema, pulmonary oedema, hypoxia and fibrinolysis.

Presentation

Symptoms of TURP syndrome may be obscured by general anaesthesia, but include burning sensations of the hands and face followed by nausea, vomiting and headache, ultimately leading to coma, convulsions or cardiac arrest. Signs include bradycardia and hypertension.[4]

Other problems of TURP syndrome

Dilutional hyponatraemia may prolong the action of non-depolarising relaxants, and cause QRS widening and T-wave inversion. Bacteraemia may confuse the clinical picture.

Prevention of TURP syndrome

Ensure that the irrigating fluid is not too high above the patient (less than 70 cm) and limit the duration of procedure, preferably to less than 30 minutes. Ideally the syndrome should be prevented by close observation of the patient and monitoring the serum sodium. Regional techniques allow observation of early symptoms.

Treatment of TURP syndrome

A sodium level below 120 mmol/L should be treated even if there are no clinical featutres. The fully established syndrome is more difficult to manage. Treatment includes mannitol, loop diuretics (e.g. furosemide [frusemide]), water restriction and hypertonic saline with central venous pressure monitoring, inotropic agents or even dialysis.

Abdominal prostatectomy

The patients for abdominal prostatectomy may be old and frail. Preoperative assessment needs particular care. There may be significant blood loss and heat loss. Relaxation is required. General anaesthesia with IPPV is often used. Caudal or lumbar extradural analgesia (7–15 mL of plain 0.5% bupivacaine for the latter) is a useful supplement because it provides relaxation and reduces bleeding.

Retropubic prostatectomy

This approach is used to remove a large benign prostate. General anaesthesia as for abdominal prostatectomy or intradural block alone with 2–3 mL heavy or plain 0.5% bupivacaine are satisfactory.

Radical prostatectomy

Radical prostatectomy is performed for prostatic cancer. The prostate and adjacent lymph nodes are removed. Patients may have undergone preoperative radiotherapy and bleeding can be difficult to control. Invasive monitoring is common, including direct arterial and central venous pressures. The operation may be long. Temperature monitoring, an active warm air system, warmed fluids and a breathing system humidifier are used.

Circumcision

Babies and children may be given intravenous or inhalation induction and spontaneous respiration maintained using oxygen, nitrous oxide and volatile agent. Spontaneous respiration is generally used in adults too. Laryngeal spasm may easily develop if anaesthesia is too light, and may need surgery to be interrupted, the application of continuous positive airway pressure or even suxamethonium and intubation.

Extradural sacral block with 0.5 mL/kg 0.25% bupivacaine is an extremely useful adjunct, especially in children.[5] Penile block is a good alternative, blocking the dorsal nerves with 0.25 mL/kg 0.25% bupivacaine in children or 10 mL in adults.

Surgery of the scrotum, including vasectomy

These operations may be done under local infiltration analgesia, especially vasectomy, but some surgeons prefer general anaesthesia because there is less likelihood of haematoma formation. This may be partly due to postoperative sedation and a short bed rest. Traction on the spermatic cord may result in bradycardia or even asystole. Atropine or glycopyrronium should be available, and some give it preoperatively.

Nephrectomy

Nephrectomy is performed for cancer, infection, or rarely a staghorn calculus.

Traditionally tumours were removed through an abdominal incision with the patient supine to gain rapid control of the renal vessels and prevent tumour embolisation. Modern imaging methods provide proper assessment of this risk and the operation is usually performed with the patient in a lateral position. In this position the lower lung has greater blood flow but less ventilation. This ventilation–perfusion mismatch may cause hypoxia. Use of the kidney bridge or breaking the table worsens dependent atelectasis. IPPV is essential. When the patient is turned on his or her back at the end of the operation the lower lung should be fully inflated. Use of the kidney bridge may also cause inferior vena cava obstruction and sudden severe hypotension.

Renal tumours are extremely vascular, so the anaesthetist should insert wide-bore intravenous cannulae and be prepared for torrential bleeding.

General anaesthesia with muscle relaxant, IPPV, nitrous oxide, volatile agent and opioid is usual. Both intradural and extradural analgesia up to T8 may be used, but is best combined with general anaesthesia. Thoracic paravertebral block produces excellent unilateral analgesia without as much hypotension as an extradural. A paravertebral catheter may be inserted for postoperative analgesia.[6]

Rarely, the pleura is damaged during kidney operations. The resulting collapse of the upper lung may prove dangerous unless IPPV is employed. An underwater drain may be required. Tumour embolus causing collapse and cardiac arrest is an occasional complication of operations for carcinoma of the kidney.

Postoperative breathing exercises help prevent atelectasis. Chest physiotherapy and postoperative oxygen for some days may be warranted. Good-quality postoperative analgesia helps prevent chest complications.

Total cystectomy

Significant bleeding may occur with total cystectomy, but this can be reduced by using extradural blockade. Circulatory monitoring is likely to include direct arterial and central venous pressures.

Lithotripsy and lithotomy

Renal stones can now be treated without open operation in many cases. Bacteraemia is likely and should be covered by antibiotics.

Percutaneous nephrolithotomy

Percutaneous nephrolithotomy involves the passage of a telescope into the renal pelvis under radiological control, irrigation with saline, and electrohydraulic fragmentation until the stone can be extracted. Large volumes of saline may be absorbed if the pressure in the renal pelvis is allowed to rise above 75 cmH_2O.[7] The patient is semiprone or prone, and IPPV is normally used. Sepsis is a well-recognised complication.

Extracorporeal shockwave lithotripsy

Extracorporeal shockwave lithotripsy fragments the stone with external acoustic shock waves. Modern lithotripters produce little pain and the procedure is undertaken with analgesics and sometimes light sedation. General anaesthesia is still sometimes required for children. This is only undertaken in specialised paediatric centres.

Haemodialysis

Insertion of a Scribner shunt involves the insertion of an arterial and venous cannula with a connecting link, in either the arm or the leg. For longer-term access an arteriovenous fistula may be formed, using infiltration of local anaesthetic.

Renal transplantation

Renal transplantation has become an extraordinarily successful operation. Quality of life and survival are considerably better than on dialysis. The mortality rate is low and graft survival at 1 year is around 90%. Patients who would previously have been considered too unfit are now candidates for surgery.

Preoperative considerations

Consider both the cause and the effects of the renal failure.

Common causes of renal failure

- Diabetes mellitus – these patients may also have autonomic neuropathy and gastroparesis;
- glomerulonephritis or pyelonephritis;
- polycystic kidneys;
- hypertension.

Common effects of renal failure

- Anaemia due to decreased erythropoietin production and reduced cell life. Platelet dysfunction due to abnormal aggregation;
- accelerated atheroma and hypertension;
- gluid and electrolyte imbalance, notably hyperkalaemia. Metabolic acidosis;
- hyperparathyroidism.

Some other well-known effects of renal failure, such as pericardial and pleural effusions, are characteristic of end-stage disease and are seldom seen in patients presenting for transplant.

Management

Erythropoietin is used to maintain haemoglobin at 9.5 g/dL. However, this can make hypertension worse and lead to a greater risk of clotting at the vascular access sites. Continue antihypertensive medication except for angiotensin-converting enzyme (ACE) inhibitors and angiotensin-II receptor blockers, which may cause hypotension at induction.

Fluid balance is crucial. Hypovolaemia causes graft failure. Patients are dialysed to within 0.5 kg of their ideal body weight just before surgery. Correct electrolyte imbalance. The serum potassium must be below 5.5 mmol/L.

Intraoperative considerations

The transplantation operation consists of exposing and preparing the iliac vessels, placing the new kidney, usually in the right iliac fossa, making the vascular connections and finally connecting the urinary drainage. The operation normally takes 2–3 hours. Consider the following aspects.

Care for current and future dialysis sites

Pad any arteriovenous fistula and place a blood pressure cuff on another limb. Use the contralateral hand for venous access, avoiding the antecubital fossa and forearm veins. Avoid arterial cannulae unless the need is overwhelming. If essential, use a dorsalis pedis artery.

Fluid balance

Central venous pressure monitoring is essential to manage fluid balance. A triple-lumen catheter also allows for infusion of drugs such as dopamine. Because of platelet dysfunction the internal jugular route is preferred to the subclavian. Also, if a subclavian vein clots or is compressed by haematoma the entire limb may become useless for fistula formation.

If a patient is hypovolaemic, fluid loading may be necessary before induction. Aim for a central venous pressure over 12 cmH_2O during the operation. Hypovolaemia must be avoided. Early onset of urine output is associated with good graft survival. Furosemide (frusemide), mannitol and dopamine are commonly used. Each unit will have its own protocol.

Extradural and intradural analgesia

Extradural and intradural analgesia are relatively contraindicated by the platelet dysfunction and the need to avoid hypotension, particularly because postoperative polyuria is likely.

Induction of anaesthesia

Induction of anaesthesia should be as gentle as possible. However, even if the patient is starved there may still be gastroparesis owing to autonomic neuropathy and anxiety. If this is suspected the usual procedures for preventing regurgitation should be followed, including rapid sequence induction. All patients are intubated and ventilated.

Muscle relaxants

Suxamethonium causes a rise in serum potassium. If it has not been possible to ensure a normal potassium level preoperatively and rapid sequence induction is needed, use rocuronium. Most non-depolarising relaxants are acceptable, except for pancuronium. Atracurium is commonly used because its elimination also occurs by Hofmann degradation. Neuromuscular blockade must be monitored to avoid extrusion of the graft before closure of the abdomen.

Volatile agents

Most volatile agents are acceptable except for enflurane, which is about 2% metabolised with production of fluoride ions, probably in amounts that are not nephrotoxic, but prudence suggests avoidance. Isoflurane is very little metabolised (0.2%) and is often used.

Temperature

Temperature maintenance and monitoring are essential.

Postoperative considerations

Fluid balance

Careful management is essential in the early postoperative period to ensure that the survival of the new kidney is not threatened by hypovolaemia or hypotension. Arterial and central venous pressures must be monitored and urine output measured at least hourly. Polyuria is common, making fluid balance more difficult. Anuria may indicate obstruction at the anastomosis.

Analgesia

Morphine metabolites may accumulate until the kidney is functioning normally. Pethidine has no advantages and norpethidine may accumulate. Many units use patient-controlled analgesia with morphine, but in a reduced bolus dose (often 0.5 mg). Alternatively patient-controlled analgesia with fentanyl may be employed. NSAIDs reduce renal blood flow and may threaten the new kidney.

Immunosuppression

All units will have their own protocol for immunosuppression, which usually includes ciclosporin, methylprednisolone and tacrolimus.

References

1. Association of Anaesthetists of Great Britain and Ireland. Anaesthesia and peri-operative care of the elderly. London: AAGBI; 2001.
2. Association of Anaesthetists of Great Britain and Ireland. Recommendations for standards of monitoring during anaesthesia and recovery. London: AAGBI; 1998.
3. Rodgers A, Walker N, Schug S, et al. Reduction of postoperative mortality and morbidity with epidural or spinal anaesthesia: results from overview of randomised trials. Br Med J 2000; 321:1493–1497.
4. Gravenstein D. Transurethral resection of the prostate (TURP) syndrome: a review of the pathophysiology and management. Anesth Analg 1997; 84:438–446.
5. Armitage EN. Regional anaesthesia in paediatrics. Clin Anesthiol 1985; 3:553–562.
6. Richardson J, Lönnqvist PA. Thoracic paravertebral block. Br J Anaesth 1998; 81:230–238.
7. Sugai K, Sugai Y, Azuma Y, et al. Vascular absorption of irrigation solution in percutaneous nephro-ureterolithotomy. Br J Anaesth 1988; 61:516–517.

CHAPTER **5.17**

VASCULAR SURGERY

For the Cheyenne Indians, joy was conveyed by the expression that 'the heart soars like a bird'. Why is it then that the hearts of anaesthetists do anything but soar when news reaches them of the ruptured aortic aneurysm in casualty, or the critically ischaemic leg that requires revascularisation? What is it about anaesthesia for vascular surgery, particularly emergency vascular surgery, that elicits a groan of collective depression more heartfelt than attends contemplation of any other surgical specialty? Perhaps it is because such cases are difficult, prolonged, labour-intensive and unpredictable, with outcomes that can be gloomy. Yet anaesthetists need not be so depressed, because they do have the skills to attenuate some of the hazards for these high-risk patients undergoing high-risk surgery. The challenge starts with preoperative evaluation.

PREOPERATIVE EVALUATION

The purpose of preoperative assessment is to gauge whether a patient has the physiological reserve to cope with the potential surgical insult, and to determine whether any improvement is possible before operation. Given that elective surgery is often prophylactic, it is also important to give patients some idea of the level of operative risk they face. Unfortunately, the ideal of being able to identify individuals specifically at risk remains elusive. As a generalisation it is probably true that major vascular procedures threaten haemodynamic stability more than any other, and fatal adverse effects are primarily cardiac. However, the various cardiac risk indices (Goldman, Detsky, Eagle) have low specificity, and are of limited value in predicting serious perioperative cardiac events. Factors that have been shown to have some consistent impact on operative mortality include coronary artery disease (as manifest by recent myocardial infarction, unstable angina and arrhythmias), increasing age and chronic renal impairment.[1] Pulmonary disease, unless it is severe, appears to exert little influence as a predictor of adverse outcome.

Specific cardiac investigations

Dipyridamole–thallium scanning

Intravenous thallium (a radioactive potassium analogue) enters myocardial cells in concentrations proportional to myocardial blood flow, thereby identifying ischaemic areas. This effect is enhanced by dipyridamole (an antiplatelet drug that is also a coronary vasodilator). Blood flow through normal vessels increases and causes a coronary steal effect, with flow to ischaemic areas being further reduced. Delayed scanning following discontinuation of the infusion identifies areas of reversible, as opposed to permanent, ischaemia. The test is one of the more specific available.

Cardiac ejection fraction

The ability of the cardiac ejection fraction (EF) to predict adverse perioperative cardiac events has not been established. A low EF does not supervene until left ventricular (LV) function is severely impaired, but still it has not consistently been shown to be an independent risk factor. Some studies have reported good results in patients with an EF below 35% (normal is ≈65%), and this matches the anecdotal experience of many clinicians. It may also reflect the limitations of two-dimensional echocardiography as a measurement technique.

Stress echocardiography

A dobutamine infusion (10–40 μg/kg/min) mimics the effect of exercise (and by extension surgical stress) on the myocardium. This has a relatively good predictive value.

PREOPERATIVE PREPARATION

Goal-directed therapy may benefit some patients by optimising preoperative cardiac function and oxygen delivery by the use of fluids and inotropes.[2] The technique is resource intensive. Selected patients may also benefit from perioperative β-adrenoceptor blockade.[3]

GENERAL CONSIDERATIONS

Blood loss

Major blood loss may occur during most vascular procedures, but is particularly associated with aortic aneurysm repair. There may be leaks at the anastomoses, back-bleeding from lumbar arteries, or difficulty in identifying the aneurysm sac before aortic cross-clamping. Clinical features of progressive blood loss are well known, but consideration should be given to blood transfusion when loss exceeds 10 mL/kg i.e. 15% of total blood volume (70 mL/kg).

Intraoperative cell-saver devices are efficient, provide blood rapidly, and save the equivalent of up to 10 units hourly should massive transfusion be necessary. Prospective trials in major vascular patients have shown, however, that they do not reduce the requirement for allogenic blood.

Coagulation failure may also result in continuous ooze, which can be impossible to stop without infusion of blood products. Transfusion laboratories are reluctant to release these in the absence of proven coagulation derangements. Fresh frozen plasma (FFP), which should contain over 70% of the activity of the donor unit, is indicated when the prothrombin time (PT) or activated partial thromboplastin time (APTT) is 1.5 times normal. Cryoprecipitate may be required when fibrinogen falls below 1.0 g/L, as can occur in disseminated intravascular coagulation (DIC) following massive transfusion. The empirical dose is 1 unit/5 kg body weight. Platelets may also be needed (1 unit/10 kg), each unit of concentrate raising the platelet count by $5–10 \times 10^9$/L. Platelet numbers give no information about platelet function. Thromboelastography (TEG) can be used in theatre to assess coagulation status (including platelet function), but each determination takes 30 minutes.

Renal function

The influence of chronic renal insufficiency on surgical outcome is procedure dependent. An infrarenal aortic cross-clamp will cause an immediate reduction in renal blood flow of 40%. There may be evidence of persistent impairment even 6 months later. Intraoperative biochemical tests are not practical, and so despite the absence of any established relationship between intraoperative oliguria and postoperative renal failure, the only method available for monitoring renal function is measurement of urine output. It is assumed that a urine output of 0.5 mL/kg/h (1 mL/kg/h during the period of cross-clamping) indicates adequate renal blood flow.

Principles of management during major surgery include maintenance of intravascular volume and cardiac output (using inotropes as appropriate). More specific therapy includes mannitol and loop diuretics. Mannitol infusion (0.25–0.5 g/kg), initiated before cross-clamping, acts as an osmotic diuretic, improves renal cortical blood flow and acts as a scavenger of free radicals, which are released into the circulation when the clamp is removed. Loop diuretics (furosemide [frusemide]) are also renal vasodilators (mediated via prostaglandin E). 'Renal-dose' dopamine (1–3 μg/kg/min) traditionally has been used for its renoprotective effect, although there is no evidence to suggest that it is better than volume expansion alone.

TECHNICAL CONSIDERATIONS

Temperature maintenance

Heat loss is a potential problem due to prolonged surgery and major evaporative losses via exposed body cavities. Hypothermia may confer some benefit by decreasing the oxygen requirement of potentially ischaemic tissues (such as those distal to a vascular clamp), but any advantage is offset by the significant problems of depressed cardiac function, increased blood viscosity and peripheral circulatory compromise. Delayed wound healing and increased infection rates may also complicate the postoperative course. Core temperature should be measured continuously (tympanic membrane, oesophagus). Heat loss should be minimised by maintaining the ambient temperature (usually 22–24°C), by warming and humidifying inspired gases, by warming infused fluids, and by using a forced-air warming blanket. As the head accounts for 10% of heat loss a reflective silver foil hat should be used.

Intraoperative monitoring

Electrocardiography

Although the electrocardiogram (ECG) is used routinely it remains a mediocre indicator of myocardial ischaemia. Every anaesthetist will have seen at least one impeccable ECG trace in a patient who has no pulse. The optimal configuration for detection of ischaemia using a single lead is the CM5 (it is unusual in the UK to use a multi-lead configuration).

Arterial blood pressure monitoring

All but the simplest vascular cases will require direct intra-arterial blood pressure (IABP) measurement. The information gained from IABP is not confined solely to numbers. The slope of the systolic upstroke gives some indication of myocardial contractility, and the dP/dt_{max}, the maximum rate of rise of LV pressure, can be calculated. The position of the dicrotic notch on the downstroke of the waveform reflects systemic vascular resistance (SVR). If there is peripheral vasoconstriction the dicrotic notch is high; with vasodilatation it moves lower down the curve. Systolic pressure variation of more than 10 mmHg during intermittent positive-pressure ventilation (IPPV) suggests at least a 10% reduction in circulating volume.

Central venous pressure measurement

Central venous pressure (CVP) monitoring is essential in cases in which fluid losses or fluid shifts will be substantial (as in aortic surgery and some peripheral revascularisation procedures). It is not indicated for routine carotid endarterectomy. The CVP is the hydrostatic pressure generated by the blood within the right atrium (RA) or the great veins of the thorax. It provides an indication of volaemic status (the venous capacitance system being a large compliant reservoir for two-thirds of the total blood volume) and also reflects right ventricular (RV) function. In major surgery the CVP is most useful if it is transduced continuously.

Pulmonary artery catheterisation

A pulmonary artery (PA) catheter gives direct information about the function of the LV, which in patients with impaired myocardial function cannot be inferred from the CVP. The role of the PA catheter in general remains contentious, but in the context of vascular surgery it is likely to be of modest benefit only in high-risk patients.[4] Their intraoperative use (not common in the UK) is likely to be superseded by noninvasive monitors.

Transoesophageal echocardiography

Modern transoesophageal echocardiography (TOE) probes allow 180° views of the heart, and the absence of large tissue masses between the probe and the myocardium produces well-defined ultrasound images, allowing the determination of LV preload and function and the diagnosis of acute LV dysfunction and myocardial ischaemia.

Transoesophageal Doppler ultrasonography

Transoesophageal Doppler ultrasonography is noninvasive and allows estimations of volaemic status and cardiac function. It has the advantage of requiring less operator expertise than TOE and is considerably easier to use.

Temperature

Heat loss is significant during major surgery and core temperature should be monitored continuously.

POSTOPERATIVE CARE

The investment of time and effort in these difficult cases is futile unless there is provision for optimal postoperative care. This can take place on a general ward, but many vascular patients will need care in a high-dependency unit (HDU) or an intensive therapy unit (ITU), depending on the level of support required.

Many of the principles of postoperative care are generic, involving haemodynamic and respiratory stabilisation, good oxygenation, normothermia and good analgesia. The problems specific to particular vascular procedures are outlined below, but this is a group of patients with a high probability of cardiovascular disease and in whom surgery may be prolonged. They are more likely to require postoperative ventilation, invasive monitoring, complex analgesic regimens and circulatory manipulation with vasoactive infusions. Oxygen therapy should be continued for at least 5 postoperative nights even in uncomplicated cases because of the risk of circadian hypoxaemia.[5]

SPECIFIC OPERATIONS

Carotid endarterectomy

Transient ischaemic attacks in patients with carotid artery atheroma have been described as 'fragments borrowed from the stroke that is yet to come', and in patients who are symptomatic the benefits of surgery are clear. In patients without symptoms the risk–benefit analysis is less straightforward. The annual stroke rate following successful endarterectomy is less than 1%, yet with optimal medical care the rate is still only around 2%.[6] Surgery is only justified therefore, if the operative hazards remain low. The anaesthetist should help ensure that the decision to operate is vindicated by minimising perioperative complications.

One decision that has to be taken is whether the procedure should be carried out under general anaesthetic (GA) or local anaesthetic (LA). The broad advantages and disadvantages of each are summarised in Box 5.17.1. The definitive answer awaits the outcome of the GALA (GA versus LA) multicentre trial.

Carotid endarterectomy involves removal of the atheromatous plaque following clamping of the common and internal carotid arteries, after which the pressure in the stump on the cerebral side of the circulation can be transduced directly. Should the stump pressure be low (<50 mmHg), indicating cerebral hypoperfusion, then the surgeon may insert a shunt (necessary in fewer than 10%). If the patient is awake, his or her mental state will provide a good index of cerebral oxygenation. The overall mortality rate is 3–4%, and neurological deficit (due to embolus, thrombus, dissection or hypoperfusion) occurs in up to 5% of patients. Cardiovascular instability, manifest by reflex hypotension and bradycardia, may persist for 12–24 hours, owing to increased pressure at the carotid sinus that was previously damped by the atheromatous plaque. Some patients develop a cerebral hyperperfusion syndrome due to increased blood flow through the recanalised vessel. Symptoms settle within about 7 days as cerebral autoregulation is restored, but in the meantime hypertension should be treated, as must cerebral oedema should it supervene.

The nerves to the carotid bodies may be lost during carotid endarterectomy, but consequent loss of hypoxic ventilatory drive is rarely significant. Wound haematoma and airway compression are potential mechanical complications of the procedure.

General anaesthesia for carotid endarterectomy

There is no evidence of benefit associated with any specific general anaesthetic technique. Anaesthesia need not be complex, but its focus must be the maintenance of global cerebral oxygenation. It is commonly based on a balanced anaesthetic technique following tracheal intubation, preferably with an armoured tube, with ventilation to normocarbia. Once the

Box 5.17.1
General versus local anaesthesia for carotid endarterectomy
General anaesthesia
Advantages
Reduction in cerebral metabolic rate
Autoregulatory cerebral blood flow curve shifts to left
Disadvantages
Cerebral status difficult to monitor
Multiple drugs (with generic complications)
Pressor response to laryngoscopy
Potential delayed awakening
Local anaesthesia
Advantages
Effective monitoring of cerebral status
Rapid restoration of postoperative function
Cardiovascular stability more likely
Higher mean arterial pressure (and stump pressure)
Disadvantages
Prolonged immobility uncomfortable
Higher cerebral and cardiac oxygen demand

carotid clamp is applied, the mean arterial pressure (MAP) should be maintained by up to 20% higher than normal, to ensure adequate collateral cerebral flow.

Carotid sinus manipulation can cause profound reflex bradycardia and hypotension. Vagolytic drugs may restore the rate, but at the expense of myocardial oxygen demand. Alternatively, the surgeon can attenuate the reflex by infiltration of local anaesthetic.

Wakening needs to be rapid to allow accurate neurological assessment.

Postoperative pain can be managed without opiates, particularly if the wound is infiltrated before extubation with local anaesthetic.

Local anaesthesia for carotid endarterectomy

The main advantage of local anaesthesia for carotid endarterectomy is that cerebral status is easy to monitor. There is no interference with cerebral autoregulation, and the requirement for vasoactive drugs is less. Cardiovascular stability may be easier to achieve throughout the procedure, a higher MAP being reflected in higher cerebral perfusion pressure, and there is rapid restoration of postoperative function.

The main disadvantage rests with the discomfort and restlessness that may attend prolonged immobility in an unnatural position. Cerebral oxygen consumption does not fall (cerebral metabolic rate decreases under general anaesthesia) and a higher pulse and blood pressure during surgery result in higher myocardial oxygen demand than otherwise would be the case. The procedure is usually carried out under superficial and deep cervical plexus block (although cervical epidural anaesthesia has also been used (see Ch. 4.2)).

Abdominal aortic surgery

Elective abdominal aortic aneurysm repair

Abdominal aortic surgery carries a high risk (mortality rate 2–8%) and patients commonly have significant co-morbidity. Up to 10% will have renal impairment, 30% will be hypertensive and over 60% will have significant ischaemic heart disease. Surgery can be prolonged, blood loss can be substantial, and aortic clamping and release comprise major physiological insults.

Invasive intra-arterial and CVP monitoring is essential, and TOE or oesophageal Doppler are useful. The insertion of large-bore cannulae is routine, and there must be provision for the rapid infusion of fluid.

Extradural analgesia can be used intraoperatively, but its greater value lies in its capacity to extend optimal analgesia well into the postoperative period. It is important to ensure that the epidural is sited at an appropriate level. A thoracic epidural alone may be insufficient for an aortobifemoral reconstruction in which both groins are opened as well as the abdomen. An additional lumbar epidural will effectively overcome this problem, although a two-catheter technique does make the postoperative analgesic regimen more complicated.

Otherwise the anaesthetic technique should aim to maintain haemodynamic stability throughout. This is difficult during aortic clamping and release. As the aorta is clamped there is a large rise in proximal SVR, together with immediate distal ischaemia. The sudden increase in afterload increases LV end-systolic wall tension, which in a healthy myocardium is associated with an increase in contractility (the Anrep effect), but which in a diseased heart may cause LV dysfunction. These effects can be attenuated by offloading the ventricle with a vasodilator such as glyceryl trinitrate (starting at 0.5 μg/kg/min), meanwhile optimising preload with fluids. In patients with partial aortic atheromatous occlusion, an extensive distal collateral circulation may provide some protection against these effects. Preoperative radiology may predict in which patients this is true. The release of the aortic clamp is also critical.

During the period of distal ischaemia anaerobic metabolism produces lactate, vasoactive substances and metabolic acidosis. Inflammatory mediators can also be released into the systemic circulation. Reactive hyperaemia in the distal vascular tree leads to effective hypovolaemia with a decrease in venous return. The net result may be severe hypotension, which may be further compounded if there is blood loss through an insecure anastomosis. These problems can be pre-empted by judicious fluid loading during the period of cross-clamping (keeping the CVP at around 12–15 mmHg) and by rapid fluid resuscitation should hypotension persist.

A large midline incision is not always used. The incision can be transverse, and a minimal retroperitoneal approach has also been described allowing patient discharge at a mean of 3.6 days.[7] POSSUM scoring is useful for predicting outcomes with some accuracy, although it may tend to over-predict mortality in infrarenal aneurysm repair.[8,9]

Endovascular (endoluminal) abdominal aortic aneurysm repair

In a subgroup of patients in whom the anatomy is favourable, open repair can be avoided by siting an aortic stent graft across the aneurysm sac (endovascular abdominal aortic aneurysm repair [EVAR]). Access to the diseased aorta is via an arteriotomy in the femoral artery. The graft is inserted under radiological control. Conversion to open repair is required in around 2% of cases. The procedure can be carried out under local infiltration, or under general or regional anaesthesia with direct IABP monitoring. Further invasive monitoring is not usually necessary. Early and midterm outcomes are better than with traditional open repair,[10] but this is not yet proven at long-term follow-up.

Emergency abdominal aortic aneurysm repair

Emergency abdominal aortic aneurysm repair is a very high-risk procedure with an operative mortality that may exceed 80%. The extreme urgency of the situation should not obscure a rational analysis of the value of proceeding to surgery. Laparotomy and resuscitation may have to be simultaneous – rapid cross-clamping of the aorta may be all that lies between the patient and death.

The patient should be anaesthetised in theatre on the operating table. Retroperitoneal bleeding can be tamponaded and the patient may appear to stabilise. This tamponading effect disappears as soon as abdominal muscle tone is abolished by muscle relaxants, and so the anaesthetist must be prepared for sudden decompensation. Direct IABP and CVP monitoring should have been established, but in the extreme situation this may have to wait. It is, in any event, difficult to insert an arterial cannula into a vessel that is barely pulsating. Once the aorta is clamped then anaesthesia can proceed as for elective aortic repair. Surgery is likely to be prolonged, and blood loss substantial.

Most patients are haemodynamically unstable for several hours and will require postoperative intensive care. Adverse prognostic indicators include sustained or severe preoperative hypotension, base deficit on presentation, massive blood transfusion, long clamp time, suprarenal clamping and prolonged surgery. Advanced age alone should not disbar a patient from theatre, but some studies have identified age as an independent risk factor for increased mortality and major postoperative complications.[11]

Lower limb revascularisation

Peripheral vascular disease is associated with generalised systemic atherosclerosis (patients with intermittent claudication have a mortality two to four times greater than those who do not have claudication).

Revascularisation procedures are carried out for critical ischaemia – when the patient has symptoms at rest and the survival of the limb is threatened. They include femoropopliteal and femorodistal bypass grafts (mortality rate ≈3%) and femorofemoral crossover and axillobifemoral grafts (aiming to improve blood flow into the iliac or femoral vessels).

Surgery is frequently lengthy, can involve significant blood loss, and with the exception of trauma cases is usually performed in patients with significant systemic occlusive arterial disease. Arterial clamping often has little effect because the circulation is already significantly occluded.

Reperfusion on release of the clamp is associated with problems analogous to those encountered in aortic surgery. These are usually less pronounced and can be managed by ensuring a modestly supranormal circulating volume during clamping. CVP and IABP monitoring is useful.

Anaesthesia can have a significant influence on flow through the graft. Driving pressure (blood pressure) should be maintained, should a haematocrit of 30–35% which will limit blood viscosity. Flow can further be enhanced by preventing peripheral vasoconstriction (caused by pain and cold) and by maximising peripheral vasodilation via a lumbar epidural (providing both good analgesia and a sympathetic block).

Acute ischaemia

Acute ischaemia is most usually embolic, affecting the lower limbs more than the upper, and the most common cause is atrial fibrillation. Unless there is rapid surgical intervention the limb is gravely at risk. Intra-arterial thrombolysis (with streptokinase or tissue plasminogen activator) may avoid surgical intervention, which can usually be initiated under local anaesthesia. Simple arterial embolectomy may be all that is necessary, but an anaesthetist is required both to monitor these high-risk patients and to provide general anaesthesia should more extensive surgery be required.

Varicose vein surgery

Venous surgery is included here for completeness, but it shares few of the problems of arterial surgery. Venous 'disease' is not associated with systemic atheroma, and although some patients are elderly, requiring surgery because of chronic dependent venous ulcers, many are young and otherwise fit.

Traditional procedures such as saphenofemoral junction ligation, stripping of the long saphenous vein and multiple avulsions are being superseded by procedures targeted at the incompetent perforators. Access to some of these may require prone positioning, but anaesthesia is otherwise straightforward. Newer techniques such as VNUS, ultrasound-directed radiofrequency ablation can substantially prolong surgery.

References

1. Geraghty PJ, Sicard GA. Abdominal aortic aneurysm repair in high-risk and elderly patients. J Cardiovasc Surg 2003; 44:543–547.
2. Wilson J, Woods I, Fawcett J, et al. Reducing the risk of major elective surgery: randomised controlled trial of preoperative optimisation of oxygen delivery. Br Med J 1999; 318:1099–1103.
3. Mangano DT, Layug EL, Wallace A, et al. for the Multicenter Study of Ischaemia Research Group. Effect of atenolol on mortality and cardiovascular morbidity after non-cardiac surgery. N Engl J Med 1996; 335:1713–1720.
4. Pulmonary Artery Catheter Consensus Conference Participants. Pulmonary artery catheter consensus conference: consensus statement. Crit Care Med 1997; 25:910–925.
5. Reeder MK, Goldman MD, Loh L, et al. Postoperative hypoxaemia after major abdominal vascular surgery. Br J Anaesth 1992; 68:23–26.
6. Prevention of disabling and fatal strokes by successful carotid endarterectomy in patients without recent neurological symptoms: randomised controlled trial. MRC Asymptomatic Carotid Surgery Trial (ACST) Collaborative Group. Lancet 2004; 363:1491–1502.
7. Mukherjee D. 'Fast–track' abdominal aortic aneurysm repair. Vasc Endovasc Surg 2003; 37:329–334.
8. Copeland GP, Jones D, Walters M. POSSUM: a scoring system for surgical audit. Br J Surg 1991; 78:356–360.
9. Shuhaiber JH, Hankins M, Robless P, et al. Comparison of POSSUM with p-POSSUM for prediction of mortality in infrarenal aneurysm repair. Ann Vasc Surg 2002; 16:736–741.

10. Zeebregts CJ, Geelkerken RH, van der Palen J, et al. Outcome of abdominal aortic aneurysm repair in the era of endovascular treatment. Br J Surg 2004; 91:563–568.

11. Vemuri C, Wainess RM, Dimick JB, et al. Effect of increasing patient age on complication rates following intact abdominal aortic aneurysm repair in the United States. J Surg Res 2004; 118:26–31.

Section 6

Non-acute pain

CHAPTER **6.1**

NON-ACUTE PAIN

Pain is defined as 'an unpleasant sensory and emotional experience associated with actual or potential tissue damage, or described in terms of such' (International Association for the Study of Pain [IASP] definition).

Chronic pain is pain that persists beyond a reasonable time in which one would expect the pain from an acute injury to settle. Three months is commonly taken as the time after which a pain becomes chronic. The origin of the pain can be from ongoing tissue damage, such as arthritis or cancer (nociceptive), or as a result of nerve injury (neuropathic) or the pain can be of unknown origin. For all pain types, both the pre-existing psychological make-up of the patient and the psychological response to ongoing pain can make an important contribution to the clinical picture.

THE PAIN CLINIC

Pain clinics are usually headed by anaesthetists in conjunction with other specialties, including rheumatology, neurology, neurosurgery, psychiatry and other disciplines, including nursing, physiotherapy, occupational therapy and clinical psychology. They are generally run as a multidisciplinary team.

The role of the pain clinic in patient care can be summed up as:

- to decrease subjective pain experience;
- to increase general level of activity;
- to decrease drug consumption;
- to return the patient to employment or full quality of life;
- to reduce further use of health care resources.

Facilities required for a successful pain clinic should include a dedicated space for the multidisciplinary team to work together. This should include dedicated office space, consulting rooms, space for group-based pain management, and one-to-one treatments such as transcutaneous electrical nerve stimulation (TENS) and physiotherapy. Access to X-ray imaging in a suitable room with monitoring and resuscitation is also required: many pain clinics make use of the day-surgery unit, which is ideally suited for nerve blocks.

Essential pain clinic equipment will include suitable imaging, suitable monitoring for sedation, a radiofrequency lesion generator, a cryoprobe machine and a peripheral nerve stimulator. Access to inpatient beds is an excellent option for those requiring complex medication changes, or therapies requiring prolonged drug administration via complex routes (e.g. epidural or intrathecal).

Pain clinics have been shown to be effective, both for nerve block treatments[1] and for psychologically based therapies.[2,3]

THE PAIN PATIENT

Chronic pain is common, affecting an estimated 20–30% of the population. As the pain clinic approach is that of symptom control, referrals should ideally come from other specialties, where previous diagnostic work-up has been completed and after appropriate surgical and medical therapy. The most common referral is for back pain, mostly via rheumatology and orthopaedic clinics. Other routes of referral are from general medical and surgical firms, as well as neurology and the palliative care service. Some general practice referrals can be accepted as long as complex diagnostic work-up is not required.

The patient will have already tried a variety of analgesic drugs, usually with only modest success. Others may be using benzodiazepines and antidepressants. Most will have tried physiotherapy and alternative therapies, often with limited success. Anxiety and depression are common in chronic pain patients, and it is often unclear whether these are primary or secondary to persistent pain. Other emotions include anger and blame. Post-traumatic stress disorder commonly follows chronic pain due to trauma.[4] Litigation for personal injury or medical negligence is increasingly common. The patient may be in receipt of benefits for unemployment and disability.

ASSESSMENT OF PAIN

Important aspects of pain assessment are as follows:

- site of the pain. Body maps indicate the extent of pain, and often request the patient to identify the primary pain site. Total body pain is a surprisingly common presentation;
- severity of pain using visual analogue pain scales (VAS 100 mm continuous line), numerical rating scale (scale of 0–10) or categorical rating (mild/moderate/severe);
- duration of pain;

- cause of pain, and diagnosis if known. Pain of unknown aetiology is common. Precipitating episode (surgery, trauma) or spontaneous onset;
- past history of pain – previous investigations, surgery, injections and other pain clinic treatments;
- pattern of pain – continuous, intermittent or flare-up pattern;
- what makes the pain worse?
- what makes the pain better?
- medications, TENS and other therapies. How effective are they?
- what words does the patient use to describe the pain?
- ask about depression and anxiety – sleep pattern, mood, fatigue, tearfulness, guilt feelings, future outlook, and any past history of depression, how treated and if successful;
- current levels of activity and employment. What does the pain stop the patient doing? How far can he or she walk or drive? Is the patient independent for dressing and bathing?
- home situation. Who is at home? Are they all well? Is the patient a carer or does he or she have a carer?
- is litigation active?

Commonly used pain questionnaires are the Brief Pain Inventory and the McGill Pain Questionnaire. Many others have been devised for research purposes, but are occasionally useful for clinical practice (Beck Depression Inventory, Hospital Anxiety and Depression [HAD] Scale, Somatic Perception Questionnaire). Patient pain diaries are commonly used by pain clinics.

Pain clinics are not intended for diagnostic assessment. If the pain clinician is at all unclear of the explanation for symptoms re-referral to an appropriate specialist is in order. Many complex pain problems, however, elude a diagnosis, in spite of extensive investigations. Many pain clinics run joint clinics with other specialties, especially rheumatology, orthopaedics, maxillofacial surgery and psychiatry. Missed pathology, however, remains a problem and the pain clinician should always bear this in mind.

GENERALISED PAIN PATTERNS

Neuropathic pain

Neuropathic pain is initiated or caused by a primary lesion in the nervous system, which can be central (e.g. multiple sclerosis) or peripheral (e.g. painful peripheral neuropathy).

Neuralgia is pain in the distribution of a nerve or nerves, including trigeminal and post-herpetic neuralgia and scar pain.

Painful polyneuropathies are usually symmetrical and distal, affecting the feet and sometimes the hands, including diabetic and ischaemic neuropathy. These conditions may present with or without paraesthesia, hypoaesthesia, hyperalgesia (excessive pain with noxious stimulus) and allodynia (touch is perceived as pain).

The mechanism of neuropathic pain is different from that of nociceptive pain. Peripheral mechanisms involve abnormal C-fibre function, which can become sensitised to sympathetic stimulation. Axon sprouts develop where primary afferent neurones have been damaged. These may show abnormal sensitivity to mechanical, noradrenergic and thermal stimulation, and may also fire independently of any sensory input. Adjacent neurones may develop abnormal connections, which may be recruited into the exaggerated response to stimuli. Central mechanisms involve changes in the long-term excitability of dorsal horn cells. These are mediated through the *N*-methyl-D-aspartate (NMDA) subtype of glutamate receptor, known as 'wind-up'. Damage to peripheral or central neurones can lead to loss of coordination of neuronal inhibitory processes. These processes are known as peripheral and central sensitisation.

Treatment of neuropathic pain is as follows:[5]

- tricyclic antidepressants are the drugs of first choice with most neuropathic pains. Commonly used examples are dothiepin, amitriptyline, doxepin, nortriptyline, imipramine (at daily doses of 25–75 mg) orally. Sedation is a problem, but lower doses are generally well tolerated;
- anticonvulsants, including gabapentin, lamotrigine, carbamazepine, phenytoin, pregabalin and clonazepam, are often effective second-line drugs. Sedation and ataxia may limit their use;
- sodium-channel blockers lidocaine (lignocaine) (intravenous and topical) and mexiletine (orally) can be effective;
- opioids (transdermal, oral, intrathecal) can be effective in some cases of neuropathic pain;
- capsaicin cream has been used on affected areas of skin, but its effectiveness is still uncertain;
- non-steroidals (oral and topical) have been effective in some studies, but not others;
- ketamine (intravenous and epidural) is effective, but its route of administration limits its use;
- clonidine (topical, oral, epidural) is also useful, but side-effects include sedation and hypotension;
- lumbar sympathectomy (chemical or radiofrequency) is often used to treat ischaemic leg pain, but it is unclear whether it works by improving blood flow or by reducing neuropathic pain;

- Electrical stimulation (spinal cord or peripheral nerve stimulation) has been used successfully for some forms of neuropathic pain.[6]

Post-herpetic neuralgia

Post-herpetic neuralgia is one of the more common forms of neuropathic pain seen in pain clinics. The herpes zoster virus causes an acute painful attack with skin lesions, that gradually resolve over several weeks. In a small percentage of cases chronic pain and associated numbness occur in the area of the scar. Clinical symptoms are pain, dysaesthesia, paraesthesia, allodynia, and paroxysms of lancinating pain. The most common sites are the cranial nerves and the thoracic dermatomes. Early recognition and prompt treatment with an antiviral agent can be effective in preventing the development of post-herpetic neuralgia. Treatment is as for other neuropathic pain. Response to treatment is unpredictable and a few patients will be left with severe intractable pain, especially the elderly.

Phantom pain

Phantom pain occurs following amputation of limbs, but has also been described following mastectomy and anterior–posterior bowel resection. The aetiology is unclear. Most patients experience transient phantom sensations following amputation, but only some patients experience phantoms as painful. Prophylactic treatment may be effective. Establishing epidural analgesia before amputation is claimed to diminish the incidence of phantom limb pain, but this remains unproven.[7] Other problems, such as painful neuroma and muscle spasms, can complicate the management of amputation pain. Treatment is as for other neuropathic pains.

Central (post-stroke) pain

Central (post-stroke) pain, also known as thalamic pain, occurs occasionally after a stroke, usually of the cerebral cortex. There may be an associated sensory deficit. There is usually a background steady pain and occasionally an intermittent or lancinating pain.[8]

Scar pain

Scar pain can occur after any operation, but is most common after thoracotomy, inguinal hernia repair and mastectomy. It is due to neuroma formation where nerves have regenerated in an abnormal manner.

Treatment is by local infiltration of the neuroma or the nerve supplying the area. If unsuccessful in the long term, cryoanalgesia or radiofrequency lesioning of the scar can be considered.

Complex regional pain syndromes

The term complex regional pain syndrome (CRPS) type I and type II is used to describe a syndrome of pain and sudomotor or vasomotor instability.

CRPS type I (reflex sympathetic dystrophy)

CRPS type I (reflex sympathetic dystrophy) is defined as a syndrome that usually starts after a noxious event, is not limited to the distribution of a single peripheral nerve, and is disproportionate to the inciting event. The diagnosis requires:

- pain, allodynia, or hyperalgesia disproportionate to the injury;
- evidence at some time of oedema, changes in skin blood flow, or abnormal sudomotor activity in the region of the pain;
- no other condition that would otherwise account for the degree of pain and dysfunction.

CRPS type II (causalgia)

CRPS type II (causalgia) is defined as a syndrome that starts after a nerve injury, and is not necessarily limited to the distribution of the injured nerve. The diagnostic criteria are the same as for CRPS I.

Difference from neuropathic pain

The difference between CRPS and neuropathic pain is that CRPS diagnosis requires evidence of oedema, cutaneous blood flow changes or abnormal sudomotor activity.

Treatment

Treatment of CRPS is as follows:

- medical therapies as for neuropathic pain (above);
- intravenous regional sympathetic blockade using guanethidine (10–20 mg) in prilocaine on three or more occasions. Although this is still commonly used, doubt has recently been cast on the effectiveness of this therapy;
- intravenous regional techniques using ketanserin, bretylium or ketorolac (30 mg) have been shown to be effective, but are probably not widely used;
- oral corticosteroids have been shown to be effective, but again are probably not widely used;
- TENS may be helpful;
- physiotherapy should be combined with pain-relieving treatments in an attempt to restore function. Specialist hand physiotherapists are worth seeking out here because the residual dysfunction can be significant. Hand rehabilitation may need to be prolonged;
- spinal cord stimulation is occasionally used for this condition;[9]
- sympathetic blocks (lumbar chemical or radiofrequency sympathectomy or cervical/thoracic sympathectomy via percutaneous

radiofrequency or diathermy using a transthoracic approach) have been used, but their effectiveness is as yet unproven.

Muscle and soft tissue pain

Fibromyalgia

Fibromyalgia is a chronic pain disorder characterised by diffuse musculoskeletal pain, stiffness, tenderness, fatigue and sleep disturbance. It occurs most commonly in women in the 20–40-year age group. Patients may describe their symptoms as total body pain, and the most striking feature on clinical examination is widespread muscle tenderness on palpation. Fibromyalgia is similar in presentation to chronic fatigue syndrome (ME), but in the latter, fatigue rather than pain is the predominant presenting symptom.

Treatment of fibromyalgia is as for many pain syndromes. Regular analgesia can be helpful. Low-dose tricyclic antidepressants can help restore sleep patterns, and in addition have analgesic properties. Pain management programmes may be helpful. Physiotherapy based on pacing physical activity is more likely to be successful than fitness programmes. Prognosis is generally guarded, although the natural history of this condition is not well described.[9]

Myofascial pain syndrome

Myofascial pain syndrome is a regional pain disorder characterised by a local area of deep muscle tenderness called a trigger point, and a reference zone of pain, which is worsened by palpation of the trigger point. Each muscle group has characteristic trigger points and pain patterns. The most common muscles groups seen in the pain clinic with identifiable myofascial pain patterns are quadratus lumborum, gluteals, quadriceps femoris, levator scapulae and trapezius.

Treatment is by avoidance of perpetuating factors such as repetitive muscle use, trigger point injection, and a technique called a 'spray and stretch', which involves stretching the affected muscle group. Prognosis is generally good.[10]

Pain of advanced cancer

Pain occurs in 70% of patients with advanced cancer. Problems related to advanced cancer are dealt with mostly by palliative care services, but there is often an overlap with pain clinics. Clinical features of cancer pain syndromes are as follows:

- bone metastases from lung, breast or prostate produce multiple pain sites, which are worse on movement;
- invasion of hollow viscus (stomach, colon) by tumour produces colicky abdominal pain, which is worse with eating and improved by vomiting;

- liver metastases from bowel, lung or breast produce upper quadrant abdominal pain and hepatomegaly;
- bladder spasm from bladder or prostate cancer produces colicky suprapubic pain. Infection or blood clots may need specific treatment;
- ureteric colic can occur with carcinoma of the ureter or bladder and will produce loin pain radiating to the groin;
- chest wall or rib pain occurs with carcinoma of the lung and mesothelioma;
- abdominal metastases occur with carcinoma of the ovary and colon, and result in diffuse abdominal pain and tenderness;
- neuropathic pain occurs when nerves are damaged by tumour, as occurs in Pancoast's syndrome or invasion of the sacral plexus;
- headache occurs when tumours result in raised intracranial pressure, and when cranial nerves are involved, such as trigeminal neuralgia associated with meningioma and acoustic neuroma;
- spinal cord involvement can result from spinal metastases and can result in radicular pain as well as progressive sensory and motor deficit and sphincter dysfunction;
- painful muscle spasm can result from bony metastases and following hemiplegia;
- infection of fungating tumours produces severe pain.

Treatment of pain of advanced cancer includes active treatments such as radiotherapy (which is especially effective for bony metastases), chemotherapy, hormone manipulation, orthopaedic correction of pathological fractures, surgical correction of bowel obstruction and neurosurgical decompression of cranium or spinal cord. Dexamethasone is commonly used to reduce painful tissue oedema.

World Health Organization analgesic ladder

Analgesic therapies are based on the World Health Organization (WHO) analgesic ladder, which involves a progression from a non-opioid analgesic such as paracetamol to weak opioid preparations such as codeine-paracetamol mixtures to strong opioid such as morphine.

When pain of advanced cancer is not adequately treated by active treatments (see above) or weak opioids the following options can be used:

- morphine, given orally as an elixir (which is fast acting but relatively short in duration), tablets (which are also fast acting), or slow-release tablets given either once or twice a day. Most patients manage on doses up to 200 mg/day, although some patients may require much higher doses. Oral diamorphine can be used as an alternative, but is not generally available outside the UK;

- methadone orally given 8–12-hourly and oxycodone can be a useful alternative when morphine becomes less effective (known as opioid rotation);
- fentanyl patches and buprenorphine patches with 72-hours' duration have become a popular alternative, especially when vomiting precludes the oral route;
- diamorphine given subcutaneously by syringe driver is a commonly used technique for patients with vomiting, dysphagia and coma. Antiemetics such as cyclizine are often added when vomiting is a problem, and midazolam can also be added to treat terminal anxiety and distress;
- co-analgesics are often added to augment opioids, and examples include non-steroidal anti-inflammatory drugs (NSAIDs), tricyclic antidepressants and other drugs used to treat neuropathic pain (see above);
- epidural catheter analgesia using bupivacaine plus diamorphine by continuous infusion can be used when oral opioid analgesia is unsuccessful. It can be used in the hospice as well as at home, but will require a large-volume (250 mL) portable pump and good coordination of staff;
- intrathecal catheter analgesia using diamorphine, clonidine and bupivacaine gives more widespread and better-quality analgesia than the epidural route. These can be tunnelled and externalised and connected to a portable pump; fully implantable systems are also available;
- other catheter techniques, such as interpleural, brachial and lumbar plexus infusions using bupivacaine, have been used.

Neurolytic techniques

A number of neurolytic techniques are in common practice for pain of advanced cancer.

Coeliac plexus block

Coeliac plexus block using alcohol or phenol is widely used for carcinoma of pancreas, but is also useful for pain emanating from stomach, liver and small intestine. The coeliac plexus transmits the majority of pain fibres from the upper abdomen via the splanchnic nerves and sympathetic trunks to T5–T12. The plexus lies anterior to the aorta at the level of T12/L1 vertebrae. It can be approached either posteriorly through the crura of the diaphragm or directly through the aorta, or anteriorly through the liver or stomach. The technique is usually done under X-ray fluoroscopy, but can be ultrasound or computed tomography (CT) guided. Side-effects include transient pain on injection, hypotension and diarrhoea.[11]

Splanchnic nerve block

Splanchnic nerve blocks using phenol or alcohol are performed above the diaphragm at T11/T12, and used for a similar indication as coeliac plexus blocks.

Chemical sympathectomy

Chemical sympathectomy, either lumbar of presacral, can be used for refractory lower limb or pelvic pain.

Cordotomy

Cordotomy done via radiofrequency of the spinothalamic tract at level of C2 vertebrae is used mostly for mesothelioma, which can be resistant to many other therapies.[12]

Intrathecal neurolysis

Intrathecal neurolysis using phenol or alcohol is an occasionally used technique for trunk pain. It carries the complication of sphincter and motor paralysis. Epidural neurolysis has also been described, but results are variable.

CHRONIC PAIN BY ANATOMICAL LOCATION

Headache

Migraine

Migraine is periodic unilateral headache. The pain is described as throbbing. Associated symptoms include nausea, vomiting and diarrhoea. Photophobia is common, as is a visual aura, which may precede the pain. Duration is usually about 4 hours, but can be longer. Occasionally focal neurological deficits occur. Treatment is to abort the current attack and to prevent the occurrence of migraine in the future.

Abortive therapies include:

- sumatriptan – a 5-hydroxytryptamine (5-HT_1) analogue, given parenterally; rizatriptan can be taken orally;
- high-dose aspirin, NSAIDs and antiemetics (metoclopramide) can also be effective;
- ergotamine was the drug of first choice in the past, but is contraindicated in coronary and cerebrovascular disease;
- nerve blocks, including sphenopalatine ganglion block, have been used to terminate an attack.

Prophylactic treatment includes:

- avoidance of trigger factors (alcohol, stress, sleep disturbance, certain drugs);

- pizotifen – a 5-HT and histamine antagonist;
- β-adrenergic antagonists – e.g. propranolol and metoprolol;
- calcium-channel antagonist – e.g. verapamil;
- serial sphenopalatine ganglion blocks have been described.

Cervicogenic headache

Cervicogenic headache is predominantly unilateral, often with neck and arm pain. There are signs of cervical spondylosis with pain on movement and a limited range of movement. Pain typically starts at the back of the head, but may also involve the face, whereas migraine mostly starts at the front of the head, often centred behind the eye. There is a close anatomical relationship between upper cervical neurones and the trigeminal spinal nucleus. When the C2 nerve root is involved the headache is over the occiput and can be relieved by greater occipital nerve block. Injection of cervical facet joints can relieve pain in some circumstances and are diagnostic for radiofrequency cervical facet denervation.

Myofascial pain syndromes involving posterior cervical muscles groups and sternomastoid can present as headache and can respond to injection and stretching (see above, p. 825).

Face pain

Temporomandibular joint dysfunction

Temporomandibular joint dysfunction is a common chronic pain syndrome, more often seen in maxillofacial units It is characterised by pain arising from the joints with joint noises and trismus. The pain radiates widely to the temporal, mastoid and occipital areas as well as the neck. The pain arises from arthritic changes in the joint and muscle spasm. There will be palpable and audible clicking and limited jaw opening. Auriculotemporal nerve block may be diagnostic. Treatment options are:

- reassurance and simple analgesia, including NSAIDs;
- low-dose tricyclic antidepressants;
- local anaesthetic injections into the joint and associated muscle groups (masseter, temporalis and lateral pterygoid) – to relieve muscle spasm;
- psychological therapies, including biofeedback – have been used to teach muscle relaxation;
- botulinum toxin has been injected in small doses into the affected muscle groups – this remains unproven;
- occasionally arthroscopy and surgery – this is reserved for severe, refractory cases.

Facial neuralgias

Facial neuralgias involve the trigeminal, glossopharyngeal and superior laryngeal nerves. The following are examples:

- mental nerve compression in the bony canal of the mandible can occur in Paget's disease, and may require surgical decompression. In elderly edentulous patients the nerve can become exposed as the mandible resorbs and may need to be repositioned;
- following tooth extraction, particularly third molar extraction, the mandibular nerve can be traumatised, resulting in peripheral neuropathic pain (see above). Mandibular nerve blocks may be helpful temporarily and may lead on to cryotherapy of the affected nerve;
- post-herpetic neuralgia can occur in the various divisions of the trigeminal nerve and can represent a great therapeutic challenge (see below);
- intracranial neuralgias can result from lesions such as meningioma and acoustic neuroma that involve the cranial nerves as they exit the skull.

Atypical face pain

Atypical face pain is a common presentation in pain clinics. It is important that a thorough diagnostic work-up is performed to exclude oral and maxillofacial pathology. Investigations may include an orthopantogram and facial and maxillary CT imaging. Atypical face pain is continuous chronic face pain that occurs in the absence of demonstrable pathology. The aetiology is unknown. Treatment options are:

- low-dose tricyclic antidepressants – dothiepin 25–75 mg orally at night;
- low-dose phenothiazines, trifluoperazine, can be added to the tricyclics;
- TENS can be useful;
- acupuncture is used for this condition;
- the value of psychological therapies is unknown.

Temporal arteritis

Temporal arteritis is an important condition to recognise. It can present as acute temporal pain, often with a tender inflamed temporal artery. Diagnosis is usually made by a high erythrocyte sedimentation rate (ESR). It is important to recognise and treat this condition promptly with high-dose corticosteroids (prednisolone up to 60 mg/day), because delay can result in involvement of the ophthalmic artery and blindness.

Trigeminal neuralgia

Trigeminal neuralgia is not a specific disease but a symptom, often caused by pathology involving the fifth cranial nerve. A loop of artery has been observed to impinge upon the nerve and surgical reposition of the artery can alleviate symptoms. The causative link, however, remains speculative. Trigeminal neuralgia can also occur in multiple sclerosis, aneurysm, and with cerebellopontine angle tumours (acoustic neuroma, meningioma). Most cases remain idiopathic.

Clinical features

Clinical features of trigeminal neuralgia are as follows:

- episodic recurrent unilateral face pain described as a sudden high-intensity jab or electric shock;
- duration is just a few seconds, with repetitive bursts over minutes. Frequent episodes may occur over several weeks, followed by prolonged pain-free intervals;
- occurs in the mandibular and maxillary divisions of the trigeminal nerve; ophthalmic pain is less common;
- pain is triggered by stimulation of face, lips or mouth, and patients will avoid stimulation;
- cranial nerve examination is usually normal. If a trigeminal neurological deficit is found, magnetic resonance imaging (MRI) is indicated to exclude underlying pathology.

Treatment options

Treatment options for trigeminal neuralgia are as follows:

- carbamazepine up to 1000 mg/day. Most cases will respond to this therapy alone. Side-effects are sedation and ataxia, which may limit its use in the elderly. Bone marrow suppression and liver and renal impairment occur with prolonged therapy and will require monitoring;
- second-line drug therapy includes phenytoin, baclofen, clonazepam and oxcarbazepine;
- radiofrequency trigeminal ganglion thermocoagulation is performed in many pain clinics. It involves placing an insulated needle through the foramen ovale under fluoroscopy. Placement is assessed by stimulation down the needle, using both motor (muscles of mastication) and sensory testing. When the correct dermatome is located a radiofrequency heat lesion (75°C for 60 seconds) is performed in the trigeminal ganglion. Some numbness will occur in the face, but this is usually self-limiting. This is probably the technique of choice when medical therapy fails;[13]
- injection of glycerol into the trigeminal ganglion is also used, but less commonly than thermocoagulation;
- cryotherapy of the peripheral branches of the trigeminal nerve, especially mental and infraorbital nerves, is commonly performed in

maxillofacial units. This is a useful short-term procedure, but repeated freezing becomes difficult because of scarring;

- microvascular decompression is a neurosurgical technique that is recommended in younger patients. It does have a mortality and morbidity rate, which are generally not seen with the percutaneous techniques, but long-term results may be better.

Neck pain

Whiplash injury

Whiplash injury is common and occurs after deceleration injury to the cervical spine. Most whiplash injuries settle spontaneously within 3 months regardless of treatment. Those that persist beyond 3 months tend to become chronic. Pre-existing neck problems, including spondylosis, and speed of impact contribute to chronicity.

Structures involved in whiplash injuries are the cervical facet (zygapophyseal) joints and the intervertebral discs. The pain is predominantly unilateral as rotation of the spine to either side often occurs during injury. There may also be marked muscle spasm secondary to facet joint injury.

Patients may also complain of headaches, arm pain and numbness, especially in the medial fingers, reflecting trauma to the nerves that contribute to the ulnar nerve where they cross the first rib.

Treatment options

The following are treatment options for whiplash injury:

- regular analgesia and TENS;
- radiofrequency cervical facet denervation of the affected facet joints. This is done percutaneously under fluoroscopy and involves thermocoagulation of the posterior ramus of the cervical nerves, usually C3–C5. The levels may need to be determined by selective diagnostic facet joint blocks;
- physiotherapy and muscle stretching may be needed following cervical facet denervation.[14]

Cervical radiculopathy

Cervical radiculopathy can occur with cervical disc prolapse or due to cervical spondylosis, often precipitated by minor trauma, if the intervertebral foramen is already narrowed by osteophytes. The pain is typically dermatomal and neuropathic, and often described as burning or lancinating. Treatment options are as follows:

- cervical epidural or nerve root injections via the intervertebral foramen;
- radiofrequency partial dorsal root ganglion rhizolysis via the foramen. This will require repeated diagnostic nerve blocks to determine the correct level;

- surgical decompression is occasionally required, but this is done infrequently.[15]

Thoracic pain

Costochondritis

Costochondritis presents as pain in the anterior chest wall. Involved sites are tender to palpation without inflammation. It is a benign, usually self-limiting disorder that may respond to simple analgesia, but may require infiltration of tender points with local anaesthetic and corticosteroid or repeated cryoanalgesia.

Osteoporotic crush fractures

Osteoporotic crush fractures commonly present to pain clinics. Osteoporosis alone tends not to be painful, but spontaneous crush fractures of the thoracic vertebrae occur with advanced osteoporosis. It usually occurs in elderly women or in those on prolonged corticosteroid therapy. There is a sudden onset of thoracic back pain, often with unilateral thoracic root pain.

The diagnosis is confirmed by plain radiograph. Recent fractures are 'hot' on bone scan and STIR sequence on MRI. It is important to exclude malignancy (myeloma) as a possible cause.

Prophylactic treatment (bisphosphonates, oral calcium) is aimed at preventing the progression of the disease, but can also improve pain associated with the crush fracture. The pain tends to diminish spontaneously over several months, but can be severe.

Treatment consists or oral analgesia, TENS, thoracic epidural injection at the level of the fracture and nerve root injection for root pain. More recently the percutaneous technique of vertebroplasty has been introduced. This involves placing a needle into the compressed vertebral body. Small volumes (1–4 mL) of bone cement are injected under fluoroscopy. Initial results look promising.[17]

Postmastectomy and post-thoracotomy pain

Postmastectomy and post-thoracotomy pain is common after surgery, although the frequency may be relatively underappreciated by surgeons. These are neuropathic pains and the treatment is described above (see p. 822).

Abdominal pain

Abdominal wall pain

Abdominal wall pain is characterised by local tender points in the abdominal wall, particularly in the rectus abdominis muscle. Carnett's sign is elicited by asking the patient to tense the abdominal wall by lifting the legs off the couch or to attempt to sit from the supine position. Aggravation of pain confirms the muscle as the site of pain. Exclusion of other causes of abdominal pain is essential, the diagnosis being one of exclusion.

Treatment is by repeated injection of tender points with local anaesthetic and corticosteroid or cryoanalgesia.

A common variation of this is pain after inguinal hernia repair, which usually responds to a series of injections around the ilioinguinal and iliohypogastric nerves. Cryoanalgesia may also be useful here.

Pelvic pain

Pelvic pain can be caused by a variety of gynaecological, urological and gastroenterological diseases, but referral to pain clinics will be for pelvic pain of unknown aetiology, following extensive investigation, medical treatment and previous surgery. Initial treatment should be simple regular analgesia, tricyclic antidepressants at low dose and psychological therapies (see below, p. 838). Some nerve blocks may be useful, including sacral nerve blocks and presacral sympathectomy.[16]

Back pain and sciatica

Mechanical back pain

Mechanical back pain is endemic in our society, and is perhaps best viewed as a design fault rather than a disease. Peak incidence is at age 45–55 years and the most common abnormality is degenerative disc disease and facet osteoarthritis, although these changes are found widely in this age group. The pain is typically worse on movement and better with rest, and may interfere with employment at a time when return to work may become difficult.

There is a substantial disability due to back pain, which has grown in recent years, partly related to changes in benefits and a propensity for litigation.

Initial assessment is based on history and examination. Routine radiographs of the spine provide relatively little useful information, and CT and MRI scans are probably best reserved for those being considered for spinal surgery or for those with 'red flags' (new onset, >55 years old, trauma, non-mechanical pain, systemically unwell).

Anatomy

Back pain emanates from four possible sites in the spine:

- lumbar facet joints are thought to account for about 30% of back pain, increasing with age. These joints may be injured by violent rotation of the spine, such as a sporting injury or trauma. The pain is often one-sided and aggravated by extension and rotation of the spine. Diagnostic facet joint injections with local anaesthetic can provide useful information;

- muscle pain is a common cause of back pain. Muscle groups may be painful to palpation and muscle spasm may be visible on examination. The most commonly affected muscles are quadratus lumborum and the gluteals;
- lumbar discs can be painful. Disc degeneration is commonly seen in radiographs and MRI scans of patients with back pain. Provocative discography involves injecting individual discs in an attempt to reproduce pain, but the validity of this has been questioned. Small tears can occur in the annulus of lumbar discs. These are observed as high-intensity zones on T_2-weighted MRI scans. These are thought to account for some back pain and also for leg pain if the tear is adjacent to a lumbar nerve root;
- spinal nerve roots can produce leg pain when trapped by a prolapsed intervertebral disc. If the L5 or S1 nerve roots are affected the patient experiences posterior leg pain to the foot, known as sciatica. The ankle jerk may be diminished in S1 entrapment. L3 and L4 entrapment results in anterior thigh pain. A diminished knee jerk is indicative of an L4 lesion. Spinal stenosis occurs as part of the ageing process and, combined with disc degeneration, can produce critical narrowing of the spinal canal. In the elderly this will present as unilateral leg pain with claudication. There is usually an absence of neurological signs in the leg.

Treatment options

Treatment options for back pain include the following:

- simple regular analgesia;
- physiotherapy including hydrotherapy and exercise regimens can be helpful. Increasingly physiotherapy departments are creating structured outpatient programmes based on exercise, fitness and education. They may have input from occupational therapy and psychology to create a multidisciplinary team;
- TENS;
- facet joint treatment includes lumbar facet joint injections with local anaesthetic, and depot corticosteroids (methylprednisolone, triamcinolone) are widely used, but are unproven as long-term therapy.[18] Radiofrequency lumbar facet denervation involves thermocoagulation of the medial branch of the posterior ramus of L3–S1. Long-term outcomes appear to be reasonable;[19]
- muscle pain can be treated as for myofascial pain syndromes (see above, p. 825). Hydrotherapy can also be useful. Rehabilitation of the spine with an indwelling epidural catheter can also enable refractory muscle pain to settle;[20]

- lumbar disc pain is more difficult to treat successfully. Local anaesthetic injection into the disc can be helpful in the short term. Two intradiscal pain relief techniques have been developed. Intradiscal electrothermal therapy[21] (IDET) involves placing a heating coil in the nucleus of the disc. The second technique involves placement of a radiofrequency probe in the posterior annulus of the disc. Both techniques involve prolonged heating (10 minutes or more) of the disc in an attempt to inactivate nociceptors within the disc.[22] In theory, interruption of the sympathetic outflow at L2 should interfere with the pain pathways from the lumbar disc.[23] This can be achieved by dorsal root ganglion rhizotomy, but experience is limited. Spinal surgeons will consider spinal fusion for isolated disc degeneration, using either a bone graft or instrumented fusion. Long-term results are variable;
- nerve root compression by a prolapsed intervertebral disc is best treated initially by lumbar epidural. This treatment is generally considered effective, although agreement is not universal.[24] Epidural injections are usually done with local anaesthetic and depot corticosteroid (methylprednisolone, triamcinolone). The caudal approach is commonly performed by orthopaedic surgeons and rheumatologists, although the technical failure rate is probably high. Loss of resistance techniques enable closer access to the site of the lesions and perhaps allow lower volumes to be injected. Previous surgery will necessitate a transforaminal approach under fluoroscopy. Microdiscectomy is commonly performed for prolapsed intervertebral disc, but usually after failure of epidural techniques. Surgical decompression of spinal stenosis is sometimes performed for intractable spinal claudication.

Coccydynia

Coccydynia describes pain in the region of the coccyx, usually worse on sitting. It may follow a fall that results in a fracture of the coccyx, but there may also not be a history of trauma.

Treatment options

Treatment options available for coccydynia include the following:

- regular simple oral analgesia;
- rubber cushions – may help distribute weight from the coccyx;
- infiltration of the sacral nerve roots via the sacral hiatus with local anaesthetic and corticosteroid. This may need to be done on several occasions, and is generally successful;
- sacral cryoanalgesia around the coccyx and sacral nerve routes can be a useful long-term therapy in refractory cases;
- occasionally coccygectomy is attempted, but success is not guaranteed.

Postspinal surgery pain

Postspinal surgery pain (failed back syndrome) represents a great challenge for pain clinicians. The incidence of persistent pain following spinal surgery is probably in the region of 30–40%. The cause is unclear. There is not always a good link between observed spinal pathology and the patient's symptoms. Advances in MRI scanning have led to an 'explosion of the false positive' because up to 70% of the normal asymptomatic population have lumbar disc bulges without symptoms.

Patients present as having either persistent back pain or leg pain as the predominant complaint, although the two often coexist.

Scarring has been demonstrated around nerve roots following spinal surgery. The nerve root can become tethered and any spinal movement can result in traction on the nerve. It is thought that complicated changes (known as peripheral and central sensitisation) occur within the central nervous system as a consequence of nerve injury, which results in chronic pain (see 'Neuropathic pain' above, p. 821). There may be some residual compression of the nerve roots not adequately relieved by surgery. Facet joint disruption can occur and may lead to persistent back pain, with secondary arthritic changes. Paraspinal muscle atrophy can occur if the posterior ramus has been injured as part of the disease process or as a consequence of surgery. This leads to loss of functional support of the spine and mechanical stresses on other structures.

Treatment options

Treatment options for failed back syndrome are as follows:

- simple regular analgesia;
- if leg pain is predominant it is worth treating as neuropathic pain, especially if a neurological deficit is present (see above, p. 821);
- nerve root blocks of the affected level can be achieved by directing a needle through the intervertebral foramen. Injection of local anaesthetic and corticosteroid around the nerve root can provide useful symptomatic relief;
- lumbar facet denervation has been used successfully for persistent low back pain;[19]
- physical reactivation through a graded exercise regimen can be used alone or to follow on from injection therapy. This is best done within a multidisciplinary setting with input from physiotherapy, occupational therapy and clinical psychology. An epidural catheter may allow physical rehabilitation to occur when pain is limiting;[25]
- pain management programmes based on cognitive–behavioural therapy can be useful ways to enable patients to better manage their symptoms and disability (see below);

- implanted pain-relieving devices, such as spinal cord stimulation and implanted intrathecal pumps, can be considered in patients whose pain and disability is not relieved by noninvasive techniques.

PSYCHOLOGICAL THERAPIES AND PAIN MANAGEMENT PROGRAMMES

Psychological therapies

Psychological therapies have much to offer chronic pain patients. The best place for them is uncertain. Some clinicians prefer patients to be exposed to a psychological approach from the start, whereas others prefer to finish appropriate drug therapy, injection therapy, physiotherapy and possibly surgery first.

Psychological therapies can be either on an individual basis or as part of a group programme. A number of conditions may be worth treating with psychological therapies alone – examples include fibromyalgia and irritable bowel syndrome.

Psychological therapies include the following:

- operant conditioning works by removing secondary gain that may be obtained by maintaining pain behaviour. Gain can be positive, such as getting attention or permission to rest, or negative as when pain allows avoidance of unpleasant situations. The technique works by eliminating reward for pain behaviour and reinforcing well behaviour;
- behavioural therapy involves manipulating the environment by taking analgesia on a time-determined basis, physical pacing, social feedback based on achievement not pain, education about the nature of pain and relaxation training;
- cognitive therapy involves changing negative thoughts to more positive ones, coping skills training by stress management, relaxation and imagery, and improving problem-solving skills;
- biofeedback is the use of increased awareness of physiological changes (heart rate, muscle tension) to enhance the learning of relaxation techniques. This may be particularly helpful for patients with increased muscle tension;
- hypnosis can be particularly helpful for pain. It involves relaxation, substitution of another sensory modality that is more acceptable (warmth), displacement of perceived site pain to a more peripheral body part and dissociation to a more pleasant location (e.g. a sunny day at the beach).

Pain management programmes

Pain management programmes have become increasingly well established in pain clinics. They are run by multidisciplinary teams involving clinical psychologists, physiotherapists and occupational therapists.

General principles involve physical reactivation based on physical pacing, rationalisation of drug consumption, teaching goal setting, improving coping strategies, education, and reducing illness behaviour. Programmes are either inpatient or outpatient and are run on a group basis over several weeks. They are not designed to treat pain directly, but help patients to manage their symptoms better. Many patients come to terms with their chronic pain and decide to stop being patients by no longer seeking medical assistance.[26]

References

1. Davies HTO, Crombie IK, Brown JH, Martin C. Diminishing returns or appropriate treatment strategy? – an analysis of short-term outcomes after pain clinic treatment. Pain 1997; 70:203–208.
2. Flor H, Fydrich T, Turk DC. Efficacy of multidisciplinary pain treatment centers: a meta-analytic review Pain 1992; 49:221–230.
3. Kingery WS. A critical review of controlled clinical trials of peripheral neuropathic pain and complex regional pain syndromes. Pain 1997; 73:123–39.
4. North RB, Ewend MB, Lawton MT, Piantadosi S. Spinal cord stimulation for chronic, intractable pain: Superiority of "multi-channel" devices. Pain 1991; 44: 119–130.
5. Bach S, Noreng MF, Tjéllden NU. Phantom limb pain in amputees during the first 12 months following limb amputation, after preoperative lumbar epidural blockade. Pain 1988; 33:297–301.
6. Andersen G, Vestergaard K, Ingeman-Nielsen M, Jensen TS. Incidence of central post-stroke pain. Pain 1995; 61:1:87–193.
7. Nagaro T, Amakawa K, Yamauchi Y, Tabo E, Kimura S, Arai T. Percutaneous cervical cordotomy and subarachnoid phenol block using fluoroscopy in pain control of costopleural syndrome. Pain 1994; 58:325–30.
8. Barnsley L, Lord S, Bogduk N. Whiplash injury. Pain 1994; 58:283–307.
9. Wallis BJ, Lord SM, Bogduk N. Resolution of psychological distress of whiplash patients following treatment by radiofrequency neurotomy: a randomised, double-blind, plaecbo-controlled trial. Pain 1997; 73:15–22.
10. Castagnera L, Maurette P, Pointillart V, Vital JM, Erny P, Sénégas J. Long-term results of cervical epidural steroid injection with and without morphine in chronic cervical radicular pain. Pain 1994; 58: 239–43.
11. Wesselmann U, Burnett AL, Heinberg LJ. The urogenital and rectal pain syndromes. Pain 1997; 73:269–94.

12. North RB, Han M, Zahurak M, Kidd DH. Radiofrequency lumbar facet denervation: analysis of prognostic factors. Pain 1994; 57:77–83.
13. Koes BW, Scholten RJPM, Mens JMA, Bouter LM. Efficacy of epidural steroid injections for low-back pain and sciatica: a systematic review of randomized clinical trials. Pain 1995; 63:279–88.
14. Williams AC deC, Richardson PH, Nicholas MK, Pither CE, Harding VR, Ridout KL, Ralphs JA, Richardson IH, Justins DM, Chamberlain JH. Inpatient vs. outpatient pain management: results of a randomised controlled trial. Pain 1996; 66:13–22.
15. Griffiths DPG, Noon JM, Campbell FA, Price CM. Clinical governance and chronic pain: towards a practical solution. Anaesthesia 2003; 58:243–248.
16. Dolin, SJ, Stephens JP. Pain clinics and liaison psychiatry. Anaesthesia 1998; 53:317–319.
17. McQuay H, Moore A. An evidence based resource for pain relief. Oxford: Oxford University Press, 1998.
18. Wolfe F. Fibromyalgia: the clinical syndrome. Rheumatic diseases clinics of North America 1989; 15:1–29.
19. Travell J. Simons DG, Cummings B. Myofascial Pain and Dysfunction: The Trigger Point Manual. Baltimore: Lippincott Williams & Wilkins, 1983.
20. Schug SA, Burrel R, Payne J, Tester P. Pre-emptive epidural analgesia may prevent phantom limb pain. Regl Anesth 1995; 20:256.
21. Eisenberg E, Carr DB, Chalmers TC. Neurolytic celiac plexus block for treatment of cancer pain: a meta-analysis. Anesth Analg 1995; 80:290–295.
22. Sweet W, Wespic. Controlled thromcoagulation of trigeminal ganglion and rootlets for differential destruction of pain fibers. J Neurosurg 1981; 36:1129–1131.
23. Lord SM, Barnsley L, Wallis BJ, McDonald GJ, Bogduk N. Percutaneous Radio-Frequency Neurotomy for Chronic Cervical Zygapophyseal-Joint Pain. New Engl J Med 1996; 335:1721–1726.
24. Carette S, Marcoux S, Truchon R, Grondin C, Gagnon J, Allard Y, Latulippe M. A controlled trial of corticosteroid injections into facet joints for chronic low bak pain. New England Journal of Medicine 1991; 325:1002–1007.
25. Diamond TH, Champion B, Clark WA. Management of acute osteoporotic vertebral fractures: a non-randomized trial comparing percutaneous vertebroplasty with conservative therapy. Am J Med 2003; 114:257–65.
26. Vervest ACM, Stolker RJ. The treatment of cervical pain syndromes with radiofrequency procedures. The Pain Clinic 1991; 4:103–112.
27. Gallagher J, Petriccione di Vadi PL, Wedley JR, Hamann W, Ryan P, Chikanza I, Kirkham B, Price R, Watson MS, Grahame R, Wood S. Radiofrequency facet joint denervation in the treatment of low back pain: a prospective controlled double-blind study to assess its efficacy. The Pain Clinic 1994; 7:193–198.
28. Karasek M Bogduk N. Twelve-Month Follow-Up of a Controlled Trial of Intradiscal Thermal Anuloplasty for Back Pain Due to Internal Disc Disruption. Spine 2000; 25:2601–2607.

29. Saal JA, Saal JS. Intradiscal Electrothermal Treatment for Chronic Discogenic Low Back Pain: A Prospective Outcome Study with Minimum 1-Year Follow-Up. Spine 2000; 25:2622–2627.
30. Lippitt A. The facet joint and its role in spine pain. Management with facet joint injections. Spine 1984; 9:746–750.
31. Nakamura SI, Takahashi K, Takahashi Y, Yamagata M, Moriya H. The afferent pathways of discogenic low-back pain. Evaluation of L2 spinal nerve infiltration J Bone Joint Surg 1996; 78B:606–612.
32. Dolin SJ, BaconRA, Drage M. Rehabilitation of chronic low back pain using continuous epidural analgesia. Disability and rehabilitation 1998; 20:151–157.

Further reading

Dolin S, Padfield N. Pain medicine manual. Oxford: Butterworth–Heinemann; 2004.

McQuay H, Moore A. An evidence based resource for pain relief. Oxford: Oxford University Press; 1998.

Wall PD, Melzack R. Textbook of pain. 3rd edn. Edinburgh: Churchill Livingstone; 1994.

World Health Organization. Cancer pain relief and palliative care: report of a WHO expert committee. Geneva: WHO; 1990.

Section 7

Training and standards in anaesthesia

CHAPTER **7.1**

TRAINING AND STANDARDS IN ANAESTHESIA

Maintenance of patient safety is the prime responsibility of all clinical staff[1] and this can be interpreted as meaning that all care should be delivered only by established experts. This is clearly a utopian concept, but remains central to most health care delivery systems. Expertise itself is a volatile entity, and can only be maintained by practice and the continuous learning and reassessment of skills. The more expert one becomes the more comprehensively other experience and skills attenuate. Imagine asking a paediatric cardiac anaesthetist to manage an adult day-case operating list, for example. With this expectation comes a dual responsibility. Practitioners are personally responsible for ensuring that they are up-to-date, and their senior colleagues have the final responsibility for ensuring that this is indeed the case.

TRAINING IN ANAESTHESIA

One of the means to achieve these ends lies in the training of doctors throughout their careers, and the assessment that this has actually resulted in learning. For this reason, the duties of a doctor include the teaching of other clinical staff,[2] and increasingly their assessment and appraisal. This process requires a clear understanding of what to teach, how to do so effectively, how to identify the outcomes from that teaching, and what to do if there are problems with such learning. The details of this process vary across countries in some respects, but the fundamentals are transferable.

Background

The specialties of anaesthesia, pain management and critical care require a comprehensive understanding of basic science to underpin the clinical care of patients. This science changes, often rapidly, over the years. Equally, the concepts behind clinical care and the therapeutic agents available change almost as rapidly. The sheer volume of information being generated is beyond anyone's ability to read, let alone digest. This has led to a dependence, sometimes reluctant, on information technology and the internet. The effectiveness of this varies with individuals and also from time to time.

The standards to which training has to aspire, and against which assessment is judged, are usually determined by national organisations (e.g. colleges, boards or faculties). The standards they set are also national and are tested by a system of examinations and clinical assessments that confirm that a particular doctor has achieved the appropriate level to be allowed to practise without supervision.

The training for anaesthesia begins on the very first day of medical school and extends until retirement from clinical practice. The skills, knowledge and attitudes that develop over this time vary, and assessments of competence that are appropriate for a trainee are inadequate when applied to an expert practitioner.

Who should teach?

Not all clinicians are good teachers in tutorials or lectures, and although training can improve their performance, for some it is impossible. Others excel in this arena, but are less able in a one-to-one setting. Good teachers realise that they are doing more than imparting knowledge. They are role models for behaviour and attitudes. Professionalism, enthusiasm, integrity and compassion are all remembered and imitated by the trainees. One high-quality teacher may inspire generations of trainees to take that career choice. The reverse is, sadly, equally true.

Qualities of a good trainer (and trainee) include:

- enthusiasm;
- knowledge;
- self-directed learning skills;
- good communication skills;
- clinical expertise;
- mutual respect for trainees, colleagues and patients;
- good sense of humour;
- modesty;
- flexibility;
- honesty.

Undergraduate training

Undergraduate training varies across medical schools and countries, but in the UK the curriculum has moved from a problem-based system to one led more by clinical cases. The drive remains to develop the students' ability to assess a problem and use available materials to resolve the scientific or clinical aspects, but more direct tutoring and directed learning allows a focus on important issues within limited contact time.

The current timescale from entry to graduation is 5 years, although this is being reduced for mature entrants to 3 or 4 years. There is usually a preclinical period and then 3 years of clinical training. Amalgamation of nursing and medical training for the early years and specialisation in the latter ones have been proposed, but are still untested on a wide scale. The duration of dedicated training in anaesthesia and critical care is usually between 2 and 8 weeks in the final 2 years of medical school. This is not the only possible exposure to anaesthetists as undergraduate teachers.

Preclinical teaching

The use of clinical staff with expertise in cardiorespiratory physiology has provided anaesthetists with an opportunity to be at the forefront of early medical training. Their theoretical understanding can be underpinned with clinical cases to give the student an appropriate context that will enhance recall once on the wards. Later opportunities arise in neurological, resuscitation and locomotor modules. The pure scientists remain indispensable because there is always a need for precise, contemporary advice on complex issues that may often be beyond clinicians.

The early clinical years

The basic training in clinical skills becomes more intensive once the students arrive in a clinical area, whether general practice or hospital. The use of part task or integrated simulators to establish and assess the acquisition of these clinical skills before using them on patients is rapidly being seen as the only ethical method of instruction. Venous access and simple examination have been taught this way for years, but the diagnosis of medical emergencies, fluid therapy and working as part of a team are all now taught on low-fidelity simulators. At another level, the assessment and treatment of acute pain should be one of the core skills of all doctors. Pain teams often deliver this training.

Later clinical training

Critical care and anaesthesia provide the environment for learning how to manage acutely ill patients. This has been incorporated into the final years as a medical student and the first 2 years following qualification. Advanced airway and vascular access skills are frequently taught, but effective and concurrent diagnosis and treatment is also a well-established training element.

Postgraduate training

Background

In the UK it takes 7 years to completely train a specialist anaesthetist. This is currently the longest training in the world. There are pressures to reduce this to 5 years or less, but dilution of experience because of shift working and reduced clinical time militate against this. The UK training is competency based and defines the core skills, knowledge and attitudes necessary for satisfactory progress through the training grades. The competency training guide is reviewed frequently and amended in line with changes in clinical practice. Competency-based training cannot be related to a set timescale for training, and the current duration of training will be too short for some trainees and too long for others.

It is possible to identify the ability of trainees to acquire knowledge by testing with short answers and MCQ papers within months of starting anaesthesia, but it takes time for a consistent exposure to clinical areas and skills, which is essential to even out training opportunities across groups of trainees. Only when this has happened, about 18 months in the UK, can a national assessment be made, which is often by formal examination, such as the primary fellowship examination. Concurrent assessment in the workplace ensures that all competencies have been developed before further, more advanced training takes place. This may become a simple progression, without interviews, towards specialist accreditation. A further assessment against national standards is made before the trainee can move on to higher or more specialised training.

Theoretical aspects

Postgraduate trainees are thought of as adult learners and to have matured from the directed to the self-directing models of education. This is simplistic, because a trainee may mature well in one area of learning and yet be poorly developed in others. They may have a motor inability (e.g. unable to perform high-dexterity tasks such as epidural placement, or an attitudinal one where their approach to complex stressful situations is to become aggressive and obstructive). Others function very well when given a task to perform, yet fail if they are expected to identify that such a task is necessary. These aspects evolve over different timescales and there is no evidence that the length of time it takes to become competent predicts long-term performance.

We have therefore to try to define what we expect the final product to be able to do (i.e. set standards for practice, and then match performance to those targets). The standard of a competent practitioner is usually obvious to an observer, but often defies description when one attempts to create a task list that covers the competency. Several descriptive schemes have been devised to help – learning, competent, skilled, master is one such scheme.

Postgraduate training then develops into several complementary activities:

- theoretical teaching;
- practical skills acquisition;
- development of non-anaesthetic skills;[3]
- assessment of progress.

The context in which learning takes place and the 'state' of the learner both have a profound influence on recall of that learning. Context here means the environment where the training takes place. Clearly if we work in an operating theatre the best place to learn the skills is in theatre. Recall is then better than if the learning had occurred at home. Remembering is also more efficient if the learner is in the same state as they were when actively learning.

Teaching in clinical areas has many advantages and an equal number of potential problems. The operating theatre, intensive care unit and more remote sites such as the emergency department or radiology suite are where most trainees will be learning and practising. They will therefore provide the most appropriate context for learning clinical and applied scientific skills. They also allow the teacher to act as role model for professional and attitudinal development.

The topic to be discussed needs to be clear and ideally agreed before the list starts. The use of the patients to provide examples of how basic science is applied or how clinical conditions can be managed embeds the knowledge clearly.

There are obvious concerns with teaching in clinical areas as follows.

The patient's care

There is usually a patient to look after who requires the same standard of care as if no teaching was taking place. Who has responsibility for the care of the patient should be clarified before teaching, and explicit thresholds for stopping or handing over care need to be identified. This is important because trainees (and other staff, such as surgeons and radiologists) need to understand that despite the apparent distraction of teaching, due care is being delivered to the patient.

Team dynamics

The majority of anaesthetic activity is within one team or another, usually leading it or helping direct it. These skills have to be learnt by most people and errors will occur during the early stages of this process. Providing a good role model is essential, and, where effective, it will be mimicked by the trainees. This core skill is often easily overlooked when you have worked within the team for many years and the initial integration process has been forgotten. Dealing with stressed surgeons or nursing staff is essential, especially when making judgements within emergency lists.

Sadly, some staff are very dependent on a small number of colleagues and become overly intrusive in the anaesthetic management when someone else takes the case. This may be the surgeon, who then tries to control both the operation and the anaesthetic, or who becomes aggressive or patronising. The role of the trainer can be difficult in this eventuality. In severe cases he or she may decide to abandon teaching other than to observe the interpersonal dynamics of the situation.

Leadership

The anaesthetic team has only one leader, and usually all information regarding the patient, changes in surgical procedure, estimation of blood loss etc. goes to that person. If the trainee is delivering the care for a specific case confusion can occur and mistakes have happened. Introducing this difficulty to the team, for example 'Alex is going to be managing this patient's anaesthetic', ensures that simple but essential information arrives with the responsible anaesthetist rather than the most senior one.

Access to monitoring

The areas around many operating theatre tables or intensive care beds are crowded. Having one or more people in the area can obscure the view of the patient and their monitors. A determined control of the space, for example 'I need to see the patient and those monitors, so sit over there', may be necessary. Other tasks, such as record taking and drug prescription, should also be retained by the trainer, and teaching delivered during natural gaps in the recording process.

Development of non-anaesthetic skills

Non-anaesthetic skills are skills that are not primarily part of the necessary clinical skills but which are essential to the safe care of patients. They include situation awareness, decision making, task management and team working:

- situation awareness incorporates information gathering and assimilation from which a prediction can be made that can alter subsequent actions;
- decisions are made in differing ways from person to person: some mentally weigh the risks whereas others act intuitively. The latter often occurs only after many years of experience and reflection. Simply doing large numbers of cases without review does not lead to this;
- task management is the balance between knowing what to do and being able to do it. Information is necessary, as is an understanding of the resources available to complete the job, for example caring for an elderly patient with a fractured hip as an emergency;
- finally, team working is the ability to complete a task effectively as part of a team, irrespective of the role played in that team.

Practical aspects of assessment

There are several important elements in the practicality of training. These include the assessment of training, both formative and summative. Appraisal, record keeping (important for medicolegal reasons) and revalidation are all equally important for the established practitioner as well as the trainee.

Formative assessment describes the ongoing feedback of performance as part of a training scheme. These assessments are relatively informal and are integral to the process by which learners can identify their strengths and also their weaknesses, leading to a more effective learning process.

Summative assessment on the other hand is a formal, often high-stakes, examination of aspects of practice that determines future training or even a career change.

Assessment in the workplace

The majority of assessment in the workplace takes place in the operating theatres or intensive care wards. This is because the acquisition of skills and behaviours is best observed in a clinical setting, although over time the use of simulators may also prove a suitable alternative.

The robustness of the process depends on several factors, but repeating the observation frequently, observing a wide range of clinical settings, and using several professionals to perform the observations make it more likely that an accurate assessment will be made.

The most robust assessment is that made by several professionals observing a range of activities over a significant period of time.

In current practice assessment takes place in the clinical setting or workplace, and as part of testing to a national standard in the national speciality examinations.

Assessments should be:

- fair;
- valid
- reliable;
- practical in real life;
- at an appropriate level;
- believable.

It is usually more effective to assess a whole task and decide on the outcome rather than trying to fragment the task into its components. Scoring tick boxes has two fundamental flaws – they do not describe the integration necessary to complete the task, and they are rarely effectively validated for reliability and reproducibility. However, when performance is poor, breaking the task into component parts may be useful as a way of identifying where the problem lies.

Workplace assessments are high-stakes events for the trainees, but even more so when needed for established specialists. They must therefore be appropriate to their purpose.

Specialist or expert performance may be difficult to assess because often the actions and outcomes are subtle and may be missed. It is easier to assess trainees at a basic level because their performance and responses are more clearly displayed.

Simulator-based assessment, whether part task, low-fidelity or more comprehensive high-fidelity simulators, are often used for the assessment of novice practitioners (e.g. in advanced cardiac support skills), but are of unproven value in assessing the performance of more expert practitioners.

Assessment of competency of a trainee

The basis of a competency-based training programme is that the competencies are testable in a practical and reliable manner in the clinical setting. The curriculum defines what they are, and often by when they should have been acquired. What is less clear is how to test for them in practice.

There are some simple guidelines for such assessments, and they should be:

- organised in advance;
- appropriate to the stage of training;
- clear as to their purpose;
- with an acceptable assessor;
- immediately followed by feedback on performance;
- accompanied by a written description of the aims and outcome.

The clinical experience necessary to achieve competence varies. Most learners take about 20 attempts at procedures to become competent, and until then supervision has to be 'immediate'. Further practice improves performance and it may take many more procedures to develop expertise. Assessment before this level of experience has been achieved is pointless and destructive for all involved. The keeping of a logbook should prevent this happening.

Poor performance

Unacceptable performance should be discussed immediately and a remedial course of action suggested. If this is in a key area relating to patient safety, a decision on the appropriate level of supervision has to be made, recorded and acted upon. Clinical governance and ethics allow no other course of action, especially if patient safety is potentially compromised.

National examinations

The role of national summative assessments is under review, but currently serves two purposes:

- the first is to test to a defined standard using valid, reliable and reproducible methodologies: criterion referencing. Those who succeed gain recognition of this and can then progress onwards through their higher training;

- the second function, which is still being developed, is to review the standard of a training scheme or school of anaesthesia. The proportion of candidates who pass reflects on the effectiveness of the local training. It is likely that this will have greater emphasis as training becomes seamless and only local peer referencing is possible, rather than the criterion-based assessment of a national examination.

Individual elements in the testing process have different functions and vary in the most appropriate time to be used:

- objective structured clinical examinations (OSCE) are reliable for testing during an early phase of training, medical school to the early anaesthetic years. They are less suitable for advanced training, where a debate on the higher levels of judgement and professionalism is not possible in such a structured process;
- MCQ examinations test knowledge, which underpins the ability to reach the higher domains of practice. They are best used as entry points to the other forms of examination, although they are still directly linked in the UK at present;
- oral or viva voce examinations have been criticised for their unreliability and poor reproducibility, but schemes that use previously selected topics that are mapped across a range of subjects with defined starter questions address some of these concerns. The ability to explore the higher domains of judgement, understanding and also communication skills remains within the ambit of oral examinations.

Centrally held examinations are expensive to organise, but this is balanced by a loss of reliability if they are franchised around the country, where each sitting is essentially a unique examination and therefore has an intrinsic unreliability.

Assessment of higher skills

Senior trainees and established practitioners cannot be assessed using a simple 'one-size-fits-all' approach because the experience and expertise become increasingly individual and finally leads to the ultimate expert – one who knows everything about almost nothing, and nothing about everything else. Assessment then becomes dependent on the observation of practice over many cases, for example a review of case notes, gathering the opinions of the rest of the team involved including management and surgeons, and possibly a review as part of a team in a high-fidelity simulation facility. The latter is problematic because most simulators insert a problem into a routine case, whereas the most realistic scenarios are of complex patients being managed uneventfully.

This sequence of assessments is currently used for all higher trainees (with the exception of the simulator). It is also being developed by the UK

General Medical Council (GMC) for its review of clinical practice, the Fitness to Practise panel. However, there is little evidence to support the validity or reliability of the assessment of experienced practitioners using medical simulators.

STANDARDS OF PRACTICE IN ANAESTHESIA

Appraisal

Appraisal is a confidential review of progress, expectations and plans for the future between two parties, one of whom is reviewing their progress over time, and the other usually has some control over the resources necessary to continue the former's development. Appraisal is not only an essential tool in training, but has now become established for all permanent clinical staff as well. Indeed, it may to become the cornerstone of revalidation in the UK.

The skills necessary to perform appraisal have to be learnt by most people. The preparation time for an appraisal takes at least twice as long as the appraisal. It should also include a post-appraisal review to confirm that the records of the process are accurate and agreed. It may take 2–3 hours per appraisal and can rarely be shortened. The appraisee has to spend even more time completing the documentation necessary for this event.

The GMC model of appraisal has a series of identified areas for review, which can be used for trainees as well. These include a review of the previous year's agreed aims and objectives, and then a discussion under the headings listed in Box 7.1.1.

Following the appraisal the agreed plan of activity for the next year is formulated and any necessary resources identified. This process remains confidential. The only exception is the simple information that an appraisal

Box 7.1.1

Suggested topics to be discussed at appraisal

Good medical practice
- Good medical care
- Maintaining good medical practice
- Working relationships with colleagues
- Relations with patients
- Teaching and training

Probity

Health

Management activity

Research

has taken place and its outcome was satisfactory. For the vast majority of trainees this document is also available to the assessment process (RITA, record of in-training assessment) and is used to plan their next year's training.

It is clear that if there is a failure either to take part in an appraisal or to make the expected progress, further action will be necessary. This may well fall outside the boundaries of confidentiality. For example, there may need to be a period of retraining, or repeated and focused training, or even advice to change specialty or career. There are robust appeal mechanisms in place for such events, which require that clear documentation of the assessment process should be available, with the evidence that supported the decision, but the appraisal documentation itself remains confidential.

There is more of a conflict of interest when permanent medical staff are appraised than for trainees. This is because the process is usually between a clinical manager and a clinician, so the employing hospital trust's imperatives are always going to be part of the agenda. This may result in the appraisal becoming a form of performance review. The ability to select from a range of appraisers may help with this concern, although having the attention of a senior member of the department may allow changes that would otherwise prove difficult (e.g. changes in job plans).

Part of the good medical practice and probity sections of appraisal rely on evidence of good practice. Where there is concern more detailed evidence will be sought. Often this is a review of a selection of case records or critical incidents. This often hinges on record keeping, one of the core skills in anaesthetic and critical care practice.

Record keeping

One of a doctor's key responsibilities in any clinical situation is to keep contemporary records of findings, treatments and outcomes. This is vital in anaesthesia and intensive care and in any critical incidents that may occur. It is considered an essential duty by the GMC and is of obvious medicolegal importance. Sadly, this aspect of training is often undervalued and happens by default.

Case and anaesthetic records should have the characteristics listed in Box 7.1.2.

Current paper records will be replaced by electronic systems (the timing of this change in the UK has been set by national policy, but it is still a few years from becoming reality). Electronic patient records (EPR) do have disadvantages as well as their clear advantages of accuracy and timeliness. Artefacts are common and usually clinically insignificant. The annotation of an electronic record whenever such artefacts are identified is time consuming and distracting. However, the ability to network such data will allow observation and assessment of the conduct of an anaesthetic in a way that is impossible at present.

Box 7.1.2 Requirements for case records and anaesthetic records

Contemporary

Correct time and date

Accurate

Clarity and a logical approach

Readable

Concise

Details of:
- History
- Clinical findings
- Diagnosis
- Investigations
- Specific therapies ordered
- Outcome
- Further care

Signature

Anaesthetic records should follow this model, but also include:

Date and details of pre-assessment
- Clinical findings on history and examination
- Investigation results
- Planned procedure
- Information given to the patient, and any other discussion

Details of relevant information
- Anaesthetics and any associated problems
- Age
- Body mass index
- Allergies

Anaesthetic care
- Supervising consultant
- Drugs administered
- Monitoring used
- Detailed physiological record
- Fluid balance
- Timing of events (e.g. induction, incision)

Postoperative instructions
- Oxygen
- Analgesia
- Fluid therapy
- Monitoring
- Further specific nursing care (e.g. for patients with epidurals in place)

Signature

External regulatory assessments – revalidation

Revalidation has become the norm in most health care systems, and takes several forms between countries. At its most intensive each practitioner has to be re-examined on a rolling basis every 5–10 years. Certification is dependent on this academic success. Others use a detailed logbook of procedures performed and an audit of defined outcomes set against normalised outcomes from a large pool of similar practitioners. This is often repeated every 2–5 years. The problem with the former approach is designing a series of tests that is effective in correctly identifying expertise and specialisation rather than basic factual recall.

Currently in the UK the GMC has outlined its proposals for revalidation, which will be repeated every 5 years and apply to every practising doctor – trainees, community and hospital specialists, and the partly retired. For the first time not only will registration be necessary, but a licence to practise will also be needed. The details and timing of this process are under review.

The underlying process will be appraisal based, with supplemental information that may be gathered directly or by questionnaire (including patients' views). The most likely event is that a senior member of the hospital trust or department will attest that the doctor meets their clinical governance responsibilities and has satisfactorily completed their annual appraisals. Every doctor will have to maintain a portfolio of evidence to support their revalidation that will not only contain their appraisal forms, but also supplements that include continuing education and professional development (CEPD) activity, self-audit outcomes and patient contact information, both praise and complaints.[4] Further developments will undoubtedly be added as the process gathers momentum.

Controversies

There are three areas where training and standards are under threat at present.

What is a specialist?

Following from the very first sentence in this chapter, patient care has to be delivered by a specialist in that area of practice. Does this equate to a consultant, and does this mean that a consultant is equally expert across all of their activity? Clearly that is unlikely. Should we develop into single-specialty practitioners where there is a dedicated training programme that results in a narrow-based but skilled practitioner? This model is undergoing trial in urology at present. Higher speciality training has been reduced from 5 to 3 years to produce an 'office urologist'. Underlying this is the government's drive to produce thousands of specialists for the NHS in a very short timeframe.

The need of patients in most hospitals is for an anaesthetist who has a broad and comprehensive training and who can safely manage the majority of clinical problems encountered. This takes a long time, currently 7 years, and although single-subspecialty training would be faster it would poorly serve most hospitals and their patients.

Does the delivery of anaesthesia care have to be solely by consultants? Again, this is not the case at present, and is unlikely to change very quickly. What is important is that there is appropriate supervision and the availability of a consultant. There are models being developed for non-anaesthetic practitioners who are expected to perform at the level of an advanced senior house officer. The pragmatic key to patient safety appears to be excellence of supervision.

Are training and experience the same?

The procedures for admittance to the GMC's Specialist Register are about to be revised to allow experience to count towards training. Does servicing the same list for many years lead to expertise? The answer lies in the attitude of the anaesthetist. Where a questioning approach has been maintained and current concepts are reviewed and balanced against their own management, it is hard to say this is anything other than acting as a specialist. Again there is little room for argument if there is self-audit and comparison with nationally published standards with equitable results. It is not expertise, however, nor is it evidence of training having taken place if there is a simple routine of performing the same technique regardless of external concepts or patient factors.

Can performing anaesthesia within a limited series of clinical lists over years equate to a broad higher training in subspecialities? The simple answer is no, but provided the anaesthetist does not change their clinical activity then the above arguments still apply. The problem becomes most difficult if specialist status is achieved and the doctor applies for a different post. How can an advisory appointments panel judge their training and experience? The threat that Foundation Trusts in the UK would not need external assessors appointed by the Royal College makes this scenario of great concern when such doctors do change hospitals, especially if there is a manpower shortage.

Who pays for training?

Historically, training was paid for by trainees working inhumane numbers of hours each week to maintain the service. This has been sensibly reduced to a sane level, but the work still has to be done. Changes have occurred, with some non-medical roles being taken over by technicians or nurse practitioners. However, the workload of the permanent medical staff has increased at a time when new contractual restrictions have been accepted. Clinical flexibility to teach and train is now dependent on management agreement, and usually appropriate funding.

Scrutiny of the role of the medical training establishment is likely to become even more intense. Bodies such as the Royal Colleges have to be much more open in promoting the value of their expertise in setting standards, the assessment of training outcomes and the validation of local training schemes. They have usually worked independently on behalf of their members and fellows, but belatedly are being asked to develop service level agreements, with costings, for their work as agents of the national training bodies. This funding may redress some of the local management disquiet with many Faculty or Royal College activities.

At the same time training itself is being re-moulded and innumerable initiatives are being promoted, for example Modernising Medical Careers (MMC), Hospital at Night and Seamless Training, which all change the boundaries of who is where, and when they are available for teaching and training. The costs of these initiatives are large – over £100 million per year – at a time when postgraduate training budgets have been frozen or even reduced.

The time for finally having a properly funded, organised and accountable training system has arrived, but there are great discrepancies between the costs of training and the money available. Several countries have approached this problem by charging trainees for their training, but none appear to have solved it. This charge may be as an annual, tax-deductible registration fee, or by locking in a period of service in their institution after training has ended. This has several problems. Legal action when a trainee fails because 'the system let them down' is one obvious threat.

In conclusion, the setting, teaching and maintenance of standards of practice in anaesthesia and critical care are essential to protect the patient. Erosion of these standards is only countered by a continuous striving for excellence in teaching, in recruiting and training first-class doctors, in keeping current with all developments in understanding and practice, and in maintaining lifelong learning.

References

1. Good medical practice. May 2001 General Medical Council UK. www.gmc-uk.org/standards/good.htm.
2. The doctor as teacher. Sept 1999 General Medical Council UK. www.gmc-uk.org/med_ed/teach.htm.
3. Fletcher G, McGeorge R, Flin R, Glavin R, Maran N. The role of non-technical skills in anaesthesia: a review of current literature. Br J Anaesth 2002; 88:418–429.
4. Personal folder. A specialty specific supplement for anaesthetists. www.rcoa.ac.uk/docs/personalfolder(Sept02).pdf.

Further reading

Greaves DG, Dodds C, Kumar CM, Mets B. Clinical teaching. A guide to teaching practical anaesthesia. Lisse Netherlands: Swetz & Zeitlinger; 2003.

APPENDIX **1**

DICTIONARY OF ADULT MEDICAL DISORDERS

This is a compilation of unusual disorders seen in adults that may be of interest to the anaesthetist, mainly those not described in Chapter 1.2. The key features and anaesthetic implications are outlined for each disorder. (AV, atrioventricular; BP, blood pressure; CPAP, continuous positive airway pressure; DVT, deep venous thrombosis; ETT, endotracheal tube; GA, general anaesthetic; IPPV, intermittent positive-pressure ventilation; LMA, laryngeal mask airway; PA, pulmonary artery; SVR, systemic vascular resistance).

Name	Description	Anaesthetic implication
Achalasia	Degeneration of myenteric neural plexus Dilated oesophagus Treated by Heller's operation (myotomy)	Dysphagia Aspiration Risk of regurgitation
Acromegaly	Pituitary adenoma Excessive growth hormone	Large tongue Difficult intubation Impaired glucose tolerance
Addison's disease	Destruction of both adrenals Hyperpigmentation May be debilitated	Hypotension Hypoglycaemia Hyponatraemia
Alport's syndrome	May present in young adult	Renal failure Hypertension in pregnancy
Alveolar hypoventilation Central alveolar hypoventilation Ondine's curse	Poor central respiratory drive May be cervical cord pathology	Respiratory failure Need for postoperative support
American trypanosomiasis	See Chagas' disease	
Amyloidosis	Abnormal protein deposits Due to chronic infection, or multiple myeloma, or autoimmune disease	Large tongue May affect heart valves, conduction and ventricular function Renal failure Peripheral neuropathy

Name	Description	Anaesthetic implication
Amyotrophic lateral sclerosis Motor neurone disease	Progressive degeneration of motor neurones Commoner in men	Bulbar weakness Respiratory weakness Suxamethonium causes dangerous hyperkalaemia
Anorexia nervosa	Morbid fear of obesity Much commoner in young women Weight up to 60% below normal	Temperature loss Bradycardia and hypotension Long QT interval Heart block Delayed gastric emptying Care with fluid and electrolytes Hypoalbuminaemia
Ankylosing spondylitis Bamboo spine	Vertebral ankylosis Mainly in men May cause respiratory failure	Difficult laryngoscopy Aortic regurgitation Pulmonary fibrosis Very difficult spinal anaesthesia
Asbestosis	May develop mesothelioma May develop carcinoma of lung Lung fibrosis	Pleural effusions Respiratory failure
Autonomic hyperreflexia	In response to skin or visceral stimuli below spinal cord lesion Hypertension and tachycardia	Need deep anaesthesia or adequate regional analgesia
Behçet's syndrome	Iritis, mouth and genital ulcers Polyarthritis May be CNS lesions	May be taking corticosteroids Mouth ulcers complicate airway management
Beri-beri See Wernicke's encephalopathy	Thiamine (B_1) deficiency	Peripheral neuropathy Autonomic neuropathy High-output cardiac failure
Buerger's disease Thromboangiitis obliterans	Peripheral vascular disease Young male smokers Emphysema and bronchitis	Lung disease Difficulty measuring BP Cuff measurement over-reads
Central alveolar hypoventilation	See Alveolar hypoventilation	
Chagas' disease American trypanosomiasis	Parasitic infection in Central and South America Can cause achalasia (see above)	Cardiomyopathy Conduction abnormalities Risk of aspiration

Name	Description	Anaesthetic implication
Charcot–Marie–Tooth disease Peroneal muscular atrophy	Sensory and motor peripheral neuropathy Hereditary (dominant) Presents in teens	Phrenic nerves may be involved Avoid suxamethonium (risk of hyperkalaemia)
Christmas disease Haemophilia B	Factor IX deficiency Sex-linked recessive	Ensure factor IX >60% normal Give factor IX fraction Liaise with haematologist
Congenital analgesia	Abnormal cutaneous sensation	Maintain temperature Care with positioning
CREST syndrome Scleroderma variant	Calcinosis Raynaud's phenomenon Sclerodactyly Telangiectasia	Regurgitation risk Lesions in heart and lungs
Creutzfeldt–Jakob disease	Progressive loss of coordination Ataxia Variant disease caused by prions	Poor nutrition Use disposable instruments for airway management
Crohn's disease	Inflammatory bowel disease Young adults Causes diarrhoea and fistulae	May be severely toxic Anaemia May be taking corticosteroids
Dermatomyositis Polymyositis	Proximal muscle weakness Arthritis May affect lungs	Regurgitation risk Poor mouth opening Anaemia Sensitive to relaxants
Eaton–Lambert syndrome	See Myasthenic syndrome	
Eosinophilic granuloma	Adult version of histiocytosis X Localised lung lesion	Anaemia May be taking corticosteroids
Erythema multiforme See also Stevens–Johnson syndrome	Papules and bullae on skin and mucous membranes Sulphonamides can be the cause	Laryngeal oedema at extubation
Factor V Leiden mutation	Resistance to anticoagulant effect of protein C	High risk of DVT and PE
Fibrosing alveolitis Hamman–Rich syndrome	Cyanosis, cor pulmonale	Respiratory failure May be taking corticosteroids

Name	Description	Anaesthetic implication
Gaisböck's syndrome	Polycythaemia due to reduction in plasma volume Seen in men Smokers, obese, hypertensive	Cardiovascular disease Risk of DVT Venesection may be needed
Glomus jugulare tumours	In middle ear or posterior fossa	Very vascular tumours May secrete 5-HT
Glucagonoma	Malignant tumour of α cells in pancreas Glucagon causes diabetes mellitus	Control blood sugar and ketosis Handling releases glucagon Prone to DVT and PE
Goodpasture's syndrome	Autoimmune disease Young adults Severe lung haemorrhages Glomerulonephritis	Microcytic anaemia Hypertension Assess renal function May be immunosuppressed Large ETT facilitates suction
Gorham syndrome	Bone destruction Pathological fractures Teenagers or young adults	Cervical spine may be affected Respiratory involvement
Haemochromatosis	Iron deposits in liver, pancreas, joints, skin, heart	Liver dysfunction Diabetes mellitus, possible heart failure
Haemolytic uraemic syndrome	Haemolysis, renal failure Thrombocytopenia	Renal dysfunction Anaemia
Hamman–Rich syndrome	See Fibrosing alveolitis	
Hartnup's disease	Tryptophan malabsorption Pellagra (see below) and ataxia	Responds to nicotinamide
Henoch–Schönlein purpura	Bruising, abdominal pain Nephritis Seen in adolescents	Renal dysfunction
Hereditary spastic paraplegia	See Strumpell's disease	
Huntington's chorea	Progressive chorea Autosomal dominant inheritance	Regurgitation risk Poor nutrition May be pseudocholinesterase deficient

Name	Description	Anaesthetic implication
Hydatid disease	Infection with the dog tapeworm *Echinococcus granulosus* Cysts in liver, lungs or muscle	Rupture during excision may cause severe anaphylaxis
Hypokalaemic familial periodic paralysis	Potassium moves into muscle cells Attacks provoked by meals	Postoperative respiratory failure Arrhythmias Sensitive to relaxants
Idiopathic thrombocytopenic purpura	Autoimmune disease Often treated by splenectomy	Possible airway bleeding May be taking corticosteroids Avoid heparin, aspirin Rebound thrombosis after splenectomy
Infectious mononucleosis	Epstein–Barr virus Rarely can cause splenic rupture	Tonsils obstruct airway
Insulinoma	Hypoglycaemia after fasting and exercise May metastasise to liver	Continual glucose monitoring Hyperglycaemic rebound
Jervell & Lange-Nielsen syndrome	Autosomal recessive inheritance Nerve deafness Long QT interval	Tendency to ventricular tachycardia
Lentiginosis	Small brown skin macules	May also have hypertrophic obstructive cardiomyopathy
Leprosy	*Mycobacterium leprae* infection Peripheral neuritis Thickened nerves	Often given corticosteroids for neuritis Analgesia in limbs Muscle wasting
Lingual vein thrombosis	Severe upper airway obstruction	Awake fibreoptic intubation Heliox may be useful
Ludwig's angina	Infection of submandibular space Usually anaerobic (*Actinomyces*)	Upper airway obstruction Indurated floor of mouth Trismus, unaffected by relaxants
Lyme disease	Tick-borne *Borrelia* infection Named after Lyme, Connecticut Skin lesions	Can progress to: Meningoencephalitis Myocarditis Peripheral neuropathy

Name	Description	Anaesthetic implication
Meig's syndrome	Pleural effusion Ovarian cyst (often carcinoma)	Drain effusion May be malnourished
Mikulicz syndrome	Enlargement of salivary and lachrymal glands May be due to sarcoidosis	May make intubation difficult Avoid anticholinergic drugs
Motor neurone disease	See Amyotrophic lateral sclerosis	
Moya Moya syndrome	Stenosis or occlusion of internal carotid arteries. Collaterals at base of brain More common in Japanese	May deteriorate after anaesthesia Avoid straining (e.g. in labour) Maintain cerebral perfusion
Multiple myeloma See Waldenström's macroglobulinaemia	Bone marrow infiltration Often affects cervical spine	Anaemia Renal dysfunction Hypercalcaemia Unstable cervical spine
Myasthenic syndrome Eaton–Lambert syndrome	Autoimmune prejunctional disorder Usually with small cell lung carcinoma Weakness of proximal muscles May be associated with bulbar muscle weakness	No response to anticholinesterases Autonomic dysfunction Sensitivity to all relaxants Increased twitch during tetany
Neurofibromatosis	See Von Recklinghausen's disease	
Ondine's curse	See Alveolar hypoventilation	
Ovarian hyperstimulation syndrome	Excessive vasoactive peptides	May cause acute lung injury
Paterson–Brown–Kelly syndrome Plummer–Vinson syndrome	Oesophageal web Anaemia and angular stomatitis	Risk of regurgitation Anaemia
Paraplegia	Level of cord lesion should be known	Autonomic hyperreflexia (see above) Suxamethonium may cause dangerous hyperkalaemia if used between 1–2 days and 6–12 months after injury

Name	Description	Anaesthetic implication
Parkinson's disease	Tremor, rigidity and dyskinesia Loss of dopaminergic neurones in substantia nigra May be associated with autonomic dysfunction	Continue therapy perioperatively Risk of regurgitation Postoperative chest infection common Postoperative confusion possible
Pellagra	Niacin (nicotinamide/ nicotinic acid) deficiency Dementia, diarrhoea, dermatitis	Confusion and excitement Responds to intravenous nicotinamide
Pemphigus vulgaris	Autoimmune bullous eruption Affects skin and mucous membranes Epidermis separates with friction forces	Avoid skin traction and friction Scarring and narrowing of larynx Avoid airway trauma Small ETT may be better than LMA May be fluid and electrolyte losses
Peroneal muscular atrophy	See Charcot–Marie–Tooth disease	
Pharyngeal pouch	Usually above cricopharyngeus Can lead to aspiration during the night	Ask patient to manually empty it Cricoid pressure ineffective Use awake fibreoptic intubation
Pickwickian syndrome	Gross obesity, hypoventilation Cor pulmonale, polycythaemia	Regional anaesthesia preferred Need IPPV or CPAP after GA Avoid respiratory depressant drugs High risk of DVT
Plummer–Vinson syndrome	See Paterson–Brown–Kelly syndrome	
Pneumatosis cystoides intestinalis	Gas-filled cysts in submucosa of gut Usually in large bowel May cause bowel obstruction	Avoid nitrous oxide
Polyarteritis nodosa	Autoimmune, commoner in men Widespread effects, especially lungs, kidneys, skin, heart, CNS, joints	Evaluate lung and renal function Heart failure from coronary arteritis

Name	Description	Anaesthetic implication
Polymyositis	See Dermatomyositis	
Post-poliomyelitis syndrome	Weakness developing many years after orginal infection May affect bulbar/ respiratory muscles	Regurgitation risk Possibility of ventilatory failure
Primary pulmonary hypertension	Unknown aetiology Mainly in young women	Dangerous condition Invasive monitoring Consider PA catheter No hypoxia or cardiac depressant drugs
Pulmonary cysts (bullae)	Emphysematous space over 1 cm diameter Present with breathlessness	Minimise peak airway pressure Beware of tension pneumothorax Avoid nitrous oxide
Pulseless disease	See Takayasu's disease	
Reninoma	Very rare benign tumour of juxtaglomerular cells Young adults Autonomous secretion of renin	Hypertension Hypokalaemia Careful monitoring of CVS
Romano–Ward syndrome	Autosomal dominant inheritance Prolonged QT interval	Tendency to ventricular tachycardia
Sarcoidosis	Multisystem granulomatous disease Lung nodules and lymphadenopathy Neuropathy, including cranial nerves Eyes often affected	May have laryngeal involvement Hypercalcaemia Renal function may be impaired
Scleroderma	Lung fibrosis Raynaud's phenomenon common Rarely can affect heart and kidneys See CREST syndrome	Limited mouth opening Risk of regurgitation Hypovolaemia Difficult venous access Regional anaesthesia preferred
Scurvy	Vitamin C deficiency Bruising and petechiae	Loose teeth, swollen gums Anaemia Excessive surgical bleeding
Sheehan's syndrome	See Simmond's disease	

Name	Description	Anaesthetic implication
Simmond's disease	Hypopituitarism Due to tumour or after surgery Necrosis of anterior lobe after obstetric haemorrhage is called Sheehan's syndrome	Depends on exact hormone deficiencies Hypoglycaemia, hypothermia Water and electrolyte balance
Sjögren's syndrome	Dry eyes, diminished salivary secretion Usually with rheumatoid arthritis Multisystem involvement common	Avoid anticholinergics Humidify inspired gases Impaired airway access due to swollen salivary glands
Stevens–Johnson syndrome See Erythema multiforme	Most severe form of erythema multiforme Can be fatal	May need intravenous fluids May need intensive care
Strumpell's disease Hereditary spastic paraplegia	Progressive degeneration of spinal cord Usually only affects legs Varying inheritance pattern	Avoid suxamethonium
Systemic lupus erythematosus (SLE)	Autoimmune vasculitis, mainly women Affects skin, kidneys, heart, lungs May cause peripheral neuropathy Antiphospholipid antibodies cause thrombosis Thrombocytopenia or antibodies to clotting factors cause bleeding defect	Cardiac and renal involvement Anaemia Assess clotting status Avoid hypothermia (Raynaud's)
Syringomyelia	Cavities in spinal cord Muscle weakness and scoliosis Can cause respiratory failure	Bulbar palsy Autonomic hyperreflexia Sensitive to muscle relaxants Avoid suxamethonium (hyperkalaemia)
Takayasu's disease Pulseless disease	Mainly in Asian girls Occlusive arteritis Affects aorta and large vessels May affect cerebral arteries	Hypertension if renal arteries involved Use invasive BP monitoring Maintain cerebral perfusion Neuraxial block useful to reduce SVR

Name	Description	Anaesthetic implication
Thromboangiitis obliterans	See Buerger's disease	
Urine drinking	In psychiatric disorders	Hyponatraemia needs correction
Von Recklinghausen's disease Neurofibromatosis	Autosomal dominant inheritance Café au lait spots and neurofibromas CNS tumours (benign and malignant) Acoustic neuromas are common	Laryngeal tumours may occur Often kyphoscoliosis Relaxants may have prolonged effect 1% have associated phaeochromocytoma
Waldenström's macroglobulinaemia See Multiple myeloma	Related to multiple myeloma Presents in elderly men	Anaemia Bleeding tendency Cardiac failure
Wegener's granulomatosis	Midline granulomas Ulcers in nose, palate, larynx and trachea Large nodules in the lungs Glomerulonephritis	Assess airway by preoperative indirect laryngoscopy Intubation may cause bleeding and possible respiratory obstruction Occasionally diagnosed by the anaesthetist
Wernicke's encephalopathy See Beri-beri	Acute thiamine (B_1) deficiency Common in alcoholics	Confusion Ataxia and nystagmus Korsakoff's psychosis Treat with intravenous thiamine
Wolff–Parkinson–White syndrome	AV accessory path (bundle of Kent) Re-entrant tachycardias	Short PR interval Delta wave at start of QRS Avoid digoxin See Chapter 1.2 for treatment
Wolfram's syndrome	Autosomal recessive Pituitary diabetes insipidus Diabetes mellitus Optic atrophy and deafness	Fluid balance

Further reading

Benumof JL. Anesthesia and uncommon diseases. 4th edn. Philadelphia: WB Saunders; 1998.

Nicholson JP, Rayman G, Donaldson P, Driver IK. The anaesthetic management of a patient with a reninoma. Anaesthesia 2003; 58:466–470.

Seller CA, Ravalia A. Anaesthetic implications of anorexia nervosa. Anaesthesia 2003; 58:437–443.

Useful websites

http://www.tylermedicalclinic.com/

http://www.nlm.nih.gov/

http://www.rarediseases.org

http://www.ncbi.nlm.nih.gov/entrez

and through this website, visit OMIM (Online Mendelian Inheritance in Man)

Further reading

[illegible]

[illegible]

[illegible]

Useful websites

[illegible]

[illegible]

[illegible]

[illegible]

[illegible]

APPENDIX **2**

DICTIONARY OF PAEDIATRIC MEDICAL DISORDERS

This appendix catalogues some of the many syndromes and diseases that may present in infancy and childhood. A brief description of each syndrome is followed by a summary of the main anaesthetic implications of that syndrome. Of necessity the descriptions are brief and the reader is directed to the list of useful websites at the end of this chapter to obtain more comprehensive information. (AS, aortic stenosis; ASD, atrial septal defect; IHD, ischaemic heart disease; PDA, patent ductus arteriosus; VSD, ventricular septal defect.)

Name	Description	Anaesthetic implication
Aarskog–Scott syndrome Faciodigitogenital dysplasia	Mainly affects male infants Stunted growth, broad facial features, genital abnormalities and mild mental retardation	Intubation problems
Achondroplasia	Short-limb dwarfism Prominent forehead with protruding jaw Respiratory problems due to narrowed nasal passages	Intubation problems Extradural anaesthesia safe
Acquired neuromyotonia	See Armadillo syndrome	
Acrocephalosyndactyly	See Apert's syndrome	
Adrenogenital syndrome	Defect in adrenal synthesis of corticosteroids resulting in aldosterone and cortisol deficiency Female virilisation due to overproduction of androgens	Check electrolytes Corticosteroids if salt-losing
Aglossia–adactylia syndrome	See Möbius syndrome	

Name	Description	Anaesthetic implication
Albers–Schönberg disease Marble bone disease Osteopetrosis	Similar to osteogenesis imperfecta Brittle bones, pathological fractures Hepatosplenomegaly	Anaemia Care with positioning
Albright–Butler syndrome	Renal tubular acidosis with hypokalaemia Renal calculi	Correct electrolytes Renal impairment
Albright's osteodystrophy Pseudohypoparathyroidism	Ectopic bone formation Mental retardation	Hypocalcaemia ECG conduction defects Neuromuscular problems Convulsions
Alport syndrome	Nephritis and nerve deafness Renal failure in later life	Renal impairment
Alström syndrome	Obesity, deafness and blind by 7 years of age Diabetes mellitus and renal failure after puberty	Obesity Diabetes mellitus Renal impairment
Amyotonia congenita Kugelberg–Welander disease Werdnig–Hoffmann disease Infantile muscular atrophy	More severe infantile muscular atrophy than Welander Spinal muscular atrophy with anterior horn cell degeneration, death before puberty Chronic respiratory problems due to muscle weakness	Sensitivity to intravenous anaesthetics Avoid respiratory depressants Avoid muscle relaxants
Amyotrophic lateral sclerosis	Degeneration of motor neurones	Avoid suxamethonium (excessive potassium release) Avoid respiratory depressants
Analbuminaemia	Almost absent albumin	Sensitive to protein-bound drugs
Andersen's disease	See Glycogen storage disease IV	
Andersen's syndrome	See Cystic fibrosis	
Anderson's disease	Hereditary hypocholesterolaemic syndrome, characterised by intestinal fat malabsorption	No anaesthetic problems reported

Name	Description	Anaesthetic implication
Andre syndrome	See Otopalatodigital syndrome	
Angelman syndrome	Microcephaly	Seizures Cardiac anomalies
Angio-osteohypertrophy	See Klippel–Trenaunay syndrome	
Anhidrotic ectodermal dysplasia	See Christ–Siemens–Touraine syndrome	
Apert's syndrome Acrocephalosyndactyly	Craniosynostosis and micrognathia Congenital heart defects (e.g. VSD)	Intubation problems Raised intracranial pressure Cardiac anomalies
Armadillo syndrome Isaacs syndrome Acquired neuromyotonia	Arises in childhood or adult life Spontaneous myokymia of arms and legs with increased tone Muscle activity persists throughout sleep, but is abolished by carbamazepine and phenytoin	Muscle activity persists during general and regional anaesthesia Muscle activity suppressed by muscle relaxants
Arthrogryposis multiplex	Scoliosis, myopathy, congenital contractures Micrognathia, cervical spine and/or jaw stiffness Congenital heart disease in 10% of patients	Difficult venous access Airway problems Sensitivity to intravenous anaesthetics Cardiac anomalies Malignant hyperpyrexia risk
Asplenia	Absent spleen. Bilateral visceral right-sidedness Complex cardiovascular anomalies with cyanosis and heart failure	Cardiac anomalies
Ataxia–telangiectasia	Cerebellar ataxia Skin and conjunctival telangiectasia Defective immunity with decreased serum IgA and IgE	Recurrent chest and sinus infections Bronchiectasis

Name	Description	Anaesthetic implication
Barlow's syndrome	Click-murmur mitral valve prolapse Bradycardia resistant to atropine Arrhythmias responding to β-blockade Thromboembolism	Avoid excessive tachycardia and anxiety Antibiotic prophylaxis
Bartter syndrome	Hyperplasia of juxtaglomerular apparatus Onset in infancy or early adolescence	Electrolyte abnormalities
Beckwith syndrome Wiedemann syndrome	Infantile gigantism Macroglossia Persistent severe neonatal hypoglycaemia.	Airway problems Hypoglycaemia
Blackfan–Diamond syndrome	Congenital idiopathic red-cell aplasia. Hypersplenism Congenital cardiac defects (e.g. VSD)	Corticosteroid therapy Anaemia Thrombocytopenia Cardiac anomalies
Bloom's syndrome	Defect in DNA management	Restrict X-ray exposure
Bournville's disease	See Tuberous sclerosis	
Bowen's syndrome Cerebrohepatorenal syndrome	Hypotonia, hepatomegaly and neonatal jaundice, polycystic kidneys Hypoprothrombinaemia Associated congenital heart disease	Renal impairment Cardiac anomalies
Branched chain ketonuria	See Maple syrup urine disease	
Cardio-auditory syndrome	See Jervell & Lange–Nielsen syndrome	
Carpenter's syndrome	Cranial synostosis with small mandible Congenital heart disease — PDA and VSD	Intubation problems Cardiac anomalies
Central core myopathy	see Amyotonia congenita	
Cerebrocostomandibular syndrome	Cleft palate, micrognathia, microthorax, tracheal abnormalities, vertebral anomalies	Intubation problems Respiratory problems

Name	Description	Anaesthetic implication
Cerebrohepatorenal syndrome	See Bowen's syndrome	
CHARGE association	Micrognathia, cleft palate, choanal atresia Microphallus and cryptorchidism Congenital heart disease in 70%	Intubation problems Cardiac anomalies
Chediak–Higashi syndrome	Partial albinism Hepatosplenomegaly and immunodeficiency	Recurrent chest infections Corticosteroid therapy Thrombocytopenia
Cherubism	Macroglossia with tumerous lesions of mandible and maxilla cause airway obstruction and respiratory distress	Intubation problems Urgent tracheostomy Profuse surgical bleeding
Chondroectodermal dysplasia	See Ellis–van Creveld syndrome	
Chotzen syndrome	Craniosynostosis Renal failure	Intubation problems Renal impairment
Christ–Siemens–Touraine syndrome Anhydrotic ectodermal dysplasia	Defective thermoregulation due to absent sweat glands Heat intolerance and recurrent chest infections No hair or teeth	Intubation problems Cooling mattress Avoid atropine
Chronic granulomatous disease	Inherited disorder of leucocyte function Recurrent infections Hepatomegaly	Poor pulmonary function Strict asepsis
Cockayne's syndrome	Progressive mental and physical retardation, deafness, blindness, bony malformations	Intubation problems
Congenital myopathy	Central core disease Ventilation problem due to muscle weakness	Sensitive to muscle relaxants Malignant hyperpyrexia risk
Conradi–Hunermann syndrome	Chondrodystrophy and mental deficiency Associated congenital heart disease and renal anomalies	Airway problems Cardiac anomalies Renal impairment

Name	Description	Anaesthetic implication
Cretinism	Congenital hypothyroidism Muscle weakness may cause respiratory problems Cardiomyopathy Corticosteroid therapy may be required	Airway problems Cardiac anomalies Sensitive to intravenous anaesthetics Hypoglycaemia Electrolyte abnormalities
Cri-du-chat syndrome	Microcephaly, micrognathia and macroglossia Associated congenital heart disease (ASD and VSD) in 25% of cases	Airway problems Intubation problems Cardiac anomalies
Crouzon's disease	Craniosynostosis Cranial operations can be very bloody Coarctation of aorta	Intubation problems Postoperative respiratory obstruction
Currerino triad	Sacral agenesis, presacral mass and anorectal malformation	Avoid caudal analgesia
Cutis laxa	Elastic fibre degeneration Fragile skin, blood vessels etc. Pendulous upper airway mucosa causes respiratory obstruction Emphysema and cor pulmonale	Frequent chest infections Difficult to maintain intravenous access
Cystic fibrosis Andersen's syndrome Fibrocystic disease	Intrinsic lung disease characterised by inspissation of secretions, airway obstruction and chronic obstructive pulmonary disease Postural drainage prevents accumulation of secretions Also associated with malnutrition, liver dysfunction and bleeding tendency	Humidification Antibiotics Bronchodilators Intubation facilitates bronchial suction Hypoxia poorly tolerated Hypotension poorly tolerated Avoid dehydration Avoid atropine
Dandy–Walker syndrome	Cerebellar malformation Hydrocephalus	Airway problems
Diastrophic dwarfism	Micrognathia and short neck	Intubation problems

Name	Description	Anaesthetic implication
DiGeorge syndrome third and fourth arch syndrome	Absent thymus – immunodeficient and increased susceptibility to infection Absent parathyroids – results in hypocalcaemia and tetany Aortic arch anomalies with cardiac failure	Stridor Recurrent chest infections Susceptible to blood transfusion-induced graft-versus-host reaction
Down's syndrome Mongolism Trisomy 21	See Trisomy 21	
Dubowitz syndrome	Microcephaly and micrognathia Hypertelorism	Intubation problems
Duchenne muscular dystrophy	Commonest muscular disorder of childhood – usually die in second decade Progressive muscular weakness and scoliosis, leading to chronic respiratory failure Frequent cardiac muscle involvement, with occasional cardiac arrest	Minimal drug dosage Avoid muscle relaxants Avoid respiratory depressants Postoperative ventilatory support often necessary Cardiac problems Malignant hyperpyrexia risk
Dutch–Kentucky syndrome	See Hecht–Beals syndrome	
Dyggve–Melchior–Clausen's syndrome	Short trunk dwarfism Mental retardation, short neck, macroglossia	ntubation problems
Dysautonomia	See Familial dysautonomia	
Dystrophia myotonica	See Myotonica dystrophia	
Ebstein's anomaly	Tricuspid valve disease	Supraventricular tachycardia during induction
Edwards' syndrome	See Trisomy 18	

Name	Description	Anaesthetic implication
Ehlers–Danlos syndrome	Collagen abnormality – hypermobility of joints and fragility of skin, blood vessels and tracheal mucosa Spontaneous rupture of blood vessels associated with aneurysms Mitral regurgitation Bleeding diathesis of unknown cause	Difficult to maintain intravenous access Intubation may cause severe tracheal bruising Spontaneous pneumothorax ECG conduction abnormalities
Eisenmenger complex	Pulmonary hypertension, intracardiac shunts, hypoxia Decreases of systemic vascular resistance increase the shunt Vasoactive agents, hypercapnia and further hypoxia exacerbate pulmonary hypertension	Strong tendency to asystole Very slow equilibration with inhaled gases Ketamine may be useful
Ellis–van Creveld syndrome Chondroectodermal dysplasia	Ectodermal defects with skeletal anomalies Associated congenital heart defects (usually septal) in 50% of cases	Poor lung function Respiratory failure due to chest wall defects Cardiac anomalies
Epidermolysis bullosa	Skin and mucous membranes easily blistered, resulting in extensive scarring	Avoid skin trauma Ketamine recommended Corticosteroid therapy Check for porphyria (similar skin lesions)
Eulenberg disease	See Paramyotonia congenita	
Fabry's disease	Lipid storage disease Lipid build-up results in myocardial infarction, stroke and renal failure	As for adults with IHD Renal impairment
Faciodigitogenital dysplasia	See Aarskog–Scott syndrome	
Fallot's tetralogy	Cyanotic congenital heart disease comprising VSD, pulmonary stenosis, overriding aorta and right ventricle hypertrophy	Avoid fall in SVR which causes further desaturation
Familial dysautonomia	See Riley–Day syndrome	

Name	Description	Anaesthetic implication
Familial periodic paralysis	Muscle disease characterised by hyperkalaemia and attacks of quadriplegic paralysis	Monitor serum potassium Avoid thiopental Avoid muscle relaxants
Familial unconjugated hyperbilirubinaemia	See Gilbert's disease	
Familial xanthomatosis	See Wolman's disease	
Fanconi's anaemia	Defect in DNA regeneration	Sensitive to X-rays
Fanconi syndrome Renal tubular acidosis	Proximal tubular defect usually secondary to other disease and characterised by acidosis, potassium loss and dehydration	Correct electrolytes Correct acid–base abnormality Monitor renal function
Farber's disease Lipogranulomatosis	Sphingomyelin deposition Widespread visceral lipogranulomas involving CNS, heart and kidney	Intubation problems Cardiomyopathy Renal impairment
Favism	Glucose-6-phosphate-dehydrogenase deficiency Haemolytic anaemia Haemolysis induced by oxidant drugs (e.g. sulphonamides, aspirin)	Avoid oxidant drugs
Felty's syndrome	A form of idiopathic thrombocytopenic purpura Anaemia, neutropenia, and susceptibility to infections	Corticosteroid therapy
Femoral hypoplasia syndrome	Unusual facies with micrognathia Femurs hypoplastic or absent	ntubation problems
Fibrocystic disease	See Cystic fibrosis	
Fibrodysplasia ossificans	See Myositis ossificans	
Focal dermal hypoplasia	See Golz–Gorlin syndrome	
Forbes' disease	See Glycogen storage disease type III	

Name	Description	Anaesthetic implication
Freeman–Sheldon syndrome	Craniofacial abnormalities with microstomia and scoliosis	Intubation problems
Friedreich's ataxia	Cerebellar degeneration, progressive ataxia and myopathy Myocardial degeneration with failure and arrhythmias, respiratory failure, diabetes, and peripheral neuropathy Treatment as for amyotrophic lateral sclerosis	Atracurium safe Heart failure
G syndrome	See Opitz–Frias syndrome	
Gardner's syndrome	Multiple polyposis, bony tumours, sebaceous cysts and fibromas	No anaesthetic problems described
Gargoylism	See Mucopolysaccharidosis I	
Gaucher's disease	Cerebroside accumulation in CNS, liver, spleen etc. Pseudobulbar palsy	Pulmonary aspiration Anaemia Thrombocytopenia Neutropenia
Gilbert's disease Familial unconjugated hyperbilirubinaemia	Jaundice precipitated by minor upsets, including starvation	
Glanzmann's disease Thrombasthenia	Reduction in platelet ADP resulting in abnormal function Abnormal haemorrhage, platelet infusion rarely effective	Corticosteroid therapy
Glycogen storage disease type I Von Gierke's disease	Hepatomegaly, enlarged kidneys Severe attacks of hypoglycaemia	Monitor blood glucose Monitor acid–base balance Diazoxide for hypoglycaemia

Name	Description	Anaesthetic implication
Glycogen storage disease type II Pompe's disease	Muscle deposits, severe hypotonicity and neuromuscular weakness Macroglossia and respiratory problems due to muscle weakness Massive cardiomegaly and heart failure Rarely survive infancy	Extreme care Avoid respiratory depressants Avoid cardiac depressants Avoid muscle relaxants Airway problems
Glycogen storage disease type III Forbes' disease	Deficiency of debrancher enzyme with onset in early childhood Mild growth and mental retardation, hepatomegaly, cardiomegaly and muscle weakness	Hypoglycaemia
Glycogen storage disease type IV Andersen's disease	Glycogen deposition in liver and spleen resulting in hepatosplenomegaly and progressive liver failure	Hypoglycaemia Hepatic failure
Glycogen storage disease type V McArdle's disease	Myopathy due to glycogen accumulation in muscles Weakness, respiratory problems, and cardiomyopathy	Care with cardiac depressants Atracurium safe Avoid suxamethonium
Glycogen storage disease type VI Hers' disease	Onset in infancy and early childhood Sometimes so mild that syndrome may pass undetected Moderate growth retardation	
Glycogen storage disease type VII Tarui disease	Muscle weakness with exercise intolerance and myoglobinuria	
Goldenhar syndrome Oculo-auriculo-vertebral syndrome Hemifacial microsomia	Unilateral facial hypoplasia Small mandible, micrognathia with unilateral cleft defect unilateral maxillary hypoplasia, cervical vertebral defects Associated congenital heart defects (Fallot's and VSD) in 20% of cases	Airway problems Intubation problems Atropine-resistant bradycardia Cardiac anomalies

Name	Description	Anaesthetic implication
Golz–Gorlin syndrome Focal dermal hypoplasia	Dental and facial asymmetry and stiff neck Associated congenital heart defects (AS and ASD) Renal anomalies	Difficult airway Cardiac anomalies
Gorlin syndrome	Basal cell naevi Skeletal anomalies	No anaesthetic problems described
Groenblad–Strandberg disease Pseudoxanthoma elasticum	Degeneration of elastic tissue in skin, eyes and cardiovascular system results in fragile blood vessels with frequent rupture and bruising Thromboses	Difficult to maintain intravenous access
Guerin–Stern syndrome	Hypertension due to prorenin/renin production See also Arthrogryposis multiplex	Airway problems Cardiac problems
Guillain–Barré syndrome	Muscle weakness due to acute idiopathic progressive polyneuritis May involve cranial nerves with autonomic dysfunction, bulbar palsy, hypoventilation and unstable circulation Usually self-limiting in up to 6 weeks	Avoid suxamethonium for up to 3 months (hyperkalaemia) Plasmapheresis may be used
Haemorrhagic telangiectasia	See Osler–Weber–Rendu syndrome	
Hallermann–Streiff syndrome	Micrognathia, brittle teeth, hypoplastic nares	Intubation problems
Hallervorden–Spatz disease	Rare progressive disorder of basal ganglia occurring in late childhood and leading to death Dementia, myotonia and muscular rigidity with trismus	Intubation problems Dystonic posturing temporarily relieved by general anaesthesia
Hand–Schüller–Christian disease	See Histiocytosis X	
Hanhart syndrome	See Möbius syndrome	

Name	Description	Anaesthetic implication
Hay–Wells syndrome	Maxillary hypoplasia	Intubation problems
Hecht–Beals syndrome Dutch–Kentucky syndrome	Trismus and various skeletal abnormalities	Airway problems
Hemifacial microsomia	See Goldenhar syndrome	
Hepatolenticular degeneration Kinnier–Wilson disease	Defect in copper metabolism, hepatic failure, epilepsy, trismus, weakness	
Hermansky syndrome	Albinism and thrombasthenia Bleeding diathesis with bruising and platelet abnormality	Platelet infusion may be required
Hers' disease	See Glycogen storage disease type VI	
Histiocytosis X Hand–Schüller–Christian disease Letterer–Siwe disease	Histiocytic granulomas in bones and viscera – laryngeal and pulmonary infiltration, cor pulmonale, hepatic involvement, hypersplenism and diabetes insipidus Clinical course as for acute leukaemia	Gingivitis Intubation problems Anaemia Pancytopenia Electrolyte disturbance Corticosteroid therapy
Holt–Oram syndrome Hand–heart syndrome	Upper limb abnormalities Congenital heart disease – usually septal defects Sudden death	Cardiac anomalies
Homocystinuria	Deficiency of cystothionine synthetase Thromboembolic phenomena, lens dislocation, osteoporosis, kyphoscoliosis, mental handicap, hypoglycaemia and renal failure	Increased blood viscosity Increased platelet adhesiveness Hypoglycaemia Renal impairment
Hunter syndrome	See Mucopolysaccharidosis I	
Hurler syndrome	See Mucopolysaccharidosis I	
Hutchinson–Gilford syndrome	See Progeria	

Name	Description	Anaesthetic implication
Hypospadias dysphagia syndrome	See Opitz–Frias syndrome	
I-Cell disease	See Mucopolylipidosis II	
Ichthyosis X-linked ichthyosis	Dry, fish-like scales on the skin's surface Condition often begins in early childhood	Difficult skin fixation of intravenous cannulae etc.
Idiopathic infantile hypercalcaemia Supraventricular aortic stenosis syndrome William's–Beurin syndrome	Hypercalcaemia and mental retardation Abnormal facies with stellate blue eyes. Congenital stenosis of aortic and pulmonary valves	Airway problems Cardiac anomalies Monitor serum calcium
Infantile muscular atrophy	See Amyotonia congenita	
Isaacs syndrome	See Armadillo syndrome	
Ivemask syndrome	Asplenia, situs inversus, dextrocardia, cyanotic heart disease.	Cardiac anomalies
Jervell & Lange–Nielsen syndrome Cardio-auditory syndrome	Cardiac conduction defects, arrhythmias, prolonged QT interval and enlarged T wave Deafness	Syncope Cardiac arrest Consider pacemaker insertion
Jeune's syndrome	Lung problems due to chest wall deformity	Chronic respiratory infection
Kallman syndrome	Hypothalamic disorder associated with delayed puberty, anosmia and brittle bones	
Kartagener's syndrome	Dextrocardia, sinusitis, bronchiectasis, immunoincompetence See also Asplenia syndrome	Chronic respiratory infection
Kasabach–Merritt syndrome	Rarely survive more than a few weeks from birth Enlarging haemangioma with thrombocytopenia and haemorrhage	Blood and platelet transfusion Corticosteroid therapy
Kawasaki disease	Risk of coronary and other aneurysms Treatment with γ-globulin within 10 days	Risk of myocardial infarction

Name	Description	Anaesthetic implication
Kearns–Sayer syndrome	Mitochondrial cytopathy Cardiomyopathy Chronic external ophthalmoplegia, retinitis pigmentosa, deafness and seizures	Sudden complete heart block during anaesthesia Normal response to muscle relaxants
King–Denborough disease	Noonan syndrome-like skeletal abnormality with dysmorphic facies and myopathy	Malignant hyperpyrexia risk
Kinnier–Wilson disease	See Hepatolenticular degeneration	
Klinefelter syndrome	Chromosomal aneuploidy Crush fractures of osteoporotic vertebrae May be very large in adult life	Care with positioning
Klippel–Feil syndrome	Congenital fusion of cervical vertebrae Cleft palate, neurological defects, scoliosis and VSD may coexist	Airway problems Intubation problems Cardiac anomalies
Klippel–Trenaunay syndrome Angio-osteohypertrophy	Cleft palate, short wide neck and inability to extend neck Arteriovenous fistulae, high-output failure Thrombocytopenia	High cardiac output state Thrombocytopenia
Kneist's syndrome	Neck stiffness	Difficult intubation
Kugelberg–Welander muscular atrophy	See Amyotonia congenita	
Kwashiorkor	Pterygoid fibrosis	Intubation problems Electrolyte abnormalities Low serum cholinesterase
Larsen's syndrome	Connective tissue defect Multiple joint dislocations, unstable neck, pulmonary infections	Difficult intubation Chronic respiratory problems
Laryngomalacia	Upper airway obstruction	Airway problems
Laurence–Moon–Biedl syndrome	Obesity, polydactyly, mental retardation Associated congenital heart disease and renal failure	Cardiac anomalies Diabetes insipidus

Name	Description	Anaesthetic implication
Leber's disease	Congenital optic atrophy Idiopathic hypoventilation with sensitivity to diazepam and mild analgesics	
Leopard syndrome	Multiple leopard skin spots, hypertelorism, congenital heart disease	Severe pulmonary stenosis
Leprechaunism	Severe mental retardation Endocrine disorders including hyperinsulinism Renal tubular defects	Hypoglycaemia Renal impairment
Lesch–Nyhan syndrome	Mental retardation Hyperuricaemia Renal failure before puberty	Renal impairment
Letterer–Siwe disease	See Histiocytosis X	
Lipodystrophy	Generalised loss of all body fat Portal hypertension, hypersplenism, nephropathy Diabetes mellitus	Hepatic impairment Anaemia Pancytopenia
Lipogranulomatosis	See Farber's disease	
Lowe syndrome Oculocerebrorenal syndrome	Affects males only Mental retardation, hypotonia, renal acidosis, osteoporosis	Hypocalcaemia Renal impairment
McArdle's disease	See Glycogen storage disease type V	
McKusick–Kaufman syndrome	Hydrocolpos, syndactyly and cardiac abnormalities	Cardiac anomalies
Macroglossia, acute		Airway problems Intubation problems
Mafucci syndrome	Enchondromas, fragile bones and haemangiomas	Labile blood pressure Sensitive to vasodilator drugs Anaemia
Mandibulofacial dysostosis	See Treacher–Collins syndrome	
Maple syrup urine disease Branched chain ketonuria	Metabolic disease involving accumulation of keto- and amino-acids Severe neurological damage and respiratory disturbances	General supportive measures Blood sugar abnormalities Electrolyte abnormalities

Name	Description	Anaesthetic implication
Marble bone disease	See Albers–Schönberg disease	
Marchiafava–Michaeli syndrome	Autoimmune haemolytic anaemia with paroxysmal nocturnal dyspnoea Venous thromboembolism	Corticosteroid therapy
Marfan's syndrome Arachnodactyly	Congenital connective tissue disorder Kyphoscoliosis, pectus excavatum, joint instability Aortic, pulmonary and mitral valve involvement and dissecting aneurysms Emphysema and lung cysts	High anaesthetic risk Airway problems Pneumothorax Cardiac anomalies
Maroteaux–Lamy syndrome	See Mucopolysaccharidosis VI	
Meckel's syndrome Meckel–Gruber syndrome	Microcephaly, encephalocoele, micrognathia and cleft palate Congenital heart disease Polycystic kidneys with renal failure in infancy	Intubation problems Cardiac anomalies Renal impairment
Median cleft face syndrome	Varying degrees of cleft face Frontal lipomas	Difficult intubation
Meckel–Gruber syndrome	See Meckel's syndrome	
Metaphyseal dysplasia	See Pyle disease	
Miller–Diecker syndrome	Microcephaly Death in infancy or childhood	Airway problems Intubation problems
Möbius syndrome Hanhart syndrome Aglossia–adactylia syndrome	Rare congenital abnormality of the cranial nerves Congenital facial diplegia, micrognathia and associated limb deformity	Intubation problems Recurrent aspiration
Mongolism	See Down's syndrome	
Morquio–Ullrich syndrome	See Mucopolysaccharidosis IV	

Name	Description	Anaesthetic implication
Moschkowitz disease	A form of thrombotic thrombocytopenic purpura Neurological damage and renal disease Treated by splenectomy	Corticosteroid therapy
Mucopolylipidosis I	Like early MPS I	Airway problems
Mucopolylipidosis II I-Cell disease	Lysosomal storage disorder causing vacuolisation of bone, cartilage and fibroblasts Musculoskeletal abnormalities, including chest wall deformities – also cardiac valvular lesions Death within first decade	Airway problems Intubation problems Frequent chest infections Cardiac anomalies
Mucopolysaccharidoses (MPS)	Hereditary metabolic disorders with deposition of abnormal amounts of mucopolysaccharides in body tissues resulting in permanent progressive cellular damage	
MPS I Hurler syndrome Gargoylism	Chest infections, pulmonary hypertension, valve lesions, cardiomyopathy and heart failure Death before puberty	Upper airway obstruction Difficult intubation Frequent chest infections Cardiac anomalies
MPS II Hunter syndrome	Stiff joints, dwarfism Macroglossia with laryngeal and pharyngeal involvement and increased secretions Thoracic skeletal abnormalities Valve lesions, cardiomyopathy	Upper airway obstruction Cardiac anomalies
MPS III Sanfilippo syndrome	Mental retardation, agitation and dementia	No anaesthetic problems reported

Name	Description	Anaesthetic implication
MPS IV Morquio–Ulrich syndrome	Severe kyphoscoliotic dwarfing with atlantoaxial instability Chest wall deformity leading to respiratory and cardiac failure by second decade Aortic incompetence and cardiomyopathy	Intubation problems Cardiac anomalies Cervical spinal cord damage
MPS V Scheie syndrome	Considered to be a mild form of MPS I – can live to adulthood Hernias, joint stiffness, aortic valve involvement	See MPS I
MPS VI Maroteaux–Lamy syndrome	Myocardial involvement with heart failure by age 20 Kyphoscoliosis, chest infections and respiratory failure Hepatosplenomegaly	Anaemia Thrombocytopenia Cardiomyopathy Poor lung function
MPS VII Sly syndrome	Extreme fluid retention Moderate mental retardation, hydrocephalus Survival into teenage or young adult years	Frequent chest infections
Multiple endocrine adenomatosis (MEA) type I Wermer syndrome	Hyperparathyroidism, pancreatic and pituitary tumours Occasionally bronchial carcinoid tumours	Hypoglycaemia Hypercalcaemia Renal impairment Carcinoid
Multiple endocrine adenomatosis (MEA) type II Sipple syndrome	Phaeochromocytoma, thyroid carcinoma, parathyroid adenoma, CNS tumours, mediastinal schwannoma and Cushing's disease	Phaeochromocytoma
Multiple mucosal neuroma syndrome	MEA type IIB Marfanoid features Onset during first decade	Intubation problems
Myalgia encephalitica	Postviral weakness In extreme cases reduction of myocardial muscle	Caution with muscle relaxants

Name	Description	Anaesthetic implication
Myasthenia congenita	Like adult myasthenia gravis	Preoperative plasmapheresis Isoflurane safe
Myositis ossificans Fibrodysplasia ossificans	Bony infiltration of tendons, fascia and muscle Stiff neck, reduced thoracopulmonary compliance with respiratory failure	Airway problems Intubation problems Corticosteroid therapy
Myotonia congenita Thomsen's disease	Decreased ability to relax muscles after contraction	Avoid muscle relaxants
Myotonica dystrophia Dystrophia myotonica	Weakness and myotonia Pulmonary complications due to impaired ventilation and poor cough Cardiac involvement with conduction defects	Avoid respiratory depressants Avoid suxamethonium Non-depolarising relaxants may not relax myotonia Regional techniques may not relax myotonia Malignant hyperpyrexia risk
Nager syndrome	Abnormality of development of first and second branchial arches	Airway problems
Nemaline myopathy	Inadequate ventilation due to muscle weakness	Sensitive to non-depolarising relaxants Malignant hyperpyrexia risk
Neonatal hypoglycaemia (idiopathic)	Symptomatic hypoglycaemia, mental retardation and convulsions	Hypoglycaemia Diazoxide effective Corticosteroid therapy
Neurofibromatosis	See Von Recklinghausen's disease	
Niemann–Pick disease	Diffuse infiltration of sphingomyelin and cholesterol in CNS, lungs etc. Epilepsy, ataxia and mental retardation	Anaemia Thrombocytopenia Pulmonary insufficiency
Noack's syndrome	Craniosynostosis and digital anomalies Obesity	Intubation problems

Name	Description	Anaesthetic implication
Noonan syndrome	Male Turner syndrome Micrognathia, short, webbed neck, pectus excavatum Congenital heart disease Renal hypoplasia, hydronephrosis	Airway problems Cardiac anomalies Renal impairment
Oculo-auriculo-vertebral syndrome	See Goldenhar syndrome	
Oculocerebrorenal syndrome	See Lowe syndrome	
Ollier disease	Multiple chondromas within bones Pathological fractures	Care with positioning
Opitz–Frias syndrome Hypospadias dysphagia syndrome G syndrome	Genital and craniofacial abnormalities	Airway problems
Orofaciodigital syndrome	Cleft palate, lobed tongue, hypoplastic maxilla and mandible Hydrocephalus Polycystic kidneys	Airway problems Intubation problems Renal impairment
Osler–Weber–Rendu syndrome Haemorrhagic telangiectasia	No coagulation defect Pulmonary arteriovenous (AV) fistulae	Difficult to control bleeding Epistaxis Cardiac anomalies Recurrent chest infection
Osteogenesis imperfecta fragilitas ossium	Fragile teeth and bones, pathological fractures Respiratory problem due to chest wall deformity	Care in positioning Subcutaneous haemorrhage Malignant hyperpyrexia risk
Osteopetrosis	See Albers–Schönberg disease	
Oto-palatal-digital (OPD) syndrome Taybi syndrome Andre syndrome	Predominantly affects males Microcephaly, micrognathia and hypertelorism Two subtypes– OPD I Taybi syndrome OPD II Andre syndrome	Airway problems Intubation problems
Paramyotonia congenita Eulenberg disease	Weakness and myotonia induced by exposure to cold Derangement of serum potassium	See Myotonica dystrophia Electrolyte abnormalities

Name	Description	Anaesthetic implication
Patau syndrome	See Trisomy 13	
Pendred syndrome	Deafness and goitre	Check euthyroid Otherwise as for cretinism
Pfeiffer's syndrome	Craniostenosis, syndactyly	Airway problems Haemorrhagic surgery
Phenylketonuria	Phenylalanine hydroxylase deficiency Hypertonia, convulsions, mental retardation	Hypoglycaemia Seizures Sensitivity to CNS depressants
Pierre Robin syndrome	Micrognathia, hypoplastic mandible with glossoptosis, cleft palate and small epiglottis Respiratory obstruction tends to disappear after 2 years of age Associated congenital heart disease	Intubation problems Nurse in prone position Cardiac anomalies
Polycystic kidneys	Associated cysts in other organs Cerebral aneurysms in 15% of cases	Renal impairment
Polycystic liver	Associated cysts in other organs Hepatic impairment occurs late	
Polysplenia	Bilateral visceral left-sidedness Associated with complex congenital heart disease See also asplenia	Cardiac anomalies
Pompe's disease	See Glycogen storage disease type II	
Porphyria	Paralytic crises precipitated by wide variety of drugs Autonomic imbalance Abdominal pain	Avoid 'trigger' agents see Chapter 1.2
Potter's syndrome	Renal agenesis, typical facies and pulmonary hypoplasia Also maternal oligohydramnios	Ventilation may be impossible even if intubated

Name	Description	Anaesthetic implication
Prader–Willi syndrome	Hypotonia and absent reflexes in the neonate Later polyphagia and extreme obesity, mental retardation, hypogonadism and sometimes cardiovascular abnormalities May be very large in adult life	Obesity Airway problems Cardiac failure
Progeria Hutchinson–Gilford syndrome	Premature ageing starts 6 months to 3 years Adult cardiac disease – myocardial ischaemia, hypertension, cardiomegaly etc.	As for adults with IHD
Progressive external ophthalmoplegia (PEO)	Mitochondrial myopathy similar to Kearns–Sayer syndrome	Care with induction agents
Prune belly syndrome	Agenesis of abdominal muscles Poor cough due to muscle weakness, causes respiratory problems Renal anomalies	Recurrent respiratory infections Treat as 'full stomach' Avoid muscle relaxants Renal impairment
Pseudohaemophilia	See von Willebrand's disease	
Pseudohypoparathyroidism	See Albright's osteodystrophy	
Pseudoxanthoma elasticum	See Groenblad–Strandberg disease	
Pyle disease (Spondylo)metaphyseal dysplasia	Craniofacial abnormalities – mandibular prognathia	Airway problems
Reiger's syndrome	Similar to dystrophia myotonica and other myopathies Maxillary hypoplasia, abnormal teeth, mental retardation	See amyotonia congenita and dystrophia myotonica
Renal tubular acidosis	See Fanconi syndrome	
Rett syndrome	Affects females Dementia, autism, movement disorders and abnormal respiratory control	Cardiac anomalies

Name	Description	Anaesthetic implication
Riley–Day syndrome Familial dysautonomia	Deficiency of dopamine hydroxylase with autonomic instability and increased sensitivity to adrenergic and cholinergic drugs Hypersalivation, regurgitation, poor temperature control, and unexplained fluctuations of blood pressure	Labile blood pressure Insensitive to CO_2 Avoid respiratory depressants Reduced sensitivity to pain
Ritter disease	Fragile skin	Difficult venous access.
Robinow syndrome	Fetal face syndrome Achondroplasia	Airway problems
Romano–Ward syndrome	Congenital delay of depolarisation with prolonged QT interval	Sudden death during induction May require transvenous pacing or stellate ganglion block
Rubinstein–Taybi syndrome	Microcephaly, mental retardation Swallowing abnormality with frequent chest infections Associated congenital heart disease	Chronic lung disease Cardiac anomalies
Russell–Silver syndrome	See Silver syndrome	
Saethre–Chotzen syndrome	See Chotzen syndrome	
Sanfilippo syndrome	See Mucopolysaccharidosis III	
Scleroderma	Diffuse cutaneous stiffening with contractures	Airway problems Intubation problems Difficult venous access Corticosteroid therapy
Sebaceous naevi disease	Linear naevi from forehead to nose Hydrocephalus and mental retardation Congenital heart disease – coarctation, hypoplastic aorta	Airway problems Cardiac anomalies
Sheie disease	See Mucopolysaccharidosis V	

Name	Description	Anaesthetic implication
Shprintzen syndrome	Micrognathia, deafness and congenital cardiac abnormalities occur	Intubation problems Cardiac anomalies
Shy–Drager syndrome	Diffuse degeneration of central and autonomic nervous systems Cardiac arrhythmias Hypersensitivity to epinephrine (adrenaline) and angiotensin	Labile blood pressure Ephedrine effective
Shy–Magee syndrome	Central core disease Myopathy and myotonia	Malignant hyperpyrexia risk
Silver syndrome Russell–Silver syndrome	Short stature, skeletal asymmetry, micrognathia, macroglossia, café-au-lait spots, sweating and mental deficiency Abnormal sexual development	Airway problems Intubation problems Hypoglycaemia
Sipple syndrome	See Multiple endocrine adenomatosis type II	
Smith–Najer syndrome	Mandibulofacial dystonia	Airway problems
Smith–Lemli–Opitz syndrome	Mental retardation, micrognathia, skeletal and genital anomalies and intrinsic lung disease Hypoplasia of thymus with increased susceptibility to infection	Airway problems Intubation problems
Sotos syndrome	Non-progressive cerebral gigantism Normal intracranial pressure	Airway problems
Spondylometaphyseal dysplasia	See Pyle's disease	
Sprengel's deformity	Congenital elevation of scapula with scoliosis and torticollis Associated with Klippel–Feil syndrome	Intubation problems

Name	Description	Anaesthetic implication
Stickler's syndrome	Progressive arthro-ophthalmopathy Myopia, retinal detachment, secondary glaucoma, pain and stiffness of joints with hypotonia, kyphoscoliosis, maxillary hypoplasia, Occasional cleft palate, deafness	Intubation problems
Still's disease	Juvenile chronic polyarthritis Limited movement of jaw and of cervical spine Atlantoaxial subluxation may be present	Difficult airway Fibreoptic intubation Ketamine may be useful
Sturge–Weber syndrome	Cavernous angioma of face Intracranial calcification, convulsions and progressive neurological deficit	Cardiac problems
Supravalvular aortic stenosis syndrome	See Idiopathic infantile hypercalcaemia	
Tangier disease	Analphalipoproteinaemia Splenomegaly, low serum cholesterol and neurological abnormalities in 50% of cases Premature coronary disease	Care with muscle relaxants Anaemia Thrombocytopenia
Thrombocytopenia with absent radius (TAR) syndrome	Episodic thrombocytopenia Congenital heart disease in 30% of cases – commonly Fallot's tetralogy Death within first year in up to 40% of cases	Avoid surgery in first year Cardiac anomalies
Tarui disease	See Glycogen storage disease type VII	
Tay–Sachs disease	Gangliosidosis CNS degeneration, blindness and progressive dementia	No anaesthetic problems reported
Taybi syndrome	See Otopalatodigital syndrome	
Thomsen's disease	See Myotonia congenita	

Name	Description	Anaesthetic implication
Thrombasthenia	See Glanzmann's disease	
Tourette syndrome Gilles de la Tourette syndrome	Repetitive, rapid sudden movements (tics) and coprolalia Prolonged QT interval syndrome associated with pimozide treatment	Motor aspects may be confused with seizure-like activity
Treacher–Collins syndrome	Mandibulofacial dysostosis Micrognathia, maxillary and mandibular hypoplasia, microstomia and ear deformities, but less severe than Pierre Robin deformity Coexistent congenital heart disease	Airway problems Intubation problems Cardiac anomalies
Trisomy 4	Complete trisomy 4 is lethal	
Trisomy 6	Craniofacial abnormalities, unusually short webbed neck, flexion contractures Growth and psychomotor retardation	Airway problems Intubation problems
Trisomy 8	Dysmorphic facies, micrognathia, musculoskeletal abnormalities, congenital heart disease and hydronephrosis	Intubation problems Cardiac anomalies Renal impairment
Trisomy 13 Patau syndrome	Mental retardation Microcephaly, micrognathia and cleft palate Dextrocardia and congenital heart disease (e.g. VSD) Usually fatal by 3 years of age	Intubation problems Cardiac anomalies
Trisomy 18 Edwards' syndrome	Micrognathia, short sternum, renal malformations, clenched hands, low-set ears Associated congenital heart disease (VSD, patent ductus, pulmonary stenosis) in 95% of cases Usually die in infancy	Intubation problems Cardiac problems Renal impairment

Name	Description	Anaesthetic implication
Trisomy 21 Down's syndrome Mongolism	Microcephaly, atlantoaxial instability, hypotonia Hypersalivation Associated congenital heart disease (especially septal defects) in 50% of cases	Airway problems Intubation problems Cardiac anomalies Hypoglycaemia
Trisomy 22	Death before or shortly after birth due to severe malformations, including microcephaly and cardiac abnormalities	Cardiac anomalies Hypoglycaemia
Tuberous sclerosis Bournville's disease	Adenoma sebaceum of skin – ash leaf and café-au-laits pots Intracranial calcification, epilepsy and mental retardation Hamartomas in heart, lungs and kidneys	Cardiac anomalies Arrhythmias Renal impairment
Turner's syndrome	Micrognathia with short webbed neck Aortic and pulmonary stenosis, coarctation and aneurysms of aorta Renal anomalies	Intubation problems Cardiac anomalies Renal impairment
Urbach–Wiethe disease	Mucocutaneous hyalinosis – a type of histiocytosis Hyaline deposits in larynx and pharynx	Intubation problems
Vater syndrome	VSD and intrinsic pulmonary disease Renal failure occurs	Cardiac anomalies Renal impairment
Velocardiofacial	Cleft palate, congenital heart defects	Airway problems Cardiac anomalies
Von–Gierke's disease	See Glycogen storage disease type I	
Von–Hippel–Lindau syndrome	Haemangioblastomas in posterior fossa and spinal cord Associated with phaeochromocytoma, hepatic and renal cysts	Phaeochromocytoma risk Hepatic pathology Renal impairment

Name	Description	Anaesthetic implication
Von Recklinghausen's disease Neurofibromatosis	Tumours in all parts of CNS Fibromas of pharynx, larynx and heart Kyphoscoliosis, multiple lung cysts and renal artery dysplasia Increased incidence of phaeochromocytoma	Airway problems Cardiac problems Phaeochromocytoma risk
Von Willebrand's disease Pseudohaemophilia	Defective platelet adhesiveness with factor VIII deficiency Also capillary abnormality	Correct coagulopathy with: Tranexamic acid Desmopressin (DDAVP) Fresh frozen plasma Avoid salicylates
Weaver's syndrome	Rare developmental condition with unusual craniofacial appearance and micrognathia May be very large in adult life	Airway problems Intubation problems
Weber–Christian disease	Chronic nonsuppurative panniculitis with widespread fat necrosis including peritoneal, pericardial and meningeal Adrenal insufficiency, constrictive pericarditis	Avoid trauma to fat
Welander muscular atrophy	Peripheral muscular atrophy	Sensitive to muscle relaxants Sensitive to opiates
Werdnig–Hoffman disease	See Amyotonia congenita	
Wermer syndrome	See Multiple endocrine adenomatosis type I	
Werner syndrome	Premature ageing, diabetes mellitus, early cataracts, mental retardation in 50% of cases Hypercalcaemia, bony lesions like osteomyelitis and myocardial ischaemia, See also Progeria	Anaesthesia as for adults with IHD
Wiedemann syndrome	See Beckwith syndrome	
Williams'–Beurin syndrome	See Idiopathic infantile hypercalcaemia	

Name	Description	Anaesthetic implication
Wilson's disease	Hepatolenticular degeneration Decreased caeruloplasmin causes widespread abnormal copper deposition	Hepatic failure Muscle relaxants ineffective Renal impairment
Wilson–Mikity syndrome	Prematurity – <1500 g birth weight Severe chronic lung disease with fibrosis, possibly due to oxygen toxicity	Recurrent chest infections Corticosteroid therapy Right heart failure
Wiskott–Aldrich syndrome	Primary immunodeficiency with thrombocytopenia All have low platelet count, anaemia and clotting problems Eczema and asthma	Anaemia Thrombocytopenia Susceptible to transfusion-induced graft-versus-host reaction Susceptible to infection Cardiac anomalies
Wolf–Hirschorn syndrome	Associated with poor intrauterine growth, severe psychomotor retardation, characteristic facies, and various midline fusion abnormalities	Malignant hyperpyrexia risk
Wolman's disease Familial xanthomatosis	Adrenal calcification Resembles Niemann–Pick disease with hepatosplenomegaly, hypersplenism and clotting problems	Anaemia Thrombocytopenia
X-linked ichthyosis	See Ichthyosis	

Further reading

Bevan JC. Congenital syndromes in paediatric anaesthesia: what is important to know. Can J Anaesth 1998; 45:R3–R16.

Jones AEP, Pelton DA. An index of syndromes and their anaesthetic implications. Can Anaesth Soc J 1970; 23:207–226.

Steward DJ. Anesthetic implications of syndromes and unusual disorders. In: Steward DJ, ed. Manual of pediatric anesthesia. 4th edn. New York: Churchill Livingstone; 1995; Appendix I: 434–493.

Useful websites

http://www.nlm.nih.gov/medlineplus/encyclopedia.html

http://www.medicinenet.com

http://www.gpnotebook.co.uk

http://www.whonamedit.com

http://www.google.com

INDEX

C

E

F

N

O

T

U

V

W

X

Y

Z